Diabetes and Cardiovascular Disease
Integrating Science and Clinical Medicine

Diabetes and Cardiovascular Disease
Integrating Science and Clinical Medicine

Editors

Steven P. Marso, M.D.
Assistant Professor
Consulting Cardiologist
University of Missouri–Kansas City
Mid America Heart Institute
Saint Luke's Hospital
Kansas City, Missouri

David M. Stern, M.D.
Chief Clinical Officer
Dean, School of Medicine
Professor of Medicine and Physiology
Medical College of Georgia
Augusta, Georgia

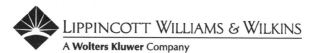

LIPPINCOTT WILLIAMS & WILKINS
A **Wolters Kluwer** Company

Philadelphia • Baltimore • New York • London
Buenos Aires • Hong Kong • Sydney • Tokyo

Acquisitions Editor: Ruth W. Weinberg
Developmental Editor: Michelle M. LaPlante
Production Editor: Frank Aversa
Manufacturing Manager: Ben Rivera
Cover Designer: Patricia Gast
Compositor: TechBooks
Printer: Maple-Press

Library of Congress Cataloging-in-Publication Data

Diabetes and cardiovascular disease: integrated science and clinical medicine / editors,
    Steven P. Marso, David M. Stern.
        p. ; cm.
    Includes bibliographical references and index.
    ISBN 0-7817-4053-3
    1. Cardiovascular system—Diseases. 2. Diabetes—Complications.   I. Marso,
        Steven P.   II. Stern, David M., M.D.
    [DNLM: 1. Cardiovascular Diseases—complications.   2. Diabetes
        Mellitus—complications.   WK 835 D533475 2004]
    RC669.D52   2004
    616.1—dc21   2003054573

To my dad, who was laconic in his lectures, led by example, and will forever be a guiding force in my life, and to my mom, who taught me the power of laughter, the importance of family, and instilled in me the love of medicine.

To my wife Janet and children Morgan, Zach, and Sam—thank you for your patience, love, and understanding throughout this latest endeavor.

Steve Marso

To my family and Ms. Claudia Edwards, who persevere with me through projects and endeavors of every kind.

David Stern

Contents

Contributing Authors

Joshua A. Beckman, M.D., M.S. *Instructor of Medicine, Department of Medicine, Harvard Medical School; Associate Attending Physician, Department of Medicine, Brigham and Women's Hospital, Boston, Massachusetts*

Deepak L. Bhatt, M.D., F.A.C.C., F.S.C.A.I. *Director, Interventional Cardiology Fellowship, Department of Cardiovascular Medicine, Cleveland Clinic Foundation, Cleveland, Ohio*

Georg Breier, M.D. *Department of Molecular Cell Biology, Max-Planck-Institute für Physiologische und Klinische Forschung, Bad Nauheim, Germany*

Cathryn A. Carroll, Ph.D. *Assistant Professor, Division of Pharmacy Practice, University of Missouri–Kansas City, Kansas City, Missouri*

Mark W. Conard, M.A. *Department of Clinical Health Psychology, University of Missouri–Kansas City; Department of Clinical Health Outcomes Research, Mid America Heart Institute, Saint Luke's Hospital, Kansas City, Missouri*

Roberto A. Corpus, M.D. *Mid America Heart Institute, Saint Luke's Hospital, Kansas City, Missouri*

Sridevi Devaraj, Ph.D. *Assistant Professor of Pathology, Laboratory for Atherosclerosis and Metabolic Research, University of California, Davis Medical Center, Sacramento, California*

Alessandro Doria, M.D., Ph.D. *Assistant Professor of Medicine, Department of Medicine, Harvard Medical School; Investigator, Research Division, Joslin Diabetes Center, Boston, Massachusetts*

Peter J. Grant, M.D., F.R.C.P. *Professor of Medicine, Academic Unit of Molecular Vascular Medicine, Leeds General Infirmary, Leeds, West Yorkshire, United Kingdom*

Hans-Peter Hammes, M.D. *Professor, Head, Fifth Medical Department, Medical School of Mannheim, University Hospital Mannheim, Mannheim, Germany*

William S. Harris, Ph.D. *Professor, Department of Medicine, University of Missouri–Kansas City; Director, Lipid Laboratory, Mid America Heart Institute, Saint Luke's Hospital, Kansas City, Missouri*

Zhiheng He, M.D., Ph.D. *Mary K. Iacocca Fellow, Department of Vascular Cell Biology and Complications, Joslin Diabetes Center, Harvard Medical School, Boston, Massachusetts*

Barry I. Hudson, Ph.D. *Postdoctoral Research Fellow, Department of Surgery, Columbia University, New York, New York*

William L. Isley, M.D. *Associate Professor, Department of Medicine, University of Missouri–Kansas City; Medical Director, Lipid and Diabetes Research Center, Saint Luke's Hospital, Kansas City, Missouri*

Ishwarlal Jialal, M.D., Ph.D.   *Professor of Pathology and Medicine, Director, Laboratory for Atherosclerosis and Metabolic Research, University of California, Davis Medical Center, Sacramento, California*

Robert Kelly, M.D.   *Cardiology Fellow, Division of Cardiology, University of North Carolina, University of North Carolina Hospital, Chapel Hill, North Carolina*

Avinash Khanna, M.D.   *Mid America Heart Institute, Saint Luke's Hospital, Kansas City, Missouri*

George L. King, M.D.   *Research Director, Joslin Diabetes Center; Professor of Medicine, Harvard Medical School, Boston, Massachusetts*

Maureen E. Knell, Pharm.D., B.C.P.S.   *Clinical Assistant Professor, School of Pharmacy, Division of Pharmacy Practice, University of Missouri–Kansas City; Clinical Pharmacist, Multi-specialty Clinic, Saint Luke's Hospital, Kansas City, Missouri*

Andrzej S. Krolewski, M.D.   *Section on Genetics and Epidemiology, Joslin Diabetes Center, Boston, Massachusetts*

Ronald E. Law, Ph.D., J.D.   *Associate Professor of Medicine, Division of Endocrinology, Diabetes, and Hypertension, David Geffen School of Medicine, University of California, Los Angeles, Los Angeles, California*

David S. Lee, M.D.   *Fellow, Department of Cardiovascular Medicine, Cleveland Clinic Foundation, Cleveland, Ohio*

Peter J. Little, Ph.D.   *Head, Cell Biology of Diabetes Laboratory, Baker Heart Research Institute; Senior Scientist, Alfred Baker Medical Unit, Alfred Hospital, Melbourne, Victoria, Australia*

Jared T. Lurk, Pharm.D.   *Adjunct Clinical Assistant Professor, Department of Pharmacy Practice, University of Missouri–Kansas City; Pharmacy Practice Resident, Department of Pharmacy, Saint Luke's Hospital, Kansas City, Missouri*

Ronald C.W. Ma, M.R.C.P.   *Medical Officer, Endocrine Division, Department of Medicine and Therapeutics, Prince of Wales Hospital, Shatin, Hong Kong, China*

Mario B. Marrero, Ph.D.   *Associate Professor, Department of Vascular Biology Center, Medical College of Georgia, Augusta, Georgia*

Steven P. Marso, M.D.   *Assistant Professor, Department of Medicine, University of Missouri–Kansas City; Consulting Cardiologist, Department of Cardiology, Mid America Heart Institute, Saint Luke's Hospital, Kansas City, Missouri*

Darren K. McGuire, M.D., M.H.Sc.   *Assistant Professor, Department of Internal Medicine, University of Texas–Southwestern Medical Center; Director, Outpatient Cardiology Services, Department of Cardiology, Parkland Hospital and Health System, Dallas, Texas*

Sunder Mudalier, M.D.   *Staff Physician, Section of Diabetes/Metabolism, Veterans Affairs, San Diego HealthCare System; Assistant Clinical Professor of Medicine, University of California, Los Angeles, California*

John D. Nachtigal, B.S.   *Research Intern, Mid America Heart Institute, Saint Luke's Hospital, Kansas City, Missouri*

Peter J. Oates, Ph.D.   *Research Advisor, Department of Cardiovascular and Metabolic Diseases, Pfizer Global Research and Development, Groton, Connecticut*

Marc S. Penn, M.D., Ph.D.   *Assistant Professor, Department of Molecular Medicine, Case Western Reserve University, Lerner Research Institute; Director, Experimental Animal Laboratory, Associate Director, Cardiovascular Medicine Training Program, Department of Cardiovascular Medicine and Cell Biology, Cleveland Clinic Foundation, Cleveland, Ohio*

Walker S. Carlos Poston, Ph.D., M.P.H., F.A.H.A.   *Associate Professor, Department of Health Psychology, University of Missouri–Kansas City; Director, Behavioral Cardiology Research, Department of Cardiovascular Research, Saint Luke's Hospital, Kansas City, Missouri*

Ravichandran Ramasamy, Ph.D.   *Assistant Professor, Division of Surgical Science, Department of Surgery, Columbia University, New York, New York*

Sunil V. Rao, M.D.   *Cardiology Fellow, Duke University Medical Center, Duke Clinical Research Institute, Durham, North Carolina*

Matthew T. Roe, M.D., M.H.S., F.A.C.C.   *Assistant Professor of Medicine, Department of Cardiology, Duke Clinical Research Institute, Duke University Medical Center, Durham, North Carolina*

Jennifer M. Roth, Pharm.D.   *Adjunct Clinical Assistant Professor, Department of Pharmacy Practice, University of Missouri–Kansas City; Pharmacy Practice Resident, Department of Pharmacy, Saint Luke's Hospital, Kansas City, Missouri*

Ann Marie Schmidt, M.D.   *Professor, Division of Surgical Science, Department of Surgery, College of Physicians and Surgeons, Columbia University, New York, New York*

Steven R. Steinhubl, M.D.   *Associate Professor, Division of Cardiology, University of North Carolina; Associate Director, Department of Cardiology, University of North Carolina Hospital, Chapel Hill, North Carolina*

David M. Stern, M.D.   *Dean, School of Medicine, Professor of Medicine and Physiology, Medical College of Georgia; Chief Clinical Officer, Medical College of Georgia Hospital, Augusta, Georgia*

Lucinda K.M. Summers, M.R.C.P., D.Phil.   *Senior Lecturer, Academic Unit of Molecular Vascular Medicine, University of Leeds; Honorary Consultant, Diabetes Center, Leeds General Infirmary, Leeds, West Yorkshire, United Kingdom*

Duncan J. Topliss, M.D., F.R.A.C.P., F.A.C.E.   *Associate Professor, Department of Medicine, Monash University; Director, Department of Endocrinology and Diabetes, Alfred Hospital, Melbourne, Victoria, Australia*

Roberto Trevisan, M.D., Ph.D.   *Honorary Professor of Diabetology, Department of Clinical and Experimental Medicine, University of Padua, Padua, Italy; Consultant, Diabetes Section, Department of Transplantation, Riuniti Hospital of Bergamo, Bergamo, Italy*

Benjamin H. Trichon, M.D.   *Fellow, Division of Cardiology, Duke University Medical Center, Durham, North Carolina*

Sonia Vega-López, Ph.D.   *Postdoctoral Fellow, Department of Pathology, University of California, Davis Medical Center, Sacramento, California*

Giancarlo F. Viberti, M.D., F.R.C.P.   *Professor, Department of Diabetes, Endocrinology, and Internal Medicine, King's College London; Honorary Consultant Physician, Department of Endocrinology and Diabetes, Guy's Hospital, London, United Kingdom*

Deepak P. Vivekananthan, M.D.   *Fellow, Department of Cardiovascular Medicine, Cleveland Clinic Foundation, Cleveland, Ohio*

James H. Warram, M.D., Sc.D.   *Instructor, Department of Epidemiology, Harvard School of Public Health; Investigator, Section on Genetics and Epidemiology, Joslin Diabetes Center, Boston, Massachusetts*

Shi-Fang Yan, M.D.   *Assistant Professor, Division of Surgical Sciences, Department of Surgery, Columbia University, New York, New York*

Preface

Caring for persons with chronic diseases, such as diabetes mellitus, is becoming an increasingly onerous task in the current era of medical delivery. Given the significant advances in biological sciences and information technology, clinicians and investigators are continually challenged to increase their fund of knowledge and apply this information in a way that will improve both the efficiency and efficacy of medical care. There is no subgroup of patients in which this paradigm is more prominent than among persons with diabetes mellitus. This group is an ever-increasing sector of our society and present commonly with cardiovascular disease states. There continues to be rapid evolution of scientific information resulting in an evolution of thought with respect to the underlying pathobiology and clinical treatments; however, it is increasingly clear that persons with diabetes present with a differential vascular biology and remain at heightened risk for cardiovascular risk in the current medical era.

Although type 1 diabetes remains an important clinical entity with numerous long-term health complications, the vast majority of patients presenting with diabetes and vascular complications have type 2 diabetes. This necessitates the need to focus solely on the underlying mechanisms of diagnosis and treatment strategies for this prevalent cohort. Diabetes mellitus currently affects 16 million persons in the United States and over 100 million persons worldwide. It is projected that these numbers will double within the next one to two decades. The increase in the worldwide prevalence of diabetes is multifactorial and likely related to complex gene-environment interactions. Important environmental determinates of developing diabetes include an increasing prevalence of obesity, sedentary lifestyle, and a westernization of worldwide diet preferences. Furthermore, there is an expected disproportionate risk in developing type 2 diabetes among certain countries and populations. For example, there will be a modest increase in type 2 diabetes mellitus among developed countries over the next 25 years. However, the prevalence of type 2 diabetes in developing countries is projected to double. Thus, in this generation, the greatest number of new cases of diabetes will be in developing nations. This will no doubt lead to unique challenges for the worldwide medical community to effectively deliver quality care.

This increasing burden is coupled with an enormous increase in biomedical information over the last 50 years. According to the Institute of Medicine's report, *Crossing the Quality Chasm: A New Health System for the 21st Century* (National Academy of Sciences, July 2001), there has been a logarithmic increase in the publication of randomized clinical trials over the last five years with a projected 10,000 published trials annually. No one can assimilate and apply all the relevant information for a complex disease state such as diabetes mellitus and vascular disease. With 49 contributors from around the world, this compendium strives to provide sufficient detail regarding this complex disease state to increase the depth of knowledge, yet relay this information in a way that is readily understandable and sufficiently concise to be clinically useful.

Stephen P. Marso, M.D.
David M. Stern, M.D.

Acknowledgments

The editors thank Deborah J. Spiers and Jose A. Aceituno for their tireless effort and substantial contribution to this project. Without their expert contribution, this book would not have been possible.

PART I

Vascular Biology

Diabetes and Cardiovascular Disease
edited by Steven P. Marso and David M. Stern
Lippincott Williams & Wilkins, Philadelphia © 2004

1

Structure and Function of the Vessel Wall

Mario B. Marrero and David M. Stern

*Associate Professor, Department of Vascular Biology Center, Medical College of Georgia;
Dean, School of Medicine, Professor of Medicine and Physiology, Medical College of Georgia,
Chief Clinical Officer, Medical College of Georgia Hospital, Augusta, Georgia*

Inappropriate cell growth and death are major pathologic processes in diabetic patients and in animal models of diabetes mellitus. In particular, dysfunction of both endothelial cells and vascular smooth muscle cells (VSMC) leads to changes in cell growth and viability that contribute to the cardiovascular complications of patients with diabetes mellitus, ranging from macrovascular atherosclerosis to microvascular angiopathy (e.g., retinopathy) (1). Similarly, glomerular mesangial cell growth and extracellular matrix production also have significant roles in the pathogenesis of diabetic nephropathy, the most common cause of end-stage renal disease (ESRD) in the United States (2). The growth of both VSMC and mesangial cells is stimulated by cytokines (e.g., transforming growth factor-β [TGF-β]) and traditional growth factors (e.g., platelet-derived growth factor [PDGF]); in addition, both cell types respond to a variety of circulating vasoactive substances. In particular, angiotensin II (Ang II), a vasoactive peptide not usually considered to be a growth factor, has been implicated as a mitogen in the setting of diabetes (3). Furthermore, hyperinsulinemia (i.e., type 2 diabetes mellitus or exogenous insulin therapy) provides a mitogenic stimulus that accentuates Ang II-mediated growth of VSMC and mesangial cells (4). Therefore, both metabolic and hormonal imbalances contribute to the pathogenesis of diabetic vascular diseases.

The most important factors that cause and advance the progression of diabetic vascular disease are hyperglycemia, insulin resistance, cytokines, and vasoactive hormones. The contributions of these factors to the development of diabetic complications depend not only on the particular vascular tissue being affected but also on the specific phase of the disease process (5). Moreover, both the environment and hereditary factors can adjust the risk and advancement of vascular complications associated with diabetes (6). Finally, the accumulation of products of glycoxidation (e.g., advanced glycation end products [AGEs]) in diabetic tissues, via their interactions with cellular receptors and direct induction of changes in tissue architecture, is likely to exacerbate the development of diabetic complications (see later chapters in this book). This introductory chapter reviews the effect of diabetes on both microvascular and macrovascular tissues and some of the theories about the contributions of hyperglycemia, AGEs, insulin resistance, cytokines, and vasoactive hormones to the development of vascular disease.

DIABETES AND MICROVASCULAR DISEASE

Microvascular abnormalities and dysfunction occur as a systemic disorder in diabetes, and the clinical and cellular expressions of microvascular disease (e.g., retinopathy, nephropathy) vary according to the structure and function of the affected tissues. For example, in nonproliferative diabetic retinopathy, loss of pericytes and formation of microaneurysms are observed. In addition, vascular barrier function is decreased and capillary closure occurs. These microvascular abnormalities lead to ischemic loci; the retina then responds to such hypoxia by increasing the expression of vascular endothelial growth factor (VEGF), thereby promoting neovascularization (7). In diabetic nephropathy, an increase in both intraglomerular pressure and extracellular matrix proteins in the glomerulus results in basement membrane thickening, mesangial expansion, and glomerular hypertrophy (8). These changes reduce glomerular filtration area and function and set the stage for progression to glomerulosclerosis. Diabetic nephropathy complicates the course of diabetes mellitus in 30% to 40% of patients and is the most common cause of ESRD in the United States (2). Diabetics account for almost 50% of all patients enrolled in the federally funded ESRD program, at a yearly cost exceeding $2 billion dollars in 1990. Diabetics with nephropathy have a 100-fold greater risk of dying relative to the nondiabetic population. The need for research into the pathogenesis, prevention, and treatment of diabetic nephropathy is highlighted by the profound financial, social, and personal impacts of this devastating complication of diabetes mellitus.

DIABETES AND MACROVASCULAR DISEASE

The impact of both insulin-dependent (type 1) and non-insulin-dependent (type 2) diabetes mellitus on the macrovasculature results from accelerated atherosclerosis and increased thrombosis, and the vessels that are affected are mainly the coronary, cerebral, and peripheral arteries. Many risk factors, some of which may exist in the prediabetic state, particularly in type 2 diabetes, are involved in the development of macrovascular disease. Some of these risk factors (e.g., hyperlipidemia, hyperinsulinemia, decreased insulin sensitivity) are associated with the insulin resistance syndrome, which has been proposed to initiate atherogenesis even before a diagnosis of type 2 diabetes can be made (9). Furthermore,

most of the macrovascular complications associated with diabetes are exacerbated by concomitant systemic hypertension (4).

The mechanisms that most likely are responsible for diabetic macrovascular complications have begun to be delineated, and it appears that metabolic and hemodynamic factors interact to stimulate the expression of cytokines and growth factors within distinct vascular beds. For example, vasoactive hormones such as Ang II and endothelin are potent stimulators of cytokines, and recent studies show that inhibitors of these vasoactive hormone pathways may confer organ protection in diabetes by inhibition of growth factor expression (10). In addition, glucose-dependent factors such as the formation of AGEs lead to overexpression of a range of cytokines and may contribute to diabetic macrovascular complications (11). It is likely that the effects of inhibitors of this pathway, at the level of AGEs, their receptors, or specific cytokines, may play a pivotal role in amelioration of diabetes. Because of the broad activity of cytokines, it is anticipated that the advent of specific inhibitors of cytokine formation or action will provide new approaches for the prevention and treatment of diabetic vascular complications (11).

Another manifestation of vascular dysfunction in patients with diabetes concerns their response to revascularization procedures. The propensity for macrovascular disease in diabetic patients reduces the efficacy of revascularization procedures, including percutaneous transluminal coronary angioplasty with stenting, as well as coronary artery bypass grafting, compared with results in nondiabetic people (5). Restenosis after percutaneous transluminal coronary angioplasty in diabetic patients is mainly a result of intimal hyperplasia (1). This is most likely a consequence of abnormal cell migration, growth, and extracellular matrix production in the diabetic vascular microenvironment.

HYPERGLYCEMIA

Hyperglycemia plays a pivotal role in the development of both microvascular and macrovascular complications. The results of the Diabetes

Complications and Control Trial (DCCT) indicate that hyperglycemia is a major contributor to microvascular disease (i.e., retinopathy and nephropathy) in type 1 diabetes. In addition, results from the DCCT together with those of other, smaller studies suggest that intensive glycemic control can reduce cardiovascular disease. On the other hand, the actual effect of hyperglycemia on the development and progression of macrovascular complications remains unclear and even somewhat controversial, particularly in type 2 diabetes. For example, macrovascular complications are increased in individuals with type 2 diabetes long before significant hyperglycemia occurs, and most studies have not shown a clear association of elevated glucose and macrovascular complications. The complicated nature of the metabolic abnormalities in type 2 diabetes and the relative roles of these associated conditions in the development of macrovascular disease make definitive conclusions somewhat difficult. Nevertheless, certain aspects of hyperglycemia, particularly elevations of postprandial glucose, are associated with macrovascular disease, and there are a number of basic mechanisms to explain these associations that could lead to the development of cardiovascular disease. These abnormalities include activation of the sorbitol pathway, oxidative stress, and generation of reactive AGEs and AGE precursors (12). Results of these events include endothelial dysfunction, altered properties of key proteins (for example, due to glycation of structural proteins), and generation of proinflammatory cytokines. These considerations suggest that hyperglycemia plays an important, but as yet not clearly defined, role in clinical macrovascular disease.

Several theories have emerged to explain how hyperglycemia directly induces activation of signaling pathways involved in diabetic vasculopathies. For example, one of the basic underlying mechanisms of diabetic nephropathy appears to involve hyperglycemia-induced production of TGF-β and extracellular matrix-associated molecules such as fibronectin (13,14). Glomerular mesangial cells cultured under hyperglycemic conditions produce TGF-β and extracellular matrix components at a significantly faster rate than do similar cells cultured under normal glucose conditions (13,14). In addition, hyperglycemia increases *de novo* synthesis of the protein kinase C (PKC) activator, diacylglycerol (15). Hyperglycemia may induce mesangial cell production of TGF-β and extracellular matrix molecules through the mechanism of chronic activation of one or more isoforms of PKC (16). However, other signaling pathways have been suggested by which hyperglycemia can stimulate similar mesangial cell activation. These include the sorbitol pathway and the mitogen-activated protein kinase (MAPK) pathway (17,18). Most recently, Amiri et al. (3) showed that exposure of VSMC to hyperglycemia results in activation of the janus kinase/signal transducers and activators of transcription (JAK/STAT) pathway. Specifically, exposure of VSMC to hyperglycemia induces tyrosine phosphorylation of JAK2 and complex formation of JAK2 with the angiotensin II AT$_1$ receptor. Amiri et al. (3) also demonstrated that hyperglycemia-induced tyrosine phosphorylation of JAK2 is accompanied by tyrosine and/or serine phosphorylation of STAT1 and STAT3 and by increased VSMC proliferation. In addition, Marrero et al. (19) demonstrated that activation of JAK2 is essential both for Ang II- and PDGF-induced MAPK pathway activation and for VSMC growth. Finally, another group recently demonstrated that activation of JAK2 and STAT proteins is a requirement for the AGE-induced production of extracellular matrix molecules in NRK-49F cells (20). Therefore, it appears that activation of JAK2 and STAT proteins in hyperglycemia might play an important role in the promotion of cell proliferation and synthesis of extracellular matrix molecules.

ADVANCED GLYCATION END PRODUCTS

Nonenzymatic glycoxidation occurs both intracellularly and extracellularly and is accelerated by oxidant stress from multiple causes, as well as elevated levels of aldoses. The ultimate result of such nonenzymatic glycoxidation of macromolecules is the formation of AGEs (11).

AGE modification can result in changes in tissue or cellular properties through the formation of crosslinks. These can modulate the function of a modified macromolecule both directly and by allowing its recognition by cellular receptors or binding sites not reactive with the native structure (11).

In view of the long duration of AGEs at sites of diabetic complications and their intimate relationship with cellular elements (as in the vascular wall, kidney, and retina), Schmidt et al. (11) reasoned that cell surface recognition sites for AGEs might be central in mediating their effects. Using an assay that detects binding activity for iodine 125-labeled albumin in tissue extracts, they fractionated lung proteins and were able to identify a polypeptide that selectively binds AGE-modified polypeptides but not the native structures. This molecule was named receptor for AGE, or RAGE, and it turned out to be a member of the immunoglobulin superfamily of cell surface molecules. As the biology of RAGE has evolved, several common themes have emerged. First, the multiligand character of RAGE is quite remarkable. Ligands of the receptor include AGEs, crossed-sheet fibrils characteristic of amyloid, amphoterin, and S100/calgranulins (21). Even within a particular ligand family, RAGE recognizes more than one species. For example, the S100/calgranulins comprise a family of more than 15 polypeptides. RAGE interacts with S100A12 and S100b (two rather divergent family members), raising the likely possibility that this receptor may interact with multiple, maybe even all, S100/calgranulins. A second salient feature of RAGE biology is the presence of more than one ligand in tissues for prolonged periods (21). For example, in diabetic tissues, both AGEs and S100/calgranulins are present at increased levels in many cases. Another unusual feature of the receptor is its apparent colocalization to sites where its ligands tend to accumulate (21). For example, where AGEs and S100/calgranulins are observed at sites of vascular lesions, higher levels of RAGE are also identified. This observation raises the possibility that the presence of ligands upregulates expression of the receptor, potentially resulting

in exaggerated RAGE-mediated cellular activation. This has been demonstrated directly with amphoterin, and it appears to be true also with AGEs, S100/calgranulins, and amyloids.

The broad consequences of RAGE-ligand interaction for cellular properties are emphasized by the spectrum of signaling mechanisms that the receptor triggers after ligand occupancy. From the JAK/STAT pathway to activation of p21ras and the MAPK family, RAGE can modulate diverse cellular functions (21). Although multiple pathways downstream of RAGE have been identified, the proximal signaling proteins that actually bind to the receptor's cytosolic tail to initiate signaling events have not yet been identified. It is important to note that the receptor's short (43 amino acids), highly charged cytosolic tail is critical for RAGE-mediated cellular activation. For example, a truncated form of RAGE lacking only the cytosolic portion (termed tail-deleted or dominant-negative RAGE) has been expressed in cells. Tail-deleted RAGE remains firmly embedded in the membrane and binds ligand analogously to wild-type RAGE, but it does not result in changes in cellular properties after ligand engagement. Cells expressing wild-type RAGE into which tail-deleted RAGE has been introduced do not demonstrate RAGE-mediated cellular activation in the presence of ligands; that is, the presence of tail-deleted RAGE results in a dominant-negative phenotype. Therefore, RAGE functions as a signal transduction receptor for its ligands, rather than simply being a binding site that tethers AGEs and other species to the cell surface.

INSULIN

Insulin is a regulatory peptide that is continuously released in varying rates by the pancreas to indirectly regulate the concentration of plasma glucose by inducing some cell types to increase glucose uptake or release. For example, insulin increases VSMC uptake of glucose. Insulin has also been found to have mitogenic properties, promoting the proliferation of various cell types, including VSMC, when present at levels commonly found in type 2 diabetics and patients with hypertension (22). Plasma insulin concentrations are 5 to 20 μU/mL in normal, fasting humans; diabetics have variable concentrations rising to as much as 250 μU/mL. When a normal human is subjected to a glucose challenge, the plasma insulin concentration increases to 75 μU/mL; in patients with type 1 diabetes it typically falls to 0 μU/mL, and in type 2 diabetes it increases to 250 μU/mL; in hypertensive patients, it increases to 175 μU/mL (23).

Insulin Signaling Pathways

Similar to many cytokine receptors, the insulin receptor (IR) is a heterotetramer of IRA and IRB subunits, each IRA possessing an inactive, cytoplasmic tyrosine kinase domain. Only one receptor need be bound to insulin for intracellular signaling to be initiated; mutual phosphorylation of the tyrosine kinase domains occurs, allowing binding and phosphorylation of a variety of intracellular proteins, including insulin receptor substrate-1 (IRS-1) (24,25). IRS-1 and other proteins bind transiently via PTB domains to the insulin receptor (26–29); once bound, they are phosphorylated on an YXXM/YMXM motif (25). Each IRS-1 can then act as a docking protein for the SH2 domains of a variety of internal signaling proteins (26,28) (Fig. 1-1), these include JAK2, STAT1, STAT3, Grb2, phosphatidyl inositol-3 kinase (PI3 kinase), and phospholipase C γ (PLC-γ). Each binding and activation event involves increased susceptibility to phosphorylation and triggers a signaling cascade. Tyrosine phosphorylation activates JAK2, which phosphorylates STAT proteins, resulting in the formation of homodimers or heterodimers that migrate to the nucleus, where they form gene activation complexes (30,31). Phosphorylated PLC-γ degrades phosphatidyl inositol bisphosphate (PIP$_2$) to produce inositol 1,4,5-triphosphate (1,4,5-IP$_3$) and diacylglycerol, which respectively trigger the release of intracellular Ca^{2+} and activate PKC. PI3 kinase converts phosphatidyl inositol to phosphatidyl inositol 3-phosphate. An IRS-1/Grb2/SOS complex activates ras (32), a small

G protein found in the chain of signaling events that leads to the activation of MAPK (33).

Insulin Resistance

Insulin resistance occurs as part of a cluster of cardiovascular-metabolic abnormalities commonly referred to as the "insulin resistance syndrome" or the "metabolic syndrome." This cluster of abnormalities may lead to the development of type 2 diabetes, accelerated atherosclerosis, hypertension, or polycystic ovary syndrome, depending on the genetic background of the individual developing the insulin resistance. Currently, insulin resistance is defined clinically as the inability of a known quantity of exogenous or endogenous insulin to increase glucose uptake and utilization in an individual as much as it does in a normal population (4). As stated previously, insulin action is the consequence of the binding of insulin to its plasma membrane receptor and the transmission of its signal throughout the cell by a series of protein-protein interactions and signaling cascades. Studies suggest that these signaling pathways are diminished in type 2 diabetes (34). Several mechanisms have been proposed as possible causes underlying the development of insulin resistance and the insulin resistance syndrome. These include (a) genetic abnormalities of one or more proteins of the insulin action cascade, (b) fetal malnutrition, and (c) increases in visceral adiposity.

It has also become clear that insulin, among its many other actions, is also a vasoactive hormone. For example, its effect in causing endothelial nitric oxide-dependent vasodilation is physiologic and dose dependent, and studies suggest that insulin's metabolic and vascular actions are closely linked. Indeed, insulin-resistant states, which by definition exhibit diminished insulin-mediated glucose uptake into peripheral tissues, also display impaired insulin-mediated vasodilation as well as impaired endothelium-dependent vasodilation (35). In addition, free fatty acids are elevated in states of insulin resistance and also cause endothelial dysfunction along with impaired insulin-mediated vasodilation (36). Thus, a picture is emerging that links insulin action

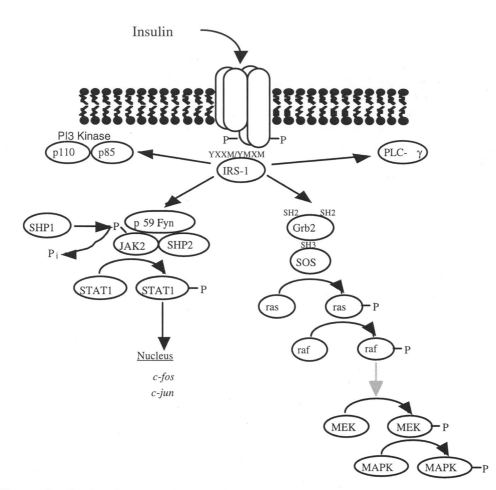

FIG. 1-1. Insulin signaling cascade. The binding of insulin to the receptor triggers its autophosphorylation at tyrosine residues. Insulin receptor substrate-1 (IRS-1) is then transiently bound and tyrosine-phosphorylated on a YXXM/YMXM motif found on PTB domains. While activated, it acts as a docking protein to proteins with an SH2 domain, known to include p59 Fyn, Grb2, phospholipase C-γ (PLC-γ) and p85 subunit of phosphatidyl inositol-3-kinase (PI3 kinase). The janus kinase/signal transducer and activator of transcription (JAK/STAT) and mitogen-activated protein kinase (MAPK) pathways are known to have the above details in connection with insulin activation.

in peripheral tissues to its action in endothelium. Moreover, recent data suggest that insulin signaling mechanisms in peripheral tissues and endothelium may be shared. Therefore, the protective action of nitric oxide and healthy endothelial function are critical to prevent atherosclerotic vascular disease.

CYTOKINES

Diabetes is associated with increased expression and action of various cytokines and growth factors. This appears to be a consequence of hyperglycemia-induced events including PKC activation, upregulation of vasoactive hormones such as endothelin and Ang II, hypoxia, and oxidative and possibly glycoxidative stress. It appears that certain cytokines play a particular role in various diabetes-induced vascular injuries. For example, TGF-β plays a pivotal role in mediating the accumulation of extracellular matrix in the kidney (37). VEGF has powerful angiogenic properties that may be responsible for retinal neovascularization (38). However, the role of cytokines in mediating microvascular and macrovascular injury at other sites remains to be determined.

Transforming Growth Factor-β

A major role for TGF-β has been suggested in a range of progressive renal diseases including diabetes mellitus (37). However, TGF-β may also be an important mediator of vascular injury at other sites in diabetes. TGF-β has been demonstrated *in vitro* to cause both hypertrophy and hyperplasia of VSMC and to favor vascular extracellular matrix production and accumulation (39). Furthermore, it has also been demonstrated that angiotensin-converting enzyme (ACE) inhibition attenuates vascular hypertrophy and prevents upregulation of the TGF-β gene and protein expression in mesenteric vessels, both short term and long term, in diabetic rats, providing *in vivo* evidence for a link between Ang II and TGF-β in blood vessels in the presence of diabetes (40). Finally, TGF-β appears to be an important mediator of various pathways implicated in the genesis of diabetic vascular complications. Indeed, several pathogenic stimuli appear to be involved in the diabetes-associated upregulation of TGF-β, including glucose-induced PKC activation, AGEs, Ang II, and cell stretch associated with hyperperfusion (41).

Vascular Endothelial Growth Factor

VEGF is one of the most potent inducers of vascular permeability and a powerful mitogen for vascular endothelial cells. Evidence suggests that VEGF plays a role in the pathogenesis of neovascularization and in the increased vascular permeability that characterizes diabetic microangiopathy (38). This cytokine has been considered to play a pivotal role in mediating proliferative diabetic retinopathy, but its role in other vascular sites in diabetes is not well characterized. Low levels of constitutive VEGF messenger RNA (mRNA) in medium-to-large arteries have been observed *in vivo* in humans, and this expression is restricted to VSMC. Similarly, various stimuli relevant to the diabetic context have been reported to increase the vascular expression

of VEGF, including hypoxia, elevated glucose concentrations, AGEs, Ang II, and TGF-β (42). The intracellular signaling pathway responsible for hyperglycemia-induced VEGF upregulation appears to involve PKC activation (43). Studies have also detected increased expression of VEGF receptors in the diabetic retina (7). A link between Ang II and VEGF is suggested by *in vitro* studies in which blockade of the AT$_1$ receptor with losartan abolished the upregulation of VEGF mRNA in cultured smooth muscle cells (44).

VASOACTIVE PEPTIDES

Angiotensin II

Cardiovascular and renal diseases are the leading causes of morbidity and mortality in patients with diabetes mellitus, and Ang II has been implicated in the pathogenesis of maladaptive growth in both cardiovascular and renal tissues in these patients (1,23,45–51). Inhibition of Ang II-induced proliferation of VSMC with ACE inhibitors and AT$_1$ receptor blockers has been shown to reduce cardiovascular disease in both diabetic patients and animal models (52,53). Several Ang II-induced cardiovascular responses (e.g., growth, contraction, Ca^{2+} signaling, AT$_1$ receptor density) are induced by hyperglycemia, and hyperglycemia correlates with an increased incidence of atherosclerosis in diabetics (1,5,51). The AT$_1$ receptor has been linked to mitogenic signaling cascades (JAK/STAT, p21ras/Raf-1/MAPK, and PLC-γ1) (54,55), and, more importantly, VSMC proliferation can be prevented by inhibition of many of these Ang II-mediated events through molecular, biochemical, and pharmacologic approaches (19,56).

Angiotensin II Signaling Pathways

The actions of Ang II are mediated through two types of cell surface receptors, AT$_1$ and AT$_2$. Most of the physiologic responses to Ang II in VSMC occur via the AT$_1$ receptor subtype (54,57). For AT$_1$ receptors, activation by Ang II results in G protein-mediated signaling, including PLC-dependent activation of PKC

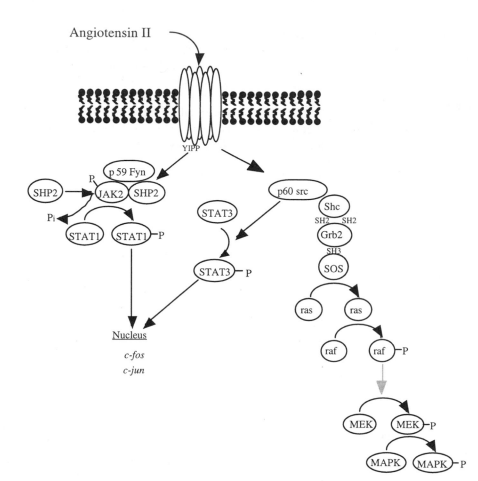

FIG. 1-2. Angiotensin II signaling cascade. The binding of angiotensin II to its AT_1 receptor requires tyrosine phosphorylation by a cytoplasmic membrane surface G protein on the YIPP motif. Once phosphorylated, it provides a transient docking site for the SH2 domain of p59 Fyn, enabling activation of the janus kinase/signal transducer and activator of transcription (JAK/STAT) pathway. The protein p60 Src is also activated by AT_1, which then activates STAT3. P60 Src also activates the mitogen-activated protein (MAP) kinase pathway, which is responsible for the serine phosphorylation of STAT1 and STAT3.

and release of calcium from intracellular stores (54). AT_1 receptors also activate signaling pathways traditionally associated with growth factor and cytokine receptors that induce the expression of early growth response genes. Signaling cascades through which Ang II induces early growth response genes, such as the *c-fos* and *c-jun* proto-oncogenes, do not in general require new protein synthesis and appear to be regulated by posttranslational modifications of preexisting transcription factors (58–61). Therefore, the Ang II-induced expression of these

early growth response genes is under the direct regulation of intracellular signal transduction pathways. Three intracellular signaling pathways have been implicated in the activation of proto-oncogenes: the JAK/STAT, p21ras/Raf-1/MAPK, and PLC-γ1 cascades (54,55,57) (Fig. 1-2). From multiple studies focusing on AT_1 receptor signal transduction pathways, it has become apparent that the temporal arrangement of agonist-stimulated signaling varies from seconds (e.g., activation of PLC-γ1 and generation of inositol phosphates) to minutes (e.g., MAPK activation) to hours (e.g., JAK/STAT pathway) (54,55). The exact mechanisms by which the AT_1 receptor is able to differentially couple to disparate signal transduction pathways are not clear but presumably involve a complex series of steps that selectively recruits, activates, and then inactivates each signaling system in a time-dependent manner.

Role of the JAK/STAT Pathway in Angiotensin II Signaling

The JAK family of cytosolic tyrosine kinases, traditionally thought to be coupled to cytokine receptors such as those for the interleukins and interferons, has four members: JAK1, JAK2, JAK3, and TYK2 (30,62). In response to ligand binding, these JAK tyrosine kinases associate with, tyrosine-phosphorylate, and activate the cytokine receptor itself. Once activated, JAKs tyrosine-phosphorylate and activate other signaling molecules, including the STAT family of nuclear transcription factors after binding of the STATs to the receptor (30,62). Thus, the JAK/STAT pathway is an important link between cell surface receptors and nuclear transcriptional events leading to cell growth.

Baker et al. showed that STAT1, STAT3, and STAT5 are tyrosine-phosphorylated in response to Ang II in cardiac fibroblasts and AT_1 receptor-transfected Chinese hamster ovary (CHO) cells (63–65). The same investigators found that Ang II exposure stimulates the phosphorylated monomeric STAT proteins to form homodimer ($STAT1_2$, $STAT3_2$, or $STAT5_2$) or heterodimer (STAT1:STAT3) complexes, referred to as SIF (*sis*-inducing factors). These SIF complexes subsequently translocate to the nucleus and interact with specific DNA motifs called SIE (*sis*-inducing elements) or PIE (prolactin-inducing element)-like elements within the *c-fos* promoter, culminating in the activation of this early growth response gene (30,62,64,65). Marrero et al. also showed that the JAK/STAT cascade can be activated by Ang II, resulting in the tyrosine phosphorylation of JAK2, STAT1, and STAT3 and the translocation of STAT1 and STAT3 to the nucleus (19,66,67). Bernstein et al. (68) previously demonstrated

that the carboxyl-terminal tail of the AT_1 receptor binds to JAK2 in an Ang II-dependent manner. In addition, Marrero et al. (19) showed that inhibition of JAK2 tyrosine phosphorylation with the pharmacologic JAK2 inhibitor, AG490, or electroporation of blocking antibodies against STAT1 or STAT3 inhibits Ang II-induced VSMC proliferation and DNA synthesis (19). These results indicate that G protein-coupled receptors, in particular the AT_1 receptor, can operate via the same intracellular tyrosine phosphorylation pathways previously linked to cytokine and growth factor receptors. Finally, Marrero et al. (69) found that the tyrosine phosphatases, SHP-1 and SHP-2, have opposing roles in Ang II-induced JAK2 phosphorylation. SHP-1 appears to be responsible for JAK2 dephosphorylation and termination of the Ang II-induced JAK/STAT cascade, whereas SHP-2 appears to have an essential role in JAK2 phosphorylation and initiation of the Ang II-induced JAK/STAT cascade leading to cell proliferation. The motif in the AT_1 receptor that is required for association with JAK2 is also required for association with SHP-2. Further, SHP-2 is also required for JAK2-Ang II AT_1 receptor association. SHP-2 may thus play a role as an adaptor protein for JAK2 association with the receptor, facilitating JAK2 phosphorylation and activation (69).

A Role for High Glucose in Angiotensin II-Mediated Responses

As previously discussed, diabetes is associated with significantly increased rates of cardiovascular complications, including atherosclerosis. However, the molecular mechanisms responsible are not very clear. For instance, it has been shown that VSMC cultured under conditions simulating hyperglycemia (25 mM glucose) proliferate more rapidly than those cultured with "physiologic" or normal levels of glucose (5.5 mM) (70,71), suggesting a possible mechanism for the accelerated vascular growth seen in diabetes. However, the specific cellular signals activated in VSMC under hyperglycemic conditions have not been completely elucidated. Amiri et al. (3)

found that hyperglycemia increases both (a) the basal and Ang II-induced VSMC proliferation, tyrosine phosphorylation, and complex formation of JAK2 with the Ang II AT_1 receptor and (b) the extent of the tyrosine and serine phosphorylation of STAT1 and STAT3. They also found that hyperglycemia alters Ang II-induced tyrosine phosphorylation and activities of SHP-1 and SHP-2 (3). These results suggest that increased and/or altered activation of tyrosine kinase (JAK2), tyrosine phosphatases (SHP-1 and SHP-2), and downstream transcription factors (STAT1, STAT3) may be key mechanisms for the increased Ang II-induced VSMC growth potential in response to hyperglycemic conditions.

High Glucose, Production of Reactive Oxygen Species, JAK2 Activation, and Growth of Vascular Smooth Muscle Cells

As previously described, hyperglycemia enhances the Ang II-induced JAK/STAT pathway (3). The molecular mechanisms responsible for augmentation of Ang II-induced activation of the JAK/STAT pathway in VSMC by hyperglycemia remain to be elucidated, but a candidate mechanism might be related to the activation of JAK2 by reactive oxygen species (ROS). For example, it has been shown that ROS stimulate the activity of JAK2 in both fibroblasts and A-431 cells (72). Furthermore, Schieffer et al. (73) demonstrated that activation of JAK2 and STAT proteins by Ang II in VSMC is significantly inhibited by the reduced nicotinamide adenine dinucleotide phosphate (NADPH) oxidase inhibitor, diphenylene iodonium, and electroporation of the NADPH oxidase neutralizing antibody, anti-p47 phox/immunoglobulin G. These data support the hypothesis that oxygen free radicals generated by NADPH oxidase ROS may contribute to the activation of JAK2 and STATs in response to Ang II (73). These findings suggest that the JAK-STAT pathway responds to intracellular ROS and that the vasoactive peptide Ang II uses ROS as a second messenger to regulate JAK2 activation.

Other studies have suggested that high glucose induces, via the polyol pathway, a rapid increase in intracellular ROS such as H_2O_2, which

stimulates intracellular signal events similar to those activated by Ang II, including stimulation of growth-promoting kinases such as JAK2 and extracellular signal-related kinase 1/2 (ERK1/2) (74–76). The polyol pathway generates ROS (H_2O_2 and O_2^-) (17,77), which can then act as signal transducers in the activation of mitogenic pathways such as the JAK/STAT signaling cascade (72). For instance, in VSMC, H_2O_2 has been shown to play an important role in regulation of cell growth (76). It has also been reported that Ang II causes a rapid increase in intracellular H_2O_2, via NADPH oxidase, which subsequently activates growth-related responses along with activation of the JAK/STAT pathway (73,76). Similar results have also been found for PDGF-induced cell proliferation, which was shown to depend on generation of H_2O_2 (72). Furthermore, PDGF uses H_2O_2 as a second messenger to regulate activation of the JAK/STAT pathway in rat fibroblasts (72). Therefore, it is reasonable to suggest that hyperglycemia augments the Ang II-induced JAK/STAT pathway and growth responses in VSMC through the reactive oxygen species H_2O_2 generated via the polyol pathway.

Advanced Glycation End Products, Reactive Oxygen Species, JAK2 Activation, and Vascular Growth

Accumulation of AGEs is accelerated in conditions associated with oxidant stress, such as diabetes mellitus. AGEs form by the interaction of aldoses with free amino groups of macromolecules as the result of a complex series of molecular events (11). AGEs have been identified in plasma, although they are more likely to be identified in tissues and intracellularly (such as in extracellular matrix, vessel walls, and other cellular elements in the diabetic kidney). The interaction of AGEs with the receptor RAGE generates ROS (H_2O_2 and O_2^-) (77,78), which can then act as signal mediators in the activation of mitogenic pathways such as the JAK/STAT signaling cascade (72). In fact, AGE-RAGE-triggered activation of NADPH oxidase has been demonstrated (78). Furthermore, it has been shown that binding of AGE to RAGE activates the JAK/STAT pathway (20). Thus, the stage is set for intracellular processes by which RAGE-mediated cellular activation can synergize with Ang II- and high glucose-induced cellular stimulation.

Activation of Protein Kinase C in Diabetes and Its Role in Glucose-Induced Stimulation of Reactive Oxygen Species Production in Vascular Smooth Muscle Cells

Recent studies have shown that activation of PKC and increased diacylglycerol levels initiated by hyperglycemia are associated with many vascular abnormalities in retinal, renal, and cardiovascular tissues (12). It has also been found that among the various PKC isoforms, the β and δ isoforms appear to be activated preferentially in the vasculatures of diabetic animals, although other PKC isoforms are also increased in the renal glomeruli and in retina (12). High glucose-induced activation of PKC has been shown to increase the production of ROS, extracellular matrix, and cytokines and to enhance contractility, permeability, and vascular cell proliferation. The synthesis and characterization of a specific inhibitor for PKC-β isoforms has confirmed the role of PKC activation in the mediation of hyperglycemic effects on vascular cells and has provided *in vivo* evidence that PKC-β activation can be responsible for abnormal ROS production and vascular growth in diabetic animals (79).

As previously discussed, several lines of experimentation have revealed that vascular cells can produce ROS through NADPH oxidase, which may be involved in vascular injury. However, the molecular activation of NADPH oxidase in diabetes remains unknown. In a recent study, the effects of glucose on ROS production in VSMC were examined (80). It was found that exposure of cultured VSMC to hyperglycemia significantly increased ROS production and that treatment of the cells with phorbol myristic acid (PMA), a PKC activator, also increased ROS production. Such hyperglycemia increased generation of ROS and was inhibited by the flavine oxidase inhibitor DPI, suggesting ROS production through PKC-dependent activation of NADPH oxidase. Furthermore, it was found that the increased ROS production caused by incubating

cultures in high glucose was completely inhibited by GF109203X, a PKC-specific inhibitor. These results suggest that hyperglycemia stimulates ROS production through PKC-dependent activation of NADPH oxidase in VSMC (80). In addition, a very recent study also showed that the PKC-βII isoform is essential for the activation of NADPH oxidase (81).

Endothelin

Role of Endothelin in Diabetes Mellitus

It has been speculated that diabetes-related endothelial activation might increase vascular production of endothelin, leading in turn to glomerular damage by augmentation of vasoconstriction, glomerular permeability, mesangial cell proliferation, and extracellular matrix production (82). In support of this proposal, it has been reported that plasma levels of endothelin and endothelin mRNA are increased both in humans with diabetes and in streptozotocin (STZ)-treated rats (83). Moreover, increased plasma endothelin levels in diabetes are associated with increased risk of microvascular complications, suggesting a possible link between endothelin and diabetes-associated microangiopathy (84,85). In addition, glucose has been shown to be a potent stimulator of endothelin production from endothelial cells (85), implying that locally released endothelin may contribute to diabetic atherosclerosis. The role of endothelin in diabetes was also supported by studies in which the ET_A receptor antagonist BQ-123 was administered to STZ-treated diabetic rats. BQ-123 was shown to prevent renal disease and to decrease production of extracellular matrix (86). Finally, endothelin was demonstrated to interfere with insulin signaling in VSMC (87). Although these studies suggest a role for endothelin in diabetic nephropathy and atherosclerosis, considerable additional work is necessary to provide support for such a link.

CONCLUSION

Diabetics account for almost 50% of all patients enrolled in the federally funded ESRD program,

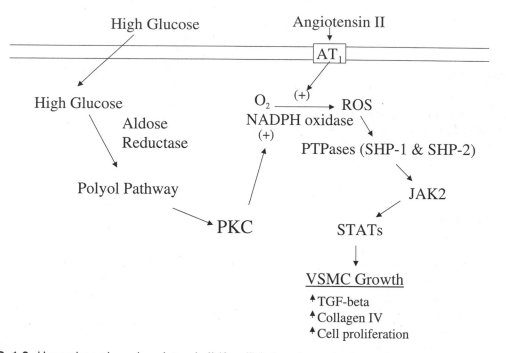

FIG. 1-3. Hyperglycemia and angiotensin II (Ang II)-induced growth of vascular smooth muscle cells (VSMC). Hyperglycemia and Ang II activate intracellular signaling processes that include the polyol pathway and the generation of reactive oxygen species, which in turn activate the janus kinase/signal transducer and activator of transcription (JAK/STAT) signaling cascade in VSMC. This signaling cascade then stimulates the proliferation and growth of VSMC.

at a cost of several billion dollars per year, and they have a 100-fold greater risk of dying compared with the nondiabetic population. The need for research into the pathogenesis, prevention, and treatment of diabetes is highlighted by the profound financial, social, and personal impacts of this devastating disease. Hyperglycemia and Ang II activate intracellular signaling processes that include the polyol pathway and the generation of ROS, which in turn trigger signaling cascades (e.g., MAPK, PLC-γ, JAK/STAT pathway) in VSMC. These signaling cascades stimulate the proliferation and growth of VSMC and mesangial cells, potentially setting the stage for cardiovascular complications such as atherosclerosis (Fig. 1-3) and diabetic nephropathy. Based on this outline of potential underlying pathophysiologic mechanisms, future work has the objective of clarifying critical cellular and molecular mechanisms of early diabetic macroangiopathy and microangiopathy, with the aim of developing improved diagnostic and therapeutic strategies.

REFERENCES

1. Wautier JL, Guillausseau PJ. Diabetes, advanced glycation endproducts and vascular disease. *Vasc Med* 1998;3:131–137.
2. Breyerj A. Diabetic nephropathy in insulin-dependent patients. *Am J Kidney Dis* 1992;20:533–547.
3. Amiri F, Venema VJ, Wang X, et al. Hyperglycemia enhances angiotensin II-induced janus-activated kinase/STAT signaling in vascular smooth muscle cells. *J Biol Chem* 1999;274:32382–32386.
4. Folli F, Saad MJ, Velloso L, et al. Crosstalk between insulin and angiotensin II signalling systems. *Exp Clin Endocrinol Diabetes* 1999;107:133–139.
5. Cosentino F, Lüscher TF. Endothelial dysfunction in diabetes mellitus. *J Cardiovasc Pharmacol* 1998;32[Suppl 3]:S54–S61.
6. Cohen RA. Dysfunction of vascular endothelium in diabetes mellitus. *Circulation* 1993;87[Suppl V]:V67–V76.
7. Lu M, Kuroki M, Amano S, et al. Advanced glycation end products increase retinal vascular endothelial growth factor expression. *J Clin Invest* 1998;101:1219–1224.

8. Amiri F, Garcia R. Renal angiotensin II receptors and protein kinase C in diabetic rats: effects of insulin and ACE inhibition. *Am J Physiol Renal Physiol* 2000;278:F603–F612.

9. Carvalho CR, Thirone AC, Gontijo JA, et al. Effect of captopril, losartan, and bradykinin on early steps of insulin action. *Diabetes* 1997;46:1950–1957.

10. Nickenig G, Böhm M. Interaction between insulin and AT_1 receptor: relevance for hypertension and arteriosclerosis. *Basic Res Cardiol* 1998;93:135–139.

11. Schmidt AM, Yan SD, Wautier JL, et al. Activation of receptor for advanced glycation end products: a mechanism for chronic vascular dysfunction in diabetic vasculopathy and atherosclerosis. *Circ Res* 1999;84:489–497.

12. Nakamura J, Kasuya Y, Hamada Y, et al. Glucose-induced hyperproliferation of cultured rat aortic smooth muscle cells through polyol pathway hyperactivity. *Diabetologia* 2001;44:480–487.

13. Oh JH, Ha H, Yu MR, et al. Sequential effects of high glucose on mesangial cell transforming growth factor-beta1 and fibronectin synthesis. *Kidney Int* 1998;54:1872–1878.

14. Kim SI, Han DC, Lee HB. Lovastatin inhibits transforming growth factor-beta1 expression in diabetic rat glomeruli and cultured rat mesangial cells. *J Am Soc Nephrol* 2000;11:80–87.

15. Derubertis FR, Craven PA. Activation of protein kinase C in glomerular cells in diabetes: mechanisms and potential links to the pathogenesis of diabetic glomerulopathy. *Diabetes* 1994;43:1–8.

16. Kapor-Drezgic J, Zhou X, Babazono T, et al. Effects of high glucose on mesangial cell protein kinase C-delta and -epsilon is polyol pathway-dependent. *J Am Soc Nephrol* 1999;10:1193–1203.

17. Ha H, Lee HB. Reactive oxygen species as glucose signaling molecules in mesangial cells cultured under high glucose. *Kidney Int* 2000;58:S19–S25.

18. Haneda M, Kikkawa R, Sugimoto T, et al. Abnormalities in protein kinase C and MAP kinase cascade in mesangial cells cultured under high glucose conditions. *J Diabetes Complications* 1995;9:246–248.

19. Marrero MB, Schieffer B, Li B, et al. Role of janus kinase/signal transducer and activator of transcription and mitogen-activated protein kinase cascades in angiotensin II- and platelet-derived growth factor-induced vascular smooth muscle cell proliferation. *J Biol Chem* 1997;272:24684–24690.

20. Huang JS, Guh JY, Chen HC, et al. Role of receptor for advanced glycation end-products (RAGE) and the JAK/STAT-signaling pathway in AGE-induced collagen production in NRK-49F cells. *J Cell Biochem* 2001;81:102–113.

21. Wendt T, Bucciarelli L, Qu W, et al. Receptor for advanced glycation endproducts (RAGE) and vascular inflammation: insights into the pathogenesis of macrovascular complications in diabetes. *Curr Atheroscler Rep* 2002;4:228–237.

22. Menon RK, Sperling MA. Insulin as a growth factor. *Endocrinol Metab Clin North Am* 1996;25:633–647.

23. Ling BN. Regulation of mesangial chloride channels by insulin and glucose: role in diabetic nephropathy. *Clin Exp Pharmacol Physiol* 1996;23:89–94.

24. White MF, Yenush L. The IRS-signaling system: a network of docking proteins that mediate insulin and cytokine action. *Curr Top Microbiol Immunol* 1998;228:179–208.

25. Avruch J. Insulin signal transduction through protein kinase cascades. *Mol Cell Biochem* 1998;182:31–48.

26. White MF, Kahn CR. The insulin signaling system. *J Biol Chem* 1994;269:1–4.

27. Eck MJ, Dhe-Paganon S, Trub T, et al. Structure of the IRS-1 PTB domain bound to the juxtamembrane region of the insulin receptor. *Cell* 1996;85:695–705.

28. Sun XJ, Wang LM, Zhang Y, et al. Role of IRS-2 in insulin and cytokine signalling. *Nature* 1995;377:173–177.

29. Sun XJ, Rothenberg P, Kahn CR, et al. Structure of the insulin receptor substrate IRS-1 defines a unique signal transduction protein. *Nature* 1991;352:73–77.

30. Schindler C, Darnell JE Jr. Transcriptional responses to polypeptide ligands: the JAK-STAT pathway. *Annu Rev Biochem* 1995;64:621–651.

31. Darnell JE Jr. STATs and gene regulation. *Science* 1997;277:1630–1635.

32. Fucini RV, Okada S, Pessin JE. Insulin-induced desensitization of extracellular signal-regulated kinase activation results from an inhibition of Raf activity independent of Ras activation and dissociation of the Grb2-SOS complex. *J Biol Chem* 1999;274:18651–18658.

33. De Fea K, Roth RA. Modulation of insulin receptor substrate-1 tyrosine phosphorylation and function by mitogen-activated protein kinase. *J Biol Chem* 1997;272:31400–31406.

34. Virkamaki A, Ueki K, Kahn CR. Protein-protein interaction in insulin signaling and the molecular mechanisms of insulin resistance. *J Clin Invest* 1999;103:931–943.

35. Ueda S, Petrie JR, Cleland SJ, et al. Insulin vasodilatation and the "arginine paradox." *Lancet* 1998;351:959–960.

36. Sobrevia L, Nadal A, Yudilevich DL, Mann GE. Activation of L-arginine transport (system y^+) and nitric oxide synthase by elevated glucose and insulin in human endothelial cells. *J Physiol* 1996;490:775–781.

37. Choi KH, Kang SW, Lee HY, et al. The effects of high glucose concentration on angiotensin II- or transforming growth factor-β-induced DNA synthesis, hypertrophy and collagen synthesis in cultured rat mesangial cells. *Yonsei Med J* 1996;37:302–311.

38. Neufeld G, Cohen T, Gengrinovitch S, et al. Vascular endothelial growth factor (VEGF) and its receptors. *FASEB J* 1999;13:9–22.

39. Satoh C, Fukuda N, Hu WY, et al. Role of endogenous angiotensin II in the increased expression of growth factors in vascular smooth muscle cells from spontaneously hypertensive rats. *J Cardiovasc Pharmacol* 2001;37:108–118.

40. Teng J, Fukuda N, Suzuki R, et al. Inhibitory effect of a novel angiotensin II type 1 receptor antagonist RNH-6270 on growth of vascular smooth muscle cells from spontaneously hypertensive rats: different anti-proliferative effect to angiotensin-converting enzyme inhibitor. *J Cardiovasc Pharmacol* 2002;39:161–171.

41. Chen S, Cohen MP, Ziyadeh FN. Amadori-glycated albumin in diabetic nephropathy: pathophysiologic connections. *Kidney Int Suppl* 2000;77:S40–S44.

42. Natarajan R, Bai W, Lanting L, et al. Effects of high glucose on vascular endothelial growth factor expression in vascular smooth muscle cells. *Am J Physiol* 1997;273:H2224–H2231.

43. Feng Y, Venema VJ, Venema RC, et al. VEGF induces nuclear translocation of Flk-1/KDR, endothelial nitric oxide synthase, and caveolin-1 in vascular endothelial cells. *Biochem Biophys Res Commun* 1999;256:192–197.

44. Zhu B, Sun Y, Sievers RE, et al. Effects of different durations of pretreatment with losartan on myocardial infarct size, endothelial function, and vascular endothelial growth factor. *J Renin Angiotensin Aldosterone Syst* 2001;2:129–133.

45. Ling BN, Matsunaga H, Ma H, et al. Role of growth factors in mesangial cell ion channel regulation. *Kidney Int* 1995;48:1158–1166.

46. Ling BN, Seal EE, Eaton DC. Regulation of mesangial cell ion channels by insulin and angiotensin II: possible role in diabetic glomerular hyperfiltration. *J Clin Invest* 1993;92:2141–2151.

47. Iyer SN, Raizada MK, Katovich MJ. AT_1 receptor density changes during development of hypertension in hyperinsulinemic rats. *Clin Exp Hypertens* 1996;18:793–810.

48. Pfeiffer A, Schatz H. Diabetic microvascular complications and growth factors. *Exp Clin Endocrinol* 1995;103:7–14.

49. Saward L, Zahradka P. Insulin is required for angiotensin II-mediated hypertrophy of smooth muscle cells. *Mol Cell Endocrinol* 1996;122:93–100.

50. Seal EE, Eaton DC, Gomez LM, et al. Extracellular glucose reduces mesangial cell ion channel responsiveness to angiotensin II. *Am J Physiol* 1995;269:F389–F397.

51. Sowers JR, Epstein M. Diabetes mellitus and associated hypertension, vascular disease, and nephropathy: an update. *Hypertension* 1995;26:869–879.

52. Volpert OV, Ward WF, Lingen MW, et al. Captopril inhibits angiogenesis and slows the growth of experimental tumors in rats. *J Clin Invest* 1996;98:671–679.

53. Goodfriend TL, Elliott ME, Catt KJ. Angiotensin receptors and their antagonists. *N Engl J Med* 1996;334:1649–1654.

54. Bernstein KE, Marrero MB. The importance of tyrosine phosphorylation in angiotensin II signaling. *Trends Cardiovasc Med* 1996;6:179–187.

55. Sayeski PP, Ali MS, Semeniuk DJ, et al. Angiotensin II signal transduction pathways. *Regul Pept* 1998;78:19–29.

56. Schieffer B, Drexler H, Ling BN, et al. G protein-coupled receptors control vascular smooth muscle cell proliferation via $pp60^{c-src}$ and $p21^{ras}$. *Am J Physiol* 1997;272:C2019–C2030.

57. Marrero MB, Paxton WG, Schieffer B, et al. Angiotensin II signalling events mediated by tyrosine phosphorylation. *Cell Signal* 1996;8:21–26.

58. Okuda M, Kawahara Y, Yokoyama M. Angiotensin II type 1 receptor-mediated activation of Ras in cultured rat vascular smooth muscle cells. *Am J Physiol* 1996;271:H595–H601.

59. Sadoshima J, Izumo S. Molecular characterization of angiotensin II-induced hypertrophy of cardiac myocytes and hyperplasia of cardiac fibroblasts: critical role of the AT_1 receptor subtype. *Circ Res* 1993;73:413–423.

60. Sadoshima J, Izumo S. Signal transduction pathways of angiotensin II induced *c-fos* gene expression in cardiac myocytes *in vitro*. *Circ Res* 1993;73:424–438.

61. Taubman MB, Berk BC, Izumo S, et al. Angiotensin II induces c-*fos* mRNA in aortic smooth muscle: role of Ca^{2+} mobilization and protein kinase C activation. *J Biol Chem* 1989;264:526–530.

62. Darnell JE Jr, Kerr IM, Stark GR. Jak-STAT pathways and transcriptional activation in response to IFNs and other extracellular signaling proteins. *Science* 1994;264:1415–1421.

63. Bhat GJ, Thekkumkara TJ, Thomas WG, et al. Activation of the STAT pathway by angiotensin II in $T3CHO/AT_{1A}$ cells: cross-talk between angiotensin II and interleukin-6 nuclear signaling. *J Biol Chem* 1995;270:19059–19065.

64. Bhat GJ, Thekkumkara TJ, Thomas WG, et al. Angiotensin II stimulates *sis*-inducing factor-like DNA binding activity: evidence that the AT_{1A} receptor activates transcription factor-Stat91 and/or a related protein. *J Biol Chem* 1994;269:31443–31449.

65. Mcwhinney CD, Dostal D, Baker K. Angiotensin II activates stat5 through Jak2 kinase in cardiac myocytes. *J Mol Cell Cardiol* 1998;30:751–761.

66. Marrero MB, Schieffer B, Bernstein KE, et al. Angiotensin-II-induced, tyrosine phosphorylation in mesangial and vascular smooth muscle cells. *Clin Exp Pharmacol Physiol* 1996;23:83–88.

67. Marrero MB, Schieffer B, Paxton WG, et al. Direct stimulation of Jak/STAT pathway by the angiotensin II AT_1 receptor. *Nature* 1995;375:247–250.

68. Ali MS, Sayeski PP, Dirksen LB, et al. Dependence on the motif YIPP for the physical association of Jak2 kinase with the intracellular carboxyl tail of the angiotensin II AT_1 receptor. *J Biol Chem* 1997;272:23382–23388.

69. Marrero MB, Venema VJ, Ju H, et al. Regulation of angiotensin II-induced JAK2 tyrosine phosphorylation: roles of SHP-1 and SHP-2. *Am J Physiol* 1998;275:C1216–C1223.

70. Natarajan R, Scott S, Bai W, et al. Angiotensin II signaling in vascular smooth muscle cells under high glucose conditions. *Hypertension* 1999;33:378–384.

71. Natarajan R, Gonzales N, Xu L, et al. Vascular smooth muscle cells exhibit increased growth in response to elevated glucose. *Biochem Biophys Res Commun* 1992;187:552–560.

72. Simon AR, Rai U, Fanburg BL, et al. Activation of the JAK-STAT pathway by reactive oxygen species. *Am J Physiol* 1998;275:C1640–C1652.

73. Schieffer B, Luchtefeld M, Braun S, et al. Role of NAD(P)H oxidase in angiotensin II-induced JAK/STAT signaling and cytokine induction. *Circ Res* 2001;87:1195–1201.

74. Berk BC, Corson MA. Angiotensin II signal transduction in vascular smooth muscle: role of tyrosine kinases. *Circ Res* 1997;80:607–616.

75. Berk BC, Duff JL, Marrero MB, et al. Angiotensin II signal transduction in vascular smooth muscle. In: Sowers J, ed. *Contemporary endocrinology of the vasculature*. Totowa, NJ: Humana Press, 1996:187–204.

76. Ushio-Fukai M, Alexander RW, Akers M, et al. Reactive oxygen species mediate the activation of Akt/protein kinase B by angiotensin II in vascular smooth muscle cells. *J Biol Chem* 1999;274:22699–22704.

77. Chappey O, Dosquet C, Wautier MP, et al. Advanced gly-cation end products, oxidant stress and vascular lesions. *Eur J Clin Invest* 1997;27:97–108.

78. Wautier M-P, Chappey O, Corda S, et al. Activation of NADPH oxidase by AGE links oxidant stress to altered gene expression via RAGE. *Am J Physiol* 2001;280:E685–E694.

79. Ishii H, Koya D, King GL. Protein kinase C activation and its role in the development of vascular complications in diabetes mellitus. *J Mol Med* 2001;76:21–31.

80. Inoguchi T, Li P, Umeda F, et al. High glucose levels and free fatty acid stimulate reactive oxygen species production through PKC-dependent activation of NAD(P)H oxidase in cultured vascular cells. *Diabetes* 2000;49:1939–1945.

81. Korchack HM, Kilpatrick LE. Roles of BII-protein kinase C and RACK1 in positive and negative signaling for superoxide anion generation in differential HL60 cells. *J Biol Chem* 2001;276:8910–8917.

82. Garcia R, Bonhomme MC, Amiri F. Vasoactive peptide receptors in the rat kidney. *Biol Res* 1998;31:217–225.

83. Hopfner RL, Misurski D, Wilson TW, et al. Insulin and vanadate restore decreased endothelin concentrations and exaggerated vascular responses to normal in the streptozotocin diabetic rat. *Diabetologia* 1998;41:1233–1240.

84. Dedov II, Shestakov MV, Kochemasova TV, et al. [Endothelial dysfunction in the development of vascular complications in diabetes mellitus]. *Ross Fiziol Zh Im I M Sechenova* 2001;87:1073–1084.

85. Ak G, Buyukberber S, Sevinc A, et al. The relation between plasma endothelin-1 levels and metabolic control, risk factors, treatment modalities, and diabetic microangiopathy in patients with type 2 diabetes mellitus. *J Diabetes Complications* 2001;15:150–157.

86. Hocher B, Schwarz A, Reinbacher D, et al. Effects of endothelin receptor antagonists on the progression of diabetic nephropathy. *Nephron* 2001;87:161–169.

87. Jiang Zy, Zhou QL, Chatterjee A, et al. Endothelin-1 modulates insulin signaling through phosphatidylinositol 3-kinase pathway in vascular smooth muscle cells. *Diabetes* 1999;48:1120–1130.

Diabetes and Cardiovascular Disease
edited by Steven P. Marso and David M. Stern
Lippincott Williams & Wilkins, Philadelphia © 2004

2

Antioxidants, Oxidative Stress, and Inflammation in Diabetes

Sridevi Devaraj, Sonia Vega-López, and Ishwarlal Jialal

Assistant Professor of Pathology, Laboratory for Artherosclerosis and Metabolic Research; Postdoctoral Fellow, Department of Pathology; Professor of Pathology and Medicine, Director, Laboratory for Atherosclerosis and Metabolic Research, University of California, Davis Medical Center, Sacramento California

Diabetes mellitus is a leading cause of morbidity and mortality, largely because of its vascular complications (1,2). Diabetic complications can be broadly classified into two types: microvascular complications (e.g., retinopathy, nephropathy) and macrovascular complications (e.g., coronary artery disease [CAD], cerebrovascular disease, peripheral vascular disease).

The most common cause of death among people with diabetes today is atherosclerotic cardiovascular disease (CVD) (3). Several studies have shown that mortality due to CAD is two to four times greater in individuals with diabetes than in nondiabetics. CVD can manifest as CAD, stroke, or peripheral vascular disease. Most studies have indicated that this excess risk for macrovascular complications cannot be explained by conventional cardiovascular risk factors such as dyslipidemia, hypertension, and smoking. Therefore, the diabetic state, *per se,* confers an increased propensity to accelerated atherogenesis.

Current concepts suggest that the earliest event in atherogenesis is endothelial cell dysfunction, manifesting as deficiencies of nitric oxide (NO) and prostacyclin. This dysfunction can be induced by various noxious insults, including dyslipidemia, diabetes, hypertension, and smoking. After endothelial dysfunction is present, mononuclear cells such as monocytes and T lymphocytes bind to the endothelium. This development is orchestrated by certain adhesion molecules such as vascular cell adhesion molecule-1 (VCAM-1), intercellular adhesion molecule (ICAM-1), and E-selectin. Once the monocytes migrate into the subendothelial space, driven by chemokines such as monocyte chemotactic protein-1 (MCP-1) and platelet endothelial cell adhesion molecule-1 (PECAM-1), they mature into resident macrophages via macrophage colony-stimulating factor (M-CSF), take up lipid largely through scavenger receptors such as scavenger receptor-A (SR-A) and CD-36, and become foam cells. This is followed by migration of smooth muscle cells to form the fibrous cap of the lesion. Plaque rupture, which is generated when lipid-laden macrophages release matrix metalloproteinases and tissue factor, results in acute coronary syndromes such as myocardial infarction and unstable angina.

PATHOPHYSIOLOGY OF DIABETIC VASCULAR DISEASE

The numerous potential mechanisms that could mediate premature atherogenesis in diabetes include dyslipidemia, a procoagulant state, hyperinsulinemia and insulin resistance syndrome, microalbuminuria, protein glycation, oxidative stress, and inflammation (4–6). This chapter focuses mainly on the roles of oxidative stress and inflammation in the genesis of diabetic macrovascular disease; other mechanisms are

TABLE 2-1. *Potential atherogenic mechanisms in diabetes*

Lipid and lipoprotein aberrations: high triglycerides, low HDL-cholesterol, small dense LDL, increased remnant lipoproteins

Procoagulant state: increased platelet aggregation, increased levels of fibrinogen, tissue factor, PAI-1

Hyperinsulinism and the metabolic syndrome

Microalbuminuria

Glycation of proteins

Oxidative stress

Inflammation

HDL, high-density lipoprotein; LDL, low-density lipoprotein; PAI-1, plasminogen activator inhibitor-1.

discussed elsewhere in this text. This chapter also reviews the effect of antioxidants on oxidative stress, inflammation, and diabetic complications. Table 2-1 summarizes the mediating mechanisms of diabetic macrovascular disease.

Glycation (nonenzymatic glycosylation) involves the nonenzymatic binding of glucose to reactive amino groups located on lysine side chains and amino-terminal amino acid residues of protein molecules (7,8). The initial products of the reaction are Schiff bases, which rearrange to form more stable Amadori products. These early glycation products are in reversible equilibrium with their precursors, and levels tend to rise and fall with ambient glucose concentrations. Amadori products are further degraded gradually into reactive carbonyls, such as 3-deoxyglucosone and methyl glyoxal, which can further react with free amino groups to form advanced glycation end products (AGEs), which are irreversible products of glycation and oxidation (9–11). The role of AGEs in diabetic macrovascular disease is detailed in a later chapter. Briefly, AGEs are recognized by specific cell surface receptors, referred to as AGE receptors or RAGEs, which are present on circulating monocytes, lymphocytes, endothelial cells, and renal mesangial cells. AGE modification of proteins results in altered structure and function, and several studies have shown a strong relationship between AGE levels and the severity of diabetic microvascular complications.

Uptake of AGE via the macrophage receptor leads to increased production of cytokines such as interleukin-1 (IL-1), tumor necrosis factor (TNF), and growth factors such as insulin-like growth factor-1 (IGF-1), resulting in proliferation of glomerular mesangial and arterial smooth muscle cells and increased glomerular synthesis of type IV collagen. Uptake of AGE by endothelial cells results in the production of endothelin-1 tissue factor, leading to thrombosis and vasoconstriction. AGEs have been shown to activate macrophages, resulting in increased chemotaxis, cholesterol ester accumulation, and quenching of NO (9–12). This implicates AGE in the defective vascular relaxation and hypertension of diabetes and aging. Infusion of AGE albumin causes activation of the transcription factor, nuclear factor κB (NFκB), a pleiotropic regulator of many "response to injury" genes (e.g., cytokines, tissue factor), the activation of which can be inhibited by pretreatment of animals with antibodies to the AGE receptor. AGE moieties formed on matrix components, such as the vessel wall and kidney, crosslink and trap a variety of plasma proteins, most notably lipoproteins and immunoglobulins. AGEs have been demonstrated to modify low-density lipoproteins (LDL) in both lipid and apolipoprotein components, and AGE-modified LDL is more atherogenic than native LDL.

OXIDATIVE STRESS

Oxidative stress plays a crucial role in atherogenesis. Several lines of evidence support a proatherogenic role for oxidized LDL (Ox-LDL) and its *in vivo* existence (13–15). Ox-LDL is not recognized by the LDL receptor but by the scavenger receptor pathway on macrophages; its uptake results in unregulated cholesterol accumulation, leading to foam cell formation. Deleterious effects of Ox-LDL include cytotoxicity and immunogenic induction. Ox-LDL can also stimulate coagulation by inducing synthesis of tissue factor and plasminogen activator inhibitor-1 (PAI-1), and it stimulates platelet aggregation by reducing expression of platelet NO synthase (NOS) (16–19). Factors that may promote oxidative stress in diabetes include antioxidant deficiencies, glycation and glyco-oxidation, and increased production of reactive oxygen species (ROS) (5,20–23).

Patients with diabetes often have a decreased antioxidant status, which promotes an increase in oxidative stress and vascular dysfunction (24–26). A decrease in antioxidant capacity has been observed in plasma of diabetic patients (27–40). In a prospective study, Salonen et al. (41) found decreased levels of natural (RRR)-α-tocopherol (RRR-AT) after the onset of non-insulin-dependent (type 2) diabetes mellitus (T2DM). Diabetic patients may have decreased concentrations of several antioxidants, including ascorbate, glutathione, and superoxide dismutase (SOD) (42–44). Valabhji et al. (45) reported that subjects with insulin-dependent (type 1) diabetes mellitus (T1DM), compared with nondiabetic individuals from a cross-sectional study, had reduced total antioxidant status, as measured by the Trolox equivalent antioxidant capacity assay, and that this reduction was associated with the presence of coronary artery calcification. In addition, reduced total antioxidant status was an independent predictor of coronary artery calcification. Furthermore, Granado et al. (46) documented that T1DM patients had lower serum retinol concentrations than sex-matched control relatives. Similarly, results from Ceriello et al. (47) showed that T2DM patients had reduced plasma antioxidant capacity (as measured by the total radical-trapping antioxidant parameter), vitamin A, thiol groups, and uric acid, compared with matched control patients. However, vitamin C levels did not differ between the groups, and vitamin E concentrations were higher in the diabetic patients. Maxwell et al. (37) reported that both T1DM and T2DM patients had reduced total antioxidant activity due to reduced urate and vitamin C levels, compared with matched control individuals. Hirsch et al. (48) measured renal clearance of ascorbic acid in diabetic patients and reported that patients with diabetic nephropathy had increased ascorbic acid renal clearance, which contributed to the observed decreased concentrations of plasma ascorbic acid.

The most common antioxidant deficiency reported in diabetes is lower levels of ascorbate in plasma and in mononuclear cells (49,50). In addition, the ratio of the oxidation product, dehydroascorbate, to ascorbate is increased in diabetic patients compared with control subjects.

Cunningham (49) showed that the ascorbate content of mononuclear leukocytes was decreased by 50% in patients with T1DM compared with controls, after correction for dietary intake of ascorbate. Also, low levels of reduced glutathione have been documented in diabetic neutrophils. Furthermore, SOD activity is decreased in monocytes and polymorphonuclear leukocytes in diabetics (42,51).

With regard to LDL oxidizability in T2DM, studies to date show divergent results due to the heterogeneity of the diabetic populations, variation in glycemic control, age differences, and extent of vascular complications (23,52–58). Whereas some studies did not find increased susceptibility of LDL to oxidation in diabetic subjects, evidence for increased LDL oxidizability was shown in at least five studies. Babiy et al. (52) demonstrated increased oxidizability of LDL in diabetic subjects after exposure of the LDL to radiation. Beaudeaux et al. (53) reported enhanced oxidative susceptibility of LDL in T2DM subjects compared with matched controls. Cominacini et al. (54) showed that LDL in both T1DM and T2DM is more susceptible to oxidation, as evidenced by a shortened lag phase of oxidation measured by fluorescence. Furthermore, Yoshida et al. (55) reported increased oxidative susceptibility of LDL in T2DM patients compared with normotriglyceridemic controls; these researchers found that the vitamin E/lipid peroxide ratio of LDL is a major determinant of LDL lag time and that diabetic subjects have a reduced ratio compared with matched controls. Also, T2DM patients have small, dense LDL, which is more prone to oxidation than large, buoyant LDL (56). In endothelial cells, Ox-LDL has been shown to decrease NO production through reductions in NOS gene expression at the transcriptional and posttranscriptional levels (59).

Glycation and gluco-oxidation can also promote formation of ROS, such as superoxide (O_2^-) and hydrogen peroxide (H_2O_2), which could in turn oxidize LDL (25,42,44,60). Increased gluco-oxidation products, such as carboxymethyl lysine, carboxymethyl hydroxylysine, and pentosidine, have been demonstrated in collagen of diabetics. *In vitro,* glycosylated collagen has been shown to catalyze the peroxidation of linoleic and arachidonic acids, mimicking the *in vivo* lipid peroxidation that occurs in the presence of diabetes (61). Glycated LDL isolated from diabetic subjects has also been found to stimulate thromboxane B_2 release as well as platelet aggregation, providing another mechanism by which it may stimulate atherosclerosis. Also, there is increased peroxidation of LDL by nonenzymatic glycated peptides, such as glycated polylysine-iron complexes (62,63). Several reports have shown that glycated LDL is more prone to oxidation than nonglycated LDL (64). Bucala and Cerami (10) showed increased AGE formation in diabetic LDL, with an increase in lipid peroxidation as evidenced by malondialdehyde (MDA) equivalents. Glycoxidation products, such as pentosidine and *N*ε-(carboxymethyl)lysine (CML), are some of the AGEs formed by oxidative reactions that have been correlated with severity of diabetic complications including CVD (25). CML has also been identified as a product of lipid peroxidation reactions to polyunsaturated fatty acids (65). In addition, CML has been identified as the major AGE epitope recognized by antibodies against AGE proteins (66).

Lipoprotein glycation and oxidation could result in lipoprotein immune complex formation. The detection of circulating autoantibodies to Ox-LDL is considered to be a biologic signature of *in vivo* LDL oxidation. Increased concentrations of autoantibodies to both oxidized, glycated LDL and glyco-oxidized LDL have been documented in diabetes. This suggests that enhanced LDL oxidation occurs *in vivo* in T2DM and that LDL glycation may represent a predisposing event that facilitates subsequent oxidative modification (57,58). The presence of these circulating immune complexes has been associated with accelerated atherosclerosis, presumably as a result of either macrophage foam cell formation in response to uptake of these complexes or stimulation of atherogenic mechanisms in cells of the arterial wall (67). When stimulated with LDL immune complexes, monocyte-macrophages have been shown to release more proatherogenic cytokines, such as IL-1 and TNF.

Direct evidence of increased oxidative stress in diabetes has also been reported. F_2-isoprostanes,

prostaglandin-like compounds formed *in vivo* from free radical-catalyzed peroxidation of arachidonic acid, are emerging as novel and direct *in vivo* measures of oxidative stress. Both plasma and urinary F_2-isoprostane levels are reported to be increased in T2DM (68–70). Another marker of increased oxidative stress in T2DM is oxidative damage to DNA. Dandona et al (71), using high-performance liquid chromatography, found that levels of 8-hydroxydeoxyguanosine (8-OHdG), an indicator of DNA damage, were significantly elevated in mononuclear cells of T1DM and T2DM patients compared with matched controls. Similarly, Leinonen et al. (72) showed that urinary levels of 8-OHdG, measured by an enzyme-linked immunosorbent assay (ELISA), were significantly elevated in T2DM patients compared with controls and were significantly associated with levels of glycated hemoglobin. Other researchers showed that T2DM patients have increased levels of nitrotyrosine, another marker of protein oxidation. Although the ELISA could not pick up values for nitrotyrosine in normal controls (less than 10 nmol/L), all of the T2DM patients studied ($n = 40$) had high levels of nitrotyrosine in plasma, thus providing evidence for the role of reactive nitrogen species in diabetes (73). In addition, the nitrotyrosine levels correlated with the levels of glycemia.

Therefore, it is evident that diabetes is associated with increased attendant oxidative stress. Figure 2-1 depicts the role of oxidative stress in diabetes, and Table 2-2 summarizes the evidence for increased oxidative stress in diabetes. Under hyperglycemic conditions, there is enhanced metabolism of glucose through the sorbitol pathway, which results in an increased ratio of reduced to oxidized nicotinamide adenine dinucleotide ($NADH/NAD^+$) with augmented production of O_2^- radicals (16,74–76). In the presence of O_2^- radicals, NO is quenched to form peroxynitrite ion ($ONOO^-$), which is a potent oxidant molecule. Peroxynitrite ion uncouples endothelial nitric oxide synthase (eNOS) by oxidizing its cofactor, tetrahydrobiopterin (BH_4), and causes eNOS to produce O_2^-, further increasing cellular oxidative stress and decreasing NO bioavailability (77–79). Moreover, under

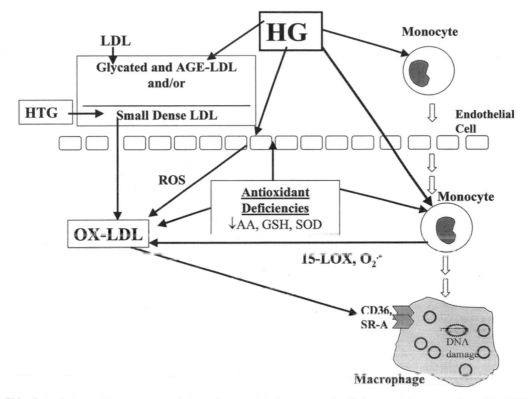

FIG. 2-1. Schematic depiction of the role of oxidative stress in diabetes. AA, ascorbic acid; AGE, advanced glycation end products; DNA, deoxyribonucleic acid; GSH, reduced glutathione; HG, high glucose; HTG, hypertriglyceridemia; LDL, low-density lipoprotein; 15-LOX, 15-lipoxygenase; O_2^-, superoxide; SOD, superoxide dismutase; SR-A, scavenger receptor-A.

hyperglycemic conditions, the diacylglycerol-sensitive protein kinase C (PKC) is activated (80), resulting in increased release of O_2^-, as documented by Inoguchi et al (81) in cultured aortic smooth muscle cells and endothelial cells.

TABLE 2-2. *Evidence for oxidative stress in diabetes*

Antioxidant deficiencies (ascorbate, reduced glutathione, superoxide dismutase)
Glycoxidation
Increased lipid peroxidation (↑LDL oxidation, ↑F2-isoprostanes, ↑autoantibodies to Ox-LDL)
Increased reactive oxygen species from monocytes and neutrophils
Increased protein oxidation (nitrotyrosine)
Increased DNA damage

LDL, low-density lipoprotein; Ox-LDL, oxidized LDL

Compared with monocytes of control subjects, those from diabetic patients secrete increased O_2^- (42–44,82,83). It has also been shown that hyperglycemia induces O_2 overproduction in bovine aortic endothelial cells *in vitro* (74,75) and that the majority of O_2^- production in these cells derives from the mitochondria. Hyperglycemia increases the inner mitochondrial membrane proton gradient as a result of overproduction of electron donors by the tricarboxylic acid cycle. This in turn causes endothelial cells to increase production of O_2^-. To determine the site of superoxide production in endothelial cells, Nishikawa et al. (74) incubated bovine aortic endothelial cells with either rotenone, a complex 1 inhibitor; thenoyltrifluoroacetone (TTFA), a complex II inhibitor; or carbonyl cyanide m-chlorophenylhydrazone (CCCP), an uncoupler of oxidative phosphorylation that abolishes the mitochondrial membrane proton gradient. In these cells, hyperglycemia-induced O_2^- production was prevented when cells were incubated with TTFA or CCCP, but not with rotenone. Furthermore, overexpression of either MnSOD (the mitochondrial form of SOD) or uncoupling protein-1 (UCP-1) completely abolished the mitochondrial proton gradient and prevented hyperglycemia-induced O_2^- formation in endothelial cells. Normalization of the levels of mitochondrial ROS prevents glucose-induced activation of PKC, formation of AGE, and sorbitol accumulation as well as NFκB activation in endothelial cells. A recent study from our laboratory provided evidence that hyperglycemia also induces increased O_2^- production in THP-1 cells, a human monocytic cell line (84). However, in contrast to ROS production inhibition in endothelial cells, the use of mitochondrial complex inhibitors did not inhibit ROS release from monocytes, suggesting that in these cells the main source of O_2^- production is not the mitochondrial respiratory chain. We further showed, using antisense oligodeoxynucleotides, that NADPH oxidase (p47phox) is essential for monocyte O_2^- production under hyperglycemia. We demonstrated that hyperglycemia induces PKC-α, which in turn activates p47phox translocation to the membranes and induces O_2^- anion release. Although we showed that PKC-β is also upregulated in monocytes under hyperglycemia, antisense oligonucleotides to PKC-β had no effect on O_2^- production, whereas antisense oligonucleotides to PKC-α inhibited O_2^- production. These data confirm that, in monocytes, PKC-α drives O_2^- production via NADPH oxidase.

INFLAMMATION

Clinical and experimental data support a major role for inflammation in atherogenesis, as evidenced by the critical functions of adhesion molecules, cytokines, and chemokines (85). The monocyte-macrophage is crucial and is the most readily accessible cell in the artery wall. ROS, such as O_2^- are increased in monocytes and neutrophils of T2DM patients (23,42–44). Studies from our laboratory show increased O_2^- levels in

lipopolysaccharide (LPS)-activated monocytes in T2DM patients with or without macrovascular complications (82). Furthermore, in support of a proinflammatory state in diabetes, we have convincingly shown that monocytic release of IL-1β and IL-6 is increased in T2DM (82, 83). Desfaits et al. (86) observed a significant increase in the levels of LPS-stimulated release of TNF-α from monocytes in T2DM. An early event in atherogenesis is the binding of monocytes to endothelial cells and their transmigration into the intima (87). *In vitro,* hyperglycemia increases binding of monocytes to human endothelial cells (88). Although increased adhesion of monocytes to endothelial cells has been reported in T2DM (89,90), this has been largely in patients with hypertriglyceridemia. Recently, we showed convincingly that T2DM patients had increased adhesion of their monocytes to human aortic endothelial cells, compared with control subjects matched for lipid level (82).

Soluble cell adhesion molecules are shed from activated cells such as endothelial cells. Increasing evidence supports the role of plasma levels of cell adhesion molecules (ICAM, VCAM, E-selectin, and P-selectin) as molecular markers of atherosclerosis (91–93). T2DM patients have increased levels of soluble adhesion molecules such as ICAM, VCAM, and E-selectin (82,94–97), as has been shown by numerous investigators. Furthermore, increased levels of ICAM and VCAM have been reported in the atherosclerotic lesions of T2DM (98). Other compelling evidence for increased inflammation in diabetes was provided by Hofmann et al. (99), who showed that diabetics with high hemoglobin A_{1C} have increased NFκB-p65 activity. They also showed a significant correlation between NFκB-p65 and hemoglobin A_{1C}.

The prototypic marker of inflammation is C-reactive protein (CRP). Numerous studies have shown that CRP levels in the highest quintile predict cardiovascular events (100–102). Pickup et al. (103) showed that IL-6 and CRP levels are increased in T2DM patients with features of the metabolic syndrome. Several studies subsequently showed that CRP levels are increased in diabetics (83,104,105). Also, IL-6, which drives the release of CRP, is increased in monocytes from diabetic patients. In addition, evidence has shown that inflammation may contribute to the pathogenesis of the diabetic syndrome. For instance, in the Women's Health Study, women in the highest quartile of high sensitivity-CRP over a 4-year period had a fourfold increased risk of diabetes, compared with women in the lowest quartile (106). This finding was confirmed by the West of Scotland Coronary Prevention Study (107).

ENDOTHELIAL DYSFUNCTION

Endothelial cells, which line the internal lumen of all the vasculature, are part of a complex system that regulates vasodilation and vasoconstriction, growth of vascular smooth muscle cells, inflammation, and hemostasis, with the end result of maintaining a proper blood supply to tissues and regulating inflammation and coagulation (107). These functions are mediated through the release of several vasoactive factors, such as NO, adhesion molecules, and prostacyclin.

Endothelial dysfunction, an early step in the development of atherosclerotic lesions, is characterized by disruption in normal function of the endothelial cells. This could result in increased macromolecule permeability, altered production of vasoactive factors and therefore abnormal vasoconstriction or vasodilation, increased prothrombotic or procoagulant activity, and/or abnormalities in regulation of the lumen of vessels (107–109). NO is one of the chemical mediators of endothelial cell function. NO is produced from L-arginine by the enzyme NOS. Once released into the subendothelial space and vascular lumen, NO is responsible for a vasodilatory response contributing to the regulation of blood pressure and for prevention of platelet adherence to endothelium and platelet aggregation (107,110,111).

Diabetes has been shown to impair endothelium-derived NO and NO-mediated vasodilation. Several mechanisms contribute to the decreased bioavailability of endothelium-derived NO in diabetes. The hyperglycemic state is a very significant contributor to vascular complications in patients with diabetes. Hyperglycemia blocks activation of eNOS and promotes activation of ROS such as O_2^- in endothelial cells. Superoxide can quench NO to form the toxic peroxynitrite, which, in turn, uncouples eNOS by oxidizing its cofactor BH_4 and causes eNOS to produce O_2^- (77). Insulin resistance in diabetic patients is associated with increased levels of free fatty acids, which activate PKC, inhibit phosphatidylinositol-3-kinase, and increase production of ROS, all of which impair NO production or decrease its bioavailability. Furthermore, peroxynitrite has been shown to decrease synthesis of prostacyclin. Decreased NO bioavailability is associated with a concomitant increase in peroxynitrite, further impairing production of subsidiary vasodilators. Also, diabetes is associated with increased production of the potent vasoconstrictor, endothelin-1. Other endothelium-derived vasoactive substances that are affected in diabetes are the vasoconstrictor prostanoids and angiotensin II. AGEs and oxidation products, which are increased in diabetes, quench endothelium-derived NO. This mechanism is thought to be an important contributor to impaired endothelial function in diabetes, because anti-AGE agents and antioxidants can inhibit it to varying degrees.

Another way in which high glucose concentrations can contribute to vascular dysfunction is through the activation of endothelial PKC, which stimulates the expression of adhesion molecules. PKC inhibition was shown to improve endothelial dysfunction in a model in which rat endothelial tissue was exposed to a hyperglycemic environment (112). In this model, it was observed that the proinflammatory action caused by incubation with D-glucose was inhibited by the addition of bisinolylmaleimide-I, a PKC inhibitor. In addition, the presence of P-selectin and ICAM on the surface of endothelial cells was decreased with bisinolylmaleimide-I.

ROLE OF ANTIOXIDANTS IN THE PREVENTION OF DIABETIC COMPLICATIONS

Because ROS are normally being formed in cells, there are scavenging antioxidants that help prevent oxidative stress. Some of the most common antioxidants are ascorbic acid, AT, carotenoids, flavonoids, uric acid, bilirubin, glutathione, N-acetyl cysteine, and lipoic acid (113). However, with regard to diabetes, the only antioxidants that have been studied in some detail are α-lipoic acid (ALA), AT, and ascorbic acid.

α-Tocopherol

AT is the most potent lipid-soluble antioxidant in plasma and LDL, and it is antiinflammatory. Studies have demonstrated decreased levels of AT in plasma and LDL fraction from diabetic patients, compared with healthy controls. Also, Gale et al. (114) showed that elderly men with low blood concentrations of cholesterol-adjusted AT were 2.5 times as likely to have carotid stenoses of greater than 30%.

AT supplementation may slow the progression of atherosclerosis by reducing oxidative stress, thereby decreasing lipid peroxidation and LDL oxidative susceptibility. Several groups have shown that AT inhibits LDL oxidation *in vitro* and *in vivo*˙ (115). At least four studies have shown that RRR-AT (800 to 1,600 IU/day) significantly reduces LDL oxidizability in T2DM patients (82,104,116,117). However, Astley et al. (118), using a lower dose of AT (400 IU/day) failed to observe a significant effect of AT on LDL oxidizability in patients with T2DM, although there was a significant decrease in controls. Therefore, it is possible that doses of RRR-AT greater than 400 IU/day would be required to decrease oxidative stress in diabetic patients. Our research has shown that AT supplementation can decrease levels of autoantibodies to Ox-LDL in T2DM patients. Further, AT supplementation (100 to 600 mg/day for 2 weeks) in short-term studies significantly decreases the *in vivo* marker of lipid peroxidation, urinary F_2-isoprostanes, by 34% to 36% in T2DM patients (69).

In addition to its antioxidant effects, AT also has effects on inflammation (119–123). At least two studies have shown that AT supplementation (more than 800 IU/day) in T2DM patients significantly reduces levels of hs-CRP, the prototypic marker of inflammation. Supplementation with 1,200 IU/day of AT significantly influenced monocyte function by decreasing the release of O_2^-, IL-1β, IL-6, and TNF-α and by

decreasing monocyte-endothelial cell adhesion *in vitro*, both in healthy controls and in T2DM patients with or without macrovascular disease (82,83,104). RRR-AT (1,200 IU/day) significantly decreased levels of soluble(s)ICAM, sVCAM and sE-selectin levels in T2DM patients with or without macrovascular complications (82). A single report showed that oral supplementation with another antioxidant, N-acetyl cysteine (1.2 mg/day), significantly decreased oxidative stress and levels of soluble VCAM-1 in T2DM (124). P-selectin mediates adhesion of platelets to endothelial cells during inflammation and thrombosis. It is contained largely in the platelet α-granules, and to some extent in the Weibel-Palade bodies of endothelial cells, and is released on activation. We showed recently that AT therapy (1,200 IU/day for 3 months) significantly reduced levels of soluble P-selectin in T2DM patients (125). Circulating levels of PAI-1 are a key regulator of fibrinolysis; elevated PAI-1 is considered to be a strong risk factor for CAD and has been shown in most reports to be elevated in T2DM (126–129). PAI-1 is also increased in coronary plaques of patients with T2DM (129). Furthermore, PAI-1 levels correlate with many variables that cosegregate with the metabolic syndrome, such as body mass index, waist-hip ratio, insulin, triglycerides, and apolipoprotein B levels. PAI-1 levels were decreased by AT in T1DM (at 1,800 IU/day) (130) and in T2DM (at 1,200 IU/day) (125). AT has been shown to inhibit smooth muscle cell proliferation *in vitro*, to inhibit platelet aggregation in diabetic patients, and to preserve endothelium-dependent vasorelaxation via inhibition of PKC (119). Table 2-3 summarizes the effects of AT on biomarkers of oxidative stress and inflammation in diabetes.

With regard to molecular mechanisms, we have explored the effects of AT on O_2^- anion release using the monocytic THP-1 cell line (84). In mechanistic studies, we showed that O_2^- anion release is driven by PKC-α and that ROS and O_2^- derive in the monocyte from NADPH oxidase and not from the mitochondrial respiratory chain. Use of antisense oligonucleotides to PKC-α obliterated the increase in ROS and O_2^- anion release under hyperglycemic conditions in monocytes, whereas antisense oligonucleotides

TABLE 2-3. *Effect of α-tocopherol on biomarkers of oxidative stress and inflammation in diabetes*

Oxidative stress	Inflammation
↓LDL oxidative susceptibility	↓Hs-CRP
↓Autoantibodies to Ox-LDL	↓Pro-inflammatory cytokines (IL-1β, TNF, IL-6)
↓Urinary F2-isoprostanes	
↓ROS (superoxide) from phagocytes	↓Monocyte adhesion to endothelium
	↓Soluble cell adhesion molecules
	↓Plasminogen activator inhibitor-1

CRP, C-reactive protein; IL, interleukin; LDL, low-density lipoprotein; Ox-LDL, oxidized LDL; ROS, reactive oxygen species; TNF, tumor necrosis factor.

to PKC-βII had no effect. AT also decreased O_2^- and PKC activity (both PKC-α and PKC-β). Therefore, this study demonstrated that the inhibitory effect of AT on O_2^- anion release in diabetic monocytes occurs via inhibition of PKC-α, which results in a decrease in NADPH oxidase activity. Other studies using different cells have implicated PKC-βII and have shown that AT also decreases PKC-βII activity. With regard to adhesion, we demonstrated in nondiabetic subjects that AT enrichment of monocytes decreases the counterreceptors, CD11b and very late antigen-4 (VLA-4), on monocytes and decreases NFκB DNA-binding activity, resulting in decreased monocyte-endothelial cell adhesion. Hofmann et al. (131) showed increased levels of NFκB DNA-binding activity in T1DM patients.

With regard to AT therapy and vascular complications in diabetics, there are limited clinical trials. Bursell et al. (130) showed in subjects with T1DM that high doses of RRR-AT (1,800 IU/day) for 4 months normalized increased retinal blood flow and hyperfiltration. In a recent study by Gaede et al. (132) of T2DM patients with microalbuminuria, combined treatment with the antioxidants vitamin C (1,250 mg/day) and RRR-AT (680 IU/day) for 4 weeks resulted in a significant reduction of 19% in albumin excretion rates. Manzella et al. (133) demonstrated in a double-blind, random-ized, placebo-controlled trial in 50 T2DM patients that supplementation with AT (600 mg/day of all rac AT) for 4 months improved the ratio of cardiac sympathetic to parasympathetic tone, indicated by a significant increase in the RR interval and improvements in low- and high-frequency components of heart rate variability. Other evidence regarding the benefit of antioxidants on biomarkers in T2DM includes a study by Paolisso et al. (134), who showed in 40 T2DM patients that supplementation with AT (600 mg/day of all rac AT) for 8 weeks was associated with a significant improvement in brachial artery reactivity, compared with placebo; also, there was an improvement in oxidative stress indices such as thiobarbituric acid-reactive substances (TBARS) and total antioxidant activity. In addition, AT supplementation (1,600 IU/day) has been shown to improve endothelial function in T2DM patients (135). Therefore, it appears that benefits are seen with AT at doses of 600 IU/day or higher, and, with regard to diabetes, that AT has effects on lipid peroxidation, platelet aggregation, inflammation, and endothelial function. Recently, in the Secondary Prevention with Antioxidants of Cardiovascular Disease in End-Stage Renal Disease (SPACE) investigation, a placebo-controlled, randomized study, a higher dose of RRR-AT (800 IU/day) resulted in an increase in plasma levels of AT and a significant reduction of 54% in the composite primary end point (136). Forty-two percent of the patients in this trial were diabetics.

Therefore, it is imperative to conduct placebo-controlled, randomized studies in diabetic patients to determine whether higher doses of AT, which decrease inflammation and oxidative stress, culminate in reduction of cardiovascular events or atherosclerosis progression.

α-Lipoic Acid

Lipoic acid is a hydrophilic and lipophilic antioxidant and therefore can partition in both aqueous and lipid environments to exert its beneficial effects. Lipoic acid and dihydrolipoate, its oxidation product, have been shown to be effective antioxidants *in vitro*. We showed in nondiabetic individuals that administration of ALA

(600 mg/day) significantly decreased oxidative stress, as measured by protein carbonyls, LDL oxidizability, and urinary F_2-isoprostanes (137). ALA has also been shown to improve NO-mediated vasodilation and to reduce the plasma concentration of MDA in diabetic patients (138). Bierhaus et al. (139) demonstrated that incubation with AGE-albumin decreased levels of reduced glutathione and ascorbic acid in bovine aortic endothelial cells, which increased oxidative stress. Supplementation of cells with ALA before AGE incubation prevented the depletion of reduced glutathione and ascorbic acid, and addition of ALA also reduced NFκB activity.

In clinical studies, ALA has been approved for the treatment of diabetic polyneuropathy. Four of the six pilot studies that have been completed showed beneficial effects on nerve function and symptoms of diabetic polyneuropathy (140–145). Five multicenter, randomized, double-blind studies of ALA in patients with diabetic and cardiac autonomic neuropathy have been conducted (146–150). In the Alpha-Lipoic Acid in Diabetic Neuropathy study (ALADIN II), ALA (600 or 1,200 mg/day for 24 months) significantly improved nerve function in patients with peripheral neuropathy. In the ALADIN study, diabetic patients with symptomatic peripheral polyneuropathy significantly benefited from infusion of ALA (greater than 600 mg/day). Treated patients had decreased symptoms compared with patients receiving placebo, as was seen in the Oral Pilot (ORPIL) study of high-dose ALA (1,800 mg/day). In ALADIN III, administration of 600 mg/day of ALA to 509 patients resulted in a significant improvement in neuropathy improvement score, compared with placebo. In the Deutsche Kardiale Autonome Neuropathie (DEKAN) study, T2DM patients with cardiac autonomic neuropathy received 800 mg/day of ALA or placebo for 4 months; two of four parameters of heart variability significantly improved with ALA therapy.

ALA (600 mg/day) has been shown to significantly reduce NFκB binding activity in mononuclear cells of diabetic patients. This effect was independent of glycemic control and degree of endothelial dysfunction and was effective at differing stages of neuropathy (99,131). ALA also has beneficial effects on insulin resistance. Several experiments *in vitro* and *in vivo,* as well as in diabetic patients, have shown improved glucose utilization (151,152) and insulin resistance with ALA (151–158). ALA appears to stimulate glucose uptake via activation of the glucose transporter, GLUT4, in the insulin signaling pathway. In T2DM, acute or chronic treatment with ALA (500 to 1,000 mg) significantly improved insulin-stimulated glucose disposal (159–162).

Therefore, ALA appears to be beneficial with regard to diabetic polyneuropathy, and it improves autonomic and peripheral function in diabetic patients. Its beneficial effect on NFκB may be associated with improvement of renal and endothelial function. Its therapeutic value is strengthened by its enhancement of insulin-stimulated glucose disposal in diabetics. However, large-scale studies need to be conducted to examine long-term safety and the translation of these effects into decreased diabetic vasculopathies.

Ascorbic Acid

Ascorbate (vitamin C) is a potent, water-soluble antioxidant that is documented to have protective effects against oxidative stress and its vascular consequences. *In vitro* studies have clearly shown that vitamin C (greater than 40 μM) inhibits LDL oxidizability induced by transition metals, free radical initiators, and human neutrophils and macrophages (163). This effect is a result of its ability to scavenge ROS and reactive nitrogen species. Several supplementation studies have shown that a vitamin C dose of 500 to 1,000 mg/day is effective in reducing LDL susceptibility to oxidation in smokers and nonsmokers (164–167). However, some studies have not shown that vitamin C protects LDL from oxidation, possibly because it is water soluble and therefore cannot partition in the LDL particle. However, Reilly et al. (168) found that urinary isoprostanes, an indicator of oxidative stress, were decreased in smokers after 5 days of vitamin C intake at a dose of 2 g/day. Vitamin C has also been shown to inhibit O_2^- production from

TABLE 2-4. *Effect of ascorbate on endothelial function in diabetes*

Reference	Study population	Treatment	Result
Ting et al (176)	10 Type 2 DM	24 mg/min infusion	↑Forearm blood flow
Timimi et al (177)	10 Type 1 DM	24 mg/min infusion	↑Forearm blood flow
Beckman et al (179)	Hyperglycemia	24 mg/min infusion	↑Brachial artery flow
Lekakis et al (180)	17 women GDM	2 g oral ascorbate	↑Brachial artery flow

DM, diabetes mellitus; GDM, gestational diabetes mellitus.

activated neutrophils (169). Ascorbate supplementation (2 g/day) decreased monocyte-endothelial cell adhesion in smokers.

In animal studies, vitamin C effectively decreased glycation of proteins such as hemoglobin and insulin in obese hyperglycemic (ob/ob) mice (170). Furthermore, Cay et al. (171) documented protective effects of intraperitoneally administered vitamin C against lipid peroxidation in red blood cells, liver, and muscle samples.

However, the most convincing evidence for the benefits of ascorbate in CVD has been its effects on endothelial function. Several studies have documented that high doses of vitamin C are effective in improving vasodilation in smokers and nonsmokers (172,173), in hypertensive patients (174,175), and in diabetics (176,177) (Table 2-4). This beneficial effect of ascorbate is most likely a result of its capacity to scavenge O_2^- radicals, conserving intracellular glutathione and potentiating intracellular NO synthesis. Duffy et al. (178) demonstrated in a randomized, double-blind, placebo-controlled study that ascorbate supplementation (500 mg/day) significantly improves blood pressure in patients with hypertension, and that these effects may be mediated by the preservation of NO by ascorbate.

CONCLUSION

Compelling evidence points to important roles for oxidative stress and inflammation in diabetic vasculopathies. Moreover, it is clear that treatment with antioxidants, especially AT, may be beneficial to ameliorate the adverse effects of oxidative stress and inflammation in diabetic patients. Further research is still needed to improve our understanding of the mechanisms by which different antioxidants may aid in the prevention of vascular dysfunction in diabetic patients. Studies examining end points of subclinical atherosclerosis (e.g., intimal medial thickness, electron beam computed tomography) are urgently needed to establish whether antioxidant supplementation can reduce atherosclerosis progression in diabetes.

REFERENCES

1. Pyorala K, Laasko M, Uusitupa M. Diabetes and atherosclerosis: an epidemiologic view. *Diabetes Metab Rev* 1987;3:463–524.
2. Everhart JE, Pettitt DJ, Knowler WC, et al. Medial arterial calcification and its association with mortality and complications of diabetes. *Diabetologia* 1988;31:16–23.
3. Bierman E. Atherogenesis in diabetes. *Atheroscl Thromb* 1992;12:647–656.
4. Calles-Escandon J, Mirza SA, Garcia-Rubi E, et al. Type 2 diabetes: one disease, multiple cardiovascular risk factors. *Coron Artery Dis* 1999;10:23–30.
5. Devaraj S, Jialal I. Oxidative stress and antioxidants. In: Bendich A, Deckelbaun RJ, eds. *Primary and secondary preventive nutrition.* Totowa, NJ: Humana Press, 2000:117–125.
6. Meigs JB, Jacques PF, Selhub J, et al. Fasting plasma homocysteine levels in the insulin resistance syndrome. *Diabetes Care* 2001;24:1403–1410.
7. Lyons TJ, Jenkins AJ. Lipoprotein glycation and its metabolic consequences. *Curr Opin Lipidol* 1997;8:174–180.
8. Brownlee M. Glycation products and the pathogenesis of diabetic complications. *Diabetes Care* 1992;15:1835–1843.
9. Bucala R, Tracey K, Cerami A. Advanced glycosylation products quench nitric oxide and mediate defective endothelium-dependent vasodilation in experimental diabetes. *J Clin Invest* 1991;87:432–438.
10. Bucala R, Cerami A. Advanced glycosylation: chemistry, biology, and implications for diabetes and aging. *Adv Pharmacol* 1992;23:1–34.
11. Bucala R, Makita Z, Koschinski T, et al. Lipid advanced glycosilation: pathway for lipid oxidation in vivo. *Proc Natl Acad Sci U S A* 1993;90:6434–6438.
12. Lopes-Virella M, Klein R, Lyons T, et al. Glycosylation of low-density lipoprotein enhances cholesteryl ester

synthesis in human monocyte-derived macrophages. *Diabetes* 1988;37:550–557.

13. Witzum J, Steinberg D. Role of oxidized low density lipoprotein in atherogenesis. *J Clin Invest* 1991;88:1785–1792.

14. Berliner J, Heinecke J. The role of oxidized lipoproteins in atherogenesis. *Free Radic Biol Med* 1992;92:127–143.

15. Devaraj S, Jialal I. Oxidized LDL and atherosclerosis. *Int J Clin Lab Res* 1996;26:178–184.

16. Oranje WA, Wolffenbuttel BH. Lipid peroxidation and atherosclerosis in type II diabetes. *J Lab Clin Med* 1999;134:19–32.

17. Bjorkerud B, Bjorkerud S. Contrary effects of lightly and strongly oxidized LDL with potent promotion of growth versus apoptosis on arterial smooth muscle cells, macrophages, and fibroblasts. *Arterioscler Thromb Vasc Biol* 1996;16:416–424.

18. Palinski W, Yla-Herttuala S, Rosenfeld ME, et al. Antisera and monoclonal antibodies specific for epitopes generated during oxidative modification of low density lipoprotein. *Arteriosclerosis* 1990;10:325–335.

19. Chen LY, Mehta P, Mehta JL. Oxidized LDL decreases L-arginine uptake and nitric oxide synthase protein expression in human platelets. *Circulation* 1996;93:1740–1746.

20. Strain J. Disturbances of micronutrient and antioxidant status in diabetes. *Proc Nutr Soc* 1991;50:591–604.

21. Baynes JW. Perspectives in diabetes: role of oxidative stress in development of complications in diabetes. *Diabetes* 1991;40:405–412.

22. Ceriello A. Oxidative stress and glycemic regulation. *Metabolism* 2000;49:27–30.

23. Rousselot DB, Bastard JP, Jaudon MC, et al. Consequences of the diabetic status on the oxidant/antioxidant balance. *Diabetes Metab* 2000;26:163–176.

24. Ohara Y, Peterson TE, Harrison DG. Hypercholesterolemia increases endothelial superoxide anion production. *J Clin Invest* 1993;91:2546–2551.

25. Baynes JW, Thorpe SR. Role of oxidative stress in diabetic complications: a new perspective on an old paradigm. *Diabetes* 1999;48:1–9.

26. Watts GF, Playford DA. Dyslipoproteinaemia and hyperoxidative stress in the pathogenesis of endothelial dysfunction in a non-insulin dependent diabetes mellitus: an hypothesis. *Atherosclerosis* 1998;141:17–30.

27. Rösen P, Naworth PP, King G, et al. The role of oxidative stress in the onset and progression of diabetes and its complications: a summary of a Congress Series sponsored by UNESCO-MCBN, the American Diabetes Association and the German Diabetes Society. *Diabetes Metab Res Rev* 2001;17:189–212.

28. Sundaram RK, Bhaskar A, Vijayalingam S, et al. Antioxidant status and lipid peroxidation in type II diabetes with and without complications. *Clin Sci* 1996;90:255–260.

29. Nourooz-Zadeh J, Rahimi A, Tajaddini-Sarmadi J, et al. Relationships between plasma measures of oxidative stress and metabolic control in NIDDM. *Diabetologia* 1997;40:647–653.

30. Leonhardt W, Hahnefeld M, Müller G, et al. Impact of concentrations of glycated hemoglobin,

31. Tsai EC, Hirsch IB, Brunzell JD, et al. Reduced plasma peroxyl radical trapping capacity and increased susceptibility of LDL to oxidation in poorly controlled IDDM. *Diabetes* 1994;43:1010–1014.

32. Chari SN, Nath N, Rathi AB. Glutathione and its redox system in diabetic polymorphonuclear leukocytes. *Am J Med Sci* 1984;287:14–15.

33. Jennings PE, Chirico S, Jones AF, et al. Vitamin C metabolites and microangiopathy in diabetes mellitus. *Diabetes Res* 1987;6:151–154.

34. Karpen CW, Cataland S, O'Dorisio TM, et al. Production of 12 HETES and vitamin E status in platelets from type 1 human diabetic subjects. *Diabetes* 1985;34:526–531.

35. Paolisso G, D'Amore A, Balbi V, et al. Plasma vitamin C affects glucose homeostasis in healthy subjects and in non-insulin-dependent diabetics. *Am J Physiol* 1994;266:E261–E268.

36. Olmedilla B, Granado F, Gilmaritnez E, et al. Reference values for retinol, tocopherol and main carotenoids in serum of control and insulin dependent diabetic Spanish subjects. *Clin Chem* 1997;43:1066–1071.

37. Maxwell SR, Thomason H, Sandler D, et al. Antioxidant status in patients with uncomplicated insulin-dependent and non-insulin-dependent diabetes mellitus. *Eur J Clin Invest* 1997;27:484–490.

38. Dyer RG, Stewart MW, Mitcheson J, et al. 7-Ketocholesterol, a specific indicator of lipoprotein oxidation, and malondialdehyde in non-insulin dependent diabetes and peripheral vascular disease. *Clin Chim Acta* 1997;260:1–13.

39. Sinclair AJ, Girling AJ, Gray L, et al. Disturbed handling of ascorbic acid in diabetic patients with and without microangiopathy during high dose ascorbate supplementation. *Diabetologia* 1997;34:171–175.

40. Srinivasan KN, Pugalendi KV, Sambandam G, et al. Diabetes mellitus, lipid peroxidation and antioxidant status in rural patients. *Clin Chim Acta* 1997;259:183–186.

41. Salonen JT, Nyyssonen K, Tuomainen TP, et al. Increased risk of non-insulin dependent diabetes mellitus at low plasma vitamin E concentrations: a four year follow up study in men. *Br Med J* 1995;311:1124–1127.

42. Kitahara M, Eyre H, Lynch R, et al. Metabolic activity of diabetic monocytes. *Diabetes* 1980;29:251–256.

43. Hill H, Hogan N, Rallison M, et al. Functional and metabolic abnormalities of diabetic monocytes. *Adv Exp Med Biol* 1980;69:621–627.

44. Hiramatsu K, Rosen H, Heinecke J, et al. Superoxide initiates oxidation of low density lipoprotein by human monocytes. *Arteriosclerosis* 1987;7:55–60.

45. Valabhji J, McColl AJ, Richmond W, et al. Total antioxidant status and coronary artery calcification in type 1 diabetes. *Diabetes Care* 2001;24:1608–1613.

46. Granado F, Olmedilla B, Gil-Martinez E, et al. Carotenoids, retinol and tocopherols in patients with insulin-dependent diabetes mellitus and their immediate relatives. *Clin Sci (Colch)* 1998;94:189–195.

47. Ceriello A, Bortolotti N, Pirisi M, et al. Total plasma antioxidant capacity predicts thrombosis-prone status

alpha-tocopherol, copper, and manganese on oxidation of low-density lipoproteins in patients with type I diabetes, type II diabetes and control subjects. *Clin Chim Acta* 1996;254:173–186.

in NIDDM patients. *Diabetes Care* 1997;20:1589–1593.

48. Hirsch IB, Atchley DH, Tsai E, et al. Ascorbic acid clearance in diabetic nephropathy. *J Diabetes Complications* 1998;12:259–263.

49. Cunningham JJ. Micronutrients as nutriceutical interventions in diabetes mellitus. *J Am Coll Nutr* 1998;17:7–10.

50. Sinclair A, Barnett A, Lunec J. Free radicals and antioxidant systems in health and disease. *Br J Hosp Med* 1990;43:334–344.

51. Nath N, Chari S, Rath A. SOD in diabetic polymorphonuclear lymphocytes. *Diabetes* 1984;33:586–589.

52. Babiy A, Gebicki J, Sullivan DR, et al. Increased oxidizability of plasma lipoproteins in diabetic patients can be decreased by probucol therapy and is not due to glycation. *Biochem Pharmacol* 1992;43:995–1000.

53. Beaudeaux J, Guillausseau P, Peynet J, et al. Enhanced susceptibility of LDL to in vitro oxidation in type 1 and 2 diabetic patients. *Clin Chim Acta* 1995;239:131–141.

54. Cominacini L, Garbin U, Pastorino A, et al. Increased susceptibility of LDL to in vitro oxidation in patients with IDDM and NIDDM. *Diabetes Res* 1994;26:173–184.

55. Yoshida H, Ishikawa T, Nakamura H. Vitamin E/lipid peroxide ratio and susceptibility of LDL to oxidative modification in non-insulin-dependent diabetes mellitus. *Arterioscler Thromb Vasc Biol* 1997;17:1438–1446.

56. Lamarche B, Lemieux I, Despres JP. The small, dense LDL phenotype and the risk of coronary heart disease: epidemiology, pato-physiology and therapeutic aspects. *Diabetes Metab* 1999;25:199–211.

57. Bellomo G, Maggi E, Poli M, et al. Autoantibodies against Ox-LDL in NIDDM. *Diabetes* 1995;44:60–66.

58. Hsu RM, Devaraj S, Jialal I. Autoantibodies to oxidized low-density lipoprotein in patients with type 2 diabetes mellitus. *Clin Chim Acta* 2002;317:145–150.

59. Liao JK, Shin WS, Lee WY, et al. Oxidized low-density lipoprotein decreases the expression of endothelial nitric oxide synthase. *J Biol Chem* 1995;270:319–324.

60. Oberley LW. Free radicals and diabetes. *Free Radic Biol Med* 1988;5:113–124.

61. Hicks M, Delbridge L, Yue DK, et al. Catalysis of lipid peroxidation by glucose and glycosylated collagen. *Biochem Biophys Res Commun* 1988;151:649–655.

62. Sakurai T, Sugioka K, Nakano M. O2 generation and lipid peroxidation during the oxidation of glycated polypeptide, glycated polylysine, in the presence of iron-ADP. *Biochem Biophys Acta* 1990;1043:17–33.

63. Sakurai T, Tsuchiya S. Superoxide production from nonenzymatically glycated protein. *Fed Eur Biochem Soc* 1988;236:406–410.

64. Li DJ, Devaraj S, Fuller CJ, et al. The effect of AT on LDL oxidation and glycation: in vitro and in vivo studies. *J Lipid Res* 1996;37:1978–1986.

65. Fu M-X, Requena JR, Jenkins AJ, et al. The advanced glycation end-product, Ne-(carboxymethyl)lysine, is a product of both lipid peroxidation and glycosylation reactions. *J Biol Chem* 1996;271:9982–9986.

66. Reddy S, Bichler J, Wells-Knecht KJ, et al. Ne-(carboxymethyl)lysine is a dominant advanced glycation end-product (AGE) antigen in tissue proteins. *Biochemistry* 1995;34:10872–10878.

67. Witzum J, Mahoney EM, Branks MJ, et al. Nonenzymatic glycation of LDL alters its biologic activity. *Diabetes* 1982;31:283–291.

68. Gopaul NK, Anggard EE, Mallet AI, et al. Plasma 8-epi-PGF2-alpha are elevated in individuals with NIDDM. *FEBS Lett* 1995;368:225–229.

69. Davi G, Ciabattoni G, Consoli A, et al. In vivo formation of 8-epi-PGF2-alpha and platelet activation in diabetes mellitus-effect of improved metabolic control and vitamin E supplementation. *Circulation* 1999;99:224–229.

70. Devaraj S, Hirany SV, Burke RF, et al. Divergence between LDL oxidative susceptibility and urinary F2-isoprostanes as measures of oxidative stress in type 2 diabetes. *Clin Chem* 2001;47:1974–1979.

71. Dandona P, Thusu K, Cook S, et al. Oxidative damage to DNA in diabetes mellitus. *Lancet* 1996;347:444–445.

72. Leinonen J, Lehtimaki T, Toyokuni S, et al. New biomarker evidence of oxidative DNA damage in patients with non-insulin-dependent diabetes mellitus. *FEBS Lett* 1997;417:150–152.

73. Ceriello A, Mercuri F, Quagliaro L, et al. Detection of nitrotyrosine in the diabetic plasma: evidence of oxidative stress. *Diabetologia* 2001;44:834–838.

74. Nishikawa T, Edelstein D, Du XL, et al. Normalizing mitochondrial superoxide production blocks three pathways of hyperglycaemic damage. *Nature* 2000;404:787–790.

75. Nishikawa T, Edelstein D, Brownlee M. The missing link: a single unifying mechanism for diabetic complications. *Kidney Int* 2000;58:S26–S30.

76. Bonnefont-Rousselot D, Bastard JP, Jaudon MC, et al. Consequences of the diabetic status on the oxidant/antioxidant balance. *Diabetes Metab* 2000;26:163–176.

77. Beckman JA, Creager MA, Libby P. Diabetes and atherosclerosis: epidemiology, pathophysiology and management. *JAMA* 2002;287:2570–2581.

78. Beckman JS, Beckman TW, Chen J, et al. Apparent hydroxyl radical production by peroxynitrite: implications for endothelial injury from nitric oxide and superoxide. *Proc Natl Acad Sci U S A* 1990;87:1620–1624.

79. Giugliano D, Ceriello A, Paolisso G. Oxidative stress and diabetic vascular complications. *Diabetes Care* 1996;19:257–267.

80. Koya D, Haneda M, Kikkawa R, et al. D-alpha-tocopherol prevents glomerular dysfunction in diabetic rats through inhibition of PKC-DAG pathway. *Biofactors* 1998;7:69–76.

81. Inoguchi T, Li P, Umeda F, et al. High glucose level and free fatty acid stimulate reactive oxygen species production through protein kinase C-dependent activation of NAD(P)H oxidase in cultured vascular cells. *Diabetes* 2000;49:1939–1945.

82. Devaraj S, Jialal I. Low-density lipoprotein postsecretory modification, monocyte function, and circulating adhesion molecules in type 2 diabetic patients

with and without macrovascular complications: the effect of α-tocopherol supplementation. *Circulation* 2000;102:191–196.

83. Devaraj S, Jialal I. AT supplementation decreases CRP and Mo IL-6 from DM-2. *Free Radic Biol Med* 2000;29:790–792.

84. Venugopal SK, Devaraj S, Yang TT, et al. Alpha tocopherol decreases superoxide anion release in THP-1 cells under hyperglycemic conditions through inhibition of PKC-a. *Diabetes* 2002;51:3049–3054.

85. Libby P, Hanson G. Biology of disease. Involvement of the immune system in atherogenesis: current knowledge and unanswered questions. *Lab Invest* 1991;64:5–13.

86. Desfaits A, Serri O, Renier G. Normalization of plasma lipid peroxides, monocyte adhesion and TNF production in NIDDM patients after gliclazide treatment. *Diabetes Care* 1998;21:487–491.

87. Ross R. Cell biology of atherosclerosis. *Annu Rev Physiol* 1995;57:791–804.

88. Kim J, Berliner J, Natarajan R, et al. Evidence that glucose increases monocyte binding to human aortic endothelial cells. *Diabetes* 1994;43:1103–1107.

89. Carantoni M, Abbasi F, Chu L, et al. Adherence of mononuclear cells to endothelium in vitro is increased in patients with NIDDM. *Diabetes Care* 1997;20:1462–1465.

90. Hoogerbrugge N, Verkerk A, Jacobs M, et al. Hypertriglyceridemia enhances monocyte binding to endothelial cells in NIDDM. *Diabetes Care* 1997;3:1122–1124.

91. Hwang S, Ballantyne CM, Sharrett AR, et al. Circulating adhesion molecules VCAM-1-1, ICAM-1-1, and E-selectin in carotid atherosclerosis and incident coronary heart disease cases: the Atherosclerosis Risk in Communities (ARIC) study. *Circulation* 1997;96:4219–4225.

92. Rohde LE, Lee RT, Jamocochian M, et al. Circulating CAMs are correlated with ultrasound measurement of carotid atherosclerosis. *Arterioscler Thromb Vasc Biol* 1998;18,1765–1770.

93. Ridker PM, Hennekens CH, Roitman-Johnson B, et al. Plasma concentration of soluble intercellular adhesion molecule-1 and risk of future myocardial infarction in apparently healthy men. *Lancet* 1998:351;88–92.

94. Albertini J-P, Valensi P, Lormeau B, et al. Soluble L-selectin level is a marker for CAD in type 2 diabetic patients. *Diabetes Care* 1999;22:2044–2048.

95. Albertini J-P, Valensi P, Lormeau B, et al. Elevated concentrations of soluble E-selectin and vascular cell adhesion molecule-1 in NIDDM: effect of intensive insulin treatment. *Diabetes Care* 1998;21,1008–1013.

96. Fasching P, Waldhausl W, Wagner OF. Elevated circulating adhesion molecules in NIDDM-potential mediators in diabetic macroangiopathy. *Diabetologia* 1996;39,1242–1244.

97. Matsumoto K, Sera Y, Abe Y, et al. Serum concentrations of soluble vascular cell adhesion molecule-1 and E-selectin are elevated in insulin-resistant patients with type 2 diabetes. *Diabetes Care* 2001;24,1697–1698.

98. Mocco J, Choudhri TF, Mack WJ, et al. Elevation of soluble intercellular adhesion molecule-1 levels in symptomatic and asymptomatic carotid atherosclerosis. *Neurosurgery* 2001;48,718–721.

99. Hofmann MA, Schiekofer S, Isermann B, et al. Peripheral blood mononuclear cells isolated from patients with diabetic nephropathy show increased activation of the oxidative-stress sensitive transcription factor NF-kappaB. *Diabetologia* 1999;42:222–232.

100. Ridker PM, Haughie P. Prospective studies of C-reactive protein as a risk factor for cardiovascular disease. *J Invest Med* 1998;46:391–395.

101. Tracy R. Inflammation in cardiovascular disease: cart, horse, or both? *Circulation* 1998;97:2000–2002.

102. Jialal I, Devaraj S. Inflammation and atherosclerosis: the value of the high-sensitivity C-reactive protein assay as a risk marker. *Am J Clin Pathol* 2001;116[Suppl]:S108–S115.

103. Pickup J, Mattock M, Chusney G, et al. NIDDM as a disease of the innate immune system: association of acute-phase reactants and interleukin-6 with metabolic syndrome X. *Diabetologia* 1997;40:1286–1292.

104. Upritchard JE, Sutherland WH, Mann JI. Effect of supplementation with tomato juice, vitamin E, and vitamin C on LDL oxidation and products of inflammatory activity in type 2 diabetes. *Diabetes Care* 2000;23:733–738.

105. Freeman DJ, Norrie J, Caslake MJ, et al. C-reactive protein is an independent predictor of risk for the development of diabetes in the west of Scotland Coronary Prevention Study. *Diabetes* 2002;51:1596–1600.

106. Ridker PM, Buring JE, Shih J, et al. Prospective study of C-reactive protein and the risk of future cardiovascular events among apparently healthy women. *Circulation* 1998;98:731–733.

107. Calles-Escandon J, Cipolla M. Diabetes and endothelial dysfunction: a clinical perspective. *Endocr Rev* 2001;22:36–52.

108. De Meyer GR, Herman AG. Vascular endothelial dysfuncion. *Prog Cardiovasc Dis* 1997;39:325–342.

109. Kario K, Matsuo T, Kobayashi H, et al. Activation of tissue factor-induced coagulation and endothelial cell dysfunction in non-insulin-dependent diabetic patients with microalbuminuria. *Arterioscler Thromb Vasc Biol* 1995;15:1114–1120.

110. Vinik AI, Erbas T, Park TS, et al. Platelet dysfunction in type 2 diabetes. *Diabetes Care* 2001;24:1476–1485.

111. Watts GF, O'Brien SF, Silvester W, et al. Impaired endothelium-dependent and independent dilatation of forearm resistance arteries in men with diet-treated non-insulin-dependent diabetes: role of dyslipidaemia. *Clin Sci* 1996;91:567–573.

112. Booth G, Stalker TJ, Lefer AM, et al. Mechanisms of amelioration of glucose-induced endothelial dysfunction following inhibition of protein kinase C in vivo. *Diabetes* 2002;51:1556–1564.

113. Schnackenberg CG. Physiological and pathophysiological roles of oxygen radicals in the renal microvasculature. *Am J Physiol Regul Integr Comp Physiol* 2002;282:R335–R342.

114. Gale CR, Ashurst HE, Powers HJ, et al. Antioxidant vitamin status and carotid atherosclerosis in the elderly. *Am J Clin Nutr* 2001;74:402–408.

115. Jialal I, Fuller CJ. Effect of vitamin E, vitamin C and beta-carotene on LDL oxidation and atherosclerosis. *Can J Cardiol* 1995;11[Suppl G]:97G–103G.

116. Fuller CJ, Chandalia M, Garg A, et al. RRR-alpha tocopherol acetate supplementation at pharmacological doses decreases LDL oxidation but not protein

glycation in patients with diabetes. *Am J Clin Nutr* 1996;63:753–759.

117. Reaven PD, Herold DA, Barnett J, et al. Effects of vitamin E on susceptibility of LDL and LDL subfractions to oxidation and on protein glycation in NIDDM. *Diabetes Care* 1995;18:807–816.

118. Astley S, Langrish-Smith A, Southon S, et al. AT supplementation and oxidative damage to DNA and plasma LDL in DM-1. *Diabetes Care* 1999;22:1626–1631.

119. Devaraj S, Jialal I. The effects of alpha tocopherol on critical cells in atherogenesis. *Curr Opin Lipidol* 1998;9:11–15.

120. Heitzer T, Herttuala S, Wild E, et al. Effect of vitamin E on endothelial vasodilator function in patients with hypercholesterolemia, chronic smoking or both. *J Am Coll Cardiol* 1999;33:122–126.

121. Motoyama T, Kawano H, Kugiyama K, et al. Vitamin E administration improves impairment of endothelium-dependent vasodilation in patients with coronary spastic angina. *J Am Coll Cardiol* 1998;32:1672–1679.

122. Faruqui R, De La Motte C, Dicorleto P. Alpha-tocopherol inhibits agonist-induced monocyte cell adherence to cultured human endothelial cells. *J Clin Invest* 1994;94:592–600.

123. Islam KN, Devaraj S, Jialal I. α-Tocopherol enrichment of monocytes decreases agonist-induced adhesion to human endothelial cells. *Circulation* 1998;98:2255–2261.

124. De Mattia G, Bravi MC, Laurenti O, et al. Reduction of oxidative stress by oral N-acetyl-L-cysteine treatment decreases plasma soluble vascular cell adhesion molecule-1 concentrations in non-obese, non-dyslipidaemic, normotensive, patients with non-insulin-dependent diabetes. *Diabetologia* 1998;41:1392–1396.

125. Devaraj S, Cabo Chan AV, Jialal I. Alpha tocopherol supplementation decreases plasminogen activator inhibitor-1 and P-selectin levels in type 2 diabetic patients. *Diabetes Care* 2002;23:324–329.

126. Sobel BE. Altered fibrinolysis and platelet function in the development of vascular complications of diabetes. *Curr Opin Endocrinol Diabetes* 1996;3:355–360.

127. Auwerx J, Bouillon R, Collen D, et al. Tissue-type plasminogen activator antigen and plasminogen activator inhibitor in diabetes mellitus. *Arteriosclerosis* 1988;8:68–72.

128. Gray RP, Yudkin JS, Patterson DL. Plasminogen activator inhibitor: a risk factor for myocardial infarction in diabetic patients. *Br Heart J* 1993;69:228–232.

129. Pandolfi A, Cetrullo D, Polishuck R, et al. Plasminogen activator inhibitor type 1 is increased in the arterial wall of type 2 diabetic subjects. *Arterioscler Thromb Vasc Biol* 2001;21:1378–1382.

130. Bursell S, Clermont AC, Aiello LP, et al. High dose alpha tocopherol supplementation normalizes retinal blood flow and creatinine clearance in patients with type I diabetes. *Diabetes Care* 1999;22:1245–1251.

131. Hofmann MA, Schiekofer S, Kanitz M, et al. Insufficient glycemic control increases NF-kB binding activity in peripheral blood mononuclear cells isolated from patients with type-1 diabetes. *Diabetes Care* 1998;21:1–7.

132. Gaede P, Poulsen HE, Parving HH, et al. Double blind randomized study of the effect of combined treatment with vitamin C and E on albuminuria in T2DM. *Diabet Med* 2001;18:756–760.

133. Manzella D, Barbieri M, Ragno E, et al. Chronic administration of pharmacologic doses of vitamin E improves the cardiac autonomic nervous system in patients with type 2 diabetes. *Am J Clin Nutr* 2001;73:1052–1057.

134. Paolisso G, Tagliamonte MR, Barbieri M, et al. Chronic vitamin E administration improves brachial reactivity and increases intracellular magnesium concentration in type II diabetic patients. *J Clin Endocrinol Metab* 2000;85,109–115.

135. Gazis A, White DJ, Page SR, et al. Effect of oral vitamin E (alpha-tocopherol) supplementation on vascular endothelial function in type 2 diabetes mellitus. *Diabet Med* 1999;16,304–311.

136. Boaz M, Smetana S, Weinstein T, et al. Secondary Prevention with Antioxidants of Cardiovascular Disease in Endstage Renal Disease (SPACE): randomized placebo controlled trial. *Lancet* 2000;356.1213–1218.

137. Marangon K, Devaraj S, Tirosh O, et al. Comparison of the effect of alpha-lipoic acid and alpha-tocopherol supplementation on measures of oxidative stress. *Free Radic Biol Med* 1999;27:1114–1121.

138. Heitzer T, Finckh B, Albers S, et al. Beneficial effects of alpha-lipoic acid and ascorbic acid on endothelium-dependent, nitric oxide-mediated vasodilation in diabetic patients: relation to parameters of oxidative stress. *Free Radic Biol Med* 2001;31:53–61.

139. Bierhaus A, Chevion S, Chevion M, et al. Advanced glycation end product induced activation of NFkB is suppressed by α-lipoic acid in cultured endothelial cells. *Diabetes* 1997;46:1481–1490.

140. Sachse G, Willms B. Efficacy of thioctic acid in the therapy of peripheral diabetic polyneuropathy. In: Gries FA, Feund HJ, Rabe F, et al., eds. *Aspects of autonomic neuropathy in diabetes.* Hormone metabolism research supplement series 9. New York. Thieme-Stratton, 1980:105–108.

141. Delcker A, Fischer P-A, Ulrich H. Randomisierte Studie Thioctsäure Gegenüber Vitamin-B-Kombinationspräparat bei patienten mit diabetischer polyneuropathie unter besonderer berücksichtigung des peripheren neurosystems. In: Borbe HO, Ulrich H, eds. *Neue biochemische, pharmakologische und klinische Erkenntnisse zur Thioctsäure.* Frankfurt: PMI Verlag, 1989:335–344.

142. Schulz B, Reichel G, Hüttl I, et al. *Zur wirksamkeit der Thioctsäuretherapie bei Typ I diabetikern.* Greifswald: Wiss Z Ernst-Moritz-Arndt-Universität Greifswald, Medizinische Reihe 1986;35:48–50.

143. Jörg J, Metz F, Scharafinski H. Zur medikamentösen behandlung der diabetischen polyneuropathie mit der Alpha-Liponsäure oder vitamin B-präparaten. *Nervenarzt* 1988;59:36–44.

144. Ziegler D, Mayer P, Mühlen H, et al. Effekte einer therapie mit a-liponsäure gegenüber vitamin B1 bei der diabetischen polyneuropathie. *Diabetes und Stoffwechsel* 1993;2:443–448.

145. Reschke B, Zeuzem S, Rosak C, et al. Hochdosierte langzeit-therapie mit thioctsäure bei der diabetischen polyneuropathie: ergebnisse einer kontrollierten randomisierten studie unter besonderer Berücksich-tigung der autonomen neuropathie. In: Borbe HO, Ulrich H,

eds. *Neue biochemische, pharmakologische und klinische erkenntnisse zurthioctsäure.* Frankfurt: PMI Verlag, 1989:318–334.

146. Ziegler D, Hanenfeld M, Ruhnau KJ, et al. The ALADIN Study Group. Treatment of symptomatic diabetic peripheral neuropathy with the antioxidant α-lipoic acid: a 3-week randomized double blind placebo controlled trial (ALADIN Study). *Diabetologia* 1995;38:1425–1433.

147. Reljanovic M, Reichel C, Rett K, et al. Treatment of diabetic polyneuropathy with the antioxidant thioctic acid (α-lipoic acid): a two-year multicenter randomized double blind placebo controlled trial (ALADIN II). *Free Radic Res* 1999;31:171–179.

148. Ruhnau KJ, Meissner HP, Finn JR, et al. Oral treatment of symptomatic diabetic polyneuropathy with the antioxidant thioctic acid (α-lipoic acid): a 3-week randomized double-blind placebo-controlled trial. *Diabet Med* 1999;16:1040–1043.

149. Ziegler D, Hanefeld M, Ruhnau KJ, et al. Treatment of symptomatic diabetic polyneuropathy with the antioxidant α-lipoic acid: a 7-month multicenter randomized controlled clinical trial (ALADIN III). *Diabetes Care* 1999;22:1296–1301.

150. Ziegler D, Conrad F, Ulrich H, et al. Effects of treatment with the antioxidant α-lipoic acid on cardiac autonomic neuropathy in NIDDM patients: a 4-month randomized controlled multicenter clinical trial (DEKAN Study). *Diabetes Care* 1997;20:369–373.

151. Jacob S, Streeper R, Fogt D, et al. The antioxidant α-lipoic acid enhances insulin-stimulated glucose metabolism in insulin-resistant rat skeletal muscle. *Diabetes* 1996;45:1024–1029.

152. Estrada D, Ewart H, Tsakiridis T, et al. Stimulation of glucose uptake by the natural coenzyme α-lipoic acid/thioctic acid. *Diabetes* 1996;45:1798–1804.

153. Haugaard N, Haugaard E. Stimulation of glucose utilization by thioctic acid in rat diaphragm incubated in vitro. *Biochim Biophys Acta* 1970;222:583–586.

154. Jacob S, Henrikson EJ, Tritschler HJ, et al. Improvement of insulin-stimulated glucose-disposal in type 2 diabetes after repeated parenteral administration of thioctic acid. *Exp Clin Endocrinol Diabetes* 1996;104:284–288.

155. Henrikson EJ, Jacob S, Streeper RS, et al. Stimulation by α-lipoic acid of glucose transporter activity in skeletal muscle of lean and obese zucker rats. *Life Sci* 1997;61:805–812.

156. Streeper RS, Henriksen EJ, Jacob S, et al. Differential effects of lipoic acid stereoisomers on glucose metabolism in insulin-resistant skeletal muscle. *Am J Physiol* 1997;273:E185–E191.

157. Strödter D, Lehmann E, Lehmann U, et al. The influence of thioctic acid on metabolism and function of the diabetic heart. *Diabetes Res Clin Pract* 1995;29:19–26.

158. Khamisi M, Potashnik R, Tirosh A, et al. Lipoic acid reduces glycemia and increases muscle GLUT 4 content in streptozotocin-diabetic rats. *Metabolism* 1997;46:763–768.

159. Rett K, Wicklmayr M, Maeker E, et al. Effect of acute infusion of thioctic acid on oxidative and non-oxidative metabolism in obese subjects with NIDDM. *Diabetologia* 1995;38:A41.

160. Jacob S, Henrikson EJ, Schiemann AL, et al. α-Lipoic acid enhances glucose disposal in patients with type 2 diabetes. *Arzneimittelforschung/Drug Research* 1995;45:872–874.

161. Jacob S, Ruus P, Herrmann R, et al. Oral administration of rac-α-lipoic acid modulates insulin sensitivity in patients with type-2 diabetes: a placebo-controlled pilot trial. *Free Radic Biol Med* 1999;27:309–314.

162. Konrad T, Vicini P, Kusterer K, et al. Alpha lipoic acid treatment decreases serum lactate and pyruvate concentrations and improves glucose effectiveness in lean and obese patients with type II diabetes. *Diabetes Care* 1999;22:280–287.

163. Jialal I, Grundy SM. Preservation of the endogenous antioxidants in low density lipoprotein by ascorbate but not probucol during oxidative modification. *J Clin Invest* 1991;87:597–601.

164. Harats D, Ben-Naim M, Dabach Y, et al. Effect of vitamin C and E supplementation on susceptibility of plasma lipoproteins to peroxidation induced by acute smoking. *Atherosclerosis* 1990;85:47–54.

165. Rifici VA, Khachadurian AK. Dietary supplementation with vitamins C and E inhibits in vitro oxidation of lipoproteins. *J Am Coll Nutr* 1993;12:631–637.

166. Fuller CJ, Grundy SM, Norkus EP, et al. Effect of ascorbate supplementation on low density lipoprotein oxidation in smokers. *Atherosclerosis* 1996;119:139–150.

167. Wen Y, Cooke T, Feely J. The effect of pharmacological supplementation with vitamin C on low-density lipoprotein oxidation. *Br J Clin Pharmacol* 1997;44:94–97.

168. Reilly M, Delanty N, Lawson JA, et al. Modulation of oxidant stress in vivo in chronic cigarette smokers. *Circulation* 1996;94:19–25.

169. Anderson R, Lukey PT. A biological role for ascorbate in the selective neutralization of extracellular phagocyte-derived oxidants. *Ann N Y Acad Sci* 1987;498:229–247.

170. Abdel-Wahab YH, O'Harte FP, Mooney MH, et al. Vitamin C supplementation decreases insulin glycation and improves glucose homeostasis in obese hyperglycemic (ob/ob) mice. *Metabolism* 2002;51:514–517.

171. Cay M, Naziroglu M, Simsek H, et al. Effects of intraperitoneally administered vitamin C on antioxidative defense mechanism in rats with diabetes induced by streptozotocin. *Res Exp Med* 2001;200:205–213.

172. Heitzer T, Just H, Munzel T. Antioxidant vitamin C improves endothelial dysfunction in chronic smokers. *Circulation* 1996;94:6–9.

173. Motoyama T, Kawano H, Kugiyama K, et al. Endothelium-dependent vasodilation in the brachial artery is impaired in smokers: effect of vitamin C. *Am J Physiol* 1997;273:H1644–H1650.

174. Solzbach U, Hornig B, Jeserich M, et al. Vitamin C improves endothelial dysfunction of epicardial coronary arteries in hypertensive patients. *Circulation* 1997;96:1513–1519.

175. Taddei S, Virdis A, Ghiadoni L, et al. Vitamin C improves endothelium-dependent vasodilation by restoring nitric oxide activity in essential hypertension. *Circulation* 1998;97:2222–2229.

176. Ting HH, Timimi FK, Boles KS, et al. Vitamin C improves endothelium-dependent vasodilation in patients with non-insulin-dependent diabetes mellitus. *J Clin Invest* 1996;97:22–28.

177. Timimi FK, Ting HH, Haley EA, et al. Vitamin C improves endothelium-dependent vasodilation in patients with insulin-dependent diabetes mellitus. *J Am Coll Cardiol* 1998;31:552–557.

178. Duffy SJ, Gokce N, Holbrook M, et al. Effect of ascorbic acid treatment on conduit vessel endothelial dysfunction in patients with hypertension.

Am J Physiol Heart Circ Physiol 2001;280:H528–H534.

179. Beckman JA, Goldfine AB, Gordon MB, et al. Ascorbate restores endothelium-dependent vasodilation impaired by acute hyperglycemia in humans. *Circulation* 2001;103:1618–1623.

180. Lekakis JP, Anastasiou EA, Papamichael CM, et al. Short-term oral ascorbic acid improves endothelium-dependent vasodilatation in women with a history of gestational diabetes mellitus. *Diabetes Care* 2000;23:1432–1434.

3

Role of Protein Kinase C Isoforms in Diabetic Vascular Dysfunction

Zhiheng He, Ronald C. W. Ma, and George L. King

Mary K. Iacocca Fellow, Department of Vascular Cell Biology and Complications, Joslin Diabetes Center, Harvard Medical School, Boston, Massachusetts; Medical Officer, Endocrine Division, Department of Medicine and Therapeutics, Prince of Wales Hospital, Shatin, Hong Kong, China; Research Director, Joslin Diabetes Center, Professor of Medicine, Harvard Medical School, Boston, Massachusetts

The major cause of mortality in diabetic patients is cardiovascular disease (1). This is thought to be a consequence, in part, of the increased incidence of atherosclerotic macrovascular disease in the diabetic state, but it is also partly due to an additional effect of diabetes in causing a variety of changes in myocardium that result in disordered cardiac remodeling, a process often referred to broadly as diabetic cardiomyopathy. In addition, diabetic microvascular disease—namely, diabetic retinopathy, neuropathy, and nephropathy—accounts for much morbidity and mortality in patients with either insulin-dependent (type 1) or non-insulin-dependent (type 2) diabetes mellitus. Although the exact mechanisms by which hyperglycemia can lead to diabetic complications are only gradually coming to light, the role of chronic hyperglycemia in initiating and exacerbating these events that lead to microvascular damage was made clear by the dramatic reduction in the development and progression of diabetic complications achieved with tight glycemic control in the Diabetes Control and Complications Trial (DCCT) (2) and in the United Kingdom Prospective Diabetes Study (UKPDS) (3). However, these two landmark studies also showed that, despite achievement of tight glycemic control with intensive treatment (which may not be possible in some patients), progression of diabetic microvascular complications still occurs. An understanding of the pathogenesis of diabetic complications is important because it may provide us with novel targets for adjuvant therapeutic interventions to prevent complications in the setting of suboptimal glycemic control. This chapter presents some of the accumulating evidence highlighting the role of protein kinase C (PKC) in the pathogenesis of diabetic macrovascular and microvascular complications and discusses potential treatment strategies based on this emerging molecular understanding of diabetic complications.

PROTEIN KINASE C

Classification and Structure of Protein Kinase C

PKC is a family of serine/threonine kinases that consists of at least 12 members (4). Structurally, this single-chain polypeptide contains an amino-terminal regulatory domain and a carboxyl-terminal catalytic domain (Fig. 3-1). Although all PKCs share high homology in primary sequence, individual members of this family bear distinctive features in structure, distribution, and substrate requirements. PKCs are traditionally classified into three groups, known as conventional PKC (cPKC), novel PKC (nPKC), and atypical PKC (aPKC).

(a) Conventional PKC (α, βI, βII, γ)

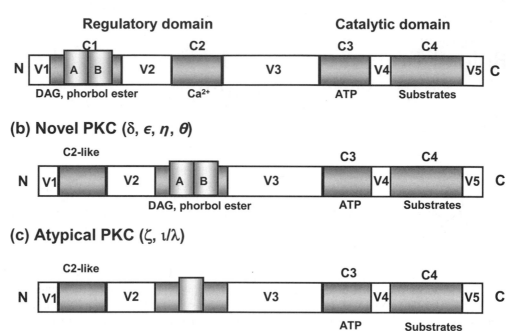

FIG. 3-1. Structure and classification of protein kinase C (PKC) family of serine/threonine kinases. PKCs can be divided into three subgroups: conventional, novel, and atypical PKCs. Structurally, all PKCs consist of an amino-terminal regulatory domain and a carboxyl-terminal catalytic domain. The regulatory domain contains two conserved regions, designated C1 and C2 in conventional PKCs (cPKCs), that include α, βI, βII, and γ isoforms. These regions are engaged in the interactions with diacylglycerol (DAG) and phorbol ester (C1), and with Ca^{2+} (C2), that are essential to the activation of cPKCs. In novel PKCs (nPKCs), which consist of δ, ϵ, η, and θ isoforms, the regulatory domain retains the DAG and phorbol ester-binding C1 domain. However, instead of having a typical C2 domain, nPKCs have a C2-like domain that is incapable of binding to Ca^{2+}, and therefore their activation does not require the presence of Ca^{2+}. Atypical PKC (aPKC) has ζ and ι/λ isoforms. Their N-terminal domain comprises half of the C1 subdomain and a C2-like domain and interacts with neither DAG, phorbol ester, nor Ca^{2+}, precluding the requirement of these factors for their full activation. All PKCs share a similar catalytic domain that contains two conserved regions, C3 and C4, that are known to serve as adenosine triphosphate (ATP)- and substrate-binding domains, respectively. Conserved domains are interspaced by five variable regions, termed V1 through V5.

cPKC represents the prototype of the PKC family and contains four isoforms: α, βI, βII, and γ. Four conserved domains are found in cPKC and designated C1 through C4; they are interspaced by five variable regions named V1 through V5 (Fig. 3-1). Domains C1 and C2 are located in the regulatory N-terminal region and confer membrane targeting regulation as well as interaction with diacylglycerol (DAG) and phorbol esters and with phosphatidylserine (PS) and Ca^{2+}. Within the C1 domain, two

tandem repeats of cysteine-rich zinc fingers have been found and are designated C1A and C1B (Fig. 3-1). These two subdomains interact with DAG and phorbol esters, respectively. The C2 site is involved in Ca^{2+}-dependent membrane binding. DAG, phorbol esters, PS, and Ca^{2+} are all activators of cPKCs. The interaction of cPKC with Ca^{2+} is unique among all PKCs, and cPKCs are also known as Ca^{2+}-dependent PKCs. The C3 and C4 subdomains are located in the C-terminal catalytic region and are engaged in interaction with adenosine triphosphate (ATP) and substrates.

nPKC is structurally similar to cPKC and contains similar C1, C3, and C4 domains (Fig. 3-1). However, instead of having a Ca^{2+}-binding C2 domain, nPKCs contain a C2-like motif that is incapable of binding to Ca^{2+}. Therefore, the activation of nPKCs does not require the presence of Ca^{2+}, although DAG and PS are needed as coactivators. This group of PKCs contains several isoforms, including δ, ϵ, η, and θ.

aPKC is structurally distinctive from all other PKCs in that its activation requires neither Ca^{2+} nor DAG, although PS can regulate its activity (5). Structurally, its N-terminal domain has a C2-like domain and half of a C1-like domain, and these differences may explain the different requirements of activators.

Activation of the Diacylglycerol-Protein Kinase C Pathway

PKC can be activated through multiple pathways in response to a wide array of stimuli, including cytokines, mechanical shears, stresses, hormones, and even glucose. With exposure to hyperglycemia in diabetes, accumulation of glycolytic intermediate glycerol-3-phosphate stimulates the *de novo* synthesis of DAG, which in turn activates specific isoforms of PKC (6). In addition, chronic hyperglycemia can also increase the production of advanced glycation end products (AGEs) and generate reactive oxygen species (ROS) (7,8), which have been shown to activate the DAG-PKC pathway (8–10). Hyperglycemia increases circulating or locally produced cytokines, growth factors, and hormones such as endothelin-1 (ET-1) (11) and angiotensin II (12,13), in some cases through a PKC-dependent pathway (11). These secreted cytokines can also activate PKCs by binding to their cell surface receptors (14–16). Diabetes is also associated with severe dyslipidemia. Increased circulating free fatty acids (FFA) have been reported to activate PKC (17–19) either directly (20) or through *de novo* synthesis of DAG in many cell types, including vascular smooth muscle cells (VSMC) (21,22) and endothelial cells (22). The activation of multiple isoforms of nPKCs, especially

PKC-θ, is considered to be important in mechanisms of insulin resistance in skeletal muscles (19,23). A simplified schematic representation of DAG-PKC activation in diabetes and related cardiovascular abnormalities is shown in Figure 3-2.

Translocation of multiple PKC isoforms and increased PKC activities have been reported in cardiovascular tissues in diabetic states. Liu et al. (24) reported that the protein contents of PKC-α, -β, -ϵ, and -ζ are increased in the homogenate fraction of hearts from diabetic rats. These increases are accompanied by a parallel upregulation of PKC activity. Malhotra et al. (25) showed a significant membrane translocation of PKC-ϵ in cardiomyocytes isolated from diabetic rats. In other studies, when cardiomyocytes were exposed to high ambient glucose, they displayed significant membrane translocations of βI, βII, δ, ϵ, and ζ isoforms of PKC that were associated with troponin I phosphorylation (16). In cultured aortic smooth muscle cells, medium containing 22 mM of glucose induced the translocation of PKC-βII (26,27). Cultured bovine aortic endothelial cells, when exposed to 25 mM glucose, showed translocation of PKC-βII and -δ isoforms to membrane pools, associated with the increased expression of vasoconstrictor ET-1 (11). Interestingly, endothelial cells from different tissues of the same species responded differently to hyperglycemia in terms of the isoforms activated. Bovine retinal endothelial cells showed translocation of PKC-α, -βII, and -δ in response to chronic hyperglycemia (11). Using an immunohistochemical approach, Kang et al. (28) showed that PKC-α is the major isoform expressed in the cardiac capillary from diabetic rats. Upregulation of PKC activities *in vivo* has been demonstrated in many tissues that are prone to diabetic macrovascular or microvascular complications, including retina (29), glomeruli (30–33), monocytes (34), aorta (6,27) and heart (6,24,31,35). In addition to the sustained activation of PKC in diabetic states, PKCs are also reported to be regulated at the levels of transcription and posttranscriptional stability in cultured cells in experimental diabetes (36,37).

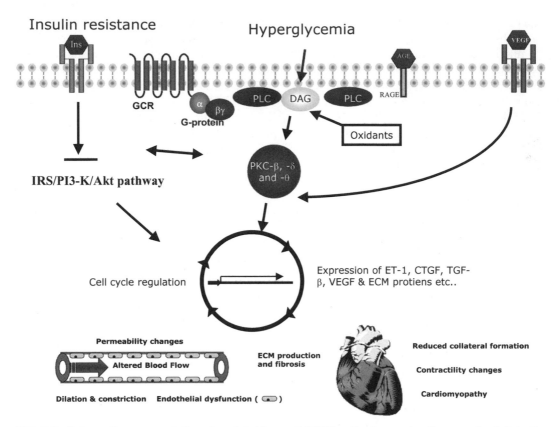

FIG. 3-2. Schematic representation of protein kinase C (PKC) activation and pathogenesis of diabetic cardiovascular complications. Activation of the diacylglycerol (DAG)-PKC pathway in cardiovascular tissues can be achieved via multiple pathways, such as the accumulation of glycolytic intermediates; activation of cell surface receptors including G protein-coupled receptors (GCR) and receptors with tyrosine kinase (RTK); and increases in oxidants and advanced glycation end products (AGEs) and their receptors (RAGEs). Activated PKC, especially the β and δ isoforms, can interact with downstream effectors such as retinoblastoma protein (pRB) and, in turn, determine the cell cycle progression of cardiovascular cells as well as the expression of multiple secreted factors such as endothelin-1 (ET-1), connective tissue growth factor (CTGF), transforming growth factor-β (TGF-β), vascular endothelial-cell growth factor (VEGF), and extracellular matrix proteins including collagens and fibronectins. Secreted ET-1 and VEGF may also activate the DAG-PKC pathway through an autocrine/paracrine route. These alterations eventually result in abnormalities of cardiovascular tissues (e.g., endothelial dysfunction), increased permeability of microvessels, reduced cardiac contractility, cardiomyocyte death, cardiac fibrosis, and reduced angiogenesis in the heart. Activation of certain PKC isoforms, especially atypical PKC-θ, plays important roles in insulin resistance that can also lead to many pathologic changes in the cardiovascular tissues.

ROLES OF PROTEIN KINASE C IN DIABETIC CARDIOVASCULAR COMPLICATIONS

Expression of Protein Kinase C in the Cardiovascular System

Multiple isoforms of PKC are expressed in cardiovascular tissues, and the expression is species dependent. Several major isoforms, including PKC-α, -βI, -βII, -δ, -ϵ and -ζ, are expressed at different levels in adult hearts (6,16,24,38–40), endothelial cells, (6,11) and VSMC (26,27,41).

Protein Kinase C Activation in Cardiovascular Disease

An increasing body of evidence suggests that PKCs play significant roles in the regulation of cardiovascular homeostasis. Because the α, βI, βII, δ, ϵ, and ζ isoforms are predominantly expressed in the adult heart, the roles of these PKCs have been extensively studied, especially in cardiac hypertrophy, preconditioning, ischemia-reperfusion injury, and infarction. Cardiac hypertrophy is the enlargement of cardiomyocyte size and mass to compensate for increases in workload (42,43). Multiple signaling pathways are activated, including PKC, mitogen-activated protein kinase (MAPK), and phosphatidyl inositol-3-kinase (PI3 kinase)/Akt (42–44). Activation of PKC-α, -βII, -δ, and -ϵ can result in hypertrophy of cardiomyocytes to different degrees both *in vitro* and *in vivo*, probably through activation of the extracellular signal-related kinase (ERK) pathway and initiation of protein translation machinery (45–47). Cardiac ischemia preconditioning is a defense mechanism against ischemic damage that is intrinsic to cardiomyocytes. It was initially reported by Murry et al. (48) in 1986. PKCs have been shown to be activated by ischemia and to play key roles in conferring cardiac protection (49). Multiple isoforms, including PKC-α, -δ, -ϵ, and -η, have been shown to translocate to the active membrane pool in different species during this process (50–52). Activation of PKC-ϵ has been reported to confer cardioprotection against ischemia insult (53–55), probably through the inhibition of apoptosis and necrosis

(54). On the other hand, activation of PKC-δ is associated with ischemia-induced cardiomyocyte apoptosis and infarction (47,56). To evaluate the role of PKC-δ in the heart, a selective peptide PKC-δ translocation inhibitor, δV, was used in a mouse model (47). Maximum suppression of PKC-δ led to early lethality (56), but when PKC translocation was slightly impaired, pathologic changes developed that were similar to those of myofibrillar cardiomyopathy, with impaired cardiac contractility, probably due to the disruption of cardiomyocyte cytoskeletal integrity (47). Interestingly, hearts from these mice conferred cardioprotection against ischemia-reperfusion injury (47,56).

Protein Kinase C in Diabetic Cardiovascular Complications

Diabetic Cardiomyopathy

It has long been noted that chronic hyperglycemia can induce structural and functional alterations in the heart. The term *diabetic cardiomyopathy* was first proposed by Rubler et al. in 1972, after the clinical encounter of a specific type of cardiomyopathy that is closely associated with diabetes (57). An increasing body of evidence has independently confirmed the existence of such cardiac complications of diabetes. Diabetic cardiomyopathy is manifested by early diastolic dysfunction, small-vessel disease, interstitial fibrosis, myocardial hypertrophy, and eventual loss of cardiac contractility and cardiomyocytes. Although it is well known that diabetic cardiomyopathy contributes to the heart failure and results in the high mortality rate observed in diabetic patients independent of coronary artery disease (58), the molecular mechanisms underlying these complications are not clear. Several theories have been proposed, including PKC activation, enhanced oxidative stress, and accumulation of AGEs (8). Among these, PKC activation no doubt plays a significant role.

As discussed earlier, hyperglycemia induces *de novo* DAG synthesis and in turn activates PKCs. In the myocardium, several isoforms of PKC are activated to the membrane fraction of the heart by hyperglycemia, including PKC-α, -βII, -δ, -ϵ, and -ζ isoforms (6,24,25,28,40). PKC-βII and -δ are the major isoforms to be activated by chronic hyperglycemia (6,40). Targeted overexpression of the βII isoform in transgenic mice resulted in a cardiac phenotype reminiscent of that seen in diabetic cardiomyopathy. Wakasaki et al. (46,59) caused overexpression of PKC-βII in mouse myocardium using an α-myosin heavy chain (MHC) promoter. Although all the transgenic animals were viable, their mortality rate was higher after 20 weeks of age. Pathologies developed in the hearts of the transgenic mice soon after birth, and with time they displayed an increased ratio of heart weight to body weight, cardiomyocyte hypertrophy, focal cardiomyocyte death, and extensive fibrosis (46,59). The structural changes unavoidably result in the loss of cardiac functions, as manifested by reduced left ventricular end diastolic dimension and reduced cardiac contractility, probably due to PKC-βII-mediated phosphorylation of troponin I, which may decrease myofilament Ca^{2+} responsiveness (60). This observation is consistent with the previous finding that PKC activation can induce phosphorylation of troponin I and T and downregulation of calcium-stimulated ATPase in actomyosin, with subsequent inhibition of cardiac sarcoplasmic reticulum Ca^{2+} accumulation, which in turn reduces cardiac contractility (61–63). Overexpression of PKC-βII resulted in extensive cardiac fibrosis, probably due to upregulation of the expression of fibrosis-promoting factors such as transforming growth factor-β1 (TGF-β1) and connective tissue growth factor (CTGF) (59). These factors can further result in the transcription and deposition of extracellular matrix components such as collagens and fibronectins (46,59). This phenomenon is consistent with the observation that collagen and fibronectin deposition is increased in myocardial tissues from diabetic humans and animals (58,64–66).

Loss of cardiomyocytes has been blamed in part for the ventricular dysfunction in diabetic hearts and is probably caused by hyperglycemia-induced cardiomyocyte apoptosis (13,67). Activation of PKC-δ is known to induce cellular apoptosis in many cell types, including neutrophils, keratinocytes, neuronal cells, fibroblasts, transformed cells, and cardiomyocytes, once activated by a wide array of stimuli (68–72). Using cultured adult rat cardiomyocytes, Shizukuda et al. (73) reported that exposure to hyperglycemia resulted in extensive PKC-δ translocation and cardiomyocyte apoptosis, which could be prevented by the addition of a PKC-δ isoform-specific translocation peptide inhibitor (73). In addition, enhancing PKC-δ activity with the use of a PKC-δ-specific peptide activator exacerbated ischemia-induced myocardial infarction (47). The exact links between hyperglycemia, PKC-δ activation, and cardiomyocyte apoptosis are not fully understood. Activation of PKC-δ could result from the increased *de novo* synthesis of DAG in cardiomyocytes exposed to hyperglycemia, as discussed earlier, or PKC-δ could be activated by the accumulation of intracellular ceramide (74), the *de novo* synthesis of which (from serine and palmitoyl-coenzyme A) can be increased by palmitate (75,76). To induce cellular apoptosis, PKC-δ has been reported to be proteolytically activated by caspase-3 (69) or by the interleukin 1β-converting enzyme/cell death abnormality (ICE/CED) 3-like cysteine protease, CPP32 (77). It has been reported that release of the catalytic domain of PKC-δ is essential to the proapoptotic effects of this kinase (78,79). Once activated, it can translocate to the membrane of mitochondria, resulting in release of cytochrome C and initiation of apoptosis (80). It can also bind to and phosphorylate p73β, which is structurally and functionally associated with the p53 tumor suppressor, and induce cellular apoptosis via a p53-mediated pathway (81). Finally, it directly serves as a lamin kinase that phosphorylates nuclear lamin B, leading to its proteolytic disassembly (82). Downregulation of PKC-δ has been shown to be associated with cell survival, which is independent of the traditional PI3 kinase/Akt cell survival signals (83). Although overexpression of PKC-δ in adult cardiomyocytes induced apoptosis when the cells were cultured in medium containing 16.5 mM of glucose (73), *in vivo* data to support the hypothesis that PKC-δ

accelerates cardiomyocyte apoptosis are not available.

Diabetic Macrovascular Diseases

Atherosclerosis is responsible for most of the mortality in diabetic patients. It occurs primarily in coronary, lower extremity, and extracranial arteries (84,85). It is manifested by vascular wall inflammation, endothelial cell damage, abnormal leukocyte adhesion, lipid deposition, and pathologic proliferation of VSMC. Although a direct link between PKC activation and atherosclerosis needs to be established through studies using a loss- or gain-of-function approach, substantial evidence has shown that activation of certain isoforms of PKC may accelerate multiple components of atherosclerosis. Hyperglycemia induces the abnormal proliferation, migration, and hypertrophy of VSMC (86). PKC, which can be activated by hyperglycemia (6,40), free fatty acids (87), or oxidized low-density lipoprotein (88,89), can also promote the proliferation of these cells. High glucose preferably increases the protein content of PKC-βI, which may be responsible for the increased cell proliferation by platelet-derived growth factor (PDGF-BB) (90,91). Using the PKC-βII-selective inhibitor, LY333531, Yasuda et al. (92) showed that high glucose-induced DNA synthesis in cultured VSMC was suppressed, suggesting that PKC-βII may play an essential role in the pathologic proliferation of VSMC in diabetes (92). PKC activation by oxidized low-density lipoprotein, which is dramatically elevated in diabetes, can phosphorylate ERK and stimulate the proliferation of VSMC (88,89). PKC inhibition, especially inhibition of the α and β isoforms, is able to prevent the death of these cells (93). Given that hyperglycemia induces the expression, translocation, and activation of PKC in these tissues (36), it is conceivable that PKC activation may play a role in the atherosclerosis of diabetes. In addition, PKC activation may directly result in endothelial dysfunction (94), increased neutrophil- and monocyte-endothelial interaction (95,96), and increased adhesion of monocytes and potentially their differentiation

to macrophages (34), which may be involved in the onset and progression of atherosclerosis.

Microvascular Complications

Roles of Protein Kinase C Isoforms in Diabetic Retinopathy

Diabetic retinopathy is the most common cause of blindness among working-age individuals; it affects more than 75% of people with diabetes lasting longer than 15 years (97). Diabetic retinopathy is diagnosed clinically by the appearance of characteristic retinal vascular lesions, exudates, and, eventually, neovascularization, which can also be detected by fluorescein angiography. One of the earliest and most specific changes in diabetic retinopathy is the loss of pericytes, the microvascular contractile cells of the retina. It is believed that pericyte loss can lead to changes in cell-to-cell interaction with retinal endothelial cells, predisposing to retinal endothelial cell proliferation and the development of microaneurysms. Retinal circulatory abnormalities appear to be an early feature of diabetic retinal microvascular pathology, because abnormalities in the retinal circulation can be detected before clinical diabetic retinopathy is evident. A reduction in retinal blood flow, as measured by video fluorescein angiography (VFA), and a reduction in arterial blood velocity, as measured with the use of laser Doppler techniques, have been noted in diabetic patients with no clinically apparent retinopathy (98,99). Similar changes in retinal blood flow have been found in rats with diabetes of short duration (100). It is believed that this alteration in retinal hemodynamics may be responsible for the development of venous dilatation, beading, and intraretinal microvascular abnormalities that represent dilated small vessels in the diabetic retina. The impairment of retinal blood flow in early stages of diabetes may be the consequence of an increased resistance to flow, secondary to the abnormal production and response to vasoactive peptides such as ET-1 (101,102) and, in other vascular tissues, nitric oxide (103). Leukocyte entrapment in the retinal microcirculation in the diabetic state may further exacerbate this flow abnormality (104).

Changes in the PKC signal transduction pathway appear to play an important part in the regulation of retinal hemodynamics. Injection of the PKC activator, phorbol dibutyrate, or the DAG kinase inhibitor, R59949, into the vitreous humor of normal rats resulted in a reduction in retinal blood flow similar to that observed in rats after 2 to 4 weeks of diabetes (29,105). One mechanism by which activation of the PKC pathway in diabetes could modulate retinal hemodynamics is by altered expression of the aforementioned vasoactive peptides. Increased membranous PKC activity and expression of ET-1 were found in cultured bovine retinal pericytes and capillary endothelial cells exposed to elevated glucose concentrations, and these changes were inhibited by a general PKC inhibitor, GF109203X, and by a MEK inhibitor, PD98059 (11). Increased expression of ET-1 messenger RNA levels was reported in retinas obtained from diabetic rats (106,107), and intravitreal injection of ET-1 in nondiabetic rats was shown to produce retinal vasoconstriction and a corresponding decrease in retinal blood flow, an effect that could be inhibited by the ET_A receptor antagonist, BQ123 (106). Several isoforms of PKC are found in the retina, and activation of PKC-βII, -ϵ, -α, and -βI isoforms has been observed in retinas of diabetic rats. In bovine retinal capillary endothelial cells, elevated glucose increased PKC-βII and PKC-δ, and overexpression of the PKC-βI and -δ isoforms by means of an adenoviral vector resulted in enhanced glucose-induced ET-1 expression (11). Development of the specific PKC inhibitor, LY333531, a bisinodoylmaleimide compound that shows selectivity for PKC-βI and -βII over PKC-α and the novel and atypical PKCs when administered over the nanomole range (31,108), has allowed confirmation of the important role of PKC-β isoforms in the pathogenesis of diabetic complications. Oral administration of LY333531 in diabetic rats was found to lead to improved retinal blood flow (31). There is recent evidence that expression of PDGF-BB is increased in cultured retinal pericytes and retinas of diabetic rats, and that this may be responsible for the increased expression of ET-1 in diabetic

retinas. The induction of ET-1 by PDGF-BB was completely suppressed by the PKC inhibitor, GF109203X, again implicating PKC in the pathogenesis of retinal hemodynamic changes (109).

Another important manifestation of diabetic vascular dysfunction is an increase in vascular permeability to circulating macromolecules. Increased albumin permeation has been noted in the eye and in vascular tissues from 3-week-diabetic rats (110). Activation of PKC by phorbol esters was shown to increase the permeability of cultured endothelial cells to macromolecules including albumin, and this effect was reduced by the inhibition of PKC (111). There is reduced cell-to-cell coupling in the retinal microvessels of streptozotocin-diabetic rats, and this effect can be induced in vitro with a PKC activator (112). One mechanism whereby PKC can modulate vascular permeability is through the phosphorylation of specific cytoskeletal proteins, which stimulates the endothelial cell contractile apparatus. In line with this idea, PKC activation has been reported to lead to phosphorylation of the cytoskeletal proteins caldesmon, vimentin, talin, and vinculin (113,114).

Progressive diabetic retinopathy is associated with neovascularization, and this is believed to involve the vascular endothelial growth factor (VEGF) (115–117). VEGF, a 45-kDa glycoprotein, is the main factor regulating hypoxia-induced angiogenesis, and it can stimulate cell growth and permeability. Increased VEGF has been detected in ocular fluids of patients with diabetic retinopathy, and the levels were noted to be higher in patients with proliferative retinopathy compared with nonproliferative retinopathy. Furthermore, VEGF concentrations were found to decline after successful laser photocoagulation, suggesting that VEGF plays a major role in mediating active intraocular neovascularization in patients with ischemic retinal diseases such as diabetic retinopathy (115). VEGF signal transduction involves activation of the PI3 kinase pathway, although VEGF can also activate phospholipase C-γ, thereby increasing DAG and resulting in PKC activation (118). Intravitreal injection of VEGF rapidly activates PKC in the retina at concentrations observed clinically, inducing membrane translocation of PKC isoforms α, βII, and δ and resulting in a threefold increase in retinal vasopermeability *in vivo*. The effect of VEGF on retinal permeability appears to be mediated predominantly by the β isoform of PKC, with more than 95% inhibition of VEGF-induced permeability achieved with intravitreal or oral administration of a PKC-β isoform-selective inhibitor (119). Support is also provided by *in vivo* studies in which transgenic mice overexpressing the PKC-βII isoform were found to have a dramatic increase in ischemia-induced retinal neovascularization, whereas a significant decrease in retinal neovascularization was observed in PKC-β isoform-null mice. The mitogenic actions of VEGF in retinal endothelial cells can be increased by overexpression of PKC-βI and -βII isoforms by means of adenoviral vectors. PKC-βII was found to be capable of associating with and phosphorylating retinoblastoma protein, a tumor suppressor that can regulate cellular proliferation, differentiation, and death (120). PKC-β-induced phosphorylation of Rb could be responsible for increasing VEGF-induced endothelial cell proliferation, as found in ischemic retinal conditions. Interestingly, it has also been shown that the hypoxia-induced increase in transcription of the transcription factor, early growth response-1 (Egr-1), and its downstream target tissue factor are also regulated by PKC-β. Therefore, PKC-β could be responsible for the hypoxia-induced vascular fibrin deposition (121,122) and could play an important role in mediating hypoxia-induced vascular occlusion.

Concomitant hypertension is known to exacerbate the neovascularization and vascular permeability seen in diabetic retinopathy. This effect may be due to stretch-induced expression of VEGF, which involves a novel mechanism that is dependent on PI3-kinase-mediated activation of PKC-ζ (123). Therefore, targeting of VEGF action with specific pharmacologic agents, such as antioxidants or PKC inhibitors, may be helpful in the treatment of diabetic retinopathy.

It can be seen that PKCs, and the PKC-β isoforms in particular, are involved in several key pathways in the pathogenesis of diabetic retinopathy—namely, decreased blood flow, increased vascular permeability, and angiogenesis. The development of an isoform-specific inhibitor allows the possibility of modulating the PKC pathway in an isoform-specific manner as an adjunct treatment for prevention of microvascular complications in diabetes (see later discussion).

Roles of Protein Kinase C Isoforms in Diabetic Nephropathy

Diabetic nephropathy is characterized by several pathologic changes: early hemodynamic alteration, with glomerular hyperfiltration; mesangial expansion and glomerular extracellular matrix accumulation, resulting ultimately in diabetic glomerulosclerosis; and progressive renal insufficiency. Several metabolic and hemodynamic factors are thought to be mediators of this injury associated with the diabetic state. The hemodynamic factors implicated in the pathogenesis of diabetic nephropathy include increased systemic and intraglomerular pressure and activation of various vasoactive hormone pathways, including the renin-angiotensin system and ET (124). These factors may interact with metabolic pathways and/or activate signaling pathways that lead to renal injury. It is not surprising that PKC, an important signaling molecule, is involved in several of these pathways leading to increased proteinuria, glomerulosclerosis, and tubulointerstitial fibrosis.

The exact mechanism underlying the renal hyperfiltration seen in diabetic patients has not been elucidated, although one possible mechanism is the increase in vasodilatory prostanoids, such as prostaglandin E_2 (PGE_2) and PGI_2, that has been noted in the kidneys of diabetic patients and in animals with glomerular hyperfiltration (125). This increase in glomerular PGE_2 appears to be caused by the activation of cytosolic phospholipase A_2 ($cPLA_2$) by PKC, which results in increased arachidonic acid release. Treatment with the specific PKC-β-isoform inhibitor, LY333531, was found to decrease PGE and arachidonic acid release caused by hyperglycemia (126). Further, it was shown in cultured glomerular mesangial cells that diabetes-induced activation of the PKC pathway via increased MAPK activity enhanced $cPLA_2$ activity, resulting in increased arachidonic acid release (127).

One of the most important glomerular pathologic changes in diabetic nephropathy is structural alteration, including glomerular hypertrophy, basement membrane thickening, and mesangial expansion resulting from the accumulation of extracellular matrix components such as collagen and fibronectin (128). Although multiple mechanisms are likely to be involved in causing mesangial expansion, much attention has been focused on the role of the cytokine, TGF-β. TGF-β can stimulate the production of extracellular matrix components such as type IV collagen, fibronectin, and laminin in cultured mesangial cells and epithelial cells (129,130). Because an increase in expression of TGF-β has been noted in glomeruli from diabetic animal models and from diabetic patients (131–133), it is believed that overexpression of TGF-β may be responsible for the development of mesangial expansion in diabetic nephropathy. PKC is involved in this enhancement of TGF-β expression in diabetes, because treatment with the PKC-β inhibitor, LY333531, was able to prevent the enhanced glomerular expression of TGF-β in diabetic rats. Inhibition of PKC-β isoforms has also been shown to prevent glomerular overexpression of extracellular matrix components such as type IV collagen and fibronectin in the glomeruli of diabetic rats and db/db mice (33,126). Treatment with LY333531 was also found to effectively reduce the albuminuria seen in animal models of type 1 (31) and type 2 (33) diabetes.

As with the changes observed in diabetic retinopathy, an increase in vascular permeability is also an early manifestation of diabetic nephropathy. VEGF, in addition to being the primary mediator of the angiogenesis observed in proliferative diabetic retinopathy, is also believed to play an important part in the vascular permeability of diabetic nephropathy. In glomeruli from diabetic and insulin-resistant rats (134,135), there is an increase in the expression of VEGF and its receptors. Treatment with neutralizing antibodies to VEGF ameliorates some of the renal changes seen in db/db mice (136). Furthermore, high glucose induced the expression of VEGF in rat mesangial cells, and this effect was inhibited by a PKC inhibitor (137). Because it has been shown in various microvascular tissues that VEGF action is mediated by PKC (118,119), it is possible that the protective effects of PKC-β inhibitor on diabetic nephropathy are partly attributable to its effects on VEGF action.

Roles of Protein Kinase C Isoforms in Diabetic Neuropathy

Diabetic neuropathy is common in diabetic patients, with a prevalence of more than 50% (138). The pathogenesis is multifactorial and is considered to be rooted in both hyperglycemia-induced pathologic changes intrinsic to neurons (139) and ischemia-induced neuronal damage resulting from decreased neurovascular blood flow (140). Because of the vascular elements, diabetic neuropathy is also considered to be a form of microvascular complications. Diabetes induces pathologic changes in the neurotrophic microvessels, reduces blood flow via reduction in endothelial- and nitric oxide-dependent vasodilatation (141,142), and alters the expression and action of vasoconstrictors such as ET-1 (143) and VEGF (144,145). This point of view is supported by studies in diabetic animal models (145). *In vivo* expression of VEGF restored blood flow in neurotrophic blood vessels as well as nerve functions in streptozotocin-induced diabetes (145). PKC activation has been known to cause similar changes in microvessels. Suppression of PKC activity in streptozotocin-diabetic rats rectified diabetes-induced impairments in nerve blood flow, conduction velocity, the sodium-potassium pump (Na^+,K^+-ATPase), and glutathione deficits (146). Furthermore, inhibition of PKC-βII activity with the use of a selective inhibitor, LY333531, restored motor nerve conduction velocity and endoneuronal blood flow that were impaired by diabetes (147–149). All of this evidence supports a role of PKC, especially the PKC-βII isoform, in the pathogenesis of diabetic neuropathy.

TARGETING THE PROTEIN KINASE C PATHWAY AS A THERAPEUTIC APPROACH FOR DIABETIC CARDIOVASCULAR COMPLICATIONS

Because pathologic activation of the DAG-PKC pathway has been unambiguously shown to regulate cardiovascular homeostasis and to play key roles in the onset and progression of cardiovascular complications, efforts have been focused on developing effective approaches to regulate PKC activities and therefore to reverse or even prevent these lethal complications. Several activators and inhibitors of PKC have been developed and have achieved some success in restoring cellular homeostasis in cell culture studies and in diabetic animal models (5). It should be noted that PKC confers isoform-dependent activities, and therefore it is essential to develop isoform-specific activators and inhibitors.

Protein Kinase C Activity Inhibitors

Many chemical PKC inhibitors have been developed and can be classified as naturally derived, indolocarbazole-derived, or bisinodolylmaleimide-derived compounds. Although these compounds confer PKC-inhibitory effects and have proved valuable in the characterization of the biologic functions of PKC, few of them demonstrate PKC isoform specificities, with the exception of a compound termed LY333531 that was developed from bisinodoylmalcimide (108). LY333531 is a PKC-βII-selective inhibitor and has been shown to ameliorate diabetes-induced PKC-βII activation and its related vascular abnormalities in cell culture (41), in animal models (31), and in clinical trials (150).

Clinical Studies Using a Protein Kinase C-β Isoform-Specific Inhibitor

Given the large body of experimental evidence indicating that various isoforms of PKC play important roles in mediating vascular changes in diabetes, and that isoform-specific inhibitors are effective in alleviating some of these changes,

clinical trials using the PKC-β-specific isoform inhibitor, LY333531, commenced several years ago. The safety and vascular effects of LY333531 were evaluated in a 1-month clinical study involving 29 patients with type 1 or type 2 diabetes of less than 10 years' duration and no or minimal retinopathy. This double-blind, placebo-controlled, randomized trial demonstrated significant improvement in retinal blood flow and mean circulation time with no change in glycemic indices (151,152). The results of a clinical trial of LY333531 in diabetic neuropathy also have been reported. A 1-year, double-blind, randomized, placebo-controlled trial with LY333531 at 32 mg or 64 mg was carried out in 205 patients with type 1 or type 2 diabetes and diabetic peripheral neuropathy. LY333531 was found to improve both symptoms of neuropathy and vibration detection threshold (153), as well as objective measures of nerve function by physician assessment (154). The Protein Kinase C Diabetic Retinopathy Study (PKC-DRS), a multinational, multicenter, placebo-controlled, randomized, double masked, four-arm clinical trial designed to evaluate the effects of LY333531 on the progression of diabetic retinopathy, is nearing completion, and its results should be available soon (155).

Peptide Inhibitors and Activators of Protein Kinase C Translocation

Activation and translocation of PKC to specific cellular compartments is associated with its biologic activities and requires the binding of specific anchoring proteins (156). Based on the fact that receptors for activated C kinases (RACKs) regulate PKC translocation and confer PKC-isoform-selective interactions (157), peptides are designed according to the protein sequence of RACKs and have been shown to inhibit the translocation of specific isoforms of PKC (47,158,159). By a similar strategy, peptide activators of specific PKC isoforms have been developed from a pseudoRACK sequence (47,56,160). These peptide inhibitors and activators have been used successfully to evaluate cardiac functions both *in vitro* and *in vivo* (47,56,158,161,162).

CONCLUSION

PKCs have been shown to play key roles in the maintenance of cardiovascular homeostasis, and sustained activation of PKCs by hyperglycemia is an important contributor to the onset and progression of diabetic cardiovascular complications. Many PKC inhibitors have been developed in attempts to reverse these pathologic processes, and at least the PKC-βII-selective inhibitor LY333531 has proved effective in clinical trials. A pressing question that needs to be addressed is what determines PKC-isoform-specific effects. The clarification of this question can facilitate the understanding and development of effective pharmacologic approaches to treat diabetic cardiovascular complications.

ACKNOWLEDGMENTS

We thank Dr. Yongjing Guo for the illustration in this chapter. This work was supported in part by National Institutes of Health grants R01 DK53105 and R01 DK59725 (G.L.K.) and by a William Randolph Hearst Fellowship provided by the Hearst Foundation (R.M.). Z.H. is the recipient of a Mary K. Iacocca fellowship. R.M. is the recipient of fellowships from the Croucher Foundation and the Hong Kong Society of Endocrinology, Metabolism and Reproduction.

REFERENCES

1. Geiss LS, Herman WH, Goldschmid MG, et al. Surveillance for diabetes mellitus—United States, 1980–1989. *MMWR CDC Surveill Summ* 1993;42:1–20.
2. The Diabetes Complications and Control Trial Research Group. The effect of intensive treatment of diabetes on the development and progression of long-term complications in insulin-dependent diabetes mellitus. *N Engl J Med* 1993;329:977–986.
3. United Kingdom Prospective Diabetes Study Group. Intensive blood-glucose control with sulphonylureas or insulin compared with conventional treatment and risk of complications in patients with type 2 diabetes (UKPDS 33). *Lancet* 1998;352:837–853.
4. Mellor H, Parker PJ. The extended protein kinase C superfamily. *Biochem J* 1998;332:281–292.
5. Way KJ, Chou E, King GL. Identification of PKC-isoform-specific biological actions using pharmacological approaches. *Trends Pharmacol Sci* 2000;21:181–187.
6. Inoguchi T, Battan R, Handler E, et al. Preferential elevation of protein kinase C isoform beta II and di-

7. Brownlee M. Biochemistry and molecular cell biology of diabetic complications. *Nature* 2001;414:813–820.
8. Sheetz MJ, King GL. Molecular understanding of hyperglycemia's adverse effects for diabetic complications. *JAMA* 2002;288:2579–2588.
9. Kim YS, Kim BC, Song CY, et al. Advanced glycosylation end products stimulate collagen mRNA synthesis in mesangial cells mediated by protein kinase C and transforming growth factor-beta. *J Lab Clin Med* 2001;138:59–68.
10. Taher MM, Garcia JG, Natarajan V. Hydroperoxide-induced diacylglycerol formation and protein kinase C activation in vascular endothelial cells. *Arch Biochem Biophys* 1993;303:260–266.
11. Park JY, Takahara N, Gabriele A, et al. Induction of endothelin-1 expression by glucose: an effect of protein kinase C activation. *Diabetes* 2000;49:1239–1248.
12. Zhang SL, Filep JG, Hohman TC, et al. Molecular mechanisms of glucose action on angiotensinogen gene expression in rat proximal tubular cells. *Kidney Int* 1999;55:454–464.
13. Fiordaliso F, Leri A, Cesselli D, et al. Hyperglycemia activates p53 and p53-regulated genes leading to myocyte cell death. *Diabetes* 2001;50:2363–2375.
14. Robin P, Boulven I, Desmyter C, et al. ET-1 stimulates ERK signaling pathway through sequential activation of PKC and Src in rat myometrial cells. *Am J Physiol Cell Physiol* 2002;283:C251–C260.
15. Seshiah PN, Weber DS, Rocic P, et al. Angiotensin II stimulation of NAD(P)H oxidase activity: upstream mediators. *Circ Res* 2002;91:406–413.
16. Malhotra A, Kang BP, Cheung S, et al. Angiotensin II promotes glucose-induced activation of cardiac protein kinase C isozymes and phosphorylation of troponin I. *Diabetes* 2001;50:1918–1926.
17. Kasahara K, Kikkawa U. Distinct effects of saturated fatty acids on protein kinase C subspecies. *J Biochem (Tokyo)* 1995;117:648–653.
18. Nishizuka Y. Protein kinase C and lipid signaling for sustained cellular responses. *FASEB J* 1995;9:484–496.
19. Schmitz-Peiffer C. Protein kinase C and lipid-induced insulin resistance in skeletal muscle. *Ann N Y Acad Sci* 2002;967:146–157.
20. Nesher M, Boneh A. Effect of fatty acids and their acyl-CoA esters on protein kinase C activity in fibroblasts: possible implications in fatty acid oxidation defects. *Biochim Biophys Acta* 1994;1221:66–72.
21. Yu HY, Inoguchi T, Kakimoto M, et al. Saturated non-esterified fatty acids stimulate de novo diacylglycerol synthesis and protein kinase C activity in cultured aortic smooth muscle cells. *Diabetologia* 2001;44:614–620.
22. Inoguchi T, Li P, Umeda F, et al. High glucose level and free fatty acid stimulate reactive oxygen species production through protein kinase C—dependent activation of NAD(P)H oxidase in cultured vascular cells. *Diabetes* 2000;49:1939–1945.
23. Griffin ME, Marcucci MJ, Cline GW, et al. Free fatty acid-induced insulin resistance is associated with

acylglycerol levels in the aorta and heart of diabetic rats: differential reversibility to glycemic control by islet cell transplantation. *Proc Natl Acad Sci U S A* 1992;89:11059–11063.

activation of protein kinase C theta and alterations in the insulin signaling cascade. *Diabetes* 1999;48:1270–1274.

24. Liu X, Wang J, Takeda N, et al. Changes in cardiac protein kinase C activities and isozymes in streptozotocin-induced diabetes. *Am J Physiol* 1999;277:E798–E804.

25. Malhotra A, Reich D, Nakouzi A, et al. Experimental diabetes is associated with functional activation of protein kinase C epsilon and phosphorylation of troponin I in the heart, which are prevented by angiotensin II receptor blockade. *Circ Res* 1997;81:1027–1033.

26. Inoguchi T, Xia P, Kunisaki M, et al. Insulin's effect on protein kinase C and diacylglycerol induced by diabetes and glucose in vascular tissues. *Am J Physiol* 1994;267:E369–E379.

27. Kunisaki M, Bursell SE, Umeda F, et al. Normalization of diacylglycerol-protein kinase C activation by vitamin E in aorta of diabetic rats and cultured rat smooth muscle cells exposed to elevated glucose levels. *Diabetes* 1994;43:1372–1377.

28. Kang N, Alexander G, Park JK, et al. Differential expression of protein kinase C isoforms in streptozotocin induced diabetic rats. *Kidney Int* 1999;56:1737–1750.

29. Shiba T, Inoguchi T, Sportsman JR, et al. Correlation of diacylglycerol level and protein kinase C activity in rat retina to retinal circulation. *Am J Physiol* 1993;265:E783–E793.

30. Lee TS, Saltsman KA, Ohashi H, et al. Activation of protein kinase C by elevation of glucose concentration: proposal for a mechanism in the development of diabetic vascular complications. *Proc Natl Acad Sci U S A* 1989;86:5141–5145.

31. Ishii H, Jirousek MR, Koya D, et al. Amelioration of vascular dysfunctions in diabetic rats by an oral PKC beta inhibitor. *Science* 1996;272:728–731.

32. Craven PA, DeRubertis FR. Protein kinase C is activated in glomeruli from streptozotocin diabetic rats: possible mediation by glucose. *J Clin Invest* 1989;83:1667–1675.

33. Koya D, Haneda M, Nakagawa H. Amelioration of accelerated diabetic mesangial expansion by treatment with a PKC beta inhibitor in diabetic db/db mice, a rodent model for type 2 diabetes. *FASEB J* 2000;14:439–447.

34. Ceolotto G, Gallo A, Miola M, et al. Protein kinase C activity is acutely regulated by plasma glucose concentration in human monocytes in vivo. *Diabetes* 1999;48:1316–1322.

35. Bowling N, Walsh RA, Song G, et al. Increased protein kinase C activity and expression of Ca2+-sensitive isoforms in the failing human heart. *Circulation* 1999;99:384–391.

36. Patel NA, Chalfant CE, Yamamoto M, et al. Acute hyperglycemia regulates transcription and posttranscriptional stability of PKCbetaII mRNA in vascular smooth muscle cells. *FASEB J* 1999;13:103–113.

37. Guo M, Wu MH, Korompai F, et al. Upregulation of PKC genes and isozymes in cardiovascular tissues during early stages of experimental diabetes. *Physiol Genomics* 2003;12:139–146.

38. Bogoyevitch MA, Parker PJ, Sugden PH. Characterization of protein kinase C isotype expression in adult rat heart: protein kinase C-epsilon is a major isotype present, and it is activated by phorbol esters, epinephrine, and endothelin. *Circ Res* 1993;72:757–767.

39. Gu X, Bishop SP. Increased protein kinase C and isozyme redistribution in pressure-overload cardiac hypertrophy in the rat. *Circ Res* 1994;75:926–931.

40. Giles TD, Ouyang J, Kerut EK, et al. Changes in protein kinase C in early cardiomyopathy and in gracilis muscle in the BB/Wor diabetic rat. *Am J Physiol* 1998;274:H295–H307.

41. Igarashi M, Wakasaki H, Takahara N, et al. Glucose or diabetes activates p38 mitogen-activated protein kinase via different pathways. *J Clin Invest* 1999;103:185–195.

42. Wagner M, Mascareno E, Siddiqui MA. Cardiac hypertrophy: signal transduction, transcriptional adaptation, and altered growth control. *Ann N Y Acad Sci* 1999;874:1–10.

43. Yamazaki T, Komuro I, Shiojima I, et al. The molecular mechanism of cardiac hypertrophy and failure. *Ann N Y Acad Sci* 1999;874:38–48.

44. Crackower MA, Oudit GY, Kozieradzki I, et al. Regulation of myocardial contractility and cell size by distinct PI3K-PTEN signaling pathways. *Cell* 2002;110:737–749.

45. Braz JC, Bueno OF, De Windt LJ, et al. PKC alpha regulates the hypertrophic growth of cardiomyocytes through extracellular signal-regulated kinase 1/2 (ERK1/2). *J Cell Biol* 2002;156:905–919.

46. Wakasaki H, Koya D, Schoen FJ, et al. Targeted overexpression of protein kinase C beta2 isoform in myocardium causes cardiomyopathy. *Proc Natl Acad Sci U S A* 1997;94:9320–9325.

47. Chen L, Hahn H, Wu G, et al. Opposing cardioprotective actions and parallel hypertrophic effects of delta PKC and epsilon PKC. *Proc Natl Acad Sci U S A* 2001;98:11114–11119.

48. Murry CE, Jennings RB, Reimer KA. Preconditioning with ischemia: a delay of lethal cell injury in ischemic myocardium. *Circulation* 1986;74:1124–1136.

49. Nakano A, Cohen MV, Downey JM. Ischemic preconditioning: from basic mechanisms to clinical applications. *Pharmacol Ther* 2000;86:263–275.

50. Ping P, Zhang J, Qiu Y, et al. Ischemic preconditioning induces selective translocation of protein kinase C isoforms epsilon and eta in the heart of conscious rabbits without subcellular redistribution of total protein kinase C activity. *Circ Res* 1997;81:404–414.

51. Mitchell MB, Meng X, Ao L, et al. Preconditioning of isolated rat heart is mediated by protein kinase C. *Circ Res* 1995;76:73–81.

52. Yoshida K, Kawamura S, Mizukami Y, et al. Implication of protein kinase C-alpha, delta, and epsilon isoforms in ischemic preconditioning in perfused rat hearts. *J Biochem (Tokyo)* 1997;122:506–511.

53. Liu GS, Cohen MV, Mochly-Rosen D, et al. Protein kinase C-epsilon is responsible for the protection of preconditioning in rabbit cardiomyocytes. *J Mol Cell Cardiol* 1999;31:1937–1948.

54. Liu H, McPherson BC, Yao Z. Preconditioning attenuates apoptosis and necrosis: role of protein kinase C epsilon and -delta isoforms. *Am J Physiol Heart Circ Physiol* 2001;281:H404–H410.

55. Saurin AT, Pennington DJ, Raat NJ, et al. Targeted disruption of the protein kinase C epsilon gene abolishes the infarct size reduction that follows ischaemic preconditioning of isolated buffer-perfused mouse hearts. *Cardiovasc Res* 2002;55:672–680.

56. Hahn HS, Yussman MG, Toyokawa T, et al. Ischemic protection and myofibrillar cardiomyopathy: dose-dependent effects of in vivo deltaPKC inhibition. *Circ Res* 2002;91:741–748.

57. Rubler S, Dlugash J, Yuceoglu YZ, et al. New type of cardiomyopathy associated with diabetic glomerulosclerosis. *Am J Cardiol* 1972;30:595–602.

58. Bell DS. Diabetic cardiomyopathy: a unique entity or a complication of coronary artery disease? *Diabetes Care* 1995;18:708–714.

59. Way KJ, Isshiki K, Suzuma K, et al. Expression of connective tissue growth factor is increased in injured myocardium associated with protein kinase C beta2 activation and diabetes. *Diabetes* 2002;51:2709–2718.

60. Takeishi Y, Chu G, Kirkpatrick DM, et al. In vivo phosphorylation of cardiac troponin I by protein kinase Cbeta2 decreases cardiomyocyte calcium responsiveness and contractility in transgenic mouse hearts. *J Clin Invest* 1998;102:72–78.

61. Noland TA Jr, Kuo JF. Protein kinase C phosphorylation of cardiac troponin I or troponin T inhibits Ca2(+)-stimulated actomyosin MgATPase activity. *J Biol Chem* 1991;266:4974–4978.

62. Liu X, Takeda N, Dhalla NS. Troponin I phosphorylation in heart homogenate from diabetic rat. *Biochim Biophys Acta* 1996;1316:78–84.

63. Rogers TB, Gaa ST, Massey C, et al. Protein kinase C inhibits Ca2+ accumulation in cardiac sarcoplasmic reticulum. *J Biol Chem* 1990;265:4302–4308.

64. Regan TJ, Lyons MM, Ahmed SS, et al. Evidence for cardiomyopathy in familial diabetes mellitus. *J Clin Invest* 1977;60:884–899.

65. Spiro MJ, Crowley TJ. Increased rat myocardial type VI collagen in diabetes mellitus and hypertension. *Diabetologia* 1993;36:93–98.

66. Roy S, Sala R, Cagliero E, et al. Overexpression of fibronectin induced by diabetes or high glucose: phenomenon with a memory. *Proc Natl Acad Sci U S A* 1990;87:404–408.

67. Fiordaliso F, Li B, Latini R, et al. Myocyte death in streptozotocin-induced diabetes in rats in angiotensin II-dependent. *Lab Invest* 2000;80:513–527.

68. Fukunaga M, Oka M, Ichihashi M, et al. UV-induced tyrosine phosphorylation of PKC delta and promotion of apoptosis in the HaCaT cell line. *Biochem Biophys Res Commun* 2001;289:573–579.

69. Pongracz J, Webb P, Wang K, et al. Spontaneous neutrophil apoptosis involves caspase 3-mediated activation of protein kinase C-delta. *J Biol Chem* 1999;274:37329–37334.

70. Villalba M. A possible role for PKC delta in cerebellar granule cells apoptosis. *Neuroreport* 1998;9:2381–2385.

71. Liu H, Zhang HY, McPherson BC, et al. Role of opioid delta1 receptors, mitochondrial K(ATP) channels, and protein kinase C during cardiocyte apoptosis. *J Mol Cell Cardiol* 2001;33:2007–2014.

72. Brodie C, Blumberg PM. Regulation of cell apoptosis by protein kinase c delta. *Apoptosis* 2003;8:19–27.

73. Shizukuda Y, Reyland ME, Buttrick PM. Protein kinase C-delta modulates apoptosis induced by hyperglycemia in adult ventricular myocytes. *Am J Physiol Heart Circ Physiol* 2002;282:H1625–H1634.

74. Sawai H, Okazaki T, Takeda Y, et al. Ceramide-induced translocation of protein kinase C-delta and -epsilon to the cytosol: implications in apoptosis. *J Biol Chem* 1997;272:2452–2458.

75. Shimabukuro M, Zhou YT, Levi M, et al. Fatty acid-induced beta cell apoptosis: a link between obesity and diabetes. *Proc Natl Acad Sci U S A* 1998;95:2498–2502.

76. Schmitz-Peiffer C, Craig DL, Biden TJ. Ceramide generation is sufficient to account for the inhibition of the insulin-stimulated PKB pathway in C2C12 skeletal muscle cells pretreated with palmitate. *J Biol Chem* 1999;274:24202–24210.

77. Ghayur T, Hugunin M, Talanian RV, et al. Proteolytic activation of protein kinase C delta by an ICE/CED 3-like protease induces characteristics of apoptosis. *J Exp Med* 1996;184:2399–2404.

78. Ren J, Datta R, Shioya H, et al. p73beta is regulated by protein kinase Cdelta catalytic fragment generated in the apoptotic response to DNA damage. *J Biol Chem* 2002;277:33758–33765.

79. Leverrier S, Vallentin A, Joubert DY. Positive feedback of protein kinase C proteolytic activation during apoptosis. *Biochem J* 2002;368:905–913.

80. Majumder PK, Pandey P, Sun X, et al. Mitochondrial translocation of protein kinase C delta in phorbol ester-induced cytochrome c release and apoptosis. *J Biol Chem* 2000;275:21793–21796.

81. Vousden KH. p53: death star. *Cell* 2000;103:691–694.

82. Cross T, Griffiths G, Deacon E, et al. PKC-delta is an apoptotic lamin kinase. *Oncogene* 2000;19:2331–2337.

83. Zhong M, Lu Z, Foster DA. Downregulating PKC delta provides a PI3K/Akt-independent survival signal that overcomes apoptotic signals generated by c-Src overexpression. *Oncogene* 2002;21:1071–1078.

84. Beckman JA, Creager MA, Libby P. Diabetes and atherosclerosis: epidemiology, pathophysiology, and management. *JAMA* 2002;287:2570–2581.

85. Lopes-Virella MF. Diabetes and atherosclerosis. In: Johnstone MT, A. V., eds. *Diabetes and cardiovascular disease.* Totowa, NJ: Humana Press, 2001:169–194.

86. Srivastava AK. High glucose-induced activation of protein kinase signaling pathways in vascular smooth muscle cells: a potential role in the pathogenesis of vascular dysfunction in diabetes [review]. *Int J Mol Med* 2002;9:85–89.

87. Chen JS, Greenberg AS, Wang SM. Oleic acid-induced PKC isozyme translocation in RAW 264.7 macrophages. *J Cell Biochem* 2002;86:784–791.

88. Velarde V, Jenkins AJ, Christopher J, et al. Activation of MAPK by modified low-density lipoproteins in vascular smooth muscle cells. *J Appl Physiol* 2001;91:1412–1420.

89. Watanabe T, Pakala R, Katagiri T, et al. Synergistic effect of urotensin II with mildly oxidized LDL on DNA synthesis in vascular smooth muscle cells. *Circulation* 2001;104:16–18.

90. Ling S, Little PJ, Williams MR, et al. High glucose abolishes the antiproliferative effect of 17beta-estradiol in human vascular smooth muscle cells. *Am J Physiol Endocrinol Metab* 2002;282:E746–E751.

91. Skaletz-Rorowski A, Waltenberger J, Muller JG, et al. Protein kinase C mediates basic fibroblast growth factor-induced proliferation through mitogen-activated protein kinase in coronary smooth muscle cells. *Arterioscler Thromb Vasc Biol* 1999;19:1608–1614.

92. Yasuda Y, Nakamura J, Hamada Y, et al. Role of PKC and TGF-beta receptor in glucose-induced proliferation of smooth muscle cells. *Biochem Biophys Res Commun* 2001;281:71–77.

93. Hall JL, Matter CM, Wang X, et al. Hyperglycemia inhibits vascular smooth muscle cell apoptosis through a protein kinase C-dependent pathway. *Circ Res* 2000;87:574–580.

94. Li D, Yang B, Mehta JL. Ox-LDL induces apoptosis in human coronary artery endothelial cells: role of PKC, PTK, bcl-2, and Fas. *Am J Physiol* 1998;275:H568–H576.

95. Omi H, Okayama N, Shimizu M, et al. Participation of high glucose concentrations in neutrophil adhesion and surface expression of adhesion molecules on cultured human endothelial cells: effect of antidiabetic medicines. *J Diabetes Complications* 2002;16:201–208.

96. Minc S, Tabata T, Wada Y, et al. Oxidized low density lipoprotein-induced LFA-1-dependent adhesion and transendothelial migration of monocytes via the protein kinase C pathway. *Atherosclerosis* 2002;160:281–288.

97. Klein R, Klein BE, Moss SE. The Wisconsin epidemiological study of diabetic retinopathy: a review. *Diabetes Metab Rev* 1989;5:559–570.

98. Bursell SE, Clermont AC, Kinsley BT, et al. Retinal blood flow changes in patients with insulin-dependent diabetes mellitus and no diabetic retinopathy. *Invest Ophthalmol Vis Sci* 1996;37:886–897.

99. Feke GT, Buzney SM, Ogasawara H, et al. Retinal circulatory abnormalities in type 1 diabetes. *Invest Ophthalmol Vis Sci* 1994;35:2968–2975.

100. Takagi C, King GL, Clermont AC, et al. Reversal of abnormal retinal hemodynamics in diabetic rats by acarbose, an alpha-glucosidase inhibitor. *Curr Eye Res* 1995;14:741–749.

101. Bursell SE, Clermont AC, Oren B, et al. The in vivo effect of endothelins on retinal circulation in nondiabetic and diabetic rats. *Invest Ophthalmol Vis Sci* 1995;36:596–607.

102. de la Rubia G, Oliver FJ, Inoguchi T, et al. Induction of resistance to endothelin-1's biochemical actions by elevated glucose levels in retinal pericytes. *Diabetes* 1992;41:1533–1539.

103. Bohlen HG, Lash JM. Topical hyperglycemia rapidly suppresses EDRF-mediated vasodilation of normal rat arterioles. *Am J Physiol* 1993;265:H219–H225.

104. Nonaka A, Kiryu J, Tsujikawa A, et al. PKC-beta inhibitor (LY333531) attenuates leukocyte entrapment in retinal microcirculation of diabetic rats. *Invest Ophthalmol Vis Sci* 2000;41:2702–2706.

105. Bursell SE, Takagi C, Clermont AC, et al. Specific retinal diacylglycerol and protein kinase C beta isoform modulation mimics abnormal retinal hemodynamics in diabetic rats. *Invest Ophthalmol Vis Sci* 1997;38:2711–2720.

106. Takagi C, Bursell SE, Lin YW, et al. Regulation of retinal hemodynamics in diabetic rats by increased expression and action of endothelin-1. *Invest Ophthalmol Vis Sci* 1996;37:2504–2518.

107. Deng D, Evans T, Mukherjee K, et al. Diabetes-induced vascular dysfunction in the retina: role of endothelins. *Diabetologia* 1999;42:1228-1234.

108. Jirousek MR, Gillig JR, Gonzalez CM, et al. (S)-13-[(dimethylamino)methyl]-10,11,14,15-tetrahydro-4,9:16,21-dimetheno-1H, 13H-dibenzo[e,k]pyrrolo [3,4-h][1,4,13]oxadiazacyclohexadecine-1,3(2H)-dione (LY333531) and related analogues: isozyme selective inhibitors of protein kinase C beta. *J Med Chem* 1996;39:2664–2671.

109. Yokota T, Ma R, Park J-Y, et al. Role of protein kinase C on the expression of platelet-derived growth factor and endothelin-1 in the retina of diabetic rats and cultured retinal capillary pericytes. *Diabetes* 2003 (in press).

110. Williamson JR, Chang K, Tilton RG, et al. Increased vascular permeability in spontaneously diabetic BB/W rats and in rats with mild versus severe streptozocin-induced diabetes: prevention by aldose reductase inhibitors and castration. *Diabetes* 1987;36:813–821.

111. Lynch JJ, Ferro TJ, Blumenstock FA, et al. Increased endothelial albumin permeability mediated by protein kinase C activation. *J Clin Invest* 1990;85:1991–1998.

112. Oku H, Kodama T, Sakagami K, et al. Diabetes-induced disruption of gap junction pathways within the retinal microvasculature. *Invest Ophthalmol Vis Sci* 2001;42:1915–1920.

113. Turner CE, Pavalko FM, Burridge K. The role of phosphorylation and limited proteolytic cleavage of talin and vinculin in the disruption of focal adhesion integrity. *J Biol Chem* 1989;264:11938–11944.

114. Werth DK, Niedel JE, Pastan I. Vinculin, a cytoskeletal substrate of protein kinase C. *J Biol Chem* 1983;258:11423–11426.

115. Aiello LP, Avery RL, Arrigg PG, et al. Vascular endothelial growth factor in ocular fluid of patients with diabetic retinopathy and other retinal disorders. *N Engl J Med* 1994;331:1480–1487.

116. Adamis AP, Miller JW, Bernal MT, et al. Increased vascular endothelial growth factor levels in the vitreous of eyes with proliferative diabetic retinopathy. *Am J Ophthalmol* 1994;118:445–450.

117. Aiello LP, Pierce EA, Foley ED, et al. Suppression of retinal neovascularization in vivo by inhibition of vascular endothelial growth factor (VEGF) using soluble VEGF-receptor chimeric proteins. *Proc Natl Acad Sci U S A* 1995;92:10457–10461.

118. Xia P, Aiello LP, Ishii H, et al. Characterization of vascular endothelial growth factor's effect on the activation of protein kinase C, its isoforms, and endothelial cell growth. *J Clin Invest* 1996;98:2018–2026.

119. Aiello LP, Bursell SE, Clermont A, et al. Vascular endothelial growth factor-induced retinal permeability is mediated by protein kinase C in vivo and suppressed by an orally effective beta-isoform-selective inhibitor. *Diabetes* 1997;46:1473–1480.

120. Suzuma K, Takahara N, Suzuma I, et al. Characterization of protein kinase C beta isoform's action on retinoblastoma protein phosphorylation, vascular endothelial growth factor-induced endothelial cell

proliferation, and retinal neovascularization. *Proc Natl Acad Sci U S A* 2002;99:721–726.

121. Yan SF, Lu J, Zou YS, et al. Hypoxia-associated induction of early growth response-1 gene expression. *J Biol Chem* 1999;274:15030–15040.

122. Yan SF, Lu J, Zou YS. Protein kinase C-beta and oxygen deprivation: a novel Egr-1-dependent pathway for fibrin deposition in hypoxemic vasculature. *J Biol Chem* 2000;275:11921–11928.

123. Suzuma I, Suzuma K, Ueki K, et al. Stretch-induced retinal vascular endothelial growth factor expression is mediated by phosphatidylinositol 3-kinase and protein kinase C (PKC)-zeta but not by stretch-induced ERK1/2, Akt, Ras, or classical/novel PKC pathways. *J Biol Chem* 2002;277:1047–1057.

124. Cooper ME. Interaction of metabolic and haemodynamic factors in mediating experimental diabetic nephropathy. *Diabetologia* 2001;44:1957–1972.

125. Craven PA, Caines MA, DeRubertis FR. Sequential alterations in glomerular prostaglandin and thromboxane synthesis in diabetic rats: relationship to the hyperfiltration of early diabetes. *Metabolism* 1987;36:95–103.

126. Koya D, Lee IK, Ishii H, et al. Prevention of glomerular dysfunction in diabetic rats by treatment with d-alpha-tocopherol. *J Am Soc Nephrol* 1997;8:426–435.

127. Haneda M, Araki S, Togawa M, et al. Mitogen-activated protein kinase cascade is activated in glomeruli of diabetic rats and glomerular mesangial cells cultured under high glucose conditions. *Diabetes* 1997;46:847–853.

128. Ziyadeh FN. The extracellular matrix in diabetic nephropathy. *Am J Kidney Dis* 1993;22:736–744.

129. MacKay K, Striker LJ, Stauffer JW, et al. Transforming growth factor-beta: murine glomerular receptors and responses of isolated glomerular cells. *J Clin Invest* 1989;83:1160–1167.

130. Nakamura T, Miller D, Ruoslahti E, et al. Production of extracellular matrix by glomerular epithelial cells is regulated by transforming growth factor-beta 1. *Kidney Int* 1992;41:1213–1221.

131. Yamamoto T, Nakamura T, Noble NA, et al. Expression of transforming growth factor beta is elevated in human and experimental diabetic nephropathy. *Proc Natl Acad Sci U S A* 1993;90:1814–1818.

132. Nakamura T, Fukui M, Ebihara I, et al. mRNA expression of growth factors in glomeruli from diabetic rats. *Diabetes* 1993;42:450–456.

133. Sharma K, Ziyadeh FN. Renal hypertrophy is associated with upregulation of TGF-beta 1 gene expression in diabetic BB rat and NOD mouse. *Am J Physiol* 1994;267:F1094–F1001.

134. Chou E, Suzuma I, Way KJ, et al. Decreased cardiac expression of vascular endothelial growth factor and its receptors in insulin-resistant and diabetic states: a possible explanation for impaired collateral formation in cardiac tissue. *Circulation* 2002;105:373–379.

135. Cooper ME, Vranes D, Youssef S, et al. Increased renal expression of vascular endothelial growth factor (VEGF) and its receptor VEGFR-2 in experimental diabetes. *Diabetes* 1999;48:2229–2239.

136. Flyvbjerg A, Dagnaes-Hansen F, De Vriese AS, et al. Amelioration of long-term renal changes in obese type 2 diabetic mice by a neutralizing vascular endothelial growth factor antibody. *Diabetes* 2002;51:3090–3094.

137. Cha DR, Kim NH, Yoon JW, et al. Role of vascular endothelial growth factor in diabetic nephropathy. *Kidney Int Suppl* 2000;77:S104–S112.

138. Dyck PJ, Kratz KM, Karnes JL, et al. The prevalence by staged severity of various types of diabetic neuropathy, retinopathy, and nephropathy in a population-based cohort: the Rochester Diabetic Neuropathy Study. *Neurology* 1993;43:817–824.

139. Eichberg J. Protein kinase C changes in diabetes: is the concept relevant to neuropathy? *Int Rev Neurobiol* 2002;50:61–82.

140. Sugimoto K, Murakawa Y, Sima AA. Diabetic neuropathy: a continuing enigma. *Diabetes Metab Res Rev* 2000;16:408–433.

141. Kihara M, Low PA. Impaired vasoreactivity to nitric oxide in experimental diabetic neuropathy. *Exp Neurol* 1995;132:180–185.

142. Maxfield EK, Cameron NE, Cotter MA. Effects of diabetes on reactivity of sciatic vasa nervorum in rats. *J Diabetes Complications* 1997;11:47–55.

143. Hopfner RL, Gopalakrishnan V. Endothelin: emerging role in diabetic vascular complications. *Diabetologia* 1999;42:1383–1394.

144. Samii A, Unger J, Lange W. Vascular endothelial growth factor expression in peripheral nerves and dorsal root ganglia in diabetic neuropathy in rats. *Neurosci Lett* 1999;262:159–162.

145. Schratzberger P, Walter DH, Rittig K, et al. Reversal of experimental diabetic neuropathy by VEGF gene transfer. *J Clin Invest* 2001;107:1083–1092.

146. Cameron NE, Cotter MA, Jack AM, et al. Protein kinase C effects on nerve function, perfusion, Na(+), K(+)-ATPase activity and glutathione content in diabetic rats. *Diabetologia* 1999;42:1120–1130.

147. Nakamura J, Kato K, Hamada Y, et al. A protein kinase C-beta-selective inhibitor ameliorates neural dysfunction in streptozotocin-induced diabetic rats. *Diabetes* 1999;48:2090–2095.

148. Cameron NE, Cotter MA. Effects of protein kinase Cbeta inhibition on neurovascular dysfunction in diabetic rats: interaction with oxidative stress and essential fatty acid dysmetabolism. *Diabetes Metab Res Rev* 2002;18:315–323.

149. Cotter MA, Jack AM, Cameron NE. Effects of the protein kinase C beta inhibitor LY333531 on neural and vascular function in rats with streptozotocin-induced diabetes. *Clin Sci (Lond)* 2002;103:311–321.

150. Beckman JA, Goldfine AB, Gordon MB, et al. Inhibition of protein kinase Cbeta prevents impaired endothelium-dependent vasodilation caused by hyperglycemia in humans. *Circ Res* 2002;90:107–111.

151. Aiello L, Bursell S, Devries T, et al. Protein kinase C-beta-selective inhibitor LY333531 ameliorates abnormal retinal hemodynamics in patients with diabetes. American Diabetes Association Annual Conference. *Diabetes* 1999;48:A19.

152. Aiello L, Bursell S, Devries T, et al. Amelioration of abnormal retinal hemodynamics by a protein kinase C-beta-selective inhibitor (LY333531) in patients with

diabetes: results of a phase 1 safety and pharmacody-
namic clinical trial. *IOVS* 1999;40:S192.

153. Vinik A, Tesfaye S, Zhang D, et al. LY333531 treatment
improves diabetic peripheral neuropathy (DPN) with
symptoms. *Diabetes* 2002;51[Suppl 2]:A79.

154. Litchy W, Dyck P, Tesfaye S, et al. Diabetic peripheral neuropathy (DPN) assessed by neurological examination (NE) and composite scores (CS) is improved
with LY333531 treatment. *Diabetes* 2002;51[Suppl
2]:A197.

155. Aiello L, Davis M, Sheetz M, et al. Design, baseline patient characteristics and high prevalence of clinically significant macular edema (CSME) in patients
with moderately severe to very severe nonproliferative diabetic retinopathy (NPDR) in the Protein Kinase
C Diabetic Retinopathy Study (PKC-DRS). *Diabetes*
2002;51[Suppl]:A209.

156. Mochly-Rosen D, Khaner H, Lopez J. Identification
of intracellular receptor proteins for activated protein
kinase C. *Proc Natl Acad Sci U S A* 1991;88:3997–
4000.

157. Mochly-Rosen D, Gordon AS. Anchoring proteins for
protein kinase C: a means for isozyme selectivity.
FASEB J 1998;12:35–42.

158. Ron D, Luo J, Mochly-Rosen D. C2 region-derived
peptides inhibit translocation and function of beta protein kinase C in vivo. *J Biol Chem* 1995;270:24180–
24187.

159. Johnson JA, Gray MO, Chen CH, et al. A protein kinase
C translocation inhibitor as an isozyme-selective antagonist of cardiac function. *J Biol Chem* 1996;271:24962–
24966.

160. Dorn GW 2nd, Souroujon MC, Liron T, et al. Sustained
in vivo cardiac protection by a rationally designed
peptide that causes epsilon protein kinase C translocation. *Proc Natl Acad Sci U S A* 1999;96:12798–
12803.

161. Pass JM, Gao J, Jones WK, et al. Enhanced PKC beta II
translocation and PKC beta II-RACK1 interactions in
PKC epsilon-induced heart failure: a role for RACK1.
Am J Physiol Heart Circ Physiol 2001;281:H2500–
H2510.

162. Balafanova Z, Bolli R, Zhang J, et al. Nitric oxide (NO) induces nitration of protein kinase Cepsilon
(PKCepsilon), facilitating PKCepsilon translocation
via enhanced PKCepsilon-RACK2 interactions: a
novel mechanism of no-triggered activation of
PKCepsilon. *J Biol Chem* 2002;277.15021–15027.

Diabetes and Cardiovascular Disease
edited by Steven P. Marso and David M. Stern
Lippincott Williams & Wilkins, Philadelphia © 2004

4

Aldose Reductase and Vascular Stress

Ravichandran Ramasamy and Peter J. Oates

Assistant Professor, Division of Surgical Science, Department of Surgery, Columbia University, New York, New York; Research Advisor, Department of Cardiovascular and Metabolic Diseases, Pfizer Global Research and Development, Groton, Connecticut

OVERVIEW

Chronic elevation of blood glucose (i.e., chronic hyperglycemia) has been identified as a primary risk factor for diabetic complications. The link between chronic hyperglycemia and diabetic complications has been well established for both insulin-dependent (type 1) and non-insulin-dependent (type 2) diabetes mellitus (1,2). The landmark United Kingdom Prospective Diabetes Study (UKPDS) demonstrated inexorable increases in the degree of hyperglycemia regardless of aggressive current therapeutic interventions (2). The UKPDS findings strongly highlight the urgent need for new and improved therapies to achieve better glucose control and to alleviate the devastating impact of complications induced by chronic hyperglycemia and/or reduced insulin action. Global efforts are underway to find more effective strategies to control hyperglycemia and the accompanying long-term diabetic complications. This chapter focuses on aldose reductase (AR), its possible link to the cardiovascular complications of diabetes mellitus, and the potential impact of pharmacologic inhibition of AR on cardiovascular complications of diabetes.

Macrovascular and Microvascular Complications of Diabetes

Cardiovascular disease represents the major cause of morbidity and mortality in patients with diabetes mellitus (3). Cardiovascular disease in diabetics has several components, including cardiac, macrovascular, and microvascular diseases, often superimposed and all accelerated by hypertension (4). Cardiac disease entities include increased sensitivity of diabetic myocardium to ischemic episodes (5) and diabetic cardiomyopathy, manifested as a subnormal functional response of the diabetic heart, independent of coronary artery disease (CAD), caused by impaired metabolism or deposition of interstitial collagen or both (6,7). Macrovascular disease in diabetics comprises pathologic processes affecting the large blood vessels and can be subdivided into several entities, notably atherosclerosis (8) with its well known sequelae, CAD, peripheral vascular disease, stroke (9), and a more rapid restenosis of large vessels in the diabetic state (10). The traditionally strong emphasis on the pathogenic role of lipid abnormalities in macrovascular disease (11,12) is now being supplemented by attention to the role of hyperglycemia-linked oxidative stress in sensitizing and/or accelerating vascular disease (13). Diabetic microvascular disease, or diabetic microangiopathy, encompasses a spectrum of functional and structural microvascular alterations in diabetic kidney, retina, and nerve that can lead to end-stage renal disease, blindness, and lower-limb amputation (14). Data indicating that lipid dysmetabolism may also contribute to the pathogenesis of diabetic microangiopathy have been inconstant but are strengthening (15–17). However, chronic hyperglycemia is still viewed as the central risk factor driving diabetic microvascular complications (1,18–20).

Hyperglycemia and Oxidative Stress in Cardiovascular Cells

Chronic hyperglycemia exerts its damaging effects on cardiovascular tissue by both intracellular and extracellular mechanisms. Extracellular mechanisms are believed to involve primarily nonenzymatic glycation reactions of extracellular molecular species and advanced glycation end products (AGEs) that result from spontaneous chemical rearrangements of glycation products (10,21,22). These derivatives can bind to preexisting glycosylated protein (23) or AGE (24) cell surface receptors. The interactions of such ligands with cell surface membrane receptors can lead to generation of reactive oxygen species such as superoxide, most likely via perturbation of reduced nicotinamide adenine dinucleotide phosphate (NADPH) oxidase (25), as described in greater detail in other chapters of this book.

Intracellular effects of chronic hyperglycemia are linked to the key observation that cardiovascular tissue, like other tissues that are particularly susceptible to diabetic complications, is at least partly independent of insulin for uptake of glucose from the extracellular environment (26,27). This property is conferred by the abundant presence of non-insulin-dependent glucose transporters such as GLUT1 in the plasma membranes of cells in cardiovascular tissue. Teleologically, this arrangement ensures that systemically critical tissues such as heart, blood vessels, and nerves are preferentially supplied with whatever glucose is available, before glucose consumption and storage by muscle and fat. However, in the presence of chronic hyperglycemia, there is an inadequate downregulation of the non-insulin-dependent transporters (28), and the cells are consequently subjected to a continuous influx of abnormally high amounts of glucose into their cytosol. Chronic elevation of cytosolic glucose or metabolic flux, a state termed "hyperglysolia" (29), has been associated with generation of excess intracellular superoxide and other mediators of oxidative stress, an insult that is now generally acknowledged to play an important role in the pathogenesis of diabetic complications (30–33).

HYPERGLYSOLIA AND OXIDATIVE STRESS IN CARDIOVASCULAR CELLS

Chronic hyperglysolia alters the biochemical homeostasis of cardiovascular cells by affecting a number of key biochemical pathways, including the polyol pathway, the cytoplasmic redox state, the pleiotropic protein kinase C (PKC) pathway, the glucosamine biosynthesis pathway, and production of intracellular glycating species (10,13,29,32,34). In some cell types, such as cultured bovine aortic endothelial cells, hyperglysolia causes enhanced glycolytic and mitochondrial oxidative metabolism (35). In other cell types, such as rat cardiac tissue, hyperglysolia causes inhibition of glycolytic rates and other significant alterations in normal metabolism of cardiovascular cells (36). Other authors in this volume focus on some of these key aspects of hyperglysolic metabolism. In this chapter, the primary emphasis is on AR, the first enzyme of the polyol pathway, which sits high in the biochemical cascade that follows the entry of excess glucose into the cytosol of cardiovascular cells.

Hyperglysolia-Linked Vascular Stress and Aldose Reductase

Polyol Pathway and the Osmotic Hypothesis

The impact of chronically elevated glucose metabolism via the polyol pathway (Fig. 4-1) has received considerable attention in the study of diabetic complications. This pathway, first described almost 50 years ago (37), comprises two oxidoreductases, AR and sorbitol dehydrogenase (SDH). In the presence of coenzyme NADPH, AR reduces glucose to sorbitol, and SDH then uses the oxidized nicotinamide adenine dinucleotide (NAD$^+$) to oxidize sorbitol to fructose. The pioneering studies of Kinoshita, Gabbay, Dvornik, and others (38) demonstrated the presence of elevated polyol pathway intermediates in diabetic rat tissues and suggested a pathogenic link to diabetic complications, particularly cataract formation. In the seminal "osmotic hypothesis" paradigm, high levels of glucose are metabolized through AR and SDH to generate high intracellular levels of polyhydroxylated sorbitol and fructose (polyols). Although

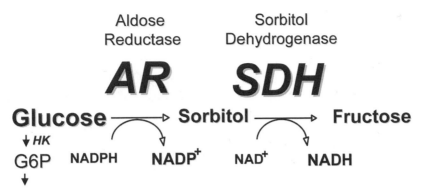

FIG. 4-1. Simple scheme illustrating metabolism of glucose via the polyol pathway. Shown here is the conversion of glucose to sorbitol by aldose reductase (AR) and reduced nicotinamide adenine dinucleotide phosphate (NADPH) and subsequent reduction of sorbitol to fructose by sorbitol dehydrogenase (SDH) and oxidized nicotinamide adenine dinucleotide (NAD+). HK, hexokinase; G6P, glucose-6-phosphate.

they are unphosphorylated, these molecules are nevertheless strongly hydrophilic and therefore penetrate lipid bilayers only relatively slowly. In the rat lens, rapid intracellular accumulation of polyols results in osmosis-driven water influx, swelling, and imbalances in ion and metabolite homeostasis, triggering formation of the "sugar cataract" (38). Data demonstrating an accelerated rate of sorbitol accumulation and cataract formation in AR-transgenic, SDH-deficient mice (39) provides clear confirmation of this mechanism for sugar cataract formation.

Polyol Pathway Metabolic Flux Hypothesis

In addition to polyol-linked osmotic stress, a potential pathogenic role for chronically high metabolic flux through the polyol pathway has long been noted (40). Some three decades of research have reemphasized that in many tissues the polyol pathway is integrally linked via its coenzymes to a variety of other metabolic pathways (Fig. 4-2). Cheng and Gonzalez (41) demonstrated that increased flux via the polyol pathway in the rat lens substantially increased turnover of NADPH. Moreover, AR and glutathione reductase, an enzyme integral to cellular antioxidant defense, were found to compete for the same pool of cytoplasmic NADPH. More recently, increased metabolic flux via the polyol pathway was shown to impair the glycolytic rate in diabetic hearts, as a result of

competition between SDH and glyceraldehyde-3 phosphate dehydrogenase (GA3PDH) for cytosolic NAD+ (36). In addition, the elegant studies of Williamson et al. (42,43) demonstrated strong linkage between polyol pathway flux and the ratio of free cytosolic NADH to NAD+, a factor critical to vascular function. Moreover, the importance of hyperglycemia-driven excess metabolic flux through the polyol pathway in relation to polyol tissue concentration has received strong emphasis from new data on human and experimental diabetic neuropathy (29).

The realization that excess metabolic flux of glucose through AR, in conjunction with possible osmotic stress in vascular tissue, affects a variety of important metabolic pathways such as oxidative stress, intracellular nonenzymatic glycation, and PKC activation (Fig. 4-2) has heightened interest in AR and the polyol pathway. This chapter summarizes some of the key data on AR and evidence linking AR to cardiovascular stress in the diabetic and nondiabetic states.

GENERAL CHARACTERISTICS OF ALDOSE REDUCTASE AND ITS GENE

Structure

Aldose reductase (E.C. 1.1.1.21), also known as AKR1B1, *ALD2,* or simply AR, is a member of the aldo-keto reductase superfamily (44) and has been extensively studied (45,46). It is

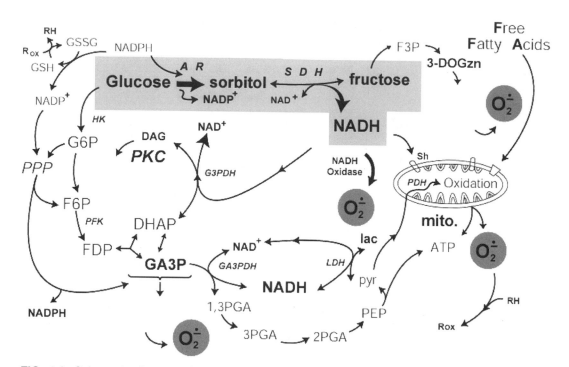

FIG. 4-2. Schematic diagram of potential detrimental metabolic effects of hyperglysolia. Cytosolic glucose *(upper left)* is metabolized typically via hexokinase (HK) to glucose-6-phosphate (G6P) and to pyruvate (pyr) and adenosine triphosphate (ATP) *(lower right)*; the pathway for glycogen synthesis is omitted for simplicity. Pyr enters cell mitochondria (mito.) and is further oxidized via pyruvate dehydrogenase (PDH), the citric acid cycle, electron transport, and oxidation phosphorylation processes (oxidation) to yield ATP (below mito.). In some cell types, hyperglysolia stimulates glycolysis, leading to increased turnover of oxidized nicotinamide adenine dinucleotide (NAD$^+$) via GA3PDH and production of pyr. Pyr undergoes mitochondrial oxidation, although under normal conditions at rest this process is limited by the availability of adenosine diphosphate (ADP), and most pyr is converted in the cytoplasm to lactate (lac) by lactate dehydrogenase (LDH), with regeneration of NAD$^+$. In many cell types, hyperglysolia stimulates metabolism through aldose reductase (AR) and sorbitol dehydrogenase (SDH) *(shaded rectangle)*, with a number of consequences, including (a) elevation of sorbitol and fructose metabolite pools (osmotic stress) *(upper center)*, (b) increased 3-deoxyglucosone (3-DOGzn), a highly reactive glycating agent (glycative stress and formation of advanced glycation end products [AGE]) *(upper right)*, and (c) increased ratio of cytosolic reduced nicotinamide adenine dinucleotide (NADH) to NAD$^+$ (reductive stress) *(center)*. Reductive stress can trigger excess production of reactive oxygen species such as superoxide (O$_2^-$) (oxidative stress), via (a) reaction of NADH with NADH oxidase (NADH Ox.) *(center)* and (b) overload of mitochondrial coenzyme shuttles (Sh) and matrix with NADH *(lower right)*. In some cases, consumption of reduced nicotinamide adenine dinucleotide phosphate (NADPH) by AR may also impair glutathione-based antioxidant defense (oxidative stress) *(upper left)*. Finally, plentiful substrate flux through HK concomitant with a high NADH/NAD$^+$ ratio can (a) cause a buildup of glyceraldehyde-3-phosphate (GA3P), a potent glycating agent (glycative stress) *(lower left)* and (b) push metabolic flow of GA3P to á-glycerophosphate, a precursor of diacylglycerol (DAG), which is an activator of protein kinase C (PKC) (protein kinase stress) *(left center)*. See text for further details. 1,3PGA, 1,3-bis-phosphoglyceric acid; 2PGA, 2-phosphoglyceric acid; 3PGA, 3-phosphoglyceric acid; DHAP, dihydroxyacetone phosphate; F3P, fructose-3-phosphate; F6P, fructose-6-phosphate; FDP, fructose-1,6-diphosphate; G3PDH, glycerol-3-phosphate dehydrogenase; GSH, reduced glutathione; GSSG, oxidized glutathione; NADP$^+$, oxidized NADPH; PEP, phosphoenolpyruvate; PFK, phosphofructokinase; PPP, pentose phosphate pathway; RH, reduced cellular molecule; Rox, oxidized form of RH. (From Oates PJ. The polyol pathway and diabetic peripheral neuropathy. In: Tomlinson DR, ed. *International review of neurobiology*. London: Academic Press, 2002:325–392.)

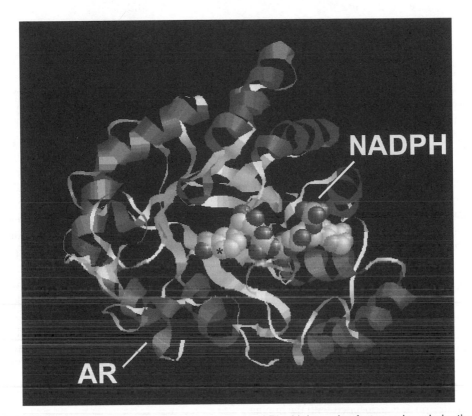

FIG. 4-3. X-ray structure of human aldose reductase (AR) with bound cofactor reduced nicotinamide adenine dinucleotide phosphate (NADPH). NADPH is shown as a space-filling model with the adenosine moiety on the right and the nicotinamide moiety on the left; carbons are gray, nitrogens blue, oxygens red, and phosphate atoms orange. AR is depicted in a ribbon diagram with α-helices shown in pink and β-sheets in yellow. The C-4 carbon of the nicotinamide ring, where the hydride transfer to substrate glucose (not shown) takes place, is marked with an asterisk. (From Protein Data Bank data of Wilson DK, et al. Science, 1992;257:81–84. Prepared by PJO with Millenium Sting, MDL Chime Pro 2.0.)

a monomeric, cytoplasmic (47,48) enzyme of approximately 35,900 Da with a triose phosphate isomerase structural motif that contains ten peripheral α-helical segments surrounding an inner barrel of β-pleated sheet segments (49) (Fig. 4-3). The enzyme preferentially and reversibly binds NADPH in an extended conformation and uses the hydride of the C-4 carbon of the nicotinamide ring of NADPH to reduce an aldehydic molecule to the corresponding alcohol (e.g., straight-chain aldehydic glucose to sorbitol) (Fig. 4-2). AR lacks structural carbohydrate, and no catalytic or structural metal ion has been detected.

As originally shown by Hers (50), AR reduces a variety of different aldehydic substrates with varying affinities. However, its "natural" substrate remains an enigma. Its catalytic center is sensitive to oxidation of a key cysteine residue, Cys 298, which when oxidized causes AR to exhibit altered properties and inhibitor sensitivity (51). The enzyme was recently reported to be catalytically altered by *S*-nitrosothiols (52) and activated by nitric oxide under ischemic conditions (53) or inhibited by exposure of rat tissues to elevated nitric oxide concentrations (54). In human tissues, AR occurs primarily as a single, reduced enzyme form (55). There is wide interindividual variability of AR levels in a particular tissue, most likely because of genetic allelic differences (see later discussion).

Aldose Reductase Gene

Localization and Structure

The human aldose reductase gene (*ALD2* or *AKR1B1*) has been mapped to locus q35 on human chromosome 7 (56). The *ALD2* gene is approximately 18 kb long and includes ten exons coding for 316 amino acids (57). The *ALD2* promoter has a TATA box (at −37), a CCAAT box (−104), and an androgen-like response element (−396 to −382) (58). At about 1,200 bp upstream of the transcription start site, there is a 132-bp region containing three osmotic response elements: OreA, OreB, and OreC (59). *ALD2* pseudogenes have also been described (60).

Polymorphisms and Risk of Diabetic Complications

Several susceptibility genes for increased severity and frequency of vascular complications have been identified, including alleles of angiotensin-converting enzyme, AR, and the non-insulin-dependent glucose transporter, GLUT1 (61). Genetic polymorphisms associated with the human *ALD2* gene have been found to be associated with diabetic complications in many, but not all, studies (62,63). The first reported microsatellite polymorphism was an $(AC)_n$ repeat region located approximately 2.1 kb upstream of the transcription start site (64). Two single-nucleotide polymorphisms (SNPs) have been detected in the basal promoter region of the *ALD2* gene, C(−106)T (64) and C(−12)G (65). In addition, a BamHI site consisting of an A-to-C substitution was reported at the 95th nucleotide of intron 8 (66). The $(AC)_n$ and C(−106)T polymorphisms are closely linked (67,68), but their effects may be distinguishable in different patient populations (63). The majority of studies have demonstrated an association between polymorphisms in the *ALD2* gene and increased risk for rapid onset or increased prevalence of diabetic complications. The so-called Z−2 $(AC)_n$ microsatellite polymorphism (i.e., $(AC)_{23}$), has been associated with high expression levels of AR (68) and with rapid progression or increased prevalence of diabetic retinopathy (64,68), diabetic nephropathy (61,69–71), and, less strongly, diabetic neuropa-

thy (72). In the last case, a relatively clear association was detected between microvascular complications and a decrease in the "protective," low AR-expressing "Z+2" allele (i.e., $(AC)_{25}$) (62). An equal (69) or even stronger (63) link with the C(−106)T promoter SNP was found in several studies.

In some studies, an association between *ALD2* alleles and risk of complications was not detected (73,74). In one study of patients with non-insulin-dependent (type 2) diabetes mellitus, although there was no association of Z−2 with proteinuria, a statistically significant association of erythrocyte AR concentration with proteinuria was found (75). The factors underlying negative findings in such studies remain to be clarified, but further examination of patient classification criteria (76) and genetic heterogeneity (e.g., additional analysis of the C(−106)T SNP versus Z−2 polymorphisms [63]) is warranted, as is analysis for potential interactions between polymorphisms of *ALD2* and *GLUT1* and genes of the antioxidant systems (62).

In Vivo Tissue Concentrations

AR is widely distributed in many tissues (77), although some tissues have richer concentrations than others. In human tissues, AR immunoreactivity is most concentrated in the inner medulla of kidney (29 μg/mg protein) (78), consonant with its role in renal osmoregulation. AR is also abundant in human sciatic nerve (5 μg/mg), lens (3 μg/mg), testis (2 μg/mg), heart (2 μg/mg), and cornea (1 μg/mg), with lesser concentrations in liver, renal cortex, stomach, spleen, lung, small intestine, and colon (0.4 to 0.8 μg/mg protein) (78). Assuming uniform distribution of AR in tissue water, the concentration of AR protein is approximately 5 μM in human muscle (79) and 10 μM in normal and short-term diabetic rat sciatic nerve (29). Because immunohistochemical staining shows that AR is not uniformly distributed within the nerve (80–82), the estimated concentration cited is likely to be an underestimate of the local concentration present in peripheral nerve. Further details about the localization of AR in cardiovascular cells are given later in this chapter.

Physiologic Functions

Specialized Tissue: Osmolyte and Fructose Biosynthesis

Despite decades of experimental studies, there have been only limited advances in elucidating the basic physiologic functions of AR. Originally discovered in seminal vesicles (37), the polyol pathway was hypothesized to be a biosynthetic route for producing fructose for the energy needs of spermatozoa. Another physiologic function for AR in a specialized tissue is the specific case of the AR-rich inner medulla of the kidney. By synthesizing intracellular sorbitol, AR forms part of a multitiered renal osmolyte system that helps protect cells in the renal inner medulla from the locally high osmotic forces associated with antidiuresis (83,84). Interestingly, pharmacologic suppression of AR activity results in upregulation of other components of the renal osmolyte system, which largely compensates for the loss of sorbitol (85).

General Function: Unknown

Despite discovery and elucidation of the specific roles of AR just mentioned, a general role for AR in cellular physiology remains unclear (86). In this regard, potential roles of sorbitol-6-phosphate (87), sorbitol-3-phosphate (88), and fructose-3-phosphate (89), formed in part via the polyol pathway activity, remain unidentified. Other possible functions that have been suggested for AR include serving as a "fuel switch" to divert excess cytoplasmic glucose away from energy metabolism and to slow glycolysis via an indirect redox effect (29); participating in the metabolism of steroids (90) and norepinephrine intermediates (91); and detoxifying aldehydes (92) or their glutathionylated derivatives (93). Because the broad substrate specificity of AR overlaps with that of ubiquitous, structurally related enzymes such as aldehyde reductase (94) and aldehyde dehydrogenase (95), it is difficult to define the role of AR simply on the basis of substrate preference. In this regard, the proposed role of AR as an antioxidant defense enzyme (96), based on experiments using supraphysiologic levels of oxidants in cell culture, will

be difficult to confirm *in vivo*. Oxidants attack cell membrane lipids and cause disturbance of membrane-mediated ionic and osmotic balance. It is well known that AR is induced by osmotic stress to help restore osmotic balance, and under such circumstances, blockade of the action of AR is detrimental (97). Moreover, specific overexpression of AR *in vivo* has been linked to increased, rather than decreased, oxidative stress (98,99). In addition, in cultured endothelial cells exposed to hyperglycemia, as well as in diabetic and galactosemic peripheral nerve and retina *in vivo*, structurally distinct AR inhibitors (ARIs) suppress and reverse (and do not accentuate) markers of aldehydic and oxidative stress (99–101).

Adding to the AR functional conundrum are data from AR knockout mice (102). Despite the fact that AR is absent from all tissues, these genetically engineered mice exhibited normal structural, biochemical, reproductive, and physiologic properties. Consistent with the known osmoregulatory function of AR, the only abnormality observed was mild polyuria, which was compensated by mild polydipsia (102). Urine and blood divalent cation concentrations were also slightly altered, but it remains unclear whether the changes were secondary to mild chronic diuresis or if AR plays a previously unsuspected role in maintaining systemic divalent cation levels (103). Nerve conduction velocity (NCV) is unaffected in normal rats by the overexpression of AR; however, in a diabetic setting, in marked contrast to the fall in NCV in wild-type mice, NCV remains completely normal in the AR knockout mouse (102). Similarly, cardiac contractile function is unaffected by pharmacologic inhibition of AR (104–106).

Aldose Reductase Inhibitors and Properties

ARIs have been sufficiently reviewed in recent literature (29,62). To date, epalrestat (Kinedak) is the only successfully commercialized ARI, and it is available in Japan only. Fidarestat (SNK-860), an analog of spirohydantoin sorbinil, is undergoing phase III neuropathy studies in Japan. Without exception, all ARIs examined have been found by x-ray crystallography to bind in the active site of AR. ARIs of the carboxylic acid class are quite selective for AR, as opposed to aldehyde reductase and other enzymes (107), but they become highly protein bound *in vivo,* which has limited their efficacy. On the other hand, hydantoin ARIs such as sorbinil are relatively nonselective, inhibiting both aldehyde reductase and AR with comparable efficacies (108), but they are much less protein bound *in vivo.*

ARIs exert antioxidant effects in biologic systems *in vitro* and *in vivo.* ARIs have been reported to blunt both hyperglycemia-induced superoxide production by cultured endothelial cells (99) and hyperglycemia-induced endothelium-dependent superoxide production by aortic rings (109); to protect reduced glutathione (GSH) tissue levels (101,110); and to normalize markers of oxidative stress in diabetic tissue, such as malondialdehyde (100) and 4-hydroxynonenal (99,110). In regard to whether ARIs are antioxidants, in general they

are inactive as (direct) antioxidants. This has been verified in several laboratories by showing a lack of ARI interference with superoxide production in xanthine oxidase assays. Another suggestion has been that ARIs of a particular chemical class, hydantoin, might have an antioxidant effect based on metal chelation (111). Although this proposal is not readily testable in an *in vivo* setting, it can be noted that all potent ARIs examined, regardless of chemical class, exert an antioxidant effect in biologic tissues and cells. For example, the ARI zopolrestat is a member of the carboxylic acid class of ARIs, a class that does not have significant direct antioxidant properties (111). Nevertheless, despite the absence of direct antioxidant activity, zopolrestat suppresses hyperglycemia-induced production of superoxide anion from vascular tissue (109) (Fig. 4-4). Most likely, the antioxidant effects of ARIs in biologic systems are linked to inhibition of excess

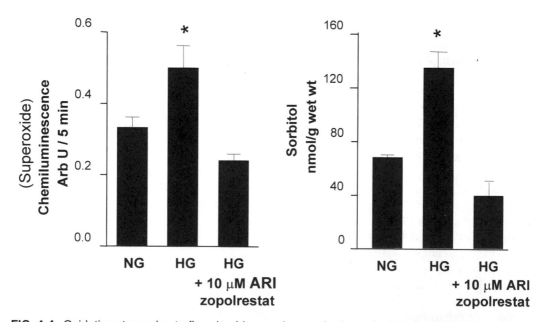

Rabbit aorta in vitro

FIG. 4-4. Oxidative stress due to flux via aldose reductase in rings of rabbit aorta. The data demonstrate the production of excess superoxide in rabbit aorta exposed *in vitro* to high glucose (HG) versus normal glucose (NG). The aldose reductase inhibitor (ARI) zopolrestat (100 μM) attenuated both sorbitol *(right panel)* and lucigen-detected superoxide production *(left panel).* (From Gupta S, et al. Hyperglycemia increases superoxide anion production in rabbit endothelium leading to decreased Na$^+$K$^+$-ATPase activity. *Am J Physiol* 2001;282:C560–C566.)

flux through AR (Fig. 4-2), which causes excess oxidation of NADPH, essential for glutathione reduction (41), as well as SDH-mediated excess production of NADH (13,31), a potential substrate for NADH oxidase and for mitochondrial metabolism (32).

ALDOSE REDUCTASE LOCALIZATION AND FUNCTIONS IN VASCULAR CELLS

Endothelial Cells

In dogs, AR was demonstrated in numerous cell types, including aortic endothelium and smooth muscle, although many other cells and tissues, including capillaries throughout the body, lacked immunoreactive AR (112). In cultured canine endothelial cells, Northern blot analysis failed to detect AR messenger RNA (mRNA) in endothelial cells (in contrast to positive findings in pericytes) (113). In rats, AR immunoreactivity was observed in arterial endothelium but not in retinal capillaries (48). In rat nerve, one study reported AR present in endothelial cells of endoneurial capillaries (113), but in another study this observation was not confirmed (81).

Studies using isolated aorta showed that the hyperglycemia-induced increase in vascular superoxide was endothelium-dependent, was inhibited by L-arginine, and was stimulated by $N\omega$-nitro-L-arginine. The ARI zopolrestat markedly blunted the hyperglycemia-induced increase in vascular superoxide (109) (Fig. 4-4). In another study (115), it was shown that zopolrestat improved the abnormal acetylcholine- and adenosine diphosphate-induced relaxation of aortas from diabetic rabbits. The ARI had no effect on the levels of cyclic guanosine monophosphate or on the increased release of thromboxane A_2 in diabetic aortas. These findings suggest that increased activity of the AR pathway in hyperglycemia is responsible, at least in part, for the abnormal endothelium-dependent relaxation in diabetic blood vessels (115).

In diabetic rat aortas, reduced production of maximal tension, particularly in response to phenylephrine, was observed at 3 months after induction of diabetes. A net 38% deficit in endothelium-dependent relaxation to acetyl-choline observed in diabetic rat aortas was prevented by ARI treatment (116). Similar observations have been made in galactosemic rats (i.e., rats experimentally fed a diet high in galactose). A 25% abnormality in endothelium-dependent relaxation was completely prevented by treatment of galactosemic rats with the ARI ponalrestat (117).

Numerous cell culture studies have examined the presence and role of AR in endothelial cells. In cultured human umbilical endothelial cells, competition between AR and nitric oxide synthase (NOS) for cofactor NADPH was suggested to be an important reason for the observed effect of high ambient glucose in blunting cellular NOS activity. Consistent with this concept, addition of the ARI, ONO-2235 (100 μM), protected NOS from inhibition by high glucose (118). However, because the Michaelis-Menten constant (K_m) for both AR and NOS is quite low and free NADPH levels were not measured, further studies are needed to confirm this possible mechanism of action of ARI effect. In cultured bovine aortic endothelial cells, the presence of AR was indicated by the detection of sorbitol after exposure of the cells to elevated ambient glucose (119). In studies of bovine retinal endothelial cells, ARIs or sorbitol dehydrogenase inhibitors (SDIs) decreased by a similar extent (approximately 40%) the transendothelial leakage induced by 24 hours of high-glucose incubation (120).

Pericytes

AR was immunohistochemically detected in pericytes in human (nondiabetic) postmortem nerve (121) and in cultured human retinal capillary pericytes (122). In cultured bovine retinal pericytes, ARI SNK-860 inhibited the glucose-induced apoptosis (123). Northern blot analysis of cultured canine retinal cells revealed the presence of AR mRNA in pericytes (but not in retinal endothelial cells) (113). Both AR and aldehyde reductase, the latter being dominant, were detected in cultured canine pericytes (113). In spontaneously diabetic BB rats, the presence of AR in the pericytes of retinal capillaries was demonstrated by immunostaining (114).

Vascular Smooth Muscle Cells

In human nondiabetic patients, AR was distributed in vascular smooth muscle cells (VSMC) of endoneurial and epineurial microvessels (121). Although AR-specific immunofluorescence was "virtually absent" in control human arterial tissue, upregulated AR expression was found to be associated with T cells, macrophages, and VSMC in areas of arteritic lesions. In the lesion zones, the presence of AR was highly correlated with that of 4-hydroxynonenal (HNE), a toxic aldehyde and downstream product of lipid peroxidation. In a temporal artery-severe combined immunodeficiency mouse chimera model, inhibition of AR increased HNE adducts twofold and the number of apoptotic cells in the arterial wall threefold (124), suggesting a protective role for AR.

A protective effect of AR inhibition was observed in cultured normal human coronary artery VSMC. In these studies, chronic high-glucose treatment for 72 hours increased intracellular oxidative stress, as directly measured by flow cytometry using carboxy-dichlorofluorescein diacetate bis-acetoxymethyl ester. The increase was significantly suppressed by 100 nM of the ARI epalrestat. The ARI also improved insulin-mediated glucose uptake and prevented high-glucose-induced migration of human coronary artery VSMC, as well as a high-glucose-driven increase in the $NADH/NAD^+$ ratio and in membrane-bound PKC activity in the human VSMC (125).

In dogs, AR was demonstrated immunohistochemically in smooth muscle of large blood vessels (112). In diabetic rats, blood flow was significantly increased in ocular tissues (anterior uvea, posterior uvea, retina, and optic nerve), sciatic nerve, kidney, new granulation tissue, cecum, and brain, and iodine 125-BSA permeation increased in all of these tissues except brain (126). The glomerular filtration rate and the 24-hour urinary albumin excretion increased 2-fold and 29-fold, respectively, in diabetic rats. Each of three structurally distinct ARIs completely prevented or markedly reduced these hemodynamic and vascular filtration changes, as well as increases in tissue sorbitol. These data were consistent with the hypothesis that (a) increases in blood flow may reflect AR-mediated redox-sensitive impaired contractile function of VSMC in resistance arterioles in various tissues of the diabetic rat, and (b) AR-mediated increases in vascular ^{125}I-BSA permeation and urinary albumin excretion in diabetic rats reflect impaired vascular barrier functional integrity in addition to increased hydraulic conductance (126). Further studies are needed to dissect possible protective effects of ARIs on VSMC contractile function from possible protective effects of ARIs on adrenergic nerves that innervate afferent arteriolar VSMC.

In diabetic rat sciatic nerve, ARIs have been well documented to correct abnormalities in endoneurial blood flow and motor nerve conduction velocity (29). Sorbinil treatment also significantly corrected a diabetes-induced deficit in acetylcholine-mediated vasodilation of epineurial vessels of the sciatic nerve (127). In rat corpus cavernosum, 10 mg/kg per day of the ARI, WAY-121509 (Wyeth-Ayerst), or 300 mg/kg per day of α-lipoic acid (AstaMedica) largely prevented a deficit in acetylcholine-induced relaxation of phenylephrine-precontracted corpus cavernosum from streptozotocin (STZ)-diabetic rats (128). These results show that a neurogenic relaxation deficit in diabetic corpus cavernosum was substantially prevented by ARI, possibly by an effect on the redox state of the tissue.

In STZ-diabetic rats treated with the ARI sorbinil, renal micropuncture studies showed lower values for single-nephron glomerular filtration rate, plasma flow, and blood flow, compared with those seen in untreated diabetic rats, and the values in the ARI-treated diabetic rats were indistinguishable from those in normal rats (129). These observations are consistent with the view that polyol pathway metabolism plays a role in glomerular hyperperfusion in diabetes and that inhibition of AR may protect VSMC tone at preglomerular and possibly postglomerular sites. The mechanism of the effect of ARIs on vascular tone probably involves regulation of cytosolic free $NADH/NAD^+$, a key regulator of vascular tone (43), although possible effects on adrenergic preglomerular nerve activity that innervates renal preglomerular arterioles merits further study.

In hyperinsulinemic Zucker diabetic fatty rats, the expression of the AR gene, compared with that of normal rats, was unchanged in VSMC of aortas, large arterioles from the brain, kidney, small intestine, and renal glomerulus. In contrast, a decrease of about 50% in glomeruli and renal VSMC AR mRNA was found in the hypoinsulinemic STZ-diabetic rat (130). Remaining tissues were unchanged in AR mRNA and were similar between the two types of diabetic rats. It should be noted that the diabetic human kidney, in contrast to the implication of these renal findings in the STZ-diabetic rat, has a 50% increase in renal cortical AR content and enhanced glomerular AR staining relative to the nondiabetic human kidney (82).

Studies of cultured rat VSMC have led to proposals of roles for AR that differ depending on the nature of the environmental stress: hyperglycemia, cytokine stimulation, or overtly toxic levels of exogenous oxidizing agents.

Rat Vascular Smooth Muscle Cells and Glucose Stress

In cultured rat aortic VSMC, exposure to 20 mmol/L of glucose significantly increased cell proliferation, PKC activity, expression of the PKC-βII isoform, and platelet-derived growth factor-β (PDGF-β) receptor protein. The ARI epalrestat and the PKC-βII inhibitor LY333531 each inhibited glucose-induced PKC activation to the same degree, but the effects of epalrestat on proliferation activities and expression of the PDGF-β receptor were more prominent than those of LY333531 (131). Epalrestat normalized the glucose-induced increased expression of membranous PKC-βII isoform. The ARI also attenuated the increase in free cytosolic NADH/NAD$^+$ ratio and protected the cellular GSH content, whereas LY333531 did not. These data indicate that in rat aortic VSMC cells PKC-β activation by glucose is dependent on increased flux through AR, probably via an indirect effect on the cytoplasmic redox state (i.e., a rise in the free NADH/NAD$^+$ ratio) (Fig. 4-2).

Similarly, the ARI zopolrestat and sodium pyruvate significantly suppressed the glucose-mediated enhancement of interleukin-1β-induced prostaglandin production and cyclooxygenase-2 expression in rat VSMC (132). These results suggest that the augmenting effect of high glucose on these end points results, at least in part, from increased glucose metabolism via the sorbitol pathway, again most likely via an impact on the cytosolic NADH/NAD$^+$ ratio (42).

Rat Vascular Smooth Muscle Cells and Cytokine Stress

Two structurally distinct ARIs, sorbinil and tolrestat, affected neither VSMC growth in the absence of TNF-α nor apoptosis, but each strongly abrogated TNF-α-stimulated rat VSMC proliferation (133). In addition, sorbinil reduced nuclear factor-κB (NF-κB) activation induced by TNF-α, basic fibroblast growth factor (bFGF), PDGF-AB, or angiotensin II stimulation of VSMC. Further, ARI treatment blocked TNF-α-stimulated phosphorylation of IκB-α, prevented the proteolytic degradation of IκB-α, and attenuated the translocation of active NF-κB dimer from the cytosol to the nucleus. Moreover, this effect was not a nonspecific side effect of ARIs, because an AR antisense oligonucleotide, but not a scrambled (control) oligonucleotide, inhibited TNF-α-induced proliferation and reduced PKC activation induced by TNF-α, bFGF, PDGF-AB, or angiotensin II, but not by phorbol 12-myristate 13-acetate (PMA) (133). These data open an exciting new chapter in the biology of AR and indicate that under normoglycemic conditions in rat VSMC, the signaling cascade for a number of proinflammatory and proliferation-inducing cytokines requires metabolic flux through AR as a prerequisite to activation of full PKC and NF-κB.

In primary cultured rat VSMC, lipopolysaccharide-mediated prostaglandin production and subsequent injurious events were mitigated by treatment of these cells with zopolrestat (134). ARI treatment almost completely blocked the stimulatory effect of glucose on prostaglandin synthesis. Sodium pyruvate, which can reverse the glucose-induced alteration in the cytosolic NADH/NAD$^+$ ratio (42), reduced the high-glucose effect on prostaglandin production.

These observations suggest that enhanced flux through the sorbitol pathway activates PKC, which increased the activities of phospholipase-A_2(PLA-2) and prostaglandin-H_2 (PGH) synthetase, resulting in the augmentation of lipopolysaccharide-induced prostaglandin production in VSMC.

Rat Vascular Smooth Muscle Cells and Toxic Exogenous Oxidative Stress

In the cultured rat VSMC line A7r5, exposure to ambient 0.1 mM hydrogen peroxide induced apoptotic cell death and increased AR expression (135). Under these conditions, the presence of the ARI ponalrestat significantly accelerated H_2O_2-induced cell death. In a similar study in the same VSMC line, the ARI sorbinil accentuated the rate of cell death induced by exogenous hydrogen peroxide or by HNE (96). These results suggest that under conditions of severe exogenous oxidative stress in A7r5 VSMC, induction of AR might represent a cellular defense mechanism, via an antioxidant mechanism (96,135) and/or the well-known osmoprotective role of AR under conditions of osmotic stress (97,133). In the latter case (i.e., under such conditions of cell death-inducing external oxidative stress), AR might act as a survival factor by producing sorbitol to help protect oxidant-damaged cells whose membranes can no longer maintain proper osmotic equilibrium (84).

Cardiac Muscle

The presence and activity of AR in cardiac myocytes of rats and rabbits has been demonstrated in several studies (53,104–106,136,137), and cardiac sorbitol and fructose tissue concentrations were shown to be significantly increased in diabetic rats compared with control rats (137). Recent studies have demonstrated that ischemia increases myocardial AR activity and that these increases are, in part, due to activation by nitric oxide (53). In bovine ventricle, AR was shown to be present and to utilize exogenous HNE as a substrate, suggesting the possibility of an oxidative stress defense function for AR (138). However, under ischemic conditions, blockade of AR with zopolrestat

or sorbinil was found to improve cardiac glucose metabolism and to dramatically reduce acute ischemia-reperfusion-induced cardiac damage in diabetic rat hearts and in nondiabetic rat and rabbit hearts (53,104–106) (see "General Function: Unknown" and later discussion).

CARDIOVASCULAR COMPLICATIONS IN DIABETES AND ALDOSE REDUCTASE

Diabetic Cardiac Ischemia

Diabetic patients with CAD have high morbidity and mortality due to cardiovascular complications, and the incidence of heart failure after myocardial infarction is significantly greater in patients with diabetes than in nondiabetic patients (139,140). Studies using diabetic animals have shown that alterations in myocardial metabolism at the myocyte level contribute to a number of biochemical and functional changes in diabetic hearts (141,142).

Specifically, impaired glucose metabolism has been implicated as a key cause for the observed cardiac dysfunction and injury after acute ischemia-reperfusion in diabetics. Investigation of the role of flux via the polyol pathway in influencing functional and metabolic recovery after acute ischemia-reperfusion in nondiabetic and diabetic rat myocardium has demonstrated that flux via AR impairs glycolysis and that this inhibition of glycolysis is probably due, in part, to consumption of NAD^+ by SDH (36,53). More importantly, it was demonstrated that ischemia increases flux via AR and that inhibition of AR in normal and diabetic rat hearts and in nondiabetic rabbit hearts strongly reduces measures of acute ischemic injury (53,104–106). The data in Figure 4-5 show a reduction in creatine kinase release in diabetic rat hearts treated with the ARI zopolrestat and a reduction in ischemic injury accompanied by beneficial changes in ATP and ion homeostasis (143). Similar reductions in ischemic injury and improved metabolic and functional recovery were observed in diabetic rat hearts treated with a structurally distinct ARI, sorbinil (unpublished data). Moreover, in a

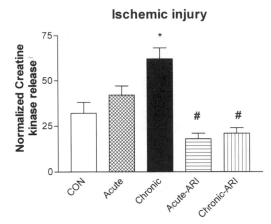

Ischemic injury

FIG. 4-5. Data demonstrating cardioprotection by the aldose reductase (AR) inhibitor zopolrestat in acute and chronic diabetic rat hearts (duration of hyperglycemia, 2 weeks and 12 weeks, respectively). Ischemic injury was assessed by measuring creatine kinase release during reperfusion. Normalized creatine kinase data is a good marker of the extent of injury due to ischemia-reperfusion in this experimental model. These data demonstrate that myocardial ischemic injury is greater with longer duration of diabetes and that acute in vitro treatment with a specific inhibitor of AR (zopolrestat, 10 μM) strongly protects both acute and chronic diabetic myocardium. Similar results were also observed with sorbinil, a member of a structurally distinct ARI class (courtesy of Ramasamy R.).

preliminary study, elevated expression and activity of human AR in transgenic mouse hearts dramatically increased acute ischemic injury compared with hearts of wild-type littermates (144). Finally, pharmacologic inhibition of AR in these transgenic mice hearts strongly reduced ischemic injury and was also associated with improved energy metabolism.

These studies indicate that AR is a key mediator of acute ischemic injury and that inhibition of AR protects acutely ischemic myocardium in nondiabetic rats and rabbits, AR-transgenic mice, and diabetic rats. The potentially important role of AR in the "late preconditioning" model in the nondiabetic hearts of rabbits, a species reported to have a tenfold lower basal AR tissue level than the rat (137), warrants further elucidation. Overall, the available animal data are consistent with the concept that the cardiopro-

tective mechanism of ARIs in the acutely ischemic heart is due primarily to their impact on the NADH/NAD$^+$ ratio and associated changes in glycolysis, ATP, and intracellular sodium and calcium regulation (143,144).

Diabetic Cardiomyopathy

Diabetic patients exhibit cardiomyopathy that is characterized by restrictive physiology (6,7). Diabetic cardiomyopathy is a distinct cause of cardiac morbidity in diabetics, independent of CAD or left ventricular hypertrophy. In a double-blind, placebo-controlled 12-month study, Johnson et al. (145) used radionuclide ventriculography to show that maximal exertional ejection fraction was improved from baseline in diabetics treated with the ARI zopolrestat, compared with placebo-treated diabetics. These promising results support further characterization of potent, well-tolerated ARIs in diabetic patients to define the impact of AR inhibition on cardiac parameters.

Diabetic Macrovascular Complications

Atherosclerosis in Diabetes

When matched for all other parameters, diabetics have a twofold increased risk of CAD (6,7). Because atherosclerosis is initiated at the level of the vascular endothelium (8), it is relevant that aortic endothelium is one of the consistently positive localizations for AR in histochemical studies (see earlier discussion). Because it is now realized that oxidative stress plays a central role in atherosclerosis (146), and that a prime source of oxidative stress is hyperglycemia (see earlier discussion), it is of interest that ARIs have been shown to strongly attenuate glucose-induced oxidative stress (i.e., glucose-induced superoxide production) in human retinal endothelial cells and bovine aortic endothelial cells (99) and in rabbit aortas (109) (Fig. 4-4). These data are consistent with a 44-month dog study showing that ARI treatment prevented hexose-induced aortic intimal thickening (147). Together, these studies support further characterization of the potential link between elevated metabolic flux through AR and the susceptibility and rate of development of macrovascular disease, particularly in diabetic patients.

Vascular Restenosis

As indicated earlier, persuasive new data indicate that AR plays a key role in VSMC proliferation and restenosis (133,147). In the same studies, it was also shown that AR expression increased in the rat carotid artery balloon injury model (147), and that AR inhibition led to a significant reduction in the neointima/media ratio after balloon injury and a decrease in the *in vivo* activation of NF-κB (133). Mechanistically, AR inhibition disrupted PKC-associated signaling, decreased transcription factor NF-κB activity, and inhibited VSMC proliferation (133). Consistent with these findings, long-term ARI treatment reduced the ratio of the aortic neointima area to media area in 44-month galactosemic dogs (147).

Diabetic Microvascular Complications

Diabetic Neuropathy

It has long been known that ARIs can improve human NCV (29,108). However, the first dose-dependent positive effects on human nerve structure and function were not demonstrated until 1999 (148). Comparison by dose (in mg/kg body weight per day) of the extent of sorbitol lowering and of NCV improvement in human nerve (148) compared with rat nerve (149) shows that the magnitude and shape of the dose-response curve for NCV response in both species were quite consistent (29). A recent analysis of the quantitative relationship between the degree of suppression of nerve sorbitol and the degree of inhibition of nerve AR strongly suggests that more potent ARIs, those that control AR flux rather than sorbitol concentration, will show improved efficacy (29). In this regard, a 12-month, double-blind, placebo-controlled study with the potent ARI, SNK-860 (fidarestat), showed impressive improvements in symptoms, as well as modest improvements in objective neuroelectrophysiologic parameters (150).

Strong support for the concept of the efficacy of a blockade of the polyol pathway was obtained in a comprehensive 5-year diabetic dog study. NCV deterioration was completely blocked with sorbinil (151), implying that flux through AR is critical to the development of the NCV deficit in the diabetic dog. The AR$^{-/-}$ mouse also provides compelling evidence of a pivotal role for AR in the pathogenesis of diabetic neuropathy. Nerve GSH and NCV were completely protected in STZ-diabetic AR$^{-/-}$ mice, in stark contrast to wild-type mice, which exhibited a substantial reduction in nerve GSH and NCV by 4 weeks after STZ treatment (152).

Diabetic Retinopathy

Diabetic retinopathy remains a major cause of loss of vision. The pathophysiologic process is complex and difficult to unravel, but there is considerable evidence that AR may play a key role (13,153). Human genetic data strongly implicate the "high AR" allele in accelerating the rate of progression of human diabetic retinopathy (see earlier discussion). On the other hand, treatment of human diabetics with the ARI sorbinil caused only a slightly slower progression rate in the microaneurysm count, a finding of uncertain clinical importance (154). Consistent with this outcome, retinal protection was not found with the use of sorbinil in an early study of diabetic and galactosemic dogs (155). However, a later study of galactose-fed dogs, which used the more potent ARI, M79175, demonstrated dose-dependent protection against pericyte degeneration and formation of microaneurysms (156). Development of diabetes-like retinopathy in galactose-fed rats was also substantially ameliorated with high doses of ARI (157). More potent drugs of this class will probably be required for success in experimental and human diabetics. At the same time, a more fundamental understanding of the nature of the pathophysiologic processes that drive retinopathy is needed. For example, one of the major scientific mysteries here is that the retinopathic disease process keeps progressing even after the initiating pathogenic insult (galactose) is removed or the hyperglycemia is brought under good control (155,156).

Diabetic Nephropathy

Diabetic nephropathy is the most common cause of end-stage renal failure in the Western world (158,159). Flux through AR has long been suggested to be involved in the development of diabetic nephropathy (160,161). In experimental models, numerous studies have demonstrated that inhibitors of AR cause partial to near-complete normalization of diabetes- or hexose-induced renal functional changes (108,161,162). Inhibition of AR in cultured human mesangial cells attenuates glucose-induced activation of PKC and TGFβ1 (34), factors that may play a central role in the pathogenesis of diabetic nephropathy (158,159). Inhibition of AR was also reported to prevent glucose-induced activation of PKC or several of its isoforms in cultured rat glomeruli (163).

Antialbuminuric effects of ARIs have been documented in rodent models in several laboratories (125,162,164,165), and several ARIs have shown positive activity on albuminuria in the clinical setting (166–168). Consistent with these data, AR inhibition has also been reported to have positive effects on diabetes-induced renal hemodynamic abnormalities in rats (reviewed in 161) and in humans (167,169). Moreover, in a recent 5-year clinical study, treatment with the ARI epalrestat was reported to prevent progression of albuminuria and of a slight but statistically significant rise in serum creatinine (168). Finally, human genetic data linking alleles associated with high expression levels of AR with enhanced susceptibility to diabetic nephropathy (62) provide clear encouragement for further studies in diabetic renal disease with potent inhibitors of AR and of polyol pathway flux.

CONCLUSION

The DCCT, UKPDS, and prior ARI studies have led to the recognition that relatively long clinical trials will be needed to demonstrate efficacy against microvascular and macrovascular complications of diabetes, and that prevention or slowing of cardiovascular disease progression in diabetic patients should be the primary expectation, not rapid reversal of disease end points. Despite some developmental setbacks over the last two decades, evidence has continued to strengthen for a strong link between the rate of progression of diabetic vascular complications and chronically elevated AR metabolism. Overall, current data on genetic polymorphisms of AR from around the world indicate an association between "high AR" alleles and diabetic vascular complications (62,63). The biochemical, genetic, and pathophysiologic data reviewed here indicate that control of excess metabolic flux through AR could play a key role in future therapeutic strategies against diabetic cardiovascular complications.

However, despite several decades of effort, no ARI is yet on the global market for treatment of the macrovascular and microvascular complications of diabetes mellitus. Numerous ARIs have failed in phase II or phase III studies due to inadequate efficacy or safety or both. Regarding efficacy, it now seems clear that clinical failure has largely been a result of lack of adequate control of hyperglysolia-driven flux through AR (29). Regarding safety, the various past ARI candidates clinically tested did not show a common pattern of side effects, suggesting compound-specific, rather than mechanism-based, toleration issues. The almost complete normalcy of the $AR^{-/-}$ mouse (102) provides strong encouragement that such a therapeutic mechanism can in principle be well tolerated.

The challenge remains for the biomedical research community to identify and develop highly potent, well-tolerated ARIs. Such agents ideally will be useful alone or in combination with other, mechanistically distinct therapies to inhibit diabetes-linked vascular stress and to slow the development of microvascular and macrovascular diabetic complications. In view of the current global epidemic of diabetes and the substantial worldwide increase in diabetes projected for the coming decades (170), the sooner we succeed, the better.

ACKNOWLEDGMENTS

This work was supported by grants from the National Institutes of Health Heart, Lung, and Blood Institute HL 61783, 68954, the Juvenile

Diabetes Research Foundation International, and Pfizer Inc. Sincere acknowledgment is given to our colleagues and friends, and particularly to our wives, Indu and Nancy, whose support has remained unbending and patience astonishing. Dr. Ramasamy is the recipient of an Established Investigator Award from the American Heart Association (0040152N).

REFERENCES

1. The Diabetes Complications and Control Trial Research Group. The effect of intensive treatment of diabetes on the development and progression of long-term complications in insulin-dependent diabetes mellitus. *N Engl J Med* 1993;329:977–986.

2. United Kingdom Prospective Diabetes Study Group. Intensive blood-glucose control with sulfonylureas or insulin compared with conventional treatment and risk of complications in patients with type 2 diabetes (UKPDS 33). *Lancet* 1998;352:837–853.

3. Reaven GM. Multiple CHD risk factors in type 2 diabetes: beyond hyperglycaemia. *Diabetes Obes Metab* 2002;4:S13–S18.

4. Jandeleit-Dahm K, Cooper M. Hypertension and diabetes. *Curr Opin Nephrol Hypertens* 2002;11:221–228.

5. Lopaschuk GD. Metabolic abnormalities in the diabetic heart. *Heart Fail Rev* 2002;7:149–159.

6. Zarich SW, Nesto RW. Diabetic cardiomyopathy. *Am Heart J* 1989;118:1000–1012.

7. Sowers JR, Epstein M, Frohlich ED. Diabetes, hypertension, and cardiovascular disease: an update. *Hypertension* 2001;37:1053–1059.

8. Beckman JA, Creager MA, Libby P. Diabetes and atherosclerosis: epidemiology, pathophysiology, and management. *JAMA* 2002;287:2570–2581.

9. Weinberger J. Prevention of ischemic stroke. *Curr Cardiol Rep* 2002;4:164–171.

10. Wendt T, Bucciarelli L, Qu W, et al. Receptor for advanced glycation endproducts (RAGE) and vascular inflammation: insights into the pathogenesis of macrovascular complications in diabetes. *Curr Atheroscler Rep* 2002;4:228–237.

11. Malloy MJ, Kane JP. A risk factor for atherosclerosis: triglyceride-rich lipoproteins. *Adv Intern Med* 2001;47:111–136.

12. Gotto AM Jr. Management of dyslipidemia. *Am J Med* 2002;112:10S–18S.

13. Tilton RG. Diabetic vascular dysfunction: links to glucose-induced reductive stress and VEGF. *Microsc Res Tech* 2002;57:390–407.

14. Ruderman NB, Williamson JR, Brownlee M. Glucose and diabetic vascular disease. *FASEB J* 1992;6:2905–2914.

15. Tesfaye S, Stevens LK, Stephenson JM, et al. Prevalence of diabetic peripheral neuropathy and its relation to glycaemic control and potential risk factors: the EURODIAB IDDM Complications Study. *Diabetologia* 1996;39:1377–1384.

16. Sjolie AK, Stephenson J, Aldington S, et al. Retinopathy and vision loss in insulin-dependent diabetes in Europe: the EURODIAB IDDM Complications Study. *Ophthalmology* 1997;104:252–260.

17. Inoguchi T, Li P, Umeda F, et al. High glucose level and free fatty acid stimulate reactive oxygen species production through protein kinase C-dependent activation of NAD(P)H oxidase in cultured vascular cells. *Diabetes* 2000;49:1939–1945.

18. Nathan DM. The pathophysiology of diabetic complications: how much does the glucose hypothesis explain? *Ann Intern Med* 1996;124:86–89.

19. Mogensen CE. Preventing end-stage renal disease. *Diabetes Med* 1998;15[Suppl 4]:S51–S56.

20. Stratton IM, Kohner EM, Aldington SJ, et al. UKPDS 50: risk factors for incidence and progression of retinopathy in type II diabetes over 6 years from diagnosis. *Diabetologia* 2001;44:156–163.

21. Brownlee M. Advanced products of nonenzymatic glycosylation and the pathogenesis of diabetic complications. In: Porte J, Sherwin RS, eds. *Diabetes mellitus*. Stamford, CT: Appleton & Lange, 1997:229–256.

22. Baynes J, Thorpe S. Role of oxidative stress in diabetic complications: a new perspective on an old paradigm. *Diabetes* 1999;48:1–9.

23. Cohen MP. Diabetes and protein glycation. JC Press: Philadelphia 1996;183–192.

24. Schmidt AM, Yan SD, Yan SF, et al. The biology of the receptor for advanced glycation end products and its ligands. *Biochim Biophys Acta* 2000;1498:99–111.

25. Wautier MP, Chappey O, Corda S, et al. Activation of NADPH oxidase by AGE links oxidant stress to altered gene expression via RAGE. *Am J Physiol* 2001;280:E685–E694.

26. Ramasamy R, Hwang YC, Whang J, et al. Protection of ischemic hearts by high glucose is mediated by the glucose transporter, GLUT-4. *Am J Physiol* 2001;281:H290–H297.

27. Depre C, Vanoverschelde JL, Taegtmeyer H. Glucose for the heart. *Circulation* 1999;99:578–588.

28. Heilig C, Brosius F III, Henry D. Glucose transporters of the glomerulus and the implications for diabetic nephropathy. *Kidney Int* 1997;60[Suppl]:S91–S99.

29. Oates PJ. The polyol pathway and diabetic peripheral neuropathy. In: Tomlinson DR, ed. *International review of neurobiology*. London: Academic Press, 2002:325–392.

30. Baynes JW. Role of oxidative stress in development of complications in diabetes. *Diabetes* 1991;40:405–412.

31. Williamson JR, Kilo C, Ido Y. The role of cytosolic reductive stress in oxidant formation and diabetic complications. *Diabetes Res Clin Pract* 1999;45:81–82.

32. Brownlee M. Biochemistry and molecular cell biology of diabetic complications. *Nature* 2001;414:813–820.

33. Spitaler MM, Graier WF. Vascular targets of redox signalling in diabetes mellitus. *Diabetologia* 2002;45:476–494.

34. Ishii H, Tada H, Isogai S. An aldose reductase inhibitor prevents glucose-induced increase in transforming growth factor-beta and protein kinase C activity in cultured human mesangial cells. *Diabetologia* 1998;41:362–364.

35. Nishikawa T, Edelstein D, Du XL, et al. Normalizing mitochondrial superoxide production blocks three pathways of hyperglycaemic damage. *Nature* 2000;404:787–790.

36. Trueblood N, Ramasamy R. Aldose reductase inhibition improves altered glucose metabolism of isolated diabetic rat hearts. *Am J Physiol* 1998;275:H75–H83.

37. Hers HG. Le méchnaisme de la transformation de glucose en fructose par les vésicules seminales. *Biochim Biophys Acta* 1956;22:202–203.

38. Kinoshita JH. A thirty year journey in the polyol pathway. *Exp Eye Res* 1990;50:567–573.

39. Lee AY, Chung SK, Chung SS. Demonstration that polyol accumulation is responsible for diabetic cataract by the use of transgenic mice expressing the aldose reductase gene in the lens. *Proc Natl Acad Sci U S A* 1995;92:2780–2784.

40. Winegrad A. Discussion. *Adv Metabol Disorders* 1973;2[Suppl]:430–432.

41. Cheng H-M, Gonzalez RG. The effect of high glucose and oxidative stress on lens metabolism, aldose reductase, and senile cataractogenesis. *Metabolism* 1986;35[Suppl 1]:10–14.

42. Williamson JR, Chang K, Frangos M, et al. Hyperglycemic pseudohypoxia and diabetic complications. *Diabetes* 1993;42:801–813.

43. Ido Y, Chang K, Woolsey TA, et al. NADH: sensor of blood flow need in brain, muscle, and other tissues. *FASEB J* 2001;15:1419–1421.

44. Jez JM, Penning TM. The aldo-keto reductase (AKR) superfamily: an update. *Chem Biol Interact* 2001;130–132:499–525.

45. Petrash JM, Tarle I, Wilson DK, Quiocho FA: Aldose reductase catalysis and crystallography: insights from recent advances in enzyme structure and function. *Diabetes* 1994;43:955–959.

46. Grimshaw CE, Bohren KM, Lai CJ, et al: Human aldose reductase: rate constants for a mechanism including interconversion of ternary complexes by recombinant wild-type enzyme. *Biochemistry* 1995;34:14356–14365.

47. Clements RS, Weaver JP, Winegrad AI: The distribution of polyol: NADP oxidoreductase in mammalian tissues. *Biochem Biophys Res Commun* 1969;37:347–353.

48. Ludvigson MA, Sorenson RL. Immunohistochemical localization of aldose reductase: I. Enzyme purification and antibody preparation: localization in peripheral nerve, artery, and testis. *Diabetes* 1980;29:438–449.

49. Rondeau J-M, Tete-Favier F, Podjarny A, et al. Novel NADPH-binding domain revealed by the crystal structure of aldose reductase. *Nature* 1992;55:469–472.

50. Hers HG. L'Aldose-reductase. *Biochim Biophys Acta* 1960;37:120–126.

51. Petrash JM, Harter TM, Devine CS, et al. Involvement of cysteine residues in catalysis and inhibition of human aldose reductase: site-directed mutagenesis of Cys-80, -298, and -303. *J Biol Chem* 1992;267:24833–24840.

52. Srivastava S, Dixit BL, Ramana KV, et al. Structural and kinetic modifications of aldose reductase by S-nitrosothiols. *Biochem J* 2001;358:111–118.

53. Hwang YC, Sato S, Tsai JY, et al. Aldose reductase activation is a key component of myocardial response to ischemia. *FASEB J* 2002;16:243–245.

54. Chandra D, Jackson EB, Ramana KV, et al. Nitric oxide prevents aldose reductase activation and sorbitol accumulation during diabetes. *Diabetes* 2002;51:3095–3101.

55. Robinson B, Hunsaker, LA, Stangebye, LA, et al. Aldose and aldehyde reductases from human kidney cortex and medulla. *Biochim Biophys Acta* 1993;1203:260–266.

56. Graham A, Heath P, Morten JEN, et al. The human aldose reductase gene maps to chromosome region 7q35. *Hum Genet* 1991;86:509–514.

57. Chung S, LaMendola J. Cloning and sequence determination of human placental aldose reductase gene. *J Biol Chem* 1989;264:14775–14777.

58. Wang K, Bohren KM, Gabbay KH. Characterization of the human aldose reductase gene promoter. *J Biol Chem* 1993;268:16052–16058.

59. Ko BCB, Ruepp B, Bohren KM, et al. Identification and characterization of multiple osmotic response sequences in the human aldose reductase gene. *J Biol Chem* 1997;272:16431–16437.

60. Bateman JB, Kojis T, Heinzmann C, et al. Mapping of aldose reductase gene sequences to human chromosomes 1, 3, 7, 9, 11, and 13. *Genomics* 1993;17:560–565.

61. Hodkinson AD, Millward BA, Demaine AG. Polymorphisms of the glucose transporter gene (GLUT1) are associated with diabetic nephropathy. *Kidney Int* 2001;59:985–989.

62. Oates PJ, Mylari BL. Aldose reductase inhibitors: therapeutic implications for diabetic complications. *Exp Opin Invest Drugs* 1999;8:2095–2119.

63. Neatmat-Allah M, Feeny SA, Savage DA, et al. Analysis of the association between diabetic nephropathy and polymorphisms in the aldose reductase gene in type 1 and type 2 diabetes mellitus. *Diabetes Med* 2001;18:906–914.

64. Ko BC, Lam KS, Wat NM, et al. An (A C)n dinucleotide repeat polymorphic marker at the 5′ end of the aldose reductase gene is associated with early-onset diabetic retinopathy in NIDDM patients. *Diabetes* 1995;44:727–732.

65. Kao YL, Donaghue K, Chan A, et al. A novel polymorphism in the aldose reductase gene promoter region is strongly associated with diabetic retinopathy in adolescents with type 1 diabetes. *Diabetes* 1999;48:1338–1340.

66. Lee SC, Wang Y, Ko GT, et al. Association of retinopathy with a microsatellite at 5′ end of the aldose reductase gene in Chinese patients with late-onset type 2 diabetes. *Ophthalmic Genet* 2001;22:63–67.

67. Kao YL, Donaghue K, Chan A, et al. An aldose reductase intragenic polymorphism associated with diabetic retinopathy. *Diabetes Res Clin Pract* 1991;46:155–160.

68. Demaine A, Cross D, Millward A. Polymorphisms of the aldose reductase gene and susceptibility to retinopathy in type 1 diabetes mellitus. *Invest Ophthalmol Vis Sci* 2000;41:4064–4068.

69. Moczulski DK, Scott L, Antonellis A, et al. Aldose reductase gene polymorphisms and susceptibility to diabetic nephropathy in type 1 diabetes mellitus. *Diabetes Med* 2000;17:111–118.

70. Shah VO, Scavini M, Nikolic J, et al. Z-2 microsatellite allele is linked to increased expression of the aldose

reductase gene in diabetic nephropathy. *J Clin Endocrinol Metab* 1998;83:2886–2891.

71. Heesom AE, Hibberd, ML, Millward A, et al. Polymorphism in the 5′-end of the aldose reductase gene is strongly associated with the development of diabetic nephropathy in type I diabetes. *Diabetes* 1997;46:287–291.

72. Heesom AE, Millward A, Demaine AG. Susceptibility to diabetic neuropathy in patients with insulin dependent diabetes mellitus is associated with a polymorphism at the 5′ end of the aldose reductase gene. *J Neurol Neurosurg Psychiatry* 1998;64:213–216.

73. Moczulski DK, Burak W, Doria A, et al. The role of aldose reductase gene in the susceptibility to diabetic nephropathy in type II (non-insulin-dependent) diabetes mellitus. *Diabetologia* 1999;42:94–97.

74. Ng DP, Conn J, Chung SS, et al. Aldose reductase (AC)n microsatellite polymorphism and diabetic microvascular complications in Caucasian type 1 diabetes mellitus. *Diabetes Res Clin Pract* 2001;52:21–27.

75. Maeda S, Haneda M., Yasuda H, et al. Diabetic nephropathy is not associated with the dinucleotide repeat polymorphism upstream of the aldose reductase (ALR2) gene but with erythrocyte aldose reductase content in Japanese subjects with type 2 diabetes. *Diabetes* 1999;48:420–422.

76. Chavers BM, Bilous RW, Ellis EN, et al. Glomerular lesions and urinary albumin excretion in type I diabetes without overt proteinuria. *N Engl J Med* 1989;320:966–970.

77. Markus HB, Raducha M, Harris H. Tissue distribution of mammalian aldose reductase and related enzymes. *Biochem Med* 1983;29:31–45.

78. Tanimoto T, Maekawa K, Okada S, et al. Clinical analysis of aldose reductase for differential diagnosis of the pathogenesis of diabetic complications. *Anal Chim Acta* 1998;365:285–292.

79. Grimshaw CE, Mathur EJ. Immunoquantitation of aldose reductase in human tissues. *Anal Biochem* 1989;176:66–71.

80. Oates PJ, Beebe DA, Ellery CA, et al. Quantitation of polyol pathway enzymes in normal and diabetic rat sciatic nerve. *Diabetologia* 2002;45[Suppl 2]:A324.

81. Powell HC, Garrett RS, Kador PF, et al. Fine-structural localization of aldose reductase and ouabain-sensitive, K(+)-dependent p-nitro-phenylphosphatase in rat peripheral nerve. *Acta Neuropathol (Berl)* 1991;81:529–539.

82. Kasajima H, Yamagishi S-I, Sugai S, et al. Enhanced in situ expression of aldose reductase in peripheral nerve and renal glomeruli in diabetic patients. *Virchows Arch* 2001;439:46–54.

83. Oates PJ, Goddu KJ. A sorbitol gradient in the rat renal medulla. *Kidney Int* 1987;31:448.

84. Burg MB, Kwon D, Kultz D. Regulation of gene expression by hypertonicity. *Annu Rev Physiol* 1997;59:437–455.

85. Burg MB. Coordinate regulation of organic osmolytes in renal cells. *Kidney Int* 1996;49:1684–1685.

86. Yabe-Nishimura C. Aldose reductase in glucose toxicity: a potential target for the prevention of diabetic complications. *Pharmacol Rev* 1998;50:21–33.

87. Srivastava SK, Ansari NH, Brown JH, et al. Formation of sorbitol 6-phosphate by bovine and human lens aldose reductase, sorbitol dehydrogenase and sorbitol kinase. *Biochim Biophys Acta* 1982;717:210–214.

88. Szwergold BS, Kappler F, Brown TR, et al. Identification of D-sorbitol 3-phosphate in the normal and diabetic mammalian lens. *J Biol Chem* 1989;264:9278–9282.

89. Szwergold BS, Kappler F, Brown TR. Identification of fructose 3-phosphate in the lens of diabetic rats. *Science* 1990;247:451–454.

90. Petrash JM, Harter TM, Murdock GL. A potential role for aldose reductase in steroid metabolism. *Adv Exp Med Biol* 1997;414:465–473.

91. Kawamura M, Kopin IJ, Kador PF, et al. Effects of aldehyde/aldose reductase inhibition on neuronal metabolism of norepinephrine. *J Autonom Nerv Sys* 1997;66:145–148.

92. Grimshaw CE. Aldose reductase: model for a new paradigm of enzymic perfection in detoxification catalysts. *Biochemistry* 1992;31:10139–10145.

93. Dixit BL, Balendiran GK, Watowich SJ, et al. Kinetic and structural characterization of the glutathione-binding site of aldose reductase. *J Biol Chem* 2000;275:21587–21595.

94. Rees-Milton KJ, Jia Z, Green NC, et al. Aldehyde reductase: the role of C-terminal residues in defining substrate and cofactor specificities. *Arch Biochem Biophys* 1998;355:137–144.

95. Vasiliou V, Pappa A, Petersen DR. Role of aldehyde dehydrogenases in endogenous and xenobiotic metabolism. *Chem Biol Interact* 2000;129:1–19.

96. Spycher SE, Tabataba-Vakili S, O'Donnell VB, et al. Aldose reductase induction: a novel response to oxidative stress of smooth muscle cells. *FASEB J* 1997;11:181–188.

97. Yancey PH, Burg MB, Bagnasco SM. Effects of NaCl, glucose, and aldose reductase inhibitors on cloning efficiency of renal medullary cells. *Am J Physiol* 1990;258:C156-C163.

98. Lee AY, Chung SS. Contributions of polyol pathway to oxidative stress in diabetic cataract. *FASEB J* 1999;13:23–30.

99. Obrosova IG, Van Huysen C, Fathallah L, et al. An aldose reductase inhibitor reverses early diabetes-induced changes in peripheral nerve function, metabolism, and antioxidative defense. *FASEB J* 2002;16:123–125.

100. Lowitt S, Malone JI, Salem AF, et al. Acetyl-L-carnitine corrects the altered peripheral nerve function of experimental diabetes. *Metabolism* 1995;44:677–680.

101. Hohman TC, Banas D, Basso M. , et al. Increased oxidative stress in experimental diabetic neuropathy. *Diabetologia* 1997;40[Suppl 1]:A549.

102. Ho HT, Chung SK, Law JW, et al. Aldose reductase-deficient mice develop nephrogenic diabetes insipidus. *Mol Cell Biol* 2000;20:5840–5846.

103. Aida K, Ikegishi Y, Chen J, et al. Disruption of aldose reductase gene (Akr1b1) causes defect in urinary concentrating ability and divalent cation homeostasis. *Biochem Biophys Res Commun* 2000;277:281–286.

104. Ramasamy R, Oates PJ, Schaefer S. Aldose reductase inhibition protects diabetic and non-diabetic rat hearts from ischemic injury. *Diabetes* 1997;46:292–300.

105. Ramasamy R, Trueblood NA, Schaefer S. Metabolic effects of aldose reductase inhibition during low-flow

ischemia and reperfusion. *Am J Physiol* 1998;275: H195–H203.

106. Tracey WR, Magee WP, Ellery CA, et al. Aldose reductase inhibition alone or combined with an adenosine A(3) agonist reduces ischemic myocardial injury. *Am J Physiol* 2000;279:H1447–H1452.

107. Mylari BL, Beyer TA, Siegel TW. A highly specific aldose reductase inhibitor, ethyl 1-benzyl-3-hydroxy-2(5H)-oxopyrrole-4-carboxylate, and its congeners. *J Med Chem* 1991;34:1011–1018.

108. Sarges R, Oates PJ. Aldose reductase inhibitors: recent developments. *Prog Drug Res* 1993;40:99–161.

109. Gupta S, Chough E, Daley J, et al. Hyperglycemia increases superoxide anion production in rabbit endothelium leading to decreased Na^+K^+-ATPase activity. *Am J Physiol* 2001;282:C560–C566.

110. Obrosova I, Lang H, Greene D. Antioxidative defense in diabetic peripheral nerve: role for aldose reductase and sorbitol dehydrogenase. *Diabetologia* 1998;41:A270.

111. Jiang ZY, Zhou QL, Eaton JW, et al. Spirohydantoin inhibitors of aldose reductase inhibit iron- and copper-catalysed ascorbate oxidation *in vitro*. *Biochem Pharmacol* 1991;42:1273–1278.

112. Kern TS, Engerman RL. Immunohistochemical distribution of aldose reductase. *Histochem J* 1984;14:507–515.

113. Sato S, Secchi EF, Lizak MJ, et al. Polyol formation and NADPH-dependent reductases in dog retinal capillary pericytes and endothelial cells. *Invest Ophthalmol Vis Sci* 1999;40:697–704.

114. Chakrabarti S, Sima AA, Nakajima T, et al. Aldose reductase in the BB rat: isolation, immunological identification and localization in the retina and peripheral nerve. *Diabetologia* 1987;30:244–251.

115. Tesfamariam B, Palacino JJ, Weisbrod RM, et al. Aldose reductase inhibition restores endothelial cell function in diabetic rabbit aorta. *J Cardiovasc Pharmacol* 1993;21:205–211.

116. Cameron NE, Cotter MA. Impaired contraction and relaxation in aorta from streptozotocin-diabetic rats: role of polyol pathway. *Diabetologia* 1992;35:1011–1019.

117. Cameron NE, Cotter MA. Contraction and relaxation of aortas from galactosaemic rats and the effects of aldose reductase inhibition. *Eur J Pharmacol* 1993;243:47–53.

118. Okuda Y, Kawashima K, Suzuki S, et al. Restoration of nitric oxide production by aldose reductase inhibitor in human endothelial cells cultured in high-glucose medium. *Life Sci* 1997;60:PL53–PL56.

119. Yorek MA, Dunlap JA. The effect of elevated glucose levels on myo-inositol metabolism in cultured bovine aortic endothelial cells. *Metabolism* 1989;38:16–22.

120. Leto G, Pricci F, Amadio L, et al. Increased retinal endothelial cell monolayer permeability induced by the diabetic milieu: role of advanced non-enzymatic glycation and polyol pathway activation. *Diabetes Metab Res Rev* 2001;17:448–458.

121. Kasajima H, Yamagishi S, Sugai S, et al. Enhanced in situ expression of aldose reductase in peripheral nerve and renal glomeruli in diabetic patients. *Virchows Arch* 2001;439:46–54.

122. Hohman TC, Nishimura C, Robison WG Jr. Aldose

reductase and polyol in cultured pericytes of human retinal capillaries. *Exp Eye Res* 1989;48:55–60.

123. Naruse K, Nakamura J, Hamada Y, et al. Aldose reductase inhibition prevents glucose-induced apoptosis in cultured bovine retinal microvascular pericytes. *Exp Eye Res* 2000;71:309–315.

124. Rittner HL, Hafner V, Klimiuk PA, et al. Aldose reductase functions as a detoxification system for lipid peroxidation products in vasculitis. *J Clin Invest* 1999;103:1007–1013.

125. Yasunari K, Kohno M, Kano H, et al. Aldose reductase inhibitor improves insulin-mediated glucose uptake and prevents migration of human coronary artery smooth muscle cells induced by high glucose. *Hypertension* 2000;35:1092–1098.

126. Tilton RG, Chang K, Pugliese G, et al. Prevention of hemodynamic and vascular albumin filtration changes in diabetic rats by aldose reductase inhibitors. *Diabetes* 1989;38:1258–1270.

127. Coppey LJ, Gellett JS, Davidson EP, et al. Effect of antioxidant treatment of streptozotocin-induced diabetic rats on endoneurial blood flow, motor nerve conduction velocity, and vascular reactivity of epineurial arterioles of the sciatic nerve. *Diabetes* 2001;50:1927–1937.

128. Cotter M, Keegan A, Cameron NE. Endothelial and autonomic relaxation of the corpus cavernosum in diabetic rats: effects of aldose reductase inhibitor and antioxidant treatments. *Eur J Clin Invest* 1998;28[Suppl 1]:A29.

129. Bank N, Mower P, Aynedjian HS, et al. Sorbinil prevents glomerular hyperperfusion in diabetic rats. *Am J Physiol* 1989;256:F1000–F1006.

130. Connors B, Lee WH, Wang G, et al. Aldose reductase and IGF-I gene expression in aortic and arteriolar smooth muscle during hypo- and hyperinsulinemic diabetes. *Microvasc Res* 1997;53:53–62.

131. Nakamura J, Kasuya Y, Hamada Y, et al. Glucose-induced hyperproliferation of cultured rat aortic smooth muscle cells through polyol pathway hyperactivity. *Diabetologia* 2001;44:480–487.

132. Lee SH, Woo HG, Baik EJ, et al. High glucose enhances IL-1beta-induced cyclooxygenase-2 expression in rat vascular smooth muscle cells. *Life Sci* 2000;68:57–67.

133. Ramana KV, Chandra D, Srivastava S, et al. Aldose reductase mediates mitogenic signaling in vascular smooth muscle cells. *J Biol Chem* 2002;277:32063–32070.

134. Fazzio A, Spycher SE, Azzi A. Signal transduction in rat vascular smooth muscle cells: control of osmotically induced aldose reductase expression by cell kinases and phosphatases. *Biochem Biophys Res Commun* 1999;255:12–16.

135. Nishinaka T, Yabe-Nishimura C. EGF receptor-ERK pathway is the major signaling pathway that mediates upregulation of aldose reductase expression under oxidative stress. *Free Radic Biol Med* 2001;31:205–216.

136. Kashiwagi A, Obata T, Suzaki M, et al. Increase in cardiac muscle fructose content in streptozotocin-induced diabetic rats. *Metabolism* 1992;41:1041–1046.

137. Shinmura K, Bolli R, Liu S-Q, et al. Aldose reductase is an obligatory mediator of the late phase of ischemic preconditioning. *Circ Res* 2002;91:240–246.

138. Srivastava S, Chandra A, Ansan NH, et al. Identification of cardiac oxidoreductase(s) involved in the metabolism of the lipid peroxidation-derived aldehyde-4-hydroxynonenal. *Biochem J* 1998;329:469–475.

139. Stone GW, Grines CL, Browne KF, et al. Predictors of in-hospital and 6-month outcome after acute myocardial infarction in the reperfusion era: the primary angioplasty in myocardial infarction (PAMI) trial. *J Am Coll Cardiol* 1995;25:370–377.

140. Jaffe AS, Spadaro JJ, Schetman R, et al. Increased congestive heart failure after myocardial infarction of moderate extent in patients with diabetes mellitus. *Am Heart J* 1984;108:31–37.

141. Young ME, McNulty P, Taegtmeyer H. Adaptation and maladaptation of the heart in diabetes. *Circulation* 2002;105:1861–1870.

142. Schaffer S. Cardiomyopathy associated with non-insulin-dependent diabetes. *Mol Cell Biochem* 1991;107:1–20.

143. Ramasamy R, Liu H, Oates PJ, et al. Attenuation of ischemia induced increases in sodium and calcium by an aldose reductase inhibitor zopolrestat. *Cardiovasc Res* 1999;42:130–139.

144. Hwang YC, Yan S, Bakr S, et al. Overexpression of human aldose reductase increases myocardial ischemic injury. *Circulation* 2001;104[Suppl]:II-227.

145. Johnson BF, Law G, Nesto R, et al. Aldose reductase inhibitor zopolrestat improves systolic function in diabetes. *Diabetes* 1999;48[Suppl 1]:0574.

146. Sorescu D, Weiss D, Lassegue B, et al. Superoxide production and expression of nox family proteins in human atherosclerosis. *Circulation* 2002;105:1429–1435.

147. Kasuya Y, Ito M, Nakamura J, et al. An aldose redutase inhibitor prevents the intimal thickening in coronary arteries of galactose-fed beagle dogs. *Diabetologia* 1999;42:1404–1409.

148. Greene DA, Arezzo JC, Brown MB, and the Zenarestat Study Group. Effect of aldose reductase inhibition on nerve conduction and morphometry in diabeticneuropathy. *Neurology* 1999;53:580–591.

149. Ao S, Shingu Y, Kikuchi C, et al. Characterization of a novel aldose reductase inhibitor, FR74366, and its effects on diabetic cataract and neuropathy in the rat. *Metabolism* 1991;40:77–87.

150. Hotta N, Toyota T, Matsuoka K, et al. , and the SNK-860 Diabetic Neuropathy Study Group. Clinical efficacy of fidarestat, a novel aldose reductase inhibitor, for diabetic peripheral neuropathy: a 52-week multicenter placebo-controlled double-blind parallel group study. *Diabetes Care* 2001;24:1776–1782.

151. Engerman RL, Kern TS, Larson ME. Nerve conduction and aldose reductase inhibition during 5 years of diabetes or galactosemia in dogs. *Diabetologia* 1994;37:141–144.

152. Ho ECM, Lam KSL, Chung SSM, et al. Aldose reductase-deficient mice are alleviated from the depletion of GSH in the peripheral nerve and MNCV deficit associated with diabetes. *Diabetes* 2001;50[Suppl 2]:A59.

153. Van den Enden MK, Nyengaard JR, Ostrow E, et al. Elevated glucose levels increase retinal glycolysis and sorbitol pathway metabolism: implications for diabetic retinopathy. *Invest Ophthalmol Vis Sci* 1995;36:1675–1685.

154. The Sorbinil Retinopathy Trial Research Group. A randomized trial of sorbinil, an aldose reductase inhibitor, in diabetic retinopathy. *Arch Ophthalmol* 1990;108:1234–1244.

155. Engerman RL, Kern TS. Aldose reductase inhibition fails to prevent retinopathy in diabetic and galactosemic dogs. *Diabetes* 1993;42:820–825.

156. Neuenschwander H, Takahashi Y, Kador PF. Dose-dependent reduction of retinal vessel changes associated with diabetic retinopathy in galactose-fed dogs by the aldose reductase inhibitor M79175. *J Ocul Pharmacol Ther* 1997;13:517–528.

157. Robison WG Jr, Jacot JL, Glover JP, et al. Diabetic-like retinopathy: early and late intervention therapies in galactose-fed rats. *Invest Ophthalmol Vis Sci* 1998;39:1933–1941.

158. Raptis AE, Viberti G. Pathogenesis of diabetic nephropathy. *Exp Clin Endocrinol Diabetes* 2001;109:S424–S437.

159. Cooper M, Gilbert R, Epstein M. Pathophysiology of diabetic nephropathy. *Metab Clin Exp* 1998;47:3–6.

160. Stribling D, Armstrong FM, Harrison HE. Aldose reductase in the etiology of diabetic complications: 2. Nephropathy. *J Diabetes Complications* 1989;3:70–76.

161. Dunlop M. Aldose reductase and the role of the polyol pathway in diabetic nephropathy. *Kidney Int* 2000;58[Suppl 77]:S3–S12.

162. Oates PJ. Diabetic nephropathy, renal hemodynamics, and aldose reductase inhibitors. *Drug Dev Res* 1994;32:104–116.

163. Keogh RJ, Dunlop ME, Larkins RG. Effect of inhibition of aldose reductase on glucose flux, diacylglycerol formation, protein kinase C, and phospholipase A-2 activation. *Metab Clin Exp* 1997;46:41–47.

164. McCaleb ML, Sredy J, Millen J, et al. Prevention of urinary albumin excretion in 6 month streptozocin-diabetic rats with the aldose reductase inhibitor tolrestat. *J Diabetes Complications* 1988;2:16–18.

165. Beyer-Mears A, Murray FT, Cruz E, et al. Comparison of sorbinil and ponalrestat (Statil) diminution of proteinuria in the BB rat. *Pharmacology* 1992;45:285–291.

166. Jennings PE, Nightingale S, Le Guen C, et al. Prolonged aldose reductase inhibition in chronic peripheral diabetic neuropathy: effects on microangiopathy. *Diabetes Med* 1990;7:63–68.

167. Passariello N, Sepe J, Marrazzo G, et al. Effect of aldose reductase inhibitor (tolrestat) on urinary albumin excretion rate and glomerular filtration rate in IDDM subjects with nephropathy. *Diabetes Care* 1993;16:789–795.

168. Iso K, Tada H, Kuboki K, et al. Long-term effect of epalrestat, an aldose reductase inhibitor, on the development of incipient diabetic nephropathy in type 2 diabetic patients. *J Diabetes Complications* 2001;15:241–244.

169. Pedersen MM, Christiansen JS, Mogensen CE. Reduction of glomerular hyperfiltration in normoalbuminuric IDDM patients by 6 mo of aldose reductase inhibition. *Diabetes* 1991;40:527–531.

170. Zimmet P, Alberti KGMM, Shaw J. Global and societal implications of the diabetes epidemic. *Nature* 2001;114:782–787.

Diabetes and Cardiovascular Disease
edited by Steven P. Marso and David M. Stern
Lippincott Williams & Wilkins, Philadelphia © 2004

5

Peroxisome Proliferator-Activated Receptors and Diabetic Vasculature

Peter J. Little, Duncan J. Topliss, Sunder Mudaliar, and Ronald E. Law

Head, Cell Biology of Diabetes Laboratory, Baker Heart Research Institute, Senior Scientist, Alfred Baker Medical Unit; Associate Professor, Department of Medicine, Monash University, Director, Department of Endocrinology and Diabetes, Alfred Hospital, Melbourne, Victoria, Australia; Staff Physician, Section of Diabetes/Metabolism, Veterans Affairs, San Diego HealthCare System, Assistant Clinical Professor of Medicine; Associate Professor of Medicine, Division of Endocrinology, Diabetes, and Hypertension, David Geffen School of Medicine, University of California, Los Angeles, Los Angeles, California

OVERVIEW AND SCOPE OF CHAPTER

Peroxisome proliferator-activated receptors (PPARs) are ligand-activated heterodimeric transcription factors that belong to the nuclear hormone receptor superfamily (1–3). Similar to the glucocorticoid receptor, the estrogen receptor, the thyroid receptor, and other hormone receptors, the PPARs play a critical role in the regulation of diverse physiologic processes mostly related to energy metabolism, although individual PPARs have distinct effects (4). Of major relevance to diabetes and its vascular complications are actions of PPARs that affect glucose metabolism, lipid oxidation, and adipocyte differentiation. Currently, two classes of medications known to modulate these receptors are available for clinical use: the fibrates, which have been used for several decades in the treatment of lipid disorders but were only recently recognized as PPARα ligands (5), and the thiazolidinediones (TZDs) or glitazones, PPARγ ligands used in the treatment of insulin resistance and the hyperglycemia of non-insulin-dependent (type 2) diabetes mellitus (6).

Dyslipidemia and hyperglycemia, the metabolic hallmarks of diabetes, are now recognized as contributing factors to athero-genesis (7). Conventional drug treatments for hyperglycemia, such as sulfonylureas and biguanides, have appreciable effects in lowering blood glucose levels, but they do not lead to a significant attenuation of cardiovascular disease. Furthermore, there is little evidence of favorable concomitant direct actions of these agents on the cardiovascular system (8), compared with the recent generations of agents for treating blood pressure, such as angiotensin-converting enzyme inhibitors and hypolipidemic drugs (e.g., statins), which have cardioprotective effects (9,10). Evidence is emerging that PPAR ligands have sustained metabolic actions to reduce hyperglycemia and correct diabetic dyslipidemia as well as direct actions to prevent the development of atherosclerosis and therefore, overall, to reduce the burden of cardiovascular disease (11). As such, the discovery of PPARs and the pharmacologic development of small molecules that bind to these receptors (ligands) may represent a turning point in the therapeutic approach to the treatment of diabetes and its complications.

This chapter reviews the role of PPARs and their therapeutic ligands in the development of macrovascular disease in diabetes. Macrovascular disease of the coronary circulation leading to ischemic heart disease is the major cause of death among persons with diabetes (12). We consider the general and diabetes-related factors that affect coronary artery disease and the role of PPARs and therapeutic agents that target these receptors in alleviating this major health burden.

PEROXISOME PROLIFERATOR-ACTIVATED RECEPTORS

Cell Biology and Distribution of PPARs

PPARs are a family of intracellular receptors for endogenous fatty acids (FAs) and FA derivatives (1–3). The initial PPAR (now called PPARα) was cloned and characterized as a novel murine orphan nuclear receptor in 1990 by Isseman and Green (13). Their work was closely followed by the identification of a further two isoforms, PPARβ/δ and PPARγ (14). PPARs are expressed at varying concentrations in a broad array of tissues, where they regulate diverse cellular processes (15). PPARs are highly expressed in metabolic tissues but also, intriguingly, in cardiovascular tissues (16,17). Unlike the majority of clinically important receptors that typically re-

side in the plasma membrane on the cell surface (e.g., insulin receptors, adrenergic receptors, angiotensin II receptors), PPARs exert their activity directly within a cell's nucleus, where they regulate gene transcription (1).

To date, three distinct types of PPARs have been identified: PPARα, PPARβ/δ (termed PPARδ in this chapter), and PPARγ. They are coded by separate genes and have similar protein structures (1,18) but differ with regard to their tissue distribution and function (4,15). PPARs contain multiple domains, including a DNA-binding domain of approximately 70 amino acids that comprises two highly conserved zinc fingers (approximately 85% similar across the group) and a carboxyl-terminal ligand-binding domain of approximately 250 amino acids that is 70% similar among the isoforms. The ligand-binding domain contains dimerization and transcriptional activation domains to give the receptors their function (Fig. 5-1).

PPARα is abundantly expressed in metabolically active tissues such as liver and was originally isolated during an investigation into the mechanism by which fibric acid derivatives such as clofibrate and gemfibrozil modulate lipid

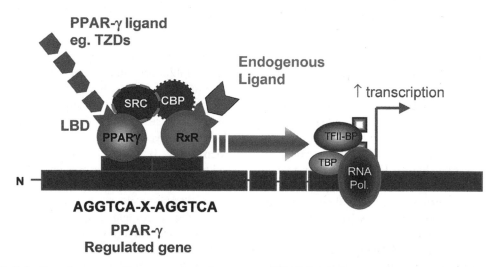

FIG. 5-1. Peroxisome proliferator-activated receptors (PPARs) are ligand-activated transcription factors that modulate the expression of genes associated with energy metabolism. Ligands such as thiazolidinediones (TZDs) bind to the ligand-binding domain of the receptor, leading to the formation of a heterodimeric complex that binds to the DNA-binding domain and alters transcription of genes. See text for details.

levels (3,13). It was found that fibric acid derivatives lead to the proliferation of peroxisomes (metabolic organelles similar in function to mitochondria) in (rat) liver cells through PPARα. Although these agents do not have these actions in human liver, this observation provided the basis for the name "peroxisome proliferator-activated receptor" that persists to this day. PPARα has also been found in skeletal muscle, adipose tissue, kidney, and heart, as well as vascular endothelial cells and smooth muscle cells (15–17). This PPAR isotype is considered to play a central role in the regulation of lipid and lipoprotein metabolism, including cellular uptake and oxidation of FAs. PPARα may also play an important role in suppressing vascular and systemic inflammation and modifying extracellular matrix (16,19). As with all PPARs, the α form is activated by both natural and synthetic molecules; endogenous activators include free fatty acids (FFA), and exogenous agents include fibrates, some TZDs, and phenylacetate and its analogs. The predominant action of PPARα is primarily catabolic, particularly enhancement of the metabolism of lipids.

PPARδ is the most widely distributed PPAR. It has been identified in virtually all tissues of the human body, although its physiologic function and natural ligands are poorly elucidated, compared with those of PPARα and PPARγ (20). Selective PPARδ ligands do not have the effects of PPARα and PPARγ ligands on glucose levels (21), but they may play a role in lipid metabolism, preadipocyte proliferation, macrophage cholesterol homeostasis, embryo implantation, and cell proliferation (3).

PPARγ is expressed abundantly in the intestine and adipose tissue; in skeletal muscle, liver, and heart; and relatively weakly in vascular smooth muscle. PPARγ has an important role in the regulation of adipocyte differentiation and glucose and lipid metabolism. PPARγ levels are highest in adipose tissue and are further increased in obese nondiabetic and type 2 diabetic patients (22). Ligands for PPARγ include FFAs, certain prostaglandin derivatives, nonsteroidal antiinflammatory agents, and the TZDs, pioglitazone and rosiglitazone. The predominant

metabolic effect of PPARγ is to enhance the action of insulin; therefore, it is anabolic.

Mechanism of Action in Regulating Gene Transcription

The activation of PPARs by endogenous ligands and therapeutic agents, although complex, has been the subject of considerable research and is reasonably well understood (23). The ligand first diffuses into the cell, where it binds to a specific site in PPARs designated the ligand-binding domain (Fig. 5-1). To function as a transcription factor, the ligand-PPAR complex must bind to another nuclear receptor, called the retinoid X receptor (RXR), forming a heterodimer. RXR has its own ligands, the retinoids. The PPAR/RXR heterodimeric complex with bound regulatory ligands attaches through its DNA-binding domain to specific DNA sequences in the regulatory (promoter) region of genes. These PPAR-response elements (PPREs) in regulatory regions of DNA consist of a direct repeat of the AGGTCA sequence separated by one or two nucleotides; binding leads to induction or repression of gene expression. Importantly, PPARs can also mediate repression of gene transcription by antagonizing nuclear factor κB (NFκB) and AP-1 signaling pathways through a process that is independent of DNA binding. The definition of the human genome allows the application of bioinformatics to identify genes that may be regulated by these PPREs. In attaching to this site, the ligand-receptor heterodimer either stimulates or inhibits the gene-directed production of specific physiologic enzymes or proteins. It is further possible that PPAR signals may interfere with other gene-based signaling systems to inhibit activity through interrelated signaling pathways (1).

PPARs in Vascular Tissues

PPARα and PPARγ are expressed in vascular tissues and vascular lesions, specifically smooth muscle, endothelial cells, and monocytes/macrophages (16,17,24). Both messenger RNA and protein (i.e., the receptor) have been detected. Although expression is at lower levels than in tissues that are more involved in metabolic regulation, the presence of the receptors allows (but does not prove) the possibility of development of therapeutic agents having actions in tissues associated with cardiovascular disease. The role of PPARs in vascular tissues, and in particular in atherosclerosis and diabetic vascular disease, is discussed later in this chapter.

PHARMACOLOGY OF PPARs RELEVANT TO DIABETES AND ITS VASCULAR COMPLICATIONS

PPARs, Lipid Metabolism, and Dyslipidemia

PPARs have profound effects on energy utilization and storage, particularly in the metabolism of glucose, FAs, and lipids. Ligands for PPARs have a marked effect on metabolic profiles and appear to represent an exciting new area for therapeutic modulation of parameters identified as cardiovascular risk factors. At this time, it is less clear that the underlying disease processes actually relate to perturbation of PPARs function, but this remains to be determined, particularly because endogenous ligands and genetic alterations of these receptors are incompletely understood.

A clear clinical outcome of treatment with PPARα ligands is a reduction in plasma triglycerides and an increase in high-density lipoprotein (HDL) cholesterol resulting from modulation of the expression of the genes regulating those processes (25). Major metabolic genes regulated by PPARα control FA uptake, FA oxidation, and lipoprotein metabolism. The uptake of FFAs and their subsequent esterification in the liver is achieved by PPARα-mediated expression of FA transport protein and acyl-coenzyme A synthase, a major enzyme regulating β-oxidation of FAs. Stimulation of carnitine palmitoyltransferase (CPT-1) in skeletal muscle and heart increases mitochondrial FA uptake and FFA oxidation. Under fasting conditions, PPARα is markedly induced to affect FA degradation and to produce ketone bodies, which serve as energy substrates for extrahepatic tissues. PPARα activity enhances the transcription of the major apolipoproteins of HDL, namely apolipoproteins A-I and A-II, leading directly to an increase

in HDL cholesterol. Triglycerides are carried in the blood in the large lipoproteins, especially very-low-density lipoprotein (VLDL). The potent triglyceride-lowering effects of fibrates are mediated by enhanced lipolysis resulting from increased expression of lipoprotein lipase and reduction of the expression of apolipoprotein C-III (4,26).

Therefore, PPARα ligands, presently the fibrates, have significant and consistent effects in decreasing plasma triglycerides and increasing HDL cholesterol, and these effects arise respectively from stimulation of lipoprotein lipase and induction of the expression of the major HDL apolipoproteins. These beneficial metabolic actions, coupled with potential direct antiatherogenic actions on blood vessels, contribute to an optimism that favorable outcomes may be observed for PPARγ ligands in clinical trials evaluating cardiovascular end points.

PPARγ ligands are highly expressed in adipose tissue, where they promote the differentiation of preadipocytes into mature fat cells (27). PPARγ ligands essentially increase energy storage, and in humans they may lead to an increase in fat mass and body weight. This produces the paradox of increased body weight (normally associated with a worsening of insulin sensitivity) together with the actual outcome in animals and humans, in whom PPARγ ligands produce a clear improvement in insulin sensitivity. The role of fat in diabetes and its vascular complications may be site specific, with visceral fat being associated with coronary heart disease (CHD), but PPARγ-mediated fat deposition may occur primarily in subcutaneous sites (26).

An early change in type 2 diabetes is an elevation of plasma FFAs; this often occurs before significant hyperglycemia is established, and indeed the elevated FFAs may contribute to the insulin-resistant state. Elevated FFAs arise from activated lipolysis in adipocytes. Insulin is antilipolytic because it activates and phosphorylates phosphodiesterase 3B, which then inactivates and dephosphorylates hormone-sensitive lipase activity (28). PPARγ ligands can restore the reduced phosphodiesterase 3B levels and increase the insulin-stimulated activity of that enzyme, leading to reduced lipolysis. The ability of PPARγ ligands to increase the uptake of FFAs and thus divert FFAs from skeletal muscle, where they may play a role in reduced insulin-stimulated glucose uptake and utilization, is thought to be a major pathway by which TZDs improve insulin sensitivity.

Therefore, PPARγ ligands activate a plethora of genes leading to lipid accumulation. These include adipocyte fatty acid binding protein, lipoprotein lipase, fatty acid translocase, fatty acid transport protein, c-Cbl-associated protein (1), and, most recently and importantly, the lipid storage enzyme, glycerol kinase (27).

PPARs and Insulin Resistance

Activation of PPARγ by TZDs selectively mimics or enhances the actions of insulin, increasing insulin-dependent glucose disposal and reducing hepatic glucose production (29). In patients with insulin resistance, this results in improved insulin sensitivity and a lowering of blood glucose levels (29). A close relationship has been shown to exist between the potency of various TZDs in binding to PPARγ and their clinical antidiabetic action. The two PPARγ ligands in clinical use today are rosiglitazone (Avandia) and pioglitazone (Actos) (6). The first clinically available TZD, troglitazone, was withdrawn from clinical use in March 2000 after reports of severe, idiosyncratic hepatotoxicity, including cases of liver transplantation and death. The toxicity of troglitazone appears to have derived from specific toxic metabolites, and therefore the property appears not to be shared by rosiglitazone and pioglitazone (29).

The improvement in cellular insulin response resulting from the administration of TZDs may occur by more than one mechanism. PPARγ is expressed at much higher levels in adipose tissue than in other organs, but it is also present in skeletal muscle. It is likely, but unproven, that activation of PPARγ in both adipose tissue and skeletal muscle contributes to the insulin-sensitizing property of TZDs. The cardinal molecular defect causing insulin resistance occurs in skeletal muscle in the insulin signaling pathway. In insulin-sensitive subjects, engagement of the insulin receptor initiates a multi-step signal emanating from the cell surface that ultimately directs a high-affinity glucose transporter (GLUT4) to move from the cytoplasm to the plasma membrane, where it extracts circulating glucose. Signaling from the insulin receptor to GLUT4 is blunted in insulin-resistant skeletal muscle. TZDs, acting through PPARγ, improve insulin action via this pathway (29).

Release of FFAs and of the cytokine, tumor necrosis factor-α (TNF-α), from adipose tissue has been implicated in the development of acquired insulin resistance. In animal models, PPARγ ligands have been shown to suppress production of FFAs and TNF-α by adipose tissue; to induce expression of adiponectin, an adipocytokine that may function to increase insulin sensitivity; and to increase the number of small adipocytes, which are more efficient than large adipocytes in glucose uptake at submaximal insulin levels (30). PPARγ, therefore, may ameliorate insulin resistance *in vivo* by modifying the expression of adipocyte genes, or by promoting adipocyte differentiation, which then conveys a metabolic or nonmetabolic signal to skeletal muscle that causes improved insulin sensitivity.

Recent data on the induction of glycerol kinase expression in adipocytes by PPARγ ligands provides a major advance in our understanding of the role of these agents in improving insulin sensitivity (27). The major pathway in adipose tissue for the storage of FFAs as triglycerides depends on the glycerol backbone derived from glucose. Rosiglitazone and pioglitazone induce the expression of glycerol kinase in adipocytes, leading to enhanced synthesis and storage of triglycerides and reduced release of FFAs. It is likely that this reduction in FFAs at least partially contributes to the improvement in insulin sensitivity (27). However, it is implicit that the basic action to improve insulin sensitivity through PPARγ is also the mechanism of increased fat mass and therefore underlies the weight-increasing action of these agents (29).

The relative importance of PPARγ expressed in skeletal muscle cells versus adipocytes in improving insulin sensitivity is not fully established. Amelioration of insulin resistance and its metabolic sequelae, however, may protect against the development and progression of atherosclerosis by normalizing diabetic dyslipidemia and other cardiovascular risk factors that are diagnostic of the insulin resistance syndrome and type 2 diabetes.

Direct Vascular Actions of PPAR Ligands

Experimental Studies on Atherosclerosis

PPARα ligands have direct actions on the vasculature that are antiatherogenic, although the contributions of these numerous activities to the clinical outcomes are not fully characterized or appreciated (16,19,31). The atherosclerotic process within a vessel wall is driven by an inflammatory response characterized by the infiltration and proliferation of inflammatory and vascular cells and by changes in the composition and properties of the extracellular matrix (16,32). PPARα ligands have antiinflammatory actions, as evidenced in the PPARα-deficient mouse, which shows a prolonged inflammatory response to inflammatory stimuli. In vascular smooth muscle cells (VSMC) and endothelial cells, fibric acid derivatives inhibit NF-κB and AP-1 proinflammatory signaling induced by interleukins. PPARα activators induce apoptosis of TNF-α-activated macrophages (3).

Vascular proteoglycans are implicated in atherogenesis through regulation of migration and proliferation of VSMC but also through binding and retention of atherogenic lipoproteins (33,34). In a transgenic mouse model with five different human apolipoproteins introduced into a C57BL6 mouse (altering the major lipoprotein component from HDL to LDL), the two isoforms that bind well to proteoglycans cause marked atherosclerosis but the three isoforms that do not bind to proteoglycans do not cause atherosclerosis, and these observations are unrelated to the binding to the LDL receptor (35). PPARα ligands can reduce the synthesis of vascular proteoglycans (19). Gemfibrozil inhibits the synthesis of proteoglycans by human VSMC (19), but more importantly, it leads to shorter glycosaminoglycan (GAG) chains, which in other situations leads to reduced lipoprotein binding (36,37). LDL from patients receiving gemfibrozil treatment also show reduced binding to proteo-

glycans, so PPARα ligands appear to have a dual complimentary role in protecting the vasculature against lipid infiltration (38).

PPARγ is expressed in all of these cell types and in general has been shown to have potentially important antiatherogenic activities of inhibiting vascular cell growth and movement, improving endothelial function, and suppressing vascular inflammatory responses (39,40). PPARγ is present in monocytes/macrophages from mice and humans and is found in macrophage foam cells in atherosclerotic lesions (41,42). Migration of monocytes into the subendothelial space is inhibited by PPARγ ligands (40). In addition, PPARγ ligands inhibit the expression of adhesion molecules on endothelial cells that trap and anchor circulating monocytes to the damaged endothelium (43). Proinflammatory gene expression by macrophages is also markedly suppressed by PPARγ ligands. In combination, these findings suggest that pharmacologic activation of PPARγ may attenuate inflammation and, hence, atherosclerosis in the vessel wall (44).

Equipotent glucose-lowering effects of troglitazone, pioglitazone, and rosiglitazone are achieved at doses that produce blood concentrations ranging from 1 to 2 μM for rosiglitazone (45), from 2 to 3 μM for pioglitazone (46), and up to 10 to 20 μM for troglitazone (47). Many of the direct vascular actions described occur at or above these concentration ranges. Potential beneficial vascular effects may arise from tissue concentration that produces effectively higher local levels than circulating drug concentrations, or from small inhibitory effects over prolonged therapeutic periods that modify vascular pathophysiology, or both. However, these possibilities require characterization in clinical trials.

Mice that have a targeted disruption in their LDL receptor gene (LDL$^{-/-}$ mice) become hypercholesterolemic and develop atherosclerosis in their vessels when they are fed a high-fat, Western-style diet in which more than 40% of the total calories are fat. The high-fat diet also causes the mice to become obese and to develop insulin resistance, hyperinsulinemia, and hyperglycemia. If this strain of mice is fed a diet rich in fructose, rather than fat, cholesterol levels become markedly elevated in the absence of

any weight gain or change in insulin sensitivity or blood glucose. Administration of troglitazone to mice on either diet reduced the amount of atherosclerosis in vessels by 30% to 40% (44). Rosiglitazone and pioglitazone have been shown to be similarly effective in suppressing atherosclerosis in various mouse models of this disease. Decreased atherosclerosis in response to PPARγ ligands was associated with a reduction in the number of macrophages present in the vessel wall and with lower levels of inflammatory markers (44).

Direct activation of PPARγ expressed by vascular cells involving mechanisms unrelated to insulin action, lipid metabolism, or glucose homeostasis may mediate the observed inhibition of atherosclerosis, because PPARγ ligands were equally effective in both insulin-resistant (diabetic) and insulin-sensitive (nondiabetic) mice. Attachment of circulating monocytes to adhesion molecules displayed by an injured endothelium and their subsequent migration into the subendothelial space (where they ingest oxidized lipids to form fatty streaks) are among the earliest events in the pathophysiologic sequelae of atherosclerosis. PPARγ ligands inhibit both of these processes *in vitro,* which may account for the reduced number of macrophages and decreased amount of fatty streaks present in vessels of mice treated with these agents. In humans receiving PPARγ ligands as insulin sensitizers, advanced plaques vulnerable to rupture most likely pose the highest risk for a cardiovascular event. Therefore, inhibition of fatty streak formation in mice by PPARγ ligands may not necessarily translate into cardiovascular protection in humans, and the results of appropriate clinical trails must be awaited to resolve this issue.

Progression of atherosclerosis is marked by the differentiation of subendothelial monocytes/macrophages into lipid-laden foam cells that organize into fatty streaks which mature into advanced plaques (48,49). Levels of PPARγ are low in monocytes but increase markedly as they differentiate into macrophages. Within the organized plaque, macrophages release procoagulant proteins such as tissue factor and secrete matrix metalloproteinases that dissolve the fibrous cap

encasing the lesion, which promotes plaque instability. PPARγ ligands have been shown to inhibit expression of both tissue factor and matrix metalloproteinases by macrophages; these actions may enhance plaque stability and facilitate lysis of clots (50).

Macrophages also regulate lipid deposition into the vessel wall through the activity of reverse cholesterol transport. Both PPARα and PPARγ ligands induce macrophage expression of the adenosine triphosphate (ATP)-binding cassette transporter A1 (ABCA1), a transporter that mediates cholesterol efflux out of the arterial wall into the circulation for its ultimate uptake and metabolism in the liver. Increasing cholesterol efflux constitutes yet another mechanism by which pharmacologic activation of PPARs may exert an antiatherosclerotic effect.

Encapsulation of an atherosclerotic plaque occurs when VSMC proliferate and migrate from the media to the intima (49). Secretion of extracellular matrix proteins by intimal VSMC results in the formation of a protective fibrous cap that entraps thrombogenic extracellular lipids within the plaque core. Activation of VSMC and macrophages causes the release of proinflammatory cytokines, matrix metalloproteinases, and various procoagulant factors. In concert, these proteins promote plaque instability and increase the probability of plaque rupture, subsequent occlusion of blood flow, and myocardial infarction. PPARα ligands potently suppress cytokine expression by VSMC, and PPARγ ligands exert a similar effect in monocytes/macrophages. Expression of matrix metalloproteinases is suppressed by PPARγ ligands, and activators of PPARα inhibit tissue factor expression (50). In combination, these data suggest that pharmacologic activation of PPARs may promote plaque stability and reduce cardiovascular mortality from myocardial infarction.

CLINICAL ASPECTS OF PPARs RELEVANT TO VASCULAR DISEASE

Diabetes and Vascular Disease

People with diabetes have at least a twofold to fourfold enhanced risk for development of CHD

compared with nondiabetic patients (7). Diabetes is an independent risk factor for CHD, and atherosclerotic disease of the coronary circulation is the underlying cause of death for almost 75% of the diabetic population (12). Enhanced macrovascular atherosclerosis similarly leads to elevated ischemic cerebral vascular disease and peripheral vascular disease, resulting in strokes and amputations, respectively (51). The diabetic vasculature can be characterized as being highly "activated," and it responds aggressively to intervention, as evidenced by the markedly accelerated restenosis rates observed after angioplasty when diabetes is present (52,53). The precarious cardiovascular state of persons with diabetes is underscored further by an increased incidence of congestive heart failure and overall postinfarction mortality (54,55). In addition, diabetes is associated with microvascular disease, which leads to nephropathy, retinopathy, neuropathy, and impotence (56). From the perspective of patient morbidity and mortality, it is clear that diabetes is a *(cardio)vascular* disease.

Multiple biochemical mechanisms underlie the accelerated vascular disease caused by the metabolic milieu of diabetes (51). Insulin resistance, defined by a defect in insulin-stimulated glucose uptake into skeletal muscle, is the chief pathologic factor in the development of type 2 diabetes, with later loss of beta-cell function contributing to the progressive nature of the disease (57). Patients with impaired glucose tolerance are at high risk for development of type 2 diabetes (58). The impaired glucose tolerance state is characterized by insulin resistance, and even in the absence of sustained hyperglycemia, persons with impaired glucose tolerance have increased risk for coronary artery disease (58). Insulin resistance, therefore, has emerged as a leading factor associated with the development and progression of atherosclerosis. Consistent with this scenario are recent data from the Insulin Resistance and Atherosclerosis Study (IRAS) identifying insulin resistance as an independent risk factor for coronary artery disease (59).

Insulin resistance frequently cosegregates with other factors that independently increase the risk for coronary artery disease: obesity, hypertension, high triglyceride levels and low HDL cholesterol levels, increased concentration of small dense LDL cholesterol (which has increased propensity for oxidation and is more proatherogenic), and increased levels of plasminogen activator inhibitor-1 (PAI-1). Persons with type 2 diabetes or poorly controlled insulin-dependent (type 1) diabetes frequently have a dyslipidemia similar to that described earlier, and many have hypertension (60).

PPARs have emerged as promising targets for pharmacologic interventions directed at protecting the diabetic vasculature (2,40). Activation of PPARγ may be beneficial by ameliorating insulin resistance and thereby reducing the risk for atherosclerosis (61). PPARα, through its important role in regulating lipid metabolism, may afford complementary vascular protection by improving the dyslipidemia commonly associated with diabetes (62,63).

Based on data from the Diabetes Complications and Control Trial (DCCT) (64,65) and the more recent United Kingdom Diabetes Prospective Study (UKPDS) (66), microvascular complications of people with diabetes may be attenuated most effectively by maintaining tight glycemic control. By improving insulin action in peripheral tissues and facilitating glucose disposal, leading to lower hemoglobin A_1C levels, TZDs and future drugs that activate PPARγ may prove effective in limiting nephropathy, retinopathy, and other microvascular complications of diabetes (67).

Normalization of diabetes-associated metabolic abnormalities through PPARs expressed in skeletal muscle, adipose tissue, and liver can indirectly lead to a healthier vasculature in persons with diabetes. PPARs are also found in most vascular cells present in the vessel wall, kidney, eye, and other tissues. Direct activation of PPARs expressed in the vasculature and the resultant physiologic effects provide another layer of mechanisms that may importantly affect the macrovascular and microvascular complications of diabetes.

Diabetes and Atherosclerosis

Atherosclerosis is a progressive vascular disease that is initiated by the trapping and retention of

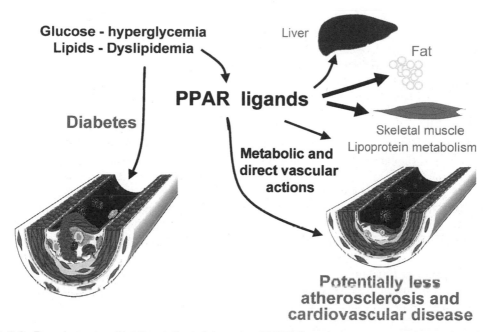

FIG. 5-2. Peroxisome proliferator-activated receptor (PPAR) ligands may prevent atherosclerosis and cardiovascular disease. PPAR ligands such as fibrates for PPARα and thiazolidinediones for PPARγ have metabolic actions to correct the dysmetabolic profile of diabetes, but they may also have direct vascular actions to prevent the development or progression of atherosclerosis. Therefore, target tissues include the major metabolic organs, lipoprotein metabolism, and the vasculature.

LDL cholesterol by proteoglycans, which results in the accumulation of cholesterol in the subintimal space (33,35). This leads to endothelial cell activation and the recruitment of circulating monocytes and T lymphocytes into the subendothelial space. These trapped monocytes then differentiate into macrophages and form foam cells after taking up oxidized LDL. With further disease progression, VSMC proliferate and migrate from the media to the intima and cause the formation of a fibrous cap. This cap encloses a lipid-rich necrotic core formed by the destruction of the foam cells (49). Further activation of the VSMC leads to secretion of proinflammatory cytokines, matrix metalloproteinases, and procoagulant factors, resulting in instability of the fibrous cap (Fig. 5-2) (68). Ultimately, the plaque ruptures, and resultant thrombosis and acute occlusion lead to myocardial infarction or stroke. Because cardiovascular events resulting from underlying atherosclerotic disease account for 75% of the mortality in the type 2 diabetic population,

it is critical to determine the impact of PPARγ-based pharmacology on plaques vulnerable to rupture.

PPARα LIGANDS AS THERAPEUTIC AGENTS

Metabolic Effects Relevant to Vascular Disease

It is clear from epidemiologic data that increased LDL cholesterol, elevated plasma triglycerides, and low HDL cholesterol are important risk factors for coronary artery disease (51,69). PPAR ligands are now known to be key regulators of lipid metabolism and thus potential modifiers of cardiovascular risk. Although the initial clinical studies of fibrates (now known to be PPARα ligands) and cardiovascular risk between 1966 and 1996 showed no benefits, several more recent studies, particularly the Veterans Affairs High-Density Lipoprotein Intervention Trial (VA-HIT) and the Bezafibrate Infarction Prevention Trial (BIP), showed that these agents improve the metabolic profile and reduce cardiovascular disease (62,70). Fibrates decrease plasma triglycerides and increase HDL cholesterol, leading to reduced cardiovascular disease. However, recent experimental studies have also pointed to the potential role of direct vascular actions in contributing to these favorable clinical outcomes (19,71), and such actions should be considered in a similar light to the better established pleiotropic actions of the statin family of cholesterol-lowering agents (10). The beneficial effect of high HDL cholesterol most likely is mediated through enhanced efflux of cholesterol from normal peripheral tissues, but also possibly from lipid-laden macrophages (foam cells) in atherosclerotic lesions, a process known as "reverse cholesterol transport." The efflux of cholesterol is mediated by the recently identified transporter, ABCA1, in an apolipoprotein A1 ([apo] A1)-dependent manner (72). HDL cholesterol esters are cleared from the circulation by uptake into the liver or transfer to VLDL and LDL particles, and ultimately excess cholesterol is cleared through excretion by the liver into bile (72,73).

The target genes of activated PPARα are mostly associated with catabolism and are specifically those associated with lipoprotein metabolism and FA uptake and oxidation (23). PPARα is principally associated with the metabolism of triglyceride-rich lipoproteins through an action mediated by increased activity of lipoprotein lipase and inhibition of apolipoprotein C-III expression (74). For example, large dietary-derived lipoproteins (chylomicrons) interact with the endothelium of muscle and fat tissues, and lipoprotein lipase activates metabolism of the triglyceride, leading to loss of triglyceride and the formation of chylomicron remnants. PPARα activation also leads to an increase in HDL cholesterol. This action derives from increased expression of the major apolipoproteins of HDL, apolipoproteins A-I and A-II. PPARα increases mitochondrial FA uptake and FA oxidation through stimulation of muscle-type CPT-1 in skeletal and cardiac muscle. Some recent evidence from animal and human studies suggests that PPARα ligands may improve glu-

cose homeostasis; however, in this case it is worth noting that the PPARα therapeutic agents are of very low affinity, and at the high doses used there is some possibility of crossover effects (i.e., to PPARγ).

Clinical Trial Results with PPARα Ligands

Early clinical trials often had diabetes as an exclusion criterion or overlooked the presence of diabetes, so results in this important area were slow to emerge. Furthermore, some early trials were often negative insofar as the potential cardioprotective role of PPARα ligands was concerned (62). More recent trials with end points of angiographic progression or major cardiovascular events have concluded with positive evidence of beneficial effects (62). Trials have been designed to focus on cardiovascular risk factors but also on easily measurable biomarkers such as LDL cholesterol, HDL cholesterol, or triglycerides. Although less well established than for the statins, there is support for the possibility that fibrates may also have direct vascular actions that contribute to favorable outcomes (18,71).

The Helsinki Heart Study was a large, randomized, double-blind trial that evaluated the effect of simultaneous elevation of HDL cholesterol and lowering of non-HDL cholesterol with gemfibrozil on the risk of CHD in 4,081 asymptomatic middle-aged men (75). After 5 years of treatment with gemfibrozil, the metabolic profile showed the expected improvements (11% increase in HDL cholesterol, 35% decrease in triglycerides, and 11% decrease in LDL cholesterol), and these were associated with a marked and significant reduction of 34% in nonfatal myocardial infarctions and CHD deaths. Similarly, the VA-HIT study used gemfibrozil in subjects in a high-risk group with known coronary artery disease but without elevated LDL cholesterol, the primary atherogenic lipoprotein (70,76). At 5.1 years, triglycerides were 31% lower and HDL cholesterol 6% higher in the gemfibrozil-treated group, and there was a significantly favorable outcome of a 22% reduction in nonfatal myocardial infarctions and deaths from coronary artery disease (70). The authors focused exclusively on the role of the lipid changes in determining the favorable outcome, but others have speculated on the contribution of direct vascular actions (18,19).

Three large studies have examined PPARα ligands with angiographic end points. The Bezafibrate Coronary Atherosclerosis Intervention Trial (BECAIT) examined the effect of bezafibrate therapy in a relatively small number of subjects (81 young male survivors of a myocardial infarction) in a randomized, placebo-controlled protocol (77). Bezafibrate therapy was associated with an appreciable and significant reduction in the extent of narrowing of segmental lesions that compromised 20% to 50% of the coronary lumen; although CHD events were not a formal end point, they were fewer in the treated group (77). The Lipid Coronary Angiography Trial (LOCAT) using gemfibrozil showed beneficial effects in a large group of 372 men who had undergone coronary artery bypass grafting (78). The only completed study to focus on type 2 diabetes was the Diabetes Atherosclerosis Intervention Study (DAIS) (63,79). A group of 418 subjects with type 2 diabetes (305 men and 113 women) were randomly assigned to treatment with fenofibrate or placebo to test the hypothesis that a correction in diabetic dyslipidemia would decrease the progression of coronary disease assessed angiographically. Fenofibrate treatment for 3 years produced a 7% decrease in LDL cholesterol, a 6% increase in HDL cholesterol, and a 29% decrease in triglycerides, compared with placebo. These results were very similar to the effects observed in the other studies described. Fenofibrate treatment was associated with a significant decrease in the progression of coronary narrowing by 40%. Therefore, there is convincing evidence that PPARα ligands, or at least gemfibrozil and fenofibrate, play a significant role in elevating CHD, particularly in patients with diabetes and the dysmetabolic lipid profile.

Numerous trials with PPARα ligands are presently underway. Unfortunately, a recent trial in diabetics of fenofibrate and the 3-hydroxy-3-methylglutaryl (HMG)-coenzyme A reductase inhibitor, cerivastatin, the Lipids in Diabetes Study (LDS), was halted because of toxicity (5). The Fenofibrate Intervention Event Lowering in Diabetes (FIELD) trial is presently being conducted in Finland, Australia, and New Zealand and will conclude in 2004–2005; it evaluates the effect of fenofibrate on coronary events in people with diabetes (5). All of these trials will add to our understanding of the range of benefits available from PPARα agents.

PPARγ LIGANDS AS THERAPEUTIC AGENTS

Metabolic Effects Related to Vascular Disease

The primary metabolic role of PPARγ is in the regulation of glucose homeostasis, with additional activity as a modulator of lipid metabolism and metabolic actions; this fact must be considered in light of those effects that derive from the correction of insulin resistance in type 2 diabetes. PPARγ is associated with diabetes by an unknown molecular mechanism that increases insulin sensitivity of diabetes-dependent tissues; PPARγ therefore reverses the particular and specific metabolic defects of diabetes and directly addresses the central metabolic issue, providing the potential for long-term management of this disease. The role of hyperglycemia as a cardiovascular risk factor has been controversial. The UKPDS showed a reduction in cardiovascular disease that did not reach statistical significance (80). However, this finding was based on the intensively treated group's having markedly increasing hyperglycemia over the course of the study, making the drawing of definitive conclusions problematic. Indeed, PPARγ ligands now provide a potential pathway to address the role of glucose in macrovascular disease through long-term maintenance and improvement in insulin sensitivity and consequently reduced hyperglycemia. The effects of hyperglycemia in microvascular complications are much more definite, and PPARγ ligands have a clear role in that situation. Because currently available PPARγ ligands may also show PPARα activity, cross-reactivity must be considered until more specific agents become available.

PPARγ plays a crucial anabolic role in energy storage and glucose homeostasis. PPARγ ligands produce a clear increase in insulin sensitivity and thus a reduction in hyperinsulinemia and hyperglycemia. Reductions of 1% to 1.5% in hemoglobin A_{1C} levels are typical of the effects observed. Multiple techniques for assessing insulin activity have been used to demonstrate the role of PPARγ ligands, including euglycemic clamp, frequently sampled intravenous or oral glucose tolerance tests, and less direct methods such as insulin tolerance tests and intravenous or oral glucose tolerance tests. The first clinical TZD PPARγ ligand, troglitazone, produced improvement in peripheral insulin action in patients with type 2 diabetes but also in other insulin resistance states, such as impaired glucose tolerance, polycystic ovary disease, and previous gestational diabetes (67).

The therapeutic ligands for PPARγ were first described in the early 1980s (81). TZDs or glitazones show a close relationship between their PPARγ ligand activity and antidiabetic actions, although this relationship is not always present (82). TZDs have been shown to favorably influence the expression of genes involved in glucose metabolism, including GLUT1, GLUT4, leptin, TNF-α, and hepatic glucokinase. Therefore, although the critical steps are unknown, relevant actions include increased glucose transporter activity leading to increased glucose uptake, activation of hepatic glucokinase and increased glucose consumption, and decreased phosphoenolpyruvate carboxykinase activity to decrease gluconeogenesis.

Like PPARα, PPARγ also plays a role in lipid metabolism. The main effect of PPARγ is in influencing the storage of FAs in adipose tissue. PPARγ, along with the C/EBP transcription factors, is part of the adipocyte differentiation program leading to the maturation of preadipocytes into fat cells. Overexpression of PPARγ in fibroblasts can direct their differentiation into an adipocyte-like phenotype (83). In the context of currently accepted models, such action would be proatherogenic. PPARγ ligands have the potential to redress the dyslipidemic profile of diabetes, which is characterized by increased hypertriglyceridemia, increased LDL cholesterol, decreased HDL cholesterol, and changes in the composition of the lipoprotein particles to a small dense form (which is more prone to oxidation and glycation and possibly more atherogenic due to greater penetration and retention in the vessel wall). There are data to suggest that TZD treatment is associated with a change in LDL particle size to one that is more buoyant and less prone to oxidation (84).

Clinical Trial Results with PPARγ Ligands

PPARγ ligands, the TZDs, have been available for clinical use only since 1999, so there are no long-term clinical trials with cardiovascular end points, as there are for PPARα (67). Clinical trials with PPARγ ligands are currently in progress. At this time, we must principally consider the effects of TZDs on well-recognized surrogate end points and emerging cardiovascular risk factors.

Diabetes is associated with a wide variety of cardiovascular risk factors that have their origin in insulin resistance. These include diabetic glucose intolerance, hyperinsulinemia, dyslipidemia, hypertension, hypercoagulability, central obesity, and low-grade inflammation; other related factors include impaired endothelial function and thrombogenicity associated with plaque rupture (85). The distinct advantage and therapeutic potential of PPARγ ligands lies in their targeting of insulin resistance and the consequent possibility that they may fully or partially alleviate the spectrum of diabetes-associated cardiovascular risk factors. The discovery of PPARγ ligands has in itself contributed appreciably to our understanding of insulin resistance.

The primary result of insulin resistance, hyperglycemia, arises from decreased glucose clearance and increased hepatic glucose production (85). Glitazones regulate genes leading to increased insulin sensitivity and subsequently to decreased plasma glucose, decreased glucose production, and increased glucose clearance (67). Glitazone treatment reduces fasting plasma glucose by 2 to 3 mM and hemoglobin A_{1C} by 0.6% to 0.7%, with possible effects as great as a 1.5% reduction in drug-naive or highly responsive subjects. The effects of rosiglitazone and pioglitazone on reducing hemoglobin A_{1C} levels are equivalent (25). Glitazones are also additive with the hypoglycemic actions of metformin, sulfonylureas, and insulin (86). The licenses for the use of these drugs are presently restricted; in most countries where the agents are available, only pioglitazone is licensed and recommended for use with insulin therapy. The hypoglycemic actions of rosiglitazone and pioglitazone take 6 to 14 weeks to reach their maximum hypoglycemic effect, and the effect is maintained for 2 years or possibly even longer (87). Unlike in animal studies, the effects of TZDs result in partial, not complete, resolution of the underlying insulin resistance. TZD treatment results in an improvement in insulin-stimulated glucose disposal of 20% to 40% in human insulin resistance states; therefore, even after treatment with the currently available agents, significant cardiovascular risk persists.

Rosiglitazone and pioglitazone raise HDL cholesterol levels and decrease FFAs (86). Only pioglitazone lowers triglyceride levels, and this may be due to an effect mediated via PPARα (86). In some studies, TZDs have been reported to raise LDL cholesterol levels. The potentially proatherogenic effects of raising LDL cholesterol are somewhat controversial, being relatively modest. The effects of increased LDL cholesterol are probably mitigated by alterations in the properties of the LDL: glitazone therapy may reverse the transition to small dense LDL particles that is present in the diabetic condition, and it may also raise the threshold for susceptibility to oxidation. However, the impact of these lipid changes on cardiovascular outcome remains speculative at this stage (51,84). Glitazones may regulate coagulation through a reduction in circulating PAI-1 levels, although the role of PAI-1 in vascular disease, and in particular in regard to the stability of atherosclerotic plaques, remains unclear (85).

Glitazones may also lead to an increase in body mass, which may be fat or fluid. The increased weight associated with fat is due to an increase in subcutaneous fat, not the visceral fat that represents a cardiovascular risk factor. Increased patient weight associated with fluid retention requires monitoring for heart failure and dilutional anemia.

The only clinical studies with cardiovascular end points have used carotid intimal medial thickness as a surrogate end point. Although intimal medial thickness represents a measure of the progression of atherosclerosis, much more sensitive issues such as plaque stability must be considered. In a study of 135 subjects with diabetes, troglitazone (400 mg/day) reduced the intimal and medial thickening in carotid arteries by 0.08 mm, compared with an increase of 0.03 mm in the control group over the same 3-month period; similar results were obtained with pioglitazone (88,89). In a further study of vascular extension within a stented coronary artery, essentially a study of VSMC proliferation, intravascular ultrasound examinations performed at baseline and at 6-month follow-up in patients with diabetes who were treated with oral troglitazone showed a statistically significant reduction in neointimal tissue mass (90). These human studies, taken along with animal studies showing reduced lipid deposition, raise the possibility that TZDs may lead the way to the development of agents that can significantly improve cardiovascular risk factors and act directly on the vascular pathophysiology of diabetes to ultimately reduce or delay the development of life-threatening complications (Fig. 5-2).

FUTURE ISSUES AND PROSPECTS

The discovery of PPARs and the recognition of therapeutic agents that interact with these receptors are rapidly and greatly expanding our knowledge and understanding of the physiology and pathophysiology of carbohydrate and lipid metabolism. This new input is extremely timely, because diseases derived from abnormalities in this area are occurring at epidemic proportions and are increasing with no respite in sight in developed countries (91). Although diet and lifestyle changes based on exercise and perhaps light weight training (92) are obviously the first line of a corrective response and are of demonstrable efficacy, resistance to the adoption of these changes appears so intransigent that there is little hope of reversing the expanding burden of disease through this approach, at least in the medium term. An expanded knowledge of the metabolic changes leading to cardiovascular disease may lead to therapeutic options but also to more targeted and therefore more successful application of lifestyle modifications.

Recent advances in medicinal chemistry have produced very specific and active PPARα agents that may be potentially exploited therapeutically (93). Interestingly, the effects of several PPARα ligands on metabolic dyslipidemia are very similar, suggesting that a maximum effect may have been reached (62); relative to the newer PPARγ ligands, the PPARα agents available are from earlier generations and have very low potency. It would be interesting to determine the effects of potent PPARα ligands in humans. One agent, the ureidofibrate GW 9578, was shown to prevent hyperinsulinemia in rodent models of insulin resistance. Because GW9578 is a highly potent PPARα ligand, it is unlikely that its effect was mediated through PPARγ (92). There may be a PPARα pathway, distinct from a PPARγ mechanism, that is capable of improving insulin sensitivity in patients with diabetes. Furthermore, in addition to effects on lipid and glucose metabolism, better direct vascular actions via PPARα may be achievable with more potent agents, with greater clinical benefit attained.

A vast array of PPARγ agents have been developed, and at least several will attain clinical status, providing a wealth of knowledge on their full utility as well as further insights into the disease process. Because the hepatotoxicity of troglitazone is not exhibited by rosiglitazone and pioglitazone, it would appear not to be a class effect; therefore, it is highly likely that a variety of new PPARγ agents will become available in the near future.

Clearly, the current development and application of combined PPARα/γ ligands with the potential to exploit the beneficial properties of each isoform in reducing triglyceride levels and increasing LDL cholesterol while at the same time directly improving insulin sensitivity, if not an overly complicated strategy, may well lead to very effective agents.

The overall increase in experimental and clinical work that has resulted from the discovery of PPARs and their therapeutically active ligands has provided tools and opportunities to enhance our knowledge of the relationship between metabolism and vascular disease. The likely outcome is that this knowledge and its practical derivatives will lead to a reduction in the increasing burden of cardiovascular disease in persons with diabetes.

ACKNOWLEDGMENTS

P.J.L. acknowledges funding from the Alfred Hospital Foundation, an Eli Lilly Pty Ltd (Australia) Endocrinology Research Grant, Diabetes Australia Research Trust grant-in-aid, and National Health and Medical Research Council Block Institute funding to the Baker Institute for the funding of research in the author's laboratory referred to in this chapter.

REFERENCES

1. Guan Y, Breyer MD. Peroxisome proliferator-activated receptors (PPARs): novel therapeutic targets in renal disease. *Kidney Int* 2001;60:14–30.
2. Kliewer SA, Xu HE, Lambert MH, et al. Peroxisome proliferator-activated receptors: from genes to physiology. *Recent Prog Horm Res* 2001;56:239–263.
3. Duval C, Chinetti G, Trottein F, et al. The role of PPARs in atherosclerosis. *Trends Mol Med* 2002;8:422.
4. Auwerx J, Schoonjans K, Fruchart JC, et al. Regulation of triglyceride metabolism by PPARs: fibrates and thiazolidinediones have distinct effects. *J Atheroscler Thromb* 1996;3:81–89.
5. Betteridge DJ, Colhoun H, Armitage J. Status report of lipid-lowering trials in diabetes. *Curr Opin Lipidol* 2000;11:621–626.
6. Fujiwara T, Horikoshi H. Troglitazone and related compounds: therapeutic potential beyond diabetes. *Life Sci* 2000;67:2405–2416.
7. Bierman EL. George Lyman Duff Memorial Lecture: Atherogenesis in diabetes. *Arterioscler Thromb* 1992; 12:647–656.
8. McVeigh GE, Brennan GM, Johnson GD, et al. Impaired endothelium-dependent and independent vasodilation in patients with type 2 (non-insulin-dependent) diabetes mellitus. *Diabetologia* 1992;35:771–776.
9. Yusuf S, Sleight P, Pogue J, et al. Effects of an angiotensin-converting-enzyme inhibitor, ramipril, on cardiovascular events in high-risk patients. The Heart Outcomes Prevention Evaluation Study Investigators. *N Engl J Med* 2000;342:145–153.
10. Gotto AM Jr, Farmer JA. Pleiotropic effects of statins: do they matter? *Curr Opin Lipidol* 2001;12:391–394.
11. Kelly DP. The pleiotropic nature of the vascular PPAR gene regulatory pathway. *Circ Res* 2001;89:935–937.
12. Pyorala K, Laakso M, Uusitupa M. Diabetes and atherosclerosis: an epidemiologic view. *Diabetes Metab Rev* 1987;3:463–524.

13. Issemann I, Green S. Activation of a member of the steroid hormone receptor superfamily by peroxisome proliferators. *Nature* 1990;347:645–650.

14. Dreyer C, Krey G, Keller H, et al. Control of the peroxisomal beta-oxidation pathway by a novel family of nuclear hormone receptors. *Cell* 1992;68:879–887.

15. Braissant O, Foufelle F, Scotto C, et al. Differential expression of peroxisome proliferator-activated receptors (PPARs): tissue distribution of PPAR-alpha, -beta, and -gamma in the adult rat. *Endocrinology* 1996;137:354–366.

16. Staels B, Koenig W, Habib A, et al. Activation of human aortic smooth-muscle cells is inhibited by PPARalpha but not by PPARgamma activators. *Nature* 1998;393:790–793.

17. Law RE, Meehan WP, Xi XP, et al. Troglitazone inhibits vascular smooth muscle cell growth and intimal hyperplasia. *J Clin Invest* 1996;98:1897–1905.

18. Neve BP, Fruchart J, Staels B. Role of the peroxisome proliferator-activated receptors (PPAR) in atherosclerosis. *Biochem Pharmacol* 2000;60:1245–1250.

19. Nigro J, Dilley RJ, Little PJ. Differential effects of gemfibrozil on migration, proliferation and proteoglycan production in human vascular smooth muscle cells. *Atherosclerosis* 2002;162:119–129.

20. Forman BM, Chen J, Evans RM. Hypolipidemic drugs, polyunsaturated fatty acids, and eicosanoids are ligands for peroxisome proliferator-activated receptors alpha and delta. *Proc Natl Acad Sci U S A* 1997;94:4312–4317.

21. Berger J, Leibowitz MD, Doebber TW, et al. Novel peroxisome proliferator activated receptor (PPAR) gamma and PPARdelta ligands produce distinct biological effects. *J Biol Chem* 1999;274:6718–6725.

22. Hotta K, Gustafson TA, Yoshioka S, et al. Relationships of PPARgamma and PPARgamma2 mRNA levels to obesity, diabetes and hyperinsulinaemia in rhesus monkeys. *Int J Obes Relat Metab Disord* 1998;22:1000–1010.

23. Torra IP, Chinetti G, Duval C, et al. Peroxisome proliferator-activated receptors: from transcriptional control to clinical practice. *Curr Opin Lipidol* 2001;12:245–254.

24. Plutzky J. Peroxisome proliferator-activated receptors in endothelial cell biology. *Curr Opin Lipidol* 2001; 12:511–518.

25. Boyle PJ, King AB, Olansky L, et al. Effects of pioglitazone and rosiglitazone on blood lipid levels and glycemic control in patients with type 2 diabetes mellitus: a retrospective review of randomly selected medical records. *Clin Ther* 2002;24:378–396.

26. Lefebvre AM, Laville M, Vega N, et al. Depot-specific differences in adipose tissue gene expression in lean and obese subjects. *Diabetes* 1998;47:98–103.

27. Guan HP, Li Y, Jensen MV, et al. A futile metabolic cycle activated in adipocytes by antidiabetic agents. *Nat Med* 2002;8:1122–1128.

28. Carey GB. Mechanisms regulating adipocyte lipolysis. *Adv Exp Med Biol* 1998;441:157–170.

29. Stumvoll M, Haring HU. Glitazones: clinical effects and molecular mechanisms. *Ann Med* 2002;34:217–224.

30. DiGirolamo M, Owens JL. Glucose metabolism in isolated fat cells: enhanced response of larger adipocytes from older rats to epinephrine and adrenocorticotropin. *Horm Metab Res* 1976;8:445–451.

31. Munro E, Patel M, Chan P, et al. Growth inhibition of human vascular smooth muscle cells by fenofibrate: a possible therapy for restenosis. *Cardiovasc Res* 1994;28:615–620.

32. Saito I, Folsom AR, Brancati FL, et al. Nontraditional risk factors for coronary heart disease incidence among persons with diabetes: the Atherosclerosis Risk in Communities (ARIC) Study. *Ann Intern Med* 2000;133:81–91.

33. Williams KJ, Tabas I. The response-to-retention hypothesis of early atherogenesis. *Arterioscler Thromb Vasc Biol* 1995;15:551–561.

34. Wight TN. The extracellular matrix and atherosclerosis. *Curr Opin Lipidol* 1995;6:326–334.

35. Skalen K, Gustafsson M, Rydberg EK, et al. Subendothelial retention of atherogenic lipoproteins in early atherosclerosis. *Nature* 2002;417:750–754.

36. Vijayagopal P, Subramaniam P. Effect of calcium channel blockers on proteoglycan synthesis by vascular smooth muscle cells and low density lipoprotein-proteoglycan interaction. *Atherosclerosis* 2001;157:353–560.

37. Tannock L, Little PJ, Wight TN, et al. Arterial smooth muscle cell proteoglycans synthesized in the presence of glucosamine demonstrate reduced binding to LDL. *J Lipid Research* 2002;43:149–157.

38. Wiklund O, Bondjers G, Wright I, et al. Insoluble complex formation between LDL and arterial proteoglycans in relation to serum lipid levels and effects of lipid lowering drugs. *Atherosclerosis* 1996;119:57–67.

39. Buchan KW, Hassall DG. PPAR agonists as direct modulators of the vessel wall in cardiovascular disease. *Med Res Rev* 2000;20:350–366.

40. Hsueh WA, Law RE. PPARgamma and atherosclerosis: effects on cell growth and movement. *Arterioscler Thromb Vasc Biol* 2001;21:1891–1895.

41. Ricote M, Huang J, Fajas L, et al. Expression of the peroxisome proliferator-activated receptor gamma (PPARgamma) in human atherosclerosis and regulation in macrophages by colony stimulating factors and oxidized low density lipoprotein. *Proc Natl Acad Sci U S A* 1998;95:7614–7619.

42. Marx N, Sukhova G, Murphy C, et al. Macrophages in human atheroma contain PPARgamma: differentiation-dependent peroxisomal proliferator-activated receptor gamma(PPARgamma) expression and reduction of MMP-9 activity through PPARgamma activation in mononuclear phagocytes in vitro. *Am J Pathol* 1998; 153:17–23.

43. Marx N, Bourcier T, Sukhova GK, et al. PPARgamma activation in human endothelial cells increases plasminogen activator inhibitor type-1 expression: PPARgamma as a potential mediator in vascular disease. *Arterioscler Thromb Vasc Biol* 1999;19:546–551.

44. Collins AR, Meehan WP, Kintscher U, et al. Troglitazone inhibits formation of early atherosclerotic lesions in diabetic and nondiabetic low density lipoprotein receptor-deficient mice. *Arterioscler Thromb Vasc Biol* 2001;21:365–371.

45. Cox PJ, Ryan DA, Hollis FJ, et al. Absorption, disposition, and metabolism of rosiglitazone, a potent thiazolidinedione insulin sensitizer, in humans. *Drug Metab Dispos* 2000;28:772–780.

46. Eckland D, Danhof M. Clinical pharmacokinetics of pioglitazone. *Exp Clin Endocrinol Diabetes* 2000;108[Suppl 2]:S234–S242.

47. Loi CM, Young M, Randinitis E, et al. Clinical pharmacokinetics of troglitazone. *Clin Pharmacokinet* 1999; 37:91–104.

48. Beckman JA, Creager MA, Libby P. Diabetes and atherosclerosis: epidemiology, pathophysiology, and management. *AMA* 2002;287:2570–2581.

49. Ross R. The pathogenesis of atherosclerosis: a perspective for the 1990s. *Nature* 1993;362:801–809.

50. Eligini S, Banfi C, Brambilla M, et al. 15-deoxy-delta12,14-Prostaglandin J2 inhibits tissue factor expression in human macrophages and endothelial cells: evidence for ERK1/2 signaling pathway blockade. *Thromb Haemost* 2002;88:524–532.

51. Chait A, Bierman E. In: Kahn CR and Weir GC, eds. *Joslin's diabetes mellitus.* Philadelphia: Lea & Febiger, 1994:648–664.

52. Kornowski R, Mintz GS, Kent KM, et al. Increased restenosis in diabetes mellitus after coronary interventions is due to exaggerated intimal hyperplasia. *Circulation* 1997;95:1366–1369.

53. Przewlocki T, Pieniazek P, Ryniewicz W, et al. Long-term outcome of coronary balloon angioplasty in diabetic patients. *Int J Cardiol* 2000;76:7–16.

54. Wilson PW. Diabetes mellitus and coronary heart disease. *Am J Kidney Dis* 1998;32:S89–S100.

55. Spector KS. Diabetic cardiomyopathy. *Clin Cardiol* 1998;21:885–887.

56. Stratton IM, Adler AI, Neil HA, et al. Association of glycaemia with macrovascular and microvascular complications of type 2 diabetes (UKPDS 35): prospective observational study. *BMJ* 2000;321:405–412.

57. Alberti KG. Treating type 2 diabetes: today's targets, tomorrow's goals. *Diabetes Obes Metab* 2001;3[Suppl 1]:S3–S10.

58. Laakso M, Lehto S. Epidemiology of risk factors for cardiovascular disease in diabetes and impaired glucose tolerance. *Atherosclerosis* 1998;137:S65–S73.

59. Howard G, O'Leary DH, Zaccaro D, et al. Insulin sensitivity and atherosclerosis: the Insulin Resistance Atherosclerosis Study (IRAS) investigators. *Circulation* 1996;93:1809–1817.

60. Sowers JR, Epstein M, Frohlich ED. Diabetes, hypertension, and cardiovascular disease: an update. *Hypertension* 2001;37:1053–1059.

61. Lebovitz HE, Banerji MA. Insulin resistance and its treatment by thiazolidinediones. *Recent Prog Horm Res* 2001;56:265–294.

62. Faergeman O. Hypertriglyceridemia and the fibrate trials. *Curr Opin Lipidol* 2000;11:609–614.

63. Barter P. Anti-atherogenic effects of fibrates in type 2 diabetes. *Curr Control Trials Cardiovasc Med* 2001;2:218–220.

64. Diabetes Complications and Control Trial. The effect of intensive treatment of diabetes on the development and progression of long-term complications in insulin-dependent diabetes. *N Engl J Med* 1993;329:977–986.

65. Diabetes Complications and Control Trial. The absence of a glycemic threshold for the development of long-term complications: the perspective of the Diabetes Control and Complications Trial. *Diabetes* 1996;45:1289–1298.

66. U.K Prospective Diabetes Study (UKPDS) Group. Intensive blood-glucose control with sulphonylureas or insulin compared with conventional treatment and risk of complications in patients with type 2 diabetes (UKPDS 33). *Lancet* 1998;352:837–853.

67. Komers R, Vrana A. Thiazolidinediones: tools for the research of metabolic syndrome X. *Physiol Rev* 1998; 47:215–225.

68. Ross R. Atherosclerosis: an inflammatory disease. *N Engl J Med* 1999;340:115–126.

69. Williams MA, Fleg JL, Ades PA, et al. Secondary prevention of coronary heart disease in the elderly (with emphasis on patients ≥75 years of age): an American Heart Association scientific statement from the Council on Clinical Cardiology Subcommittee on Exercise, Cardiac Rehabilitation, and Prevention. *Circulation* 2002;105:1735–1743.

70. Rubins HB, Robins SJ, Collins D, et al. Gemfibrozil for the secondary prevention of coronary heart disease in men with low levels of high-density lipoprotein cholesterol. *N Engl J Med* 1999;341:410–418.

71. Fruchart JC, Staels B, Duriez P. PPARS, metabolic disease and atherosclerosis. *Pharmacol Res* 2001;44:345–352.

72. Sviridov D, Nestel P. Dynamics of reverse cholesterol transport: protection against atherosclerosis. *Atherosclerosis* 2002;161:245–254.

73. Lawn RM, Wade DP, Garvin MR, et al. The Tangier disease gene product ABC1 controls the cellular apolipoprotein-mediated lipid removal pathway. *J Clin Invest* 1999;104:R25–R31.

74. Shachter NS. Apolipoproteins C-I and C-III as important modulators of lipoprotein metabolism. *Curr Opin Lipidol* 2001;12:297–304.

75. Frick MH, Elo O, Haapa K, et al. Helsinki Heart Study: primary-prevention trial with gemfibrozil in middle-aged men with dyslipidemia. Safety of treatment, changes in risk factors, and incidence of coronary heart disease. *N Engl J Med* 1987;317:1237–1245.

76. Rubins HB, Robins SJ, Iwane MK, et al. Rationale and design of the Department of Veterans Affairs High-Density Lipoprotein Cholesterol Intervention Trial (HIT) for secondary prevention of coronary artery disease in men with low high-density lipoprotein cholesterol and desirable low-density lipoprotein cholesterol. *Am J Cardiol* 1993;71:45–52.

77. Ericsson CG, Hamsten A, Nilsson J, et al. Angiographic assessment of effects of bezafibrate on progression of coronary artery disease in young male postinfarction patients. *Lancet* 1996;347:849–853.

78. Frick MH, Syvanne M, Nieminen MS, et al. Prevention of the angiographic progression of coronary and vein-graft atherosclerosis by gemfibrozil after coronary bypass surgery in men with low levels of HDL cholesterol. Lipid Coronary Angiography Trial (LOCAT) Study Group. *Circulation* 1997;96:2137–2143.

79. Steiner G. Lipid intervention trials in diabetes. *Diabetes Care* 2000;23[Suppl 2]:B49–B53.

80. Tight blood pressure control and risk of macrovascular and microvascular complications in type 2 diabetes: UKPDS 38. U.K Prospective Diabetes Study Group. *BMJ* 1998;317:703–713.

81. Sohda T, Mizuno K, Tawada H, et al. Studies on antidiabetic agents: I. Synthesis of 5-[4-(2-methyl-2-phenylpropoxy)-benzyl]thiazolidine-2,4-dione (AL-321) and

related compounds. *Chem Pharm Bull (Tokyo)* 1982; 30:3563–3573.

82. Fukui Y, Masui I, Osada S, et al. A new thiazolidinedione, NC-2100, which is a weak PPAR-gamma activator, exhibits potent antidiabetic effects and induces uncoupling protein 1 in white adipose tissue of KKAy obese mice. *Diabetes* 2000;49:759–767.

83. Nagy L, Tontonoz P, Alvarez JG, et al. Oxidized LDL regulates macrophage gene expression through ligand activation of PPARgamma. *Cell* 1998;93:229–240.

84. Crawford RS, Mudaliar SR, Henry RR, et al. Inhibition of LDL oxidation in vitro but not ex vivo by troglitazone. *Diabetes* 1999;48:783–790.

85. Haffner SM, D'Agostino R Jr, Mykkanen L, et al. Insulin sensitivity in subjects with type 2 diabetes: relationship to cardiovascular risk factors. The Insulin Resistance Atherosclerosis Study. *Diabetes Care* 1999;22:562–568.

86. Wagstaff AJ, Goa KL. Rosiglitazone: a review of its use in the management of type 2 diabetes mellitus. *Drugs* 2002;62.1005–1037.

87. O'Moore-Sullivan TM, Prins JB. Thiazolidinediones and type 2 diabetes: new drugs for an old disease. *Med J Aust* 2002;177:396.

88. Minamikawa J, Tanaka S, Yamauchi M, et al. Potent inhibitory effect of troglitazone on carotid arterial wall thickness in type 2 diabetes. *J Clin Endocrinol Metab* 1998;83:1818–1820.

89. Koshiyama H, Shimono D, Kuwamura N, et al. Rapid communication: inhibitory effect of pioglitazone on carotid arterial wall thickness in type 2 diabetes. *J Clin Endocrinol Metab* 2001;86:3452–3456.

90. Takagi T, Akasaka T, Yamamuro A, et al. Troglitazone reduces neointimal tissue proliferation after coronary stent implantation in patients with non-insulin dependent diabetes mellitus: a serial intravascular ultrasound study. *J Am Coll Cardiol* 2000;36:1529–1535.

91. Gu K, Cowie CC, Harris MI. Diabetes and decline in heart disease mortality in U.S. adults. *JAMA* 1999;281:1291–1297.

92. Dunstan DW, Daly RW, Owen N, et al. High-intensity resistance training improves glycemic control in older patients with type 2 diabetes. *Diabetes Care,* Oct;2002;25(10):1729-36.

93. Guerre-Millo M, Gervois P, Raspe E, et al. Peroxisome proliferator-activated receptor alpha activators improve insulin sensitivity and reduce adiposity. *J Biol Chem* 2000;275:16638–16642.

Diabetes and Cardiovascular Disease
edited by Steven P. Marso and David M. Stern
Lippincott Williams & Wilkins, Philadelphia © 2004

6

Receptor-Dependent Vascular Stress in Diabetes

Ann Marie Schmidt, Barry I. Hudson, Shi-Fang Yan, and David M. Stern

Professor, Division of Surgical Science, Department of Surgery, College of Physicians and Surgeons; Postdoctoral Research Fellow, Department of Surgery; Assistant Professor, Division of Surgical Sciences, Department of Surgery, Columbia University, New York, New York; Dean, School of Medicine, Professor of Medicine and Physiology, Medical College of Georgia, Chief Clinical Officer, Medical College of Georgia Hospital, Augusta, Georgia

DIABETES AND VASCULAR COMPLICATIONS: OVERVIEW

The dramatic rise in the incidence of diabetes in the United States and worldwide is mounting to near-epidemic proportions. An estimated 150 million people suffer from this disease throughout the world (1). Based on current expectations, this figure is expected to rise substantially during the 21st century. In addition to the great toll the disease exerts on quality of life in human beings, it is predicted that diabetes and its multisystem complications will continue to profoundly affect the health care system in the United States. Diabetes is characterized by two main forms: insulin-dependent (type 1) diabetes mellitus, in which progressive destruction and dysfunction of pancreatic beta-cell islets cause frank insulin deficiency and ketoacidosis requiring regular replacement, and non-insulin-dependent (type 2) diabetes mellitus, in which insulin resistance coupled with insufficient secretion leads to hyperglycemia. In addition, although children affected by diabetes typically display features of frank insulin deficiency, recent studies have highlighted the emergence of type 2 diabetes in this population, especially among adolescents (2), most likely as a consequence of obesity and physical inactivity. Despite the diverse etiologies implicated in the development of hyperglycemia, common mechanisms are responsible, at least in part, for end-organ damage and systemic complications in affected subjects.

Diabetic complications affect almost every organ system in the body. Not unexpectedly, a focal point for such outcomes lies in the vasculature. Microvascular complications are linked to retinopathy, nephropathy and renal failure, peripheral neuropathy, impotence, and impaired wound healing. In the macrovasculature, the chronic effects of diabetes lead to increased incidence and severity of myocardial infarction, stroke, and amputation of digits or limbs (3,4). Taken together, these facets of the disease portend a striking increase in morbidity and mortality in affected subjects compared with age-matched nondiabetic controls.

Epidemiologic studies have demonstrated that the effects of diabetes on the large blood vessels are less sensitive than the microvascular complications to the beneficial effects of strict control of hyperglycemia. In the original findings of the Diabetes Control and Complications Trial (DCCT), strict glycemic control significantly reduced the incidence of microvascular complications, but the incidence of macrovascular complications was not substantially affected (5). In more recent long-term trials, such as studies reported by the United Kingdom Prospective Diabetes

Study (UKPDS), tight control of hyperglycemia did not exert a profound impact on macrovascular dysfunction (3). These considerations suggest that hyperglycemia, in both its immediate and its indirect effects, synergizes with superimposed stresses in the blood vessel wall (e.g., hyperlipidemia) to augment cellular perturbation and cause irreversible vascular dysfunction. Recent studies in children have underscored the premise that the macrovascular complications of diabetes begin early in the course of the disease. For example, using advanced ultrasound technology, increased intima/media thickness of the aorta and carotid arteries was found in diabetic children compared with healthy control subjects (6). These considerations highlight the need for early, rigorous, and complementary strategies to diminish the risk of macrovascular complications and their sequelae in diabetic subjects.

The detrimental effects of diabetes on macrovascular structures are not limited to atherosclerosis. Multiple studies have suggested that the vascular response to induced mechanical injury, such as that introduced by therapeutic angioplasty in coronary artery disease, is exaggerated in diabetic subjects (7,8). After mechanical injury, diabetic blood vessels display enhanced proliferation of vascular smooth muscle cells (VSMC) and production of extracellular matrix, factors leading to early reocclusion and, sometimes, thrombosis and the emergence of clinical events. Indeed, these considerations have often led to modifications in the means by which diabetic subjects with severe coronary artery disease are managed in the clinic. Based on the results of the Bypass Angioplasty Revascularization Investigation (BARI), which showed that 5-year survival in diabetic subjects was significantly higher after multivessel bypass surgery than after percutaneous interventions (80.6% versus 65.5%, respectively), it is suggested that percutaneous intervention, in general, is a less favored therapeutic approach for revascularization in the diabetic population (9).

Taken together, these considerations highlight the importance of identifying the molecular mechanisms by which the specific impact of the direct and indirect effects of hyperglycemia on key cells implicated in atherogenesis and restenosis (e.g., endothelial cells, smooth muscle cells, inflammatory cells) distinguishes, from the outset of the diagnosis of diabetes, the diabetic subject from euglycemic control individuals with respect to vascular risk, prognosis, and response to therapy.

This chapter presents an overview of the means by which hyperglycemia may alter vascular function, thereby leading to accelerated atherosclerosis and exaggerated restenosis after vascular mechanical injury. Our work, focussed on the biology of the receptor for advanced glycation end products (AGEs) and featured in this chapter, highlights the role of this signal transduction receptor in mediating the cellular consequences of its ligands, AGEs and S100/calgranulins—both enriched in diabetic blood vessels—in the pathogenesis of complications. We propose that these observations lay the groundwork for the development of receptor antagonists targeted to the prevention and treatment of diabetes-associated complications.

GLYCOXIDATION: CELLULAR CONSEQUENCES AND RECEPTORS

AGEs are a heterogeneous group of structures that form in multiple milieus, such as hyperglycemia, oxidant stress, inflammation, neurodegenerative disorders (e.g. Alzheimer's disease), and renal failure (10–14). Although a wide range of AGE-related chemical structures are likely to be present in the vasculature and other tissues in these disease settings, specific AGE structures commonly found in diabetic tissues include carboxymethyl-lysine (CML)-protein adducts, which are the predominant AGEs present *in vivo* (15–18); carboxyethyl-lysine (CEL)-protein adducts; pentosidine-adducts, a major AGE crosslink found in diabetic tissues linked to destabilization of collagen and basement membranes (19–22); and other structures, such as pyrralines, imidazolones, methylglyoxal (also considered a precursor to the formation of a range of other AGEs); and crosslines (23–28).

It is important to note that, beyond diabetes, key insights into the rapid acceleration and production of AGEs has come from the study of renal failure. In this disorder, accelerated AGE formation is prompted by a number of mechanisms, including decreased protein turnover and sustained oxidant stress (29,30). Importantly, in renal failure, β_2-microglobulin appears especially susceptible to glycoxidation, because one outcome of its accelerated modification appears to be the development of dialysis-related amyloidosis, a destructive polyarthropathy that occurs in patients undergoing long-term hemodialysis. Accumulation of AGE-modified β_2-microglobulin amyloid, particularly in joint tissues of affected subjects, has been linked to cytokine production and activation of matrix metalloproteinases (MMPs) in dialysis-related amyloidosis (31,32). Despite the diversity of AGE structures, the formation and accumulation of these adducts is largely viewed as irreversible. Therefore, their long-term accumulation distinguishes affected tissues from normal controls, in that the impact of superimposed stresses may be magnified.

A central focus in AGE research lies in uncovering the mechanisms by which accumulation of these diverse classes of structures may be linked to the pathogenesis of complications in diabetes. Clearly, their effects may be mediated by diverse mechanisms, broadly classified as receptor-independent and receptor-dependent pathways. AGEs may have a direct impact on the structural integrity of the vessel wall and underlying basement membrane. For example, excessive crosslinking of matrix molecules such as collagen may disrupt matrix-matrix and matrix-cell interactions (33,34). Nonenzymatic glycation of intracellular molecules such as basic fibroblast growth factor may lead to impaired function of this molecule (35). AGEs have also been found to quench nitric oxide, thereby potentially affecting vascular relaxation and function (36). The impaired ability of diabetic vasculature to respond appropriately to stimuli such as acetylcholine in human subjects, as well as experimental models, has suggested that such endothelial dysfunction may, indeed, provide a window into more diffuse and widespread vascular disease and atherosclerosis (37–40).

In addition, AGEs may also exert pathogenic effects by engagement of cellular binding sites or receptors. A number of cell surface interaction sites for AGEs have been identified, including macrophage scavenger receptor (MSR) type II, OST-48, 80K-H, galectin-3, and receptor for AGE (RAGE) (41–45). These receptors have been ascribed a range of functions in diabetic tissues, including removal and detoxification of AGEs, as well as modulation of cellular properties by receptor-triggered signaling pathways on AGE engagement. Of these receptors, RAGE does not appear to contribute to removal and detoxification of AGEs. Rather, RAGE has been shown to be a signal transduction receptor for this class of molecules Although it is well established that AGEs are a heterogeneous class of structures, RAGE has been shown to mediate the effects of CML-adducts, the most prevalent AGEs identified thus far *in vivo*, via signal transduction (46). *In vitro* and *in vivo*, physiologically relevant concentrations of CML-adducts activate endothelial cells, VSMC, and macrophages; these events cause expression of a range of proinflammatory molecules and activation of nuclear factor-κB (NF-κB) (46).

In the sections that follow, the broad implications of RAGE activation in diabetic tissues for modulation of cellular properties are explored.

RAGE: A MULTILIGAND RECEPTOR OF THE IMMUNOGLOBULIN SUPERFAMILY

RAGE was first identified as a cellular binding site for AGEs with the use of bovine lung extract and an iodine 125-radiolabeled probe of *in vitro* prepared AGE-albumin (44). Multiple studies confirmed that AGEs in cell culture are bound in a dose-dependent and saturable manner, largely via engagement of RAGE, which is present on the surface of multiple cell types including endothelial cells and macrophages (44–48). Molecular cloning analyses revealed that RAGE was a member of the immunoglobulin superfamily of cell surface molecules (45). The predicted hydropathy plot for bovine RAGE indicated that the extracellular portion of the molecule was composed of 332 amino acids and consisted of one V-type immunoglobulin domain, followed by two C-type immunoglobulin domains. A series of studies on truncations of the extracellular region indicated that its ligands interacted with the V-domain of the receptor (46,49–50). The RAGE extracellular domain sequence was found to be most homologous to MUC 18 and the neural cell adhesion molecule (NCAM) (45). After the extracellular region, there is a single hydrophobic transmembrane spanning domain; this portion of the molecule is followed by a short, highly-charged cytosolic tail at the carboxyl terminus. The cytosolic domain of RAGE was found to be most homologous to the B-cell activation marker, CD20. Our studies have shown that this portion of the molecule is essential for RAGE-triggered signaling, because deletion of the cytosolic domain imparts a "dominant-negative" effect, both *in vitro* and *in vivo* (46,50) (Fig. 6-1). The gene encoding human RAGE is located on chromosome 6 in the major histocompatibility complex, specifically in the class III region (51). These observations strongly suggest the possibility that the gene for RAGE is responsive to environmental stimulation.

RAGE: PATTERNS OF EXPRESSION IN HOMEOSTASIS AND DISEASE

A number of studies have established that in homeostasis, in humans and in animal model systems, RAGE is present at low levels in the adult (52–55). RAGE messenger RNA and antigen are found in a wide range of cell types, including endothelial cells, macrophages, lymphocytes, VSMC, glomerular epithelial cells (podocytes), and neurons. During embryonic development, the expression of RAGE is increased in neurons of the central nervous system, including those within the cerebral cortex, cerebellum, and hippocampus (55). Although these findings

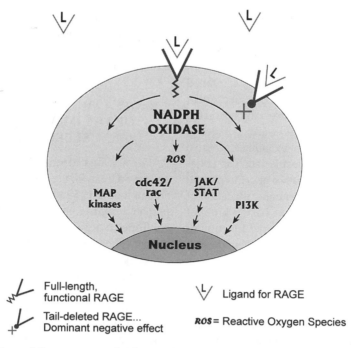

FIG. 6-1. Activation of the receptor of advanced glycation end products (RAGE) triggers multiple cell signaling pathways. Engagement of RAGE by its ligands triggers diverse signaling cascades within the cell, as indicated. Once activation occurs, a range of biologic effects may ensue, including pathways promoting amplification of inflammatory mechanisms, cell survival, or death. Studies *in vitro* and *in vivo* have shown that the cytosolic domain of RAGE is critical for RAGE-mediated modulation of cellular properties; in its absence, ligands may bind the receptor, but they are unable to effect changes in cellular properties.

initially suggested that genetic deletion of RAGE might result in embryonic lethality or in severe impairment of growth or cellular functions, especially within the brain, the recent generation of homozygous RAGE-null mice has refuted this premise (56). RAGE-null mice are viable, display normal lifespan and fertility, and appear to exhibit only phenotypic differences, compared with wild-type animals, on induction of certain stresses (e.g., femoral artery denudation injury, induction of diabetes) (56). These animals provide an excellent template with which to rigorously test the concept that activation of RAGE contributes to cellular mechanisms linked to the pathogenesis of complications in diabetes, as well as other settings.

In the presence of superimposed stresses such as diabetes, mechanical injury, inflammation, or chronic neurodegenerative disease (e.g., Alzheimer's disease), expression of RAGE is upregulated, in parallel with that of its ligands; such RAGE upregulation may be sustained for years (57–59). The striking overlapping expression of RAGE and its ligands in diabetic tissues, inflamed milieu, or brain tissue of patients with Alzheimer's disease suggests the likely possibility that ligands and receptor are located in the tissues at the "right place and right time" to initiate and/or propagate cellular dysfunction. A likely molecular basis for these observations was suggested by our first studies analyzing regulatory elements within the gene encoding RAGE (60,61). We found that two functional binding sites for NF-κB most likely mediate, at least in part, ligand-stimulated upregulation of the receptor. Ongoing studies are now dissecting promoter elements further upstream of those initially re-

ported to identify other regulatory elements as well as possible polymorphisms that might account for differences in receptor expression in populations susceptible to or resistant to disease settings relevant to RAGE, such as diabetic complications, immune and inflammatory diseases, and Alzheimer's disease. Therefore, we postulate that the enhanced formation and/or accumulation of RAGE ligands provides a mechanism to sustain cellular activation in RAGE-associated disease settings. Instead of upregulated expression of ligands causing downregulated receptor expression, here it appears that ligand upregulation generates a positive feedback loop for chronic upregulation of RAGE. In this context, recent studies have suggested that chronic activation of NF-κB may typify diabetic tissues, thus linking this transcription factor to regulation of RAGE expression as well as a range of target genes (62).

RAGE IS A MULTILIGAND RECEPTOR

In addition to AGEs, specifically CML-modified adducts of proteins and lipids, our studies have shown definitively that RAGE is a multiligand receptor (Table 6-1). In addition to its interaction with amyloid-β peptide and, in general, β-sheet fibrils that form in amyloidoses (58,59,63), RAGE interacts with amphoterin and S100/calgranulins. Amphoterin is a member of the high mobility group-1 (HMG-1) family of DNA-binding proteins that, in addition to functions within the cell, also may exist extracellularly and on the surface of cells, especially migrating cells in milieu as distinct as developing neurons and tumors (64,65). Engagement

TABLE 6-1. *Known ligands for RAGE and their potential impact in homeostasis and pathophysiologic settings.*

Ligands for RAGE	Physiologic/pathophysiologic impact
Advanced glycation end products (e.g., CML-protein adducts)	Diabetes, renal failure, amyloidoses, inflammation, oxidant stress, aging
Amyloid-β peptide and beta-sheet fibrils	Alzheimer's disease, amyloidoses
S100/calgranulins	Development, neurite outgrowth, inflammation, tumor biology
Amphoterin	Development, neurite outgrowth, inflammation, tumor biology

CML, carboxymethyl-lysine.

of RAGE on the surface of embryonic neurons is probably one axis linked to their ability to migrate within the developing nervous system, because, at least *in vitro*, blockade of RAGE, using either soluble RAGE (sRAGE, the extracellular ligand-binding domain of the receptor) or blocking F(ab')$_2$ fragments of anti-RAGE immunoglobulin G (IgG), strikingly suppressed neurite outgrowth selectively on amphoterin, but not on poly-L-lysine-coated matrices (52). In addition, amphoterin is also expressed on the surface of transformed cells to enhanced degrees, implying its potential role in tumor cell migration (66). Indeed, our studies have shown that engagement of tumor cell RAGE by amphoterin enhances cellular migration, invasion, proliferation, and generation of MMPs—processes that are linked, at least in part, to local tumor growth and distant invasion (67). *In vivo,* blockade of the receptor in rat C6 glioma cells locally implanted onto the backs of immunocompromised mice, using either sRAGE or blocking antibodies, or by genetic manipulation of the tumor cells to overexpress either sRAGE or dominant-negative (DN) RAGE (a form of the receptor in which the cytosolic domain is deleted, thereby abrogating signaling), resulted in markedly decreased tumor size, proliferation, and local invasion (67). In addition, blockade of RAGE, using sRAGE in a model of metastases in Lewis lung carcinoma, strikingly decreased the number of lung-surface metastases in a dose-dependent manner (67).

Recent observations have expanded the potential implications of amphoterin in biology. It was found that amphoterin may be released from activated macrophages, thereby leading to propagation of inflammatory responses (68,69). *In vivo*, administration of blocking antibodies to amphoterin led to enhanced survival in rodents subjected to conditions mimicking overwhelming septic shock (68). The dependence of these observations on RAGE has yet to be directly tested; it is likely, however, that RAGE serves, at least in part, as a receptor for macrophage-derived amphoterin, because the sequence is virtually identical to that of the molecule linked to neurite outgrowth.

In the context of inflammation, there is little doubt that RAGE serves as a propagation receptor for proinflammatory molecules. Specif-ically, S100/calgranulins, members of a large family (more than 15 members) of proinflammatory cytokines, have central functions within the cell, where their roles are linked to homeostatic properties (e.g., calcium binding), as well as distinct properties outside the cell. Multiple studies have suggested that S100/calgranulins exist extracellularly in multiple milieus, such as acute and chronic inflammation, developing neurons, and tumors (70–72). We tested these concepts *in vitro* and showed that interaction of S100A12 (EN-RAGE), a prototypic S100/calgranulin, activated endothelial cells, macrophages, and peripheral blood mononuclear cells (PBMC), in a manner linked to generation of cytokines and proinflammatory adhesion molecules (50). Importantly, blockade of RAGE in euglycemic mice resulted in suppression of delayed-type hypersensitivity induced by sensitization/challenge with methylated bovine serum albumin; diminished colonic inflammation in mice deficient in interleukin-10 (IL-10); and decreased phenotypic and molecular indices of arthritis in DBA/1 mice subjected to sensitization/challenge with bovine type II collagen (50,73). In these settings, RAGE is not the initiating cause of the immune/inflammatory event; rather, RAGE activation is a key mechanism associated with propagation of inflammation and sustained cellular injury. In our studies in delayed-type hypersensitivity and collagen-induced arthritis, we found that sRAGE-treated animals were able to mount an IgG response to the stimulating antigen; nevertheless, markedly decreased inflammation resulted on RAGE blockade (50,73). It is important to note that ongoing studies suggest that the interaction between S100 and RAGE on lymphocytes may represent an additional pathway of costimulation, in which triggering of this axis further prompts T-cell activation in adaptive immunity. Studies are actively underway to test these hypotheses, both *in vitro* and *in vivo*, in rodent models of allogeneic transplantation.

Based on these considerations, we hypothesized that triggers to RAGE activation in diabetes most likely include molecular species beyond AGEs. We found that, in addition to AGE structures, diabetic atherosclerotic lesions in apolipoprotein E (apoE)-deficient mice were enriched not only in AGEs but also in

S100/calgranulins (74). Given that, in multiple contexts, accelerated atherosclerosis in diabetes is probably best characterized, in part, as an exaggerated inflammatory response, it is highly plausible that in atherosclerotic plaques S100/calgranulins are not "innocent bystanders" but rather contributing facets to the biology of accelerated atherosclerosis that typifies diabetic macrovascular dysfunction.

Taken together, these considerations underlie our hypothesis that RAGE is a multiligand receptor linked to cellular/host response mechanisms in a range of disease settings in which ligand accumulation occurs. Blockade of this receptor may be a targeted strategy to suppress inflammation and diminish cellular injury in a diverse set of conditions, from diabetes to inflammation and cancer.

RAGE, OXIDANT STRESS, AND SIGNAL TRANSDUCTION

From our very earliest studies, it was apparent that a central mechanism by which RAGE activation transduces signal inside the cell is by generation of reactive oxygen intermediates (75,76). On engagement of RAGE by its ligands, activation of p21ras ensues, followed by activation of mitogen-activated protein kinases (MAPK) and nuclear translocation of the transcription factor NF-κB, resulting in transcription of target genes linked to proinflammatory mechanisms. Definitive evidence for the role of p21ras in RAGE-mediated signaling was provided by studies employing mutants of the molecule. When wild-type p21ras was substituted for a mutant in which the cysteine at residue 118 (known to be a target of reactive free radicals in p21ras) was replaced by serine, AGE-RAGE-dependent activation of extracellular signal-related kinase 1/2 (ERK1/2) was blocked (76). Recent studies have shown that a principal mechanism by which RAGE activation leads to generation of reactive oxygen intermediates is via activation of reduced nicotinamide dinucleotide phosphate (NADPH) oxidase (77). In those studies, we demonstrated that incubation of human endothelial cells with AGEs on the surface of diabetic red blood cells, or with specific AGEs (CML-modified adducts), prompted intracellular generation of hydrogen

peroxide, cell surface expression of vascular cell adhesion molecule-1 (VCAM-1), and generation of tissue factor, and that these effects could be suppressed by treatment with diphenyliodonium (DPI) but not by inhibitors of nitric oxide. Consistent with an important role for NADPH oxidase, although macrophages derived from wild-type mice expressed enhanced levels of tissue factor on stimulation with AGE, macrophages derived from mice deficient in a central subunit of NADPH oxidase, gp91phox, failed to display enhanced tissue factor in the presence of AGE (77). These findings highlighted a central role of NADPH oxidase in AGE-RAGE-mediated generation of reactive oxygen species and the altered gene expression triggered by this axis.

Since those studies, we and others have identified multiple signaling cascades that are activated on ligand-mediated stimulation of RAGE, including cdc/rac, p38 and SAPK/JNK MAPKs, phosphoinositol-3-kinase, and the janus kinase/ signal transducer and activator of transcription (JAK/STAT) pathway (67,78–81) (Fig. 6-1). At this time, intense investigation is underway to determine the most proximal intracellular molecules that engage the cytosolic domain of the receptor to trigger and sustain activation of distal pathways. Once defined, the pathways leading to RAGE-mediated altered gene expression will be fully elucidated. We speculate that both intracellular signaling and biologic outcomes linked to RAGE are dependent on the specific cell type and extent or timing of ligand accumulation. For example, the cellular consequences of RAGE activation in vascular cells such as endothelial cells may be quite distinct from those observed in neurons. Depending on the specific time and duration of RAGE ligand accumulation, outcomes may result in cellular proliferation or cell death. Studies are ongoing to better define the distinct milieus in which activation of RAGE leads to these distinct outcomes.

RAGE AND RODENT MODELS OF DIABETIC VASCULOPATHY AND ATHEROSCLEROSIS

The considerations just delineated suggested that RAGE is a signal transduction receptor for a number of ligands linked to the diabetic vascular milieu; we speculated that AGEs and S100/calgranulins, which are enriched in diabetic blood vessels, innately affect the "basal" state of activation/injury in the diabetic environment. According to our hypothesis, when endogenous and exogenous stressors are superimposed (as in the accumulation of modified lipoproteins or physical vascular injury induced by angioplasty) in the setting of heightened RAGE activation, an exaggerated host response to these stresses ensues, leading to enhanced vascular injury and, ultimately, accelerated vasculopathy.

RAGE and Diabetic Vascular Permeability

As a first test of the involvement of the ligand-RAGE axis in vascular perturbation of diabetes,

the effect of RAGE on the barrier function of diabetic vasculature was studied. Increased vascular leakage is a well-known feature of diabetic microvasculature (82–85), and it may be studied in rodent models of diabetes (86). In our initial studies, we induced diabetes in rats using the beta-cell toxin, streptozotocin (STZ). By 11 weeks after administration of the drug, diabetic animals displayed increased vascular leakage, as demonstrated by the tissue-blood isotope ratio (87). Increased vascular permeability in diabetic rats, compared with nondiabetic controls, was most evident in intestine, skin, and kidney; albumin leakage was increased in these tissues approximately 2.8-, 3-, and 2.8-fold, respectively (Fig. 6-2). Blockade of ligand-RAGE interaction was accomplished with the use of a truncated, soluble form of the receptor comprising only the

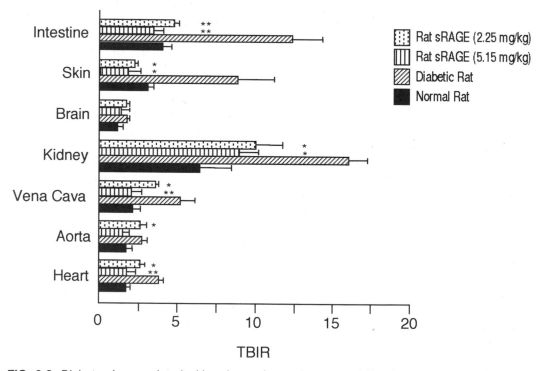

FIG. 6-2. Diabetes is associated with enhanced vascular permeability: impact of RAGE blockade. Normal rats and rats rendered diabetic with streptozotocin were studied 9 to 11 weeks after induction of diabetes. Diabetic animals were infused with soluble RAGE (sRAGE, 2.25 or 5.15 mg/kg) and the tissue-blood isotope ratio (TBIR) was assessed. The results of permeability measurements in normal animals are shown for comparison. The findings are presented as mean ± standard error of the mean (SEM). *, $p < .05$; **, $p < .01$. (Wautier JL, et al. Receptor mediated endothelial cell dysfunction in diabetic vasculopathy: soluble receptor for advanced glycation endproducts blocks hyperpermeability. *J Clin Invest* 1996;97:238–243, with permission.)

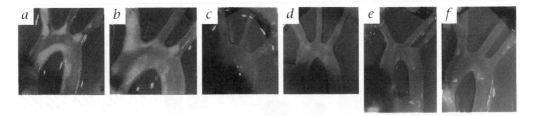

FIG. 6-3. Accelerated atherosclerosis in diabetic apolipoprotein E (apoE)-deficient mice and the impact of RAGE blockade, shown by dissection microscopy. Apo E-deficient mice were either rendered diabetic with streptozotocin (STZ) or treated with citrate buffer as control. After 6 weeks of diabetes or control treatment, the heart and aorta were dissected under microscopy and photographed (magnification, 18×). **A:** Diabetes/murine serum albumin (MSA) (80 µg/day). **B:** Diabetes/sRAGE (3 µg/day). **C:** Diabetes/sRAGE (20 µg/day). **D:** Diabetes/sRAGE (40 µg/day). **E:** Control without diabetes/MSA (40 µg/day). **F:** Control without diabetes/sRAGE (20 µg/day). MSA, ; sRAGE, soluble RAGE. (Reprinted with permission from Park L, et al. *Nature Medicine* 1998;4:1025–1031.)

extracellular domain (V-C-C'), which we have termed sRAGE. Diabetic rats treated with a single dose of sRAGE, 2.25 or 5.15 mg/kg, had plasma levels of sRAGE corresponding to about 10 to 30 and 40 to 60 µg/mL, respectively. Vascular permeability studies were then performed using the tissue-blood isotope ratio (Fig. 6-2) (87). Administration of sRAGE at the lower dose completely blocked vascular leakage in intestine and skin and largely prevented it in the kidney (approximately 60%). With the higher dose of sRAGE, hyperpermeability was suppressed completely in intestine and skin and by approximately 90% in kidney. These data were the first in which application of RAGE blockade *in vivo* demonstrated the dependence of an established vascular complication of diabetes on RAGE. The critical test of these concepts, however, was the extent to which RAGE affected chronic manifestations of diabetes, especially accelerated atherosclerosis.

RAGE and Diabetic Atherosclerosis

It is difficult to study atherosclerosis in wild-type rodents, at least in part because of their high levels of antiatherogenic high-density lipoprotein (HDL). Therefore, we employed atherosclerosis-prone mice deficient in apoE (88,89). Induction of diabetes was first accomplished with the use of STZ at 6 weeks of age in male apoE-null mice. After at least 6 weeks of established diabetes in these animals, the mouse aortas were retrieved

and were found to display increased lesions at aortic branch points and at the lesser curvature (Fig. 6-3A), compared with nondiabetic controls (Fig. 6-3E). Quantitative analysis of multiple sections demonstrated significantly increased lesion area and number in diabetic versus euglycemic apoE-null controls (55) (Fig. 6-4A and B, respectively). Histologic analysis of oil red O-stained sections revealed that more complex lesions (fibrous caps, calcification, necrosis, aneurysm formation) were evident in diabetic aortas compared with those of control mice (55) (Fig. 6-4C). Diabetic lesions displayed increased expression of RAGE and enhanced accumulation of AGEs and S100/calgranulins (55,74).

To address the impact of RAGE activation on accelerated atherosclerosis, we administered sRAGE to diabetic mice, beginning immediately at the time of documentation of diabetes and continuing for an additional 6 weeks. Analysis of aortas revealed a marked dose-dependent suppression of atherosclerotic lesion area in samples from diabetic apoE-null mice treated with sRAGE, compared with controls (Fig. 6-3B,C, and D versus A). Quantification of these findings revealed that blockade of RAGE was associated with dose-dependent suppression of accelerated atherosclerotic lesion area, number, and complexity in diabetic apoE-null mice (Figs. 6-4A–C).

Importantly, examination of the lipid and glycemic profile revealed that RAGE blockade

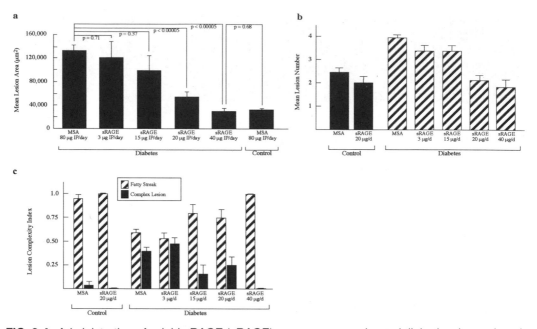

FIG. 6-4. Administration of soluble RAGE (sRAGE) suppresses accelerated diabetic atherosclerosis. **A:** Dose dependence. Diabetic or control mice were treated as indicated for 6 weeks and then killed; mean atherosclerotic lesion area was determined. There were no statistically significant differences between diabetic mice and diabetic mice treated with MSA. **B:** Effect on lesion number. Total lesion number per mouse was determined from analysis of sections 2 through 5 prepared at the aortic sinus. Mean total lesion number is reported. **C:** Effect on complexity. A lesion complexity index was calculated from the ratio of fatty streak (FS) or complex [C] lesions (defined by the presence of cholesterol clefts and necrosis or fibrous cap formation) to total lesion number. The sum of the ratio of FS/total and C/total is 1. (Reprinted with permission from Park L, et al. *Nature Medicine* 1998;4:1025–1031.)

did not exert its beneficial effects by modulation of these pathways. Administration of sRAGE did not affect levels of glycosylated hemoglobin, nor did it affect the number or profile of cholesterol or triglyceride (55). In addition, an unexpected observation in these studies was the finding that concentrations of AGEs were reduced in sRAGE-treated diabetic animals (55). We speculate that diminished AGE formation and accumulation occurred due to suppression of RAGE-mediated oxidant stress in the vessel wall. Because AGEs are formed in milieus characterized by oxidant stress, it is likely that intercepting ligand engagement of the receptor diminished local oxidant stress, which in turn diminished further AGE generation. Consistent with this concept, we observed diminished susceptibility to copper-induced oxidation of low-density lipoprotein (LDL) retrieved from sRAGE-treated

diabetic apoE-null mice, compared with vehicle-treated diabetic apoE-null mice (55).

To be certain that the impact of RAGE blockade was not limited to apoE-null mice with diabetes, we induced diabetes with STZ in mice overexpressing human apoB and in mice deficient in the LDL receptor. In both cases, induction of diabetes accelerated atherosclerosis, in a manner suppressed by blockade of RAGE (90,91). In addition, a key test of our observations was the extent to which genetically induced diabetes in apoE would modify atherosclerosis. We accomplished this aim by breeding the apoE null mouse into the db/db background; in the resulting animals, there was a striking increase in atherosclerosis at the aortic sinus that was dependent on activation of RAGE (92). Administration of sRAGE to diabetic mice from 8 to 11 weeks of age decreased atherosclerotic lesion area, in parallel with vascular levels of VCAM-1, tissue factor, and MMP-9 (92).

Finally, a key test of these concepts was the extent to which blockade of RAGE in apoE-null mice with *established* diabetes would modify the course of vascular disease. Male apoE-null mice were rendered diabetic with STZ at age 6 weeks, then maintained on normal rodent chow until age 14 weeks, after which they were treated with either vehicle or sRAGE until age 20 weeks. Blockade of RAGE stabilized lesion area, complexity, and vascular inflammation in the absence of changes in lipid profile or blood glucose.

Taken together, these findings establish a role for RAGE activation in accelerated atherosclerosis in murine models and suggest that blockade of the receptor might synergize with traditional therapies aimed at lowering blood glucose and optimizing the lipid profile to reduce vascular consequences in both new-onset and established diabetes. Future testing of these concepts in human diabetes should establish the relevance of these findings in rodent models to human clinical situations.

RAGE and Restenosis after Vascular Injury

As discussed earlier, diabetic patients subjected to revascularization procedures by percutaneous balloon-induced injury display enhanced restenosis and clinical events. These considerations necessitated the development of rodent models with which to establish the underlying molecular mechanisms and test potential therapeutic agents in these settings. Previously, a model of accelerated neointimal expansion after carotid artery injury was described in fatty Zucker rats, in which insulin resistance results in hyperglycemia (93). In parallel with increased neointimal expansion, enhanced proliferation of VSMC, as assessed by incorporation of bromodeoxyuridine (BrdU), was observed in the injured diabetic vessels (93). Evidence of an important role for RAGE activation in enhanced neointimal expansion after carotid artery injury was highlighted by the results of recent pilot studies. Fatty Zucker rats treated with sRAGE displayed decreased neointimal expansion and incorporation of BrdU after carotid artery injury,

compared with diabetic rats treated with vehicle (albumin) (94). In these experiments, no effect on levels of blood glucose were observed in diabetic rats treated with sRAGE, indicating that this axis was distinct from those associated with traditional risk factors in this model, such as increased levels of blood glucose.

RAGE activation in injured vasculature appears to be a central mechanism linked to VSMC proliferation and migration, in addition to its role in diabetic animals. In euglycemic C57BL/6 mice subjected to femoral artery denudation, administration of either sRAGE or blocking $F(ab')_2$ fragments of anti-RAGE IgG suppressed neointimal expansion in a dose-dependent manner (56). Further, pilot studies in homozygous RAGE-null mice and in transgenic mice expressing DN-RAGE selectively in VSMC (driven by the smooth muscle $22-\alpha$ (SM22-α promoter) revealed that mice deficient in RAGE function are strikingly resistant to neointimal expansion after vascular injury (56). These observations strongly suggest that RAGE is a critical regulator of VSMC function, especially after induced injury.

RAGE AND DIABETIC COMPLICATIONS

A key test of the role of RAGE in diabetic complications was addressed by applying RAGE blockade in animals with multiple distinct complications of diabetes. This section describes our findings in diabetic mice subjected to RAGE blockade and the impact of this intervention on accelerated alveolar bone loss (periodontal disease), impaired wound healing, and nephropathy.

RAGE and Diabetic Periodontal Disease

Multiple studies have shown that diabetes is associated with increased prevalence, severity, and progression of periodontal disease (95,96). To test the hypothesis that activation of RAGE contributes, at least in part, to the pathogenesis of diabetes-associated periodontitis, diabetic mice infected with the human periodontal pathogen *Porphyromonas gingivalis* were treated with sRAGE. Blockade of RAGE diminished accelerated alveolar bone loss in a dose-dependent manner, in parallel with decreased generation of proinflammatory cytokines, tumor necrosis factor-α (TNF-α), and IL-6 in gingival tissue, together with decreased levels of MMP protein antigens/activity. Furthermore, levels of gingival AGEs were decreased in mice treated with sRAGE (97).

These findings underscored the concept that exaggerated host response mechanisms in diabetic animals, typified by increased expression of proinflammatory and tissue-destructive molecules, are at least partly dependent on RAGE.

RAGE and Diabetic Wound Healing

A central consequence of diabetes is the long-term development of impaired wound healing, which leads to amputations of digits or limbs in diabetic subjects (98,99). We tested these concepts in db/db mice subjected to full-thickness excisional wounds, as a means to model chronic ulcers in these animals. Histologic analysis revealed that RAGE and two of its ligands, AGEs and S100/calgranulins, were expressed to enhanced degrees in db/db wounds after injury (100). To test the role of RAGE, sRAGE was administered by both local and intraperitoneal means. Administration of sRAGE accelerated the development of appropriately limited inflammatory cell infiltration and activation in wound foci. In parallel with accelerated wound closure at later times, blockade of RAGE suppressed levels of cytokines, TNF-α, IL-6, and MMP-2, -3, and -9. At later times, generation of thick, well-vascularized granulation tissue was enhanced, in parallel with increased levels of platelet-derived growth factor-B (PDGF-B) and vascular endothelial growth factor (VEGF) (100).

Taken together, these considerations underscore the concept that a fine balance must be struck in wound healing between appropriately limited inflammatory responses and those that, when sustained, portend ongoing tissue degradation. Our findings suggest that RAGE is at the center of a cascade of events that disturbs the equilibrium between *beneficial* and *injurious* inflammation in the diabetic wound. We speculate that chronic accumulation of AGEs within the skin and subcutaneous elements serves as a temporary "glue," delaying the entry of blood- and tissue-derived inflammatory cells such as macrophages into the wound site. Once in the wound, however, RAGE-bearing macrophages and other cellular effector cells, including endothelial cells and fibroblasts, interact with AGEs and S100/calgranulins in a sustained manner. These events prime a spiraling cascade of cellular activation and a vicious cycle of cytokine and MMP generation, mediated at least in part by delayed egress of activated inflammatory cells from the wound milieu. Blockade of RAGE restores physiologic *migration* of inflammatory cells into, and then out of, inflamed foci, as well as their limited *activation*, thereby resetting molecular cues within the wound and leading to effective inflammation and wound repair.

These findings highlight the premise that whether the diabetic setting is a wound, infected periodontium, or a hyperlipidemic blood vessel, an exaggerated inflammatory response, at least in part triggered by activation of RAGE, is a key mechanism distinguishing the diabetic milieu from that seen in euglycemia.

RAGE and Diabetic Nephropathy

An unexpected observation regarding the role of RAGE in diabetic nephropathy was that the principal site of RAGE expression in the diabetic kidney/glomerulus in human subjects or in db/db mice was the glomerular epithelial cell or podocyte (101). In contrast, no detectable RAGE expression was found in the mesangium or in endothelial cells in human or rodent models of diabetes (db/db mouse) (101,102).

To test the role of RAGE, in our first studies, sRAGE was administered to db/db mice. In parallel with decreased albuminuria and increased creatinine clearance, levels of transforming growth factor-β (TGF-β) and VEGF, expansion of the mesangium, and thickness of the glomerular basement membrane were all suppressed by blockade of RAGE (103). Studies are underway to dissect the underlying molecular pathways by which podocyte RAGE is linked to the pathogenesis of diabetes-associated nephropathy.

GENETIC VARIANTS OF RAGE: POLYMORPHISMS AND THEIR IMPLICATIONS

A key factor that is likely to affect the design of clinical trials targeting RAGE blockade is the degree to which individuals may display enhanced or reduced predilection for the development of diabetic complications based on variants in the RAGE gene. In this context, a number of studies have now reported genetic variants of the receptor, both within the coding/translated region and within regulatory elements (104–107). One particular variant of RAGE, the Gly82Ser polymorphism, is of particular interest in that it lies within the V-domain of the extracellular segment of the receptor, which places it at the site of ligand interaction. We speculated that cells bearing this variant might display altered affinity for RAGE ligands. We tested these concepts in Chinese hamster ovary cells (which do not express detectable RAGE natively) bearing either wild-type or variant RAGE (82S) and in monocytes derived from wild-type or variant RAGE-bearing subjects. Transfected Chinese hamster ovary cells or monocytes bearing the RAGE 82S allele displayed enhanced binding and cytokine/MMP generation after ligation by a prototypic S100/calgranulin, compared with cells expressing the RAGE 82G allele (108). Similar observations were made when CML-albumin was tested as a prototypic RAGE ligand. These considerations prompted the hypothesis that in the diabetic milieu, which is certainly enriched in S100/calgranulins and AGEs, enhanced interaction of these ligands with variant forms of the receptor might represent a further amplification mechanism in cellular perturbation. Alternatively, variant forms of RAGE might impart striking protection against the development of complications.

Multiple studies are underway to elucidate specific variants of RAGE whose protein products display modified ligand affinity, or, in regulatory elements, variants of the receptor that display enhanced or downregulated transcription of the RAGE gene on interfacing with critical regulatory stimuli.

HYPOTHESES AND FUTURE DIRECTIONS

In conclusion, our finding that RAGE is a multiligand member of the immunoglobulin superfamily led us to rigorously test its role in a range of disease settings in which ligand accumulation was a characteristic feature. In the setting of hyperglycemia and consequent oxidant stress, RAGE expression is enhanced, and the prolonged proximity of AGEs and S100/calgranulins (and, perhaps, amphoterins) to cells expressing RAGE sets the stage for sustained cellular activation and vascular dysfunction. Here, in stark contrast to other host response systems in which a negative feedback loop terminates cellular activation on ligand accumulation, ligand engagement of RAGE appears to recruit cellular effector mechanisms (e.g., MAPKs, NF-κB), thereby enhancing receptor expression and perpetuating cellular perturbation by upregulating a broad range of proinflammatory and tissue-destructive molecules. Therefore, it is reasonable to postulate that intercepting the spiraling cycle of ligand-RAGE interaction has the potential to interrupt cellular activation, with possibly profound impacts on a range of chronic disorders, especially the complications of diabetes. To address these hypotheses, multiple studies are ongoing in mice bearing genetic manipulations of RAGE or complete RAGE deletion. Using induction or genetic introduction of diabetes, the course of complications is being studied as a means to track the sites, times, and disease stages in which RAGE activation may have important effects. We anticipate that the results of such studies will clearly identify whether therapeutic administration of sRAGE, or perhaps low-molecular-weight antagonists of the receptor, has the potential to dramatically modify the course of diabetes and its complications in human subjects.

It is also essential to elucidate what, if any, homeostatic functions of RAGE may render its

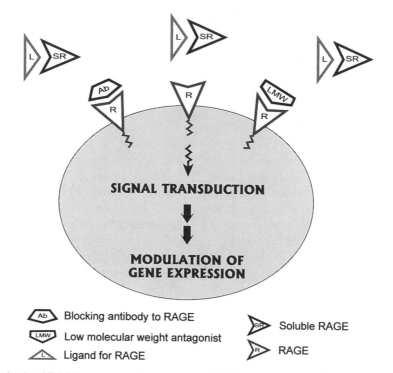

FIG. 6-5. Blockade of RAGE: therapeutic strategies. RAGE is a signal transduction receptor for ligands found to be enriched in diabetic tissues—including, but probably not limited to, advanced glycation end products (AGEs) and proinflammatory S100/calgranulins. Blockade of the receptor *in vivo* may be accomplished by administration of soluble RAGE, the extracellular ligand domain of RAGE that acts as a decoy to trap ligands and prevent their engagement and activation of the cell surface receptor. Alternatively, agents that directly block the cell surface receptor, such as blocking antibodies or low-molecular-weight antagonists, bear the potential to suppress ligand-mediated engagement and receptor activation in diabetic tissues. Strategies to target these distinct axes are under active development.

chronic inhibition ill-advised. As described earlier, RAGE-null mice are viable and fertile. However, recent studies have suggested that blockade of RAGE in euglycemic wild-type mice subjected to unilateral sciatic nerve crush impairs Wallerian degeneration and nerve fiber regeneration (109,110). These observations highlight the concept that proinflammatory mechanisms (not unexpectedly) may imbue beneficial effects in biologic systems. Chronic blockade of the receptor in the clinical setting will require careful analysis of its relative risks and potential benefits. Certainly, in the history of medicine and advances in therapeutics, this is not a unique concept. Figure 6-5 displays our current approach to blockade of the receptor in animal model systems. Modifica-

tion and refinement of these strategies is a key focus of our efforts to translate RAGE blockade from animal studies to the clinic.

Based on the evidence we have accrued to date, we propose that the striking increase in morbidity and mortality in patients with chronic diabetes, compared with euglycemic subjects, renders RAGE blockade a new strategy worthy of careful testing.

ACKNOWLEDGMENTS

This work was supported by the Surgical Research Fund and by grants from the U. S. Public Health Service and Juvenile Diabetes Research Foundation International. A.M.S. is a recipient of a Burroughs Wellcome Fund Clinical Scientist Award in Translational Research.

REFERENCES

1. King H, Aubert R, Herman W. Global burden of diabetes, 1995–2005. Prevalence, numerical estimates and projections. *Diabetes Care* 1998;21:1414–1431.
2. Fagot-Campagna A, Narayan K. Type 2 diabetes in children. *BMJ* 2001;322:377–387.
3. United Kingdom Prospective Diabetes Study (UKPDS) Group. Intensive blood-glucose control with sulphonylureas or insulin compared with conventional treatment and risk of complications in patients with type 2 diabetes. *Lancet* 1998;352:837–853.
4. Haffner SM, Lehto S, Ronnemaa T, et al. Mortality from coronary heart disease in subjects with type 2 diabetes and in nondiabetic subjects with and without prior myocardial infarction. *N Engl J Med* 1998;339:229–234.
5. The Diabetes Control and Complications Trial Research Group. The effect of intensive treatment of diabetes on the development and progression of long-term complications in insulin-dependent diabetes mellitus. *N Engl J Med* 1993;329:977–986.
6. Jarvisalo MJ, Martti L, Nanto-Salonen K, et al. Increased aortic intima-media thickness: a marker of preclinical atherosclerosis in high-risk children. *Circulation* 2001;104:2943–2947.
7. Rozenman Y, Sapoznikov D, Mosseri M, et al. Long-term angiographic follow-up of coronary balloon angioplasty in patients with diabetes mellitus: a clue to the explanation of the results of the BARI study (Balloon Angioplasty Revascularization Investigation). *J Am Coll Cardiol* 1997;30:1420–1425.
8. Abizaid A, Kornowski R, Mintz GS, et al. The influence of diabetes mellitus on acute and late clinical outcome following coronary stent implantation. *J Am Coll Cardiol* 1998;32:584–589.
9. The Bypass Angioplasty Revascularization Investigation (BARI) Investigators. Comparison of coronary bypass surgery with angioplasty in patients with multivessel disease. *N Engl J Med* 1996;335:217–225.
10. Brownlee M. Advanced glycosylation in diabetes and aging. *Annu Rev Med* 1995;46:223–234.
11. Smith MA, Taneda S, Richey P, et al. Advanced Maillard reaction end products are associated with Alzheimer disease pathology. *Proc Natl Acad Sci U S A* 1994;91:5710–5714.
12. Anderson MM, Requena JR, Crowley JR, et al. The myeloperoxidase system of human phagocytes generates N-epsilon-(carboxymethyl)lysine on proteins: a mechanism for producing advanced glycation endproducts at sites of inflammation. *J Clin Invest* 1999;104:103–113.
13. Makita Z, Yanagisawa K, Kuwajima S, et al. Advanced glycation endproducts and diabetic nephropathy. *J Diabetes Complications* 1995;9:265–268.
14. Sousa MM, Du Yan S, Fernandes R, et al. Familial amyloid polyneuropathy: receptor for advanced glycation end products-dependent triggering of neuronal inflammatory and apoptotic pathways. *J Neuroscience* 2001;21:7576–7586.
15. Schleicher E, Wagner E, Nerlich A. Increased accumulation of glycoxidation product carboxymethyllysine in human tissues in diabetes and aging. *J Clin Invest* 1997;99:457–468.
16. Ikeda K, Higashi T, Sano H, et al. Carboxymethyllysine protein adduct is a major immunological epitope in proteins modified with AGEs of the Maillard reaction. *Biochemistry* 1996;35:8075–8083.
17. Reddy S, Bichler J, Wells-Knecht K, et al. Carboxymethyllysine is a dominant AGE antigen in tissue proteins. *Biochemistry* 1995;34:10872–10878.
18. Baynes J. Role of oxidative stress in development of complications in diabetes. *Diabetes* 1991;40:405–412.
19. Ahmed MU, Brinkmann FE, Degenhardt TP, et al. N-epsilon-(carboxyethyl)lysine, a product of the chemical modification of proteins by methylglyoxal. *Biochem J* 1997;324:565–570.
20. Dyer D, Blackledge S, Thorpe S, et al. Formation of pentosidine during nonenzymatic browning of protein by glucose: Identification of glucose and other carbohydrates as possible precursors of pentosidine in vivo. *J Biol Chem* 1991;266:11654–11660.
21. Grandhee S, Monnier VM. Mechanisms of formation of the Maillard protein crosslink pentosidine: ribose, glucose, fructose and ascorbate as pentosidine precursors. *J Biol Chem* 1991;266:11649–11653.
22. Beisswenger P, Moore L, Brinck-Johnsen T, et al. Increased collagen-linked pentosidine levels and AGEs in early diabetic nephropathy. *J Clin Invest* 1993;92:212–217.
23. Miyata S, Monnier VM. Immunohistochemical detection of AGEs in diabetic tissues using monoclonal antibody to pyrraline. *J Clin Invest* 1992;89:1102–1112.
24. Tauer A, Knerr T, Niwa T, et al. In vitro formation of N(epsilon)-(carboxymethyl)lysine and imidazolones under conditions similar to continuous ambulatory peritoneal dialysis. *Biochem Biophys Res Commun* 2001;280:1408–1414.
25. Niwa T, Katsuzaki T, Miyazaki S, et al. Immunohistochemical detection of imidazolone, a novel advanced glycation end product, in kidneys and aortas of diabetic patients. *J Clin Invest* 1997;99:1272–1280.
26. Webster L, Abordo EA, Thornalley PJ, et al. Induction of TNF-alpha and IL-1 beta mRNA in monocytes by methylglyoxal- and advanced glycation endproduct-modified human serum albumin. *Biochem Soc Trans* 1997;25:250S.
27. Westwood ME, Argirov OK, Abordo EA, et al. Methylglyoxal-modified arginine residues: a signal for receptor-mediated endocytosis and degradation of proteins by monocytic THP-1 cells. *Biochim Biophys Acta* 1997;1356:84–94.
28. Ienaga K, Nakamura K, Hochi T, et al. Crosslines, fluorophores in the AGE-related cross-linked proteins. *Contrib Nephrol* 1995;112:42–51.
29. Sebekova K, Podracka L, Heidland A, et al. Enhanced plasma levels of advanced glycation end products (AGE) and pro-inflammatory cytokines in children/adolescents with chronic renal insufficiency and after renal replacement therapy by dialysis and transplantation: are they inter-related? *Clin Nephrol* 2001;56:S21–S26.
30. Shimoike T, Inoguchi T, Umeda F, et al. The meaning of serum levels of advanced glycosylation end products

in diabetic nephropathy. *Metabolism* 2000;49:1030–1035.

31. Drueke T. Beta-2-microglobulin amyloidosis and renal bone disease. *Miner Electrolyte Metab* 1991;17:261–272.

32. Miyata T, Oda O, Inagi R, et al. Beta-2-microglobulin modified with AGEs is a major component of hemodialysis-associated amyloidosis. *J Clin Invest* 1993;92:1243–1252.

33. Tanaka S, Avigad G, Brodsky B, et al. Glycation induces expansion of the molecular packing of collagen. *J Mol Biol* 1988;203:495–505.

34. Haitoglou CS, Tsilbary EC, Brownlee M, et al. Altered cellular interactions between endothelial cells and nonenzymatically glycosylated laminin/type IV collagen. *J Biol Chem* 1992;267:12404–12407.

35. Giardino I, Edelstein D, Brownlee M. Nonenzymatic glycosylation in vitro and in bovine endothelial cells alters basic fibroblast growth factor activity: a model for intracellular glycosylation in diabetes. *J Clin Invest* 1994;94:110–117.

36. Bucala R, Tracey K, Cerami A. AGEs quench nitric oxide and mediate defective endothelium-dependent vasodilation in experimental diabetes. *J Clin Invest* 1991;87:432–438.

37. Williams SB, Cucso JA, Roddy MA, et al. Impaired nitric oxide-mediated vasodilation in patients with non-insulin-dependent diabetes mellitus. *J Am Coll Cardiol* 1996;27:567–574.

38. Johnstone MT, Creager SJ, Scales KM, et al. Impaired endothelium-dependent vasodilation in patients with insulin-dependent diabetes mellitus. *Circulation* 1993;88:2510–2516.

39. De Vriese AS, Verbeuren TJ, Van de Voorde J, et al. Endothelial dysfunction in diabetes. *Br J Pharmacol* 2000;130:963–974.

40. Caballero AE, Arora S, Saouaf R, et al. Microvascular and macrovascular reactivity is reduced in subjects at risk for type 2 diabetes. *Diabetes* 1999;48:1856–1862.

41. El Khoury J, Thomas CA, Loike JD, et al. Macrophages adhere to glucose-modified basement membrane via their scavenger receptors. *J Biol Chem* 1994;269:10197–10200.

42. Vlassara H, Li YM, Imani F, et al. Galectin-3 as a high affinity binding protein for AGE: a new member of the AGE-receptor complex. *Mol Med* 1995;1:634–646.

43. Li YM, Mitsuhashi T, Wojciechowicz D, et al. Molecular identity and cellular distribution of advanced glycation endproduct receptors: relationship of p60 to OST-48 and p90 and 80K-H membrane proteins. *Proc Natl Acad Sci U S A* 1996;93:11047–11052.

44. Schmidt AM, Vianna M, Gerlach M, et al. Isolation and characterization of binding proteins for advanced glycosylation endproducts from lung tissue which are present on the endothelial cell surface. *J Biol Chem* 1992;267:14987–14997.

45. Neeper M, Schmidt AM, Brett J, et al. Cloning and expression of RAGE: a cell surface receptor for advanced glycosylation end products of proteins. *J Biol Chem* 1992;267:14998–15004.

46. Kislinger T, Fu C, Huber B, et al. N^e (carboxymethyl)lysine modifications of proteins are ligands for RAGE that activate cell signalling pathways and modulate gene expression. *J Biol Chem* 1999;274:31740–31749.

47. Schmidt AM, Yan SD, Brett J, et al. Regulation of mononuclear phagocyte migration by cell surface binding proteins for advanced glycosylation endproducts. *J Clin Invest* 1993;92:2155–2168.

48. Miyata T, Hori O, Zhang J, et al. The receptor for advanced glycation endproducts (RAGE) mediates the interaction of AGE-β_2-microglobulin with human mononuclear phagocytes via an oxidant-sensitive pathway: implications for the pathogenesis of dialysis-related amyloidosis. *J Clin Invest* 1996;98:1088–1094.

49. Schmidt AM, Yan SD, Stern D. The V-domain of receptor for advanced glycation endproducts (RAGE) mediates binding of AGEs: a novel target for therapy of diabetes. *Circulation* 1997;96[Suppl]:I-37.

50. Hofmann MA, Drury S, Fu C, et al. RAGE mediates a novel proinflammatory axis: a central cell surface receptor for S100/calgranulin polypeptides. *Cell* 1999;97:889–901.

51. Sugaya K, Fukagawa T, Matsumoto KI, et al. Three genes in the human MHC class III region near the junction with class II: gene for RAGE, PBX2 homeobox gene and a notch homolog, human counterpart of mouse mammary tumor gene int-2. *Genomics* 1994;23:408–419.

52. Hori O, Brett J, Nagashima M, et al. RAGE is a cellular binding site for amphoterin: mediation of neurite outgrowth and co-expression of RAGE and amphoterin in the developing nervous system. *J Biol Chem* 1995;270:25752–25761.

53. Brett J, Schmidt AM, Zou YS, et al. Tissue distribution of the receptor for advanced glycation endproducts (RAGE): expression in smooth muscle, cardiac myocytes, and neural tissue in addition to vasculature. *Am J Pathol* 1993;143:1699–1712.

54. Ritthaler U, Roth H, Bierhaus A, et al. Expression of RAGE in peripheral occlusive vascular disease. *Am J Pathol* 1995;146:688–694.

55. Park L, Raman KG, Lee KJ, et al. Suppression of accelerated diabetic atherosclerosis by soluble receptor for AGE (sRAGE). *Nat Med* 1998;4:1025–1031.

56. Sakaguchi T, Sousa M, Yan SD, et al. Restenosis: central role of RAGE-dependent neointimal expansion. *Circulation* 2001;104[Suppl]:II-522.

57. Schmidt AM, Yan SD, Stern D. The dark side of glucose [News and Views]. *Nat Med* 1995;1:1002–1004.

58. Yan SD, Chen X, Chen M, et al. RAGE and amyloid-β peptide neurotoxicity in Alzheimer's disease. *Nature* 1996;382:685–691.

59. Yan SD, Zhu H, Fu J, et al. Amyloid beta peptide-receptor for advanced glycation endproduct interaction elicits neuronal expression of macrophage-colony stimulating factor: a proinflammatory pathway in Alzheimer disease. *Proc Natl Acad Sci U S A* 1997;94:5296–5301.

60. Li J, Schmidt AM. Characterization and functional analysis of the promoter of RAGE. *J Biol Chem* 1997;272:16498–16506.

61. Li J, Qu X, Schmidt AM. Sp1 binding elements in the promoter of RAGE are essential for amphoterin-mediated gene expression in cultured neuroblastoma cells. *J Biol Chem* 1998;273:30870–30878.

62. Bierhaus A, Schiekofer S, Schwaninger, M, et al.

Diabetes-associated sustained activation of the transcription factor nuclear factor-kappa B. *Diabetes* 2001;50:2792–2808.

63. Yan SD, Zhu H, Zhu A, et al. Receptor-dependent cell stress and amyloid accumulation in systemic amyloidosis. *Nat Med* 2000;6:643–651.

64. Rauvala H, Merenmies J, et al. The adhesive and neurite-promoting molecule p30: analysis of the amino terminal sequence and production of antipeptide antibodies that detect p30 at the surface of neuroblastoma cells and of brain neurons. *J Cell Biol* 1987;107:2293–2305.

65. Rauvala H, Pihlaskari R. Isolation and some characteristics of an adhesive factor of brain that enhances neurite outgrowth in central neurons. *J Biol Chem* 1987;262:16625–16635.

66. Parkkinen J, Raulo E, Merenmies J, et al. Amphoterin, the 30-kDa protein in a family of HMG1-type polypeptides: enhanced expression in transformed cells, leading edge localization, and interactions with plasminogen activation. *J Biol Chem* 1993;268:19726–19738.

67. Taguchi A, Blood DC, del Toro G, et al. Blockade of amphoterin/RAGE signalling suppresses tumor growth and metastases. *Nature* 2000;405:354–360.

68. Wang H, Bloom O, Zhang M, et al. HMG-1 as a late mediator of endotoxin lethality in mice. *Science* 1999;285:248–251.

69. Andersson U, Wang H, Palmblad K, et al. High mobility group 1 protein (HMG-1) stimulates proinflammatory cytokine synthesis in human monocytes. *J Exp Med* 2000,192.565–570.

70. Schafer BW, Heinzmann CW. The S100 family of EF-hand calcium-binding proteins: functions and pathology. *Trends Biochem Sci* 1996;21:134–140.

71. Zimmer DB, Cornwall EH, Landar A, et al. The S100 protein family: history, function, and expression. *Brain Res Bull* 1995;37:417–429.

72. Donato R. S100: a multigenic family of calcium-modulated proteins of the EF-hand type with intracellular and extracellular functional roles. *Int J Biochem Cell Biol* 2001;33:637–668.

73. Hofmann MA, Drury S, Hudson BI, et al. RAGE and arthritis: the G82S polymorphism amplifies the inflammatory response. *Genes Immunity* 2002;3:123–135.

74. Kislinger T, Tanji N, Wendt T, et al. RAGE mediates inflammation and enhanced expression of tissue factor in the vasculature of diabetic apolipoprotein E null mice. *Arteriosclerosis, Thrombosis and Vascular Biology* 2001;21:905–910.

75. Yan SD, Schmidt AM, Anderson GM, et al. Enhanced cellular oxidant stress by the interaction of AGEs with their receptors/binding proteins. *J Biol Chem* 1994;269:9889–9897.

76. Lander H, Tauras J, Ogiste J, et al. Activation of RAGE triggers a MAP kinase pathway regulated by oxidant stress. *J Biol Chem* 1997;272:17810–17814.

77. Wautier MP, Chappey O, Corda S, et al. Activation of NADPH oxidase by advanced glycation endproducts (AGEs) links oxidant stress to altered gene expression via RAGE. *Am J Physiol Endocrinol Metab* 2001;280:E685–E694.

78. Huttunen HJ, Fages C, Rauvala H. Receptor for advanced glycation endproducts (RAGE)-mediated neurite outgrowth and activation of NF-kB require the cytoplasmic domain of the receptor but different downstream signaling pathways. *J Biol Chem* 1999;274:19919–19924.

79. Huang JS, Guh JY, Chen HC, et al. Role of receptor for advanced glycation end-product (RAGE) and the JAK/STAT-signaling pathway in AGE-induced collagen production in NRK-49F cells. *J Cell Biochem* 2001;81:102–113.

80. Yeh CH, Sturgis L, Haidacher J, et al. Requirement for p38 and p44/42 mitogen-activated protein kinases in RAGE-mediated nuclear factor-kappa B transcriptional activation and cytokine secretion. *Diabetes* 2001;50:1495–1504.

81. Deora AA, Win T, Vanhaesebroeck B, et al. A redox-triggered ras-effector interaction: recruitment of phosphatidylinositol 3'-kinase to ras by redox stress. *J Biol Chem* 1998;273:29923–29928.

82. Viberti G. Increased capillary permeability in diabetes mellitus and its relationship to microvascular angiopathy. *Am J Med* 1983;146.600–604.

83. Mattock M, Morrish N, Viberti G, et al. Prospective study of microalbuminuria as predictor of mortality in NIDDM. *Diabetes* 1992;41:736–741.

84. Feldt-Rasmussen B. Increased transcapillary escape rate of albumin in type 1 diabetic patients with microalbuminuria. *Diabetologia* 1996;29:282–286.

85. Nannipieri M, Rizzo L, Rapuano A, et al. Increased transcapillary escape rate of albumin in a microalbuminuric type II diabetic subject. *Diabetes Care* 1995;18:1–9.

86. Williamson J, Chang K, Tilton R, et al. Increased vascular permeability in spontaneously diabetic BB/W rats and in rats with mild versus severe streptozotocin-induced diabetes. *Diabetes* 1987;36:813–821.

87. Wautier JL, Zoukourian C, Chappey O, et al. Receptor-mediated endothelial cell dysfunction in diabetic vasculopathy: soluble RAGE blocks hyperpermeability. *J Clin Invest* 1996;97:238–243.

88. Plump AS, Smith JD, Hayek T, et al. Severe hypercholesterolemia and atherosclerosis in apolipoprotein E-deficient mice created by homologous recombination in ES cells. *Cell* 1992;71:343–353.

89. Zhang SH, Reddick RL, Piedrahita JA, et al. Spontaneous hypercholesterolemia and arterial lesions in mice lacking apolipoprotein E. *Science* 1992;258:468–471.

90. Raman KG, Lu Y, Tsai M, et al. A model of accelerated atherosclerosis in diabetic mice overexpressing of apo B: soluble receptor for advanced glycation endproducts. *FASEB J* 1998;12:A106.

91. Makker G, Fan L, Lindenberg N, et al. Suppression of accelerated atherosclerosis in diabetic LDL receptor null mice by soluble receptor for AGE (sRAGE). *Circulation* 1998;98[Suppl]:I-310.

92. Wendt TM, Bucciarelli LG, Lu Y, et al. Accelerated atherosclerosis and vascular inflammation develop in apo E null mice with type 2 diabetes. *Circulation* 2000;102[Suppl]:II-231.

93. Park SH, Marso SP, Zhou Z, et al. Neointimal hyperplasia after arterial injury is increased in a rat model of non-insulin-dependent diabetes mellitus. *Circulation* 2001;104:815–819.

94. Zhou ZM, Marso SP, Schmidt AM, et al. Blockade of receptor for AGE (RAGE) suppresses neointimal

formation in diabetic rat carotid artery injury model. *Circulation* 2000;102[Suppl]:II-246.

95. Shlossman M, Knowler WC, Pettitt DJ, et al. Type 2 diabetes mellitus and periodontal disease. *J Am Dent Assoc* 1991;121:531–536.

96. Löe H. Periodontal disease: the sixth complication of diabetes mellitus. *Diabetes Care* 1993;16:329–334.

97. Lalla E, Lamster IB, Feit M, et al. Blockade of RAGE suppresses periodontitis-associated alveolar bone loss in diabetic mice. *J Clin Invest* 2000;105:1117–1124.

98. Goodson WH, Hunt TK. Wound healing and the diabetic patient. *Surg Gynecol Obstet* 1979;149:690–698.

99. Morain WD, Colen LB. Wound healing in diabetes mellitus. *Clin Plastic Surg* 1990;17:493–501.

100. Goova MT, Li J, Kislinger T, et al. Blockade of receptor for AGE (RAGE) restores effective wound healing in diabetic mice. *Am J Pathol* 2001;159:513–525.

101. Tanji N, Markowitz GS, Fu C, et al. The expression of advanced glycation endproducts and their cellular receptor RAGE in diabetic nephropathy and nondiabetic renal disease. *J Am Soc Nephrol* 2000;11:1656–1666.

102. Ziyadeh FN, Cohen MP, Guo J, et al. RAGE mRNA expression in the diabetic mouse kidney. *Mol Cell Biochem* 1997;170:147–152.

103. Wendt TM, Tanji N, Kislinger T, et al. Blockade of receptor for AGE (RAGE) suppresses albuminuria and glomerulosclerosis in murine diabetic kidney: implications for podocyte activation in the pathogenesis of diabetic nephropathy. *Circulation* 2001;104[Suppl]:II-237.

104. Hudson BI, Stickland MH, Grant PJ. Identification of polymorphisms in the receptor for advanced glycation end products (RAGE) gene: prevalence in type 2 diabetes and ethnic groups. *Diabetes* 1998;47:1155–1157.

105. Schenk S, Schraml P, Bendik I, et al. A novel polymorphism in the promoter of the RAGE gene is associated with non-small cell lung cancer. *Lung Cancer* 2001;32:7–12.

106. Poirier O, Nicaud V, Vionnet N, et al. Polymorphism screening of four genes encoding advanced glycation end-product putative receptors: association study with nephropathy in type 1 diabetic patients. *Diabetes* 2001;50:1214–1218.

107. Hudson, BI, Stickland MH, Futers TS, et al. Effects of novel polymorphisms in the RAGE gene on transcriptional regulation and their association with diabetic retinopathy. *Diabetes* 2001;50:1505–1511.

108. Hofmann MA, Drury S, Hudson BI, et al. RAGE and arthritis: the G82S polymorphism amplifies the inflammatory response. *Genes Immunity* 2002;3:123–135.

109. Rong LL, Bernstein E, Hays AP, et al. Receptor for AGE (RAGE) and its ligands, EN-RAGEs and amphoterin, are expressed in injured peripheral nerve and modulate regeneration in a murine model of unilateral sciatic nerve crush. Abstracts of the 30th Annual Meeting of the Society of Neuroscience. Washington: Society of Neuroscience 2000;26:114.4:303.

110. Rong LL, Yan SF, Hans-Wagner D, et al. Receptor for AGE expressed in macrophages and neurons regulates peripheral nerve repair after injury. Abstracts of the 31st Annual Meeting of the Society of Neuroscience. Washington: Society of Neuroscience 2001;351.4:179.

Diabetes and Cardiovascular Disease
edited by Steven P. Marso and David M. Stern
Lippincott Williams & Wilkins, Philadelphia © 2004

7

Genetic Determinants of Late Diabetic Complications

Alessandro Doria, James H. Warram, and Andrzej S. Krolewski

Assistant Professor of Medicine, Department of Medicine, Harvard Medical School, Investigator, Research Division, Joslin Diabetes Center; Instructor, Deparment of Epidemiology, Harvard School of Public Health, Investigator, Section on Genetics and Epidemiology, Joslin Diabetes Center; Associate Professor, Department of Medicine, Harvard Medical School, Head, Section on Genetics and Epidemiology, Joslin Diabetes Center, Boston, Massachusetts

Of all the long-term complications of diabetes, nephropathy and premature cardiovascular disease (CVD) are the ones imposing the highest social and economic burden. About one of every three patients with diabetes eventually develops overt proteinuria, which progresses inexorably toward renal failure (1,2). As a result, diabetic nephropathy is the most frequent cause of renal replacement therapy in the United States. In addition, diabetic nephropathy and its related metabolic alterations accelerate the progression of atherosclerotic lesions, further increasing the already high risk of coronary artery disease (CAD) that is characteristic of diabetic patients (3–5). Relative to nondiabetic subjects, patients with diabetes have a twofold to fivefold increased risk of cardiovascular death (6,7). Therefore, a large proportion of the excess morbidity and mortality observed in diabetic patients is related to the presence of renal and/or cardiovascular complications.

Whereas the identification of specific factors involved in the initiation and progression of diabetic nephropathy and atherosclerosis (8,9) has led to clinical measures that modify the natural history of these complications (10,11), the currently available interventions (primarily the control of blood glucose, hypertension, and lipid levels) still fall short of the ultimate goal of their eradication. Potentially, such measures may result from investigations of the genetic bases underlying microvascular and macrovascular damage. Knowledge of which genes predispose to diabetic nephropathy and accelerate the atherosclerotic process leads to a better understanding of the pathogenesis of these complications. In the clinical setting, this knowledge may permit the identification of those patients who are at high risk for renal damage and early atherosclerosis. Also, new targets for drug development may emerge, especially if the genes found are novel and have not been previously implicated in the pathogenesis of nephropathy or atherosclerosis in diabetes.

This chapter reviews current knowledge of the genetic bases of nephropathy and CVD in diabetes. Specifically, we examine the evidence for the importance of genetics in the etiology of these complications and summarize studies seeking to discover the responsible susceptibility genes.

GENETIC SUSCEPTIBILITY TO DIABETIC COMPLICATIONS

The first suggestion of variable susceptibility to diabetic nephropathy emerged from analysis of the incidence rates of diabetic complications according to the duration of diabetes. If the cumulative exposure to diabetes (i.e., levels of hyperglycemia × duration of diabetes) is assumed to be the only determinant of organ damage in diabetes, one would expect a strictly increasing relationship between the incidence of complications (new cases per 100 persons per year) and the duration of diabetes. Although this roughly describes the relationship between diabetes exposure and background and proliferative retinopathy, it does not describe nephropathy (2,12,13). The incidence of proteinuria rises rapidly after an initial lag phase of 5 years from diabetes onset, peaks during the second decade, and then declines (1,2). This pattern can be explained only by postulating the existence of a *subset* of diabetic individuals who are susceptible to the development of nephropathy in the first and second decades of diabetes. Under this model, the observed decline in nephropathy incidence reflects the fact that after 20 years of diabetes most of the susceptible patients have already been affected by this complication. Evidence for a role of genetic factors in determining susceptibility to diabetic nephropathy has been derived from family studies (14). These investigations have also provided support for the existence of a similar genetic susceptibility to cardiovascular complications (15).

Familial Aggregation of Diabetic Nephropathy

Table 7-1 summarizes family studies that used sib-pairs with diabetes to determine familial aggregation of diabetic nephropathy (16–20). Most of them were cross-sectional comparisons that assessed the prevalence of diabetic nephropathy in siblings conditional on the nephropathy status of the index case. Despite different methods of ascertainment and differences in the definitions of diabetic nephropathy, all studies found familial aggregation of this complication, both in insulin-dependent (type 1) and non-insulin-dependent (type 2) diabetes mellitus. The strength of the aggregation, moreover, was remarkably similar across studies, with one exception, the study from Minnesota (16). That exception was not only the smallest study but also perhaps the one most vulnerable to an ascertainment bias that inflated the association.

The cohort study by Quinn et al. (18) was the only one that allowed estimation of familial aggregation of diabetic nephropathy using cumulative risk, which is the most informative estimate of sibling recurrence risk. The cumulative risk of diabetic nephropathy after 30 years' duration of diabetes was 71.5% in siblings of index cases with nephropathy but only 25.4% in siblings of index cases without it (18). The large difference in cumulative risk (46.1%) between these two groups of siblings could not be attributed to differences in other covariates, suggesting that a major gene effect might be responsible for familial aggregation of diabetic nephropathy (18).

The findings of familial aggregation of diabetic nephropathy are not restricted to sib-pair families. Indeed, studies of parent-offspring pairs or extended families have detected familial aggregation of renal disease (21–23). For example, Fogarty et al. (24) used 96 Caucasian families ascertained for type 2 diabetes to estimate the heritability of urinary albumin excretion measured

TABLE 7-1. *Sib-pair studies of familial clustering of diabetic nephropathy*

Reference	Population	Proband	N	Prevalence of DN in siblings (%)	Odds ratio (confidence interval)
Seaquist et al. (16)	Type 1	ESRD	26	82	24 (4.0–145)
	USA	DN−	11	17	
Borch-Johnsen et al. (17)	Type 1	DN+	20	33	4.9 (1.2–19.0)
	Denmark	DN−	29	10	
Quinn et al. (18)	Type 1	DN+	38	72[a]	2.5 (1.3–8.0)
	USA	DN−	72	25[a]	
Faronato et al. (19)	Type 2	DN+	56	47	
	Italy	DN−	78	14	3.9 (1.9–9.0)
Canani et al. (20)	Type 2	DN+	41	53	
	Brazil	DN−	49	26	3.2 (1.3–7.9)

DN, diabetic nephropathy; ESRD, end-stage renal disease.
[a]Cumulative risk after 30 years of diabetes.

as the urinary albumin-to-creatinine ratio (ACR). Among the 96 families, there were 630 individuals with type 2 diabetes and 639 nondiabetic individuals who were examined and had measurements of urinary ACR. A variance components approach was used to estimate the heritabilities and genetic correlations for urinary ACR and systolic and diastolic blood pressure after adjustment for relevant covariates. In the total collection of 6,481 pairs of relatives, heritability for urinary albumin excretion (heritability $(h^2) = 0.27$, $p < .001$) was similar to that for blood pressure (24). Among diabetic family members, the heritability was slightly higher ($h^2 = 0.31, p < .001$). This finding provides very strong evidence that urinary albumin excretion, as measured by the ACR, is a heritable trait in Caucasians with and without diabetes (24).

Moreover, significant genetic correlation was found between the ACR and both systolic blood pressure (genetic correlation coefficient (r_g) = 0.27) and diastolic blood pressure ($r_g = 0.26$) in all pairs of relatives ($p < .001$). In pairs of diabetic relatives, the r_g values were significantly higher: 0.38 for systolic and 0.52 for diastolic blood pressure. Significant genetic correlation (but not environmental correlation) between urinary albumin excretion and blood pressure, particularly in the presence of diabetes, indicates that these traits share common genetic determinants (24). A similar hypothesis was proposed previously, on the basis of studies conducted in type 1 diabetics (25–27).

To examine the finding of heritability of the ACR further, complex segregation analysis was performed on the members of these 96 families (28). Likelihood ratio tests were performed to test hypotheses related to genetic transmission. The Mendelian model with multifactorial inheritance was supported more strongly than Mendelian inheritance alone. These analyses suggested that the best model for ACR levels was multifactorial with evidence for a common major gene. When the analyses were repeated for diabetic subjects only, the evidence for Mendelian inheritance was improved, and the model of a single major locus with additional multifactorial effects was more strongly supported. The results of this study suggested that levels of urinary albumin excretion are determined by a mixture of genes with large and small effects as well as other measured covariates such as diabetes and its duration. Our results are consistent with recent data from studies of diabetic nephropathy in Pima Indians (29).

Familial Aggregation of Cardiovascular Complications

The contribution of genetic factors to the development of cardiovascular complications in diabetes was first hypothesized after the observation of strong familial aggregation of CAD in the general population. Several studies showed that the risk for death from CAD was significantly greater in first-degree relatives of individuals with CAD than in the general population (30–32). Further support for the concept of genetic susceptibility to CAD was provided by studies of monozygotic and dizygotic twins. In one of these, a follow-up study of 20,000 twins from Sweden, the cardiovascular risk for monozygotic twins of subjects who died from CAD before 55 years of age was about eight times higher than that of twins of subjects who survived after that age (33). Because the risk was lower for dizygotic twins (relative risk [RR] = 4.0), genetic factors rather than shared familial environment were deemed to be responsible for these findings (33). Based on the evidence in the general population, it was assumed that genetic factors would also be important players in the development of atherosclerosis in the presence of diabetes.

A direct demonstration of genetic susceptibility to CAD in diabetes was recently provided by Wagenknecht et al. (15). These authors used the amount of calcium deposited in the coronary arteries, as measured by computed tomography, to quantify the extent of atherosclerosis in the coronary arteries. This parameter (coronary artery calcification, or CAC) has been shown to predict future CVD events in several short-term studies (34,35). In 122 individuals with type 2 diabetes and 13 individuals without diabetes from 56 families, the age-adjusted extent of CAC was positively associated with male gender ($p = .0003$), reduced high-density lipoproteins (HDL; $p = .02$), ARC ($p = .008$), cigarette pack-years ($p = .03$), and previous vascular events ($p < .01$). After adjusting for age, sex, race, and diabetes status, CAC was found to be heritable ($h^2 = 0.50$, $p = .009$, meaning that 50% of the phenotypic variance of CAC, after removal of covariates, was due to a familial component (15). In a multivariate analysis with additional adjustment for other cardiovascular risk factors such as HDL, body mass index, and hypertension, CAC heritability was 0.40 ($p = .04$). Similar heritability estimates ($h^2 = 0.41, p = .004$) were obtained using carotid intima-medial thickness as a marker of subclinical atherosclerosis (36). Thus, strong familial factors (both genetic and environmental) were found to contribute to the variance of CAC in individuals with diabetes. Familial aggregation of traditional cardiovascular risk factors explains only a small part of this effect.

The strong association between diabetic nephropathy and CAD (3–5) and the finding that both disorders cluster in families (14,15) raise the possibility that the same genetic factors are involved in the development of both complications. To address this question, Earle et al. (37) investigated the prevalence of CVD in nondiabetic parents of 122 type 1 diabetics, 61 of whom had diabetic nephropathy. Cardiovascular disease was more often a cause of death among the parents of individuals with diabetic nephropathy (40% versus 22%, $p < .03$), and the combined morbidity and mortality from CAD was greater in this group than among the parents of normoalbuminuric subjects (31% versus 14%, $p < .01$) (37). These data indicate that a familial predisposition to CVD is related to the development of nephropathy in diabetes and that this predisposition plays an important role in causing the excess cardiovascular morbidity and mortality in diabetic patients with nephropathy. By contrast, Norgaard et al. (38) did not find an increased prevalence of CAD among parents of proteinuric patients. In this study, however, differences in CAD mortality may have been obscured by the younger age of the parents.

GENOME-WIDE STUDIES

A promising strategy for identifying genes with major influence on diabetic nephropathy or CAD is through a genome scan using genetic markers spread throughout the entire human genome at intervals of about 5 to 10 centimorgans (cM).

The marker information is used to test whether any of the chromosomal regions represented by each marker cosegregates (i.e., is linked) with nephropathy or CAD. This is accomplished by comparing the likelihood that cosegregation between a marker and the complication is due to linkage with the likelihood that this pattern is due to chance. Results are expressed as logarithm of the odds (LOD) scores, representing the base-10 logarithm of the ratio of the two likelihoods (39). A LOD of 3.0, corresponding to odds of 1,000:1 in favor of linkage, is usually taken as a significant result. With the ongoing development of new genotyping techniques and the availability of dense maps of highly polymorphic markers (microsatellites) (40), the task of performing a complete genome scan is well within the capacity of the molecular genetics laboratory. The main limitation has been in the collection of families suitable for linkage studies.

The most appropriate strategy to identify linkage between specific chromosomal regions and diabetic complications is the nonparametric approach based on the probability of allele-sharing between siblings who are concordant or discordant for diabetic nephropathy. Whereas studies of concordant sib-pairs (known as affected sib-pair analysis) have been commonly used in genetic studies (41), the less frequently used designs involving analysis of discordant sib-pairs (DSPs) seem to be more effective for studies of diabetic nephropathy and perhaps of CAD (42). A summary of the chromosomal regions that have thus far been implicated in the etiology of diabetic complications is provided in Table 7-2.

Affected Sib-pair Analysis of Diabetic Nephropathy

A genome scan for diabetic nephropathy loci has been completed in Pima Indian families with type 2 diabetes (43). The authors used a 6.4-cM scan and genotyped 98 sib-pairs concordant for type 2 diabetes and diabetic nephropathy. Nephropathy was defined as the presence of a protein-to-creatinine ratio of 500 mg/g or higher, or a urinary ARC of 300 mg/g or higher.

Four chromosomal regions with some evidence of linkage ($p < .01$, LOD > 1.18) to

TABLE 7-2. *Chromosomal regions linked with diabetic nephropathy or coronary artery disease*

Reference	Population	Trait	Chromosome	LOD score
Imperatore et al. (43)	Pima Indians, type 2 diabetes	ACR ≥300 µg/mg	3q26	1.48
			7q32-33	2.04
			9q22-32	1.12
			20p12	1.83
Moczulski et al. (45)	U.S. Caucasians, type 1 diabetes	ACR ≥100 µg/mg	3q24-25	3.1
Fogarty et al. (46)	U.S. Caucasians, type 2 diabetes	ACR ≥100 µg/mg	7q32-33	1.7
Pajukanta et al. (48)	Finnish, general population	≥50% stenosis in two or three coronary arteries	2q22-21	3.0
			Xq23-26	2.5
Harrap et al. (47)	Australian Caucasians, general population	Acute coronary syndrome	2q36-37	2.64
			3q26	1.76
			20q11-13	1.57
Lange et al. (49)	U.S. Caucasians, general population	CAC >70th percentile	6q21	2.22
			10q21	3.24

ACR, albumin-to-creatinine ratio; CAC, coronary artery calcification; LOD, logarithm of the odds.

nephropathy were identified. The strongest evidence for linkage with nephropathy was on chromosome 7q, where two adjacent markers, *D7S1804* and *D7S500*, were linked both by two-point analysis (LODs, 2.28 and 2.73, respectively) and by multipoint analysis (LOD = 2.04) (Table 7-2). Additional loci potentially linked to nephropathy were found on chromosomes 3q, 9q, and 20p (multipoint LODs, 1.48, 1.12, and 1.83, respectively) (Table 7-2). Because this study was based on sib-pairs concordant for both type 2 diabetes and diabetic nephropathy, one cannot be certain whether the positive signals were for nephropathy or for type 2 diabetes. However, a subsequent genome-wide scan for type 2 diabetes in the Pima Indian families did not show any evidence for linkage with type 2 diabetes in any of these regions (44).

Discordant Sib-pair Analysis of Diabetic Nephropathy

Several years ago we started a genome scan for diabetic nephropathy loci in type 1 diabetes. We used DSPs—that is, pairs of siblings, both with type 1 diabetes, of whom one had proteinuria or end-stage renal disease (ESRD) and the other had normoalbuminuria after at least 10 years of diabetes. Previously, we demonstrated through simulation that the DSP study design might be more effective than a concordant sib-pair design in detecting linkage for diabetic nephropathy (42). So

far, we have examined 20 chromosomes in the 96 DSPs, a sample size having about 90% power to detect a major gene effect. We have obtained evidence for linkage on chromosome 3q (45) and three other chromosomes (Krolewski et al., unpublished observations). The maximum (peak) LOD score on chromosome 3q in the type 1 DSPs was about 20 cM centromeric to the peak observed in diabetic Pima Indians with nephropathy (43).

Recently, we have developed preliminary data on linkage of candidate chromosomal regions with diabetic nephropathy in 108 Caucasian DSPs with type 2 diabetes. So far, we have genotyped our DSPs with type 2 diabetes for the markers on chromosome 7 that gave suggestive evidence of linkage in the Pima Indian group (43). We found positive evidence for linkage (maximum LOD score (MLS) = 1.7) in our DSPs at exactly the same location (46) (Table 7-2). By contrast, we found no evidence for linkage with this chromosomal region in the DSPs with type 1 diabetes.

Genome Screens for Susceptibility Loci for Coronary Artery Disease

Given the strong association between diabetic nephropathy and CAD, one can hypothesize that the loci just described may also play a role in determining predisposition to CAD in patients with diabetes. In this regard, evidence of linkage with the acute coronary syndrome (LOD = 1.8) was detected at 3q26 in a genome scan of non-diabetic sib-pairs concordant for the occurrence of the acute coronary syndrome (Table 7-2) (47). This linkage peak is placed about 20 to 30 cM telomeric of the nephropathy locus that was observed by Moczulski et al. in type 1 diabetics (45). Considering the small size of this study and its limited power to position linkage peaks precisely, it is quite possible that the two loci correspond to the same gene.

Interesting data on CAD susceptibility genes have also come from a larger genome screen performed in the genetically isolated population of Finland (Table 7-2) (48). This study included 156 families in which at least two individuals were affected with premature CAD, defined as greater than 50% stenosis in two or three coronary arteries, confirmed by coronary angiography, in individuals younger than 55 (men) or 65 (women) years of age. Although this study could not confirm the presence of a CAD susceptibility locus on 3q, two other chromosomal regions showed evidence of linkage, one on chromosome 2q21-22 (MLS = 3.0) and the other on Xq23-26 (MLS = 2.5). The locus on Xq23-26 is especially interesting. Because men are hemizygous for disease alleles on chromosome X, they have higher probability of showing the effect of recessively acting X-chromosomal susceptibility genes than do women. Therefore, the presence of a CAD gene on chromosome X may contribute to the excess cardiovascular risk that is observed in men as compared with women. Two other regions, on 6p21 and 10q21, have been linked with extent of coronary artery calcification in the general population (Table 7-2) (49).

Although studies in the general population may offer interesting clues, some of the pathways mediating the effect of diabetes on the acceleration of atherogenesis may be unique to this disorder, being induced by excess glucose. Therefore, important information could be obtained from genome screens specifically targeted to diabetic individuals. Such investigations have yet to be conducted, although studies of DSPs (i.e., a diabetic proband with CAD paired with a diabetic sibling without CAD) hold the promise of being especially powerful for this endeavor. As was shown by Rogus and Krolewski (42), the power

of DSP analysis surpasses that of affected sib-pairs when the sibling recurrence risk is greater than 50%. Epidemiologic data indicate that diabetic patients have, on average, a 30% to 40% lifetime risk of CAD (7). At the same time, studies in the general population indicate that being a sibling of a CAD proband is associated with a twofold to fourfold increase in the risk of CAD (33). It can be inferred that diabetic siblings of diabetic probands with CAD have a risk of CAD that is greater than 50%. Therefore, DSP-based genome screens appear to be especially well suited to the search for CAD susceptibility genes in diabetes, although the increase in power offered by this design might be outweighed in part by difficulties in excluding subclinical CAD in CAD-negative siblings.

EXAMINATION OF CANDIDATE GENES FOR DIABETIC NEPHROPATHY AND CORONARY ARTERY DISEASE

In addition to genome scanning, an alternative strategy currently employed by many investigators is the "candidate gene" approach. Unlike genome scans that do not require prior knowledge of the location or biology of the susceptibility gene, this approach is hypothesis-driven because it is focused on proteins that are suspected to be involved in the pathogenesis of diabetic nephropathy or atherosclerosis. Genes encoding for these proteins are screened for the presence of polymorphisms (single-nucleotide polymorphisms [SNPs], insertion or deletions, microsatellite markers), and a case-control comparison is typically carried out to evaluate whether there is a differential distribution of alleles and genotypes of these polymorphisms among unrelated diabetic patients who have developed complications (cases), compared with unrelated diabetic patients who have remained free of complications despite long duration of diabetes (controls). Because the case-control study design may not be free from bias arising from unrecognized population stratification and may potentially return a false-positive result, the transmission disequilibrium test (TDT) has also been employed in some studies to confirm positive results from case-control experiments (50).

Unlike genome scans that detect only genes having major or moderate effects, both case-control and TDT study designs permit investigation of genes exerting major to minor effects (14).

The selection of genes for examination by the candidate gene approach is based on our current understanding of the pathways whereby the hyperglycemia in diabetes translates into the manifestation of diabetic nephropathy and accelerated atherosclerosis. Although the mechanisms have yet to be fully elucidated, available data suggest a model by which cellular pathways linking glucose to tissue damage can be divided in two components: (a) pathways that are common to all insulin-independent cells and mediate the production of cellular "toxins" (e.g., reactive oxygen species, sorbitol, advanced glycation end products [AGEs]) in response to excess glucose, and (b) tissue-specific pathways that mediate (or modulate) the tissue damage induced by these toxins (e.g., excessive matrix production in kidneys, inflammation in arterial walls). Genes coding for proteins in both groups of pathways have

been intensively studied. Several of those that have received attention are highlighted in the following sections.

Candidate Genes Involved in Glucose-Induced Pathways

Recent evidence suggests that a central role in the development of diabetic complications is played by increased mitochondrial production of superoxide resulting from increased availability of intracellular glucose in insulin-independent tissues exposed to hyperglycemia (51,52). As illustrated in Figure 7-1, increased cellular levels of superoxide dramatically enhance the effects of glucose on four pathways that lead in different ways to tissue damage: (a) increased flux through the polyol pathway (53); (b) increased formation of AGEs (54); (c) activation of protein kinase C (PKC) (55); and (d) increased hexosamine pathway flux (56). In addition to enhancing these four pathways, increased oxidative stress directly promotes the development of macrovascular complications by increasing the formation of oxidized

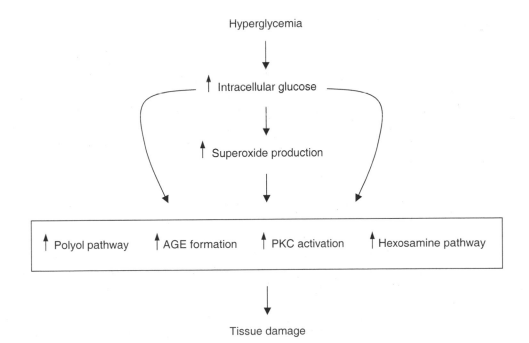

FIG. 7-1. Schematic representation of glucose-induced pathways in the etiology of diabetic complications.

low-density lipoprotein (LDL), which, through interaction with scavenger receptors, promotes the formation of foam cells and triggers inflammatory changes in the arterial wall (57–59). Two genes in these glucose-induced pathways have been at the center of intensive investigation for a role in diabetic complications: paraoxonase, an enzyme involved in the detoxification of oxidation products, and aldose reductase, the main enzyme of the polyol pathway.

Paraoxonase

Paraoxonase is a HDL-associated, Ca^{++}-dependent arylesterase that catalyzes the hydrolysis of nerve gases and toxic organophosphates such as paraoxon (a metabolic product of the widely used pesticide, parathion) (60,61). Interest in this enzyme as part of the etiology of diabetic complications dates back to 1991, when paraoxonase was reported to inhibit the copper-catalyzed oxidation of LDL (62). This effect was subsequently shown to be a result of the enzymatic removal of lipid peroxides from LDL (63). Based on this protective action against oxidative damage, genetic variability in this gene was proposed as a possible determinant of CVD, especially in diabetic patients who are at increased risk for oxidative stress (59).

The human paraoxonase gene (*PON1*) is placed on chromosome 7q21-22 and is clustered with two closely related genes, *PON2* and *PON3*, whose physiologic function is unknown. *PON1* is codominantly expressed as two isoforms resulting from a polymorphism in the coding sequence. One isoform (*PON1A*) has a glutamine at position 192 and displays low activity toward paraoxon (but high activity toward certain other organophosphates); the other isoform (*PON1B*) contains an arginine at position 192 and shows high activity toward paraoxon (64). Another coding polymorphism (Leu54Met), which is in partial linkage disequilibrium with Gln192Arg, may modulate paraoxonase activity by regulating its serum levels (65).

An association between the Arg192 allele and cardiovascular complications was first described in subjects with type 2 diabetes by Ruiz et al. (66). In a study of 171 CAD cases and 263 controls, homozygous carriers of the Arg192 allele had a 2.5-fold increased risk of CAD (95% confidence interval [CI], 1.2–5.3), compared with Gln192 homozygotes, and heterozygous carriers had intermediate risk (odds ratio [OR] = 1.6, 95% CI, 1.1–2.4) (66). Part of this effect could be attributed to the linkage disequilibrium with the Leu54Met polymorphism (65). Although the association between Arg192 and CAD has been confirmed in type 2 diabetic patients from Japan and Germany and in the U.S. general population (67,68), the contribution of *PON1* variability to CAD is still at the center of intense discussion. For instance, it is unclear whether the Gln192Arg and Leu54Met polymorphisms are themselves responsible for the association with CAD or are mere markers in linkage disequilibrium with other variants affecting *PON1* expression or activity. Several adequately powered studies have failed to observe an association between the Arg192 and/or Leu54 alleles and CAD (61,69–71). These discrepancies might reflect differences across populations in patterns of linkage disequilibrium of the Arg192 and Leu54 alleles with causal variants for which these polymorphisms are markers. The physiologic basis of the association is also uncertain, because the risk alleles at both polymorphic loci (Arg192 and Leu54) are associated with *increased* rather than decreased enzymatic activity on paraoxon (61). A possible explanation of these findings is that degradation of the artificial substrate paraoxon does not accurately reflect paraoxonase activity against physiologic substrates (72). Indeed, the Arg192 allele has been reported to be associated with *decreased* activity toward phenylacetate, which may more closely mirror the activity toward peroxidation products. On the other hand, *in vitro* studies comparing the abilities of different *PON1* alleles to protect LDL from oxidation have produced conflicting results (72,73). Another layer of complexity is added by the existence of other polymorphisms located in the *PON1* promoter (g.−107T→C) and in the coding sequence of the adjacent *PON2* gene (Cys311Ser) that also are associated with increased CAD risk, independently from Gln192Arg and Leu54Met (74–76).

Equally conflicting are the data concerning the role of *PON1* polymorphisms in diabetic nephropathy. A preliminary report described an association between renal complications and the Gln192Arg polymorphisms in type 1 diabetes (77). However, this finding concerned the Gln rather than the Arg allele. No evidence of association with nephropathy was found at this or other *PON1* polymorphic sites by Araki et al. (78) in a study of 367 patients with type 1 diabetes. Pinizzotto et al. (79) reported an association between diabetic nephropathy and a *PON2* polymorphism, but this finding has not been confirmed by subsequent studies (80).

Aldose Reductase

The excess glucose that is not utilized by insulin-dependent tissues stimulates the production of sorbitol (a sugar alcohol or polyol) and fructose in insulin-independent tissues through the polyol pathway (53). In animal models, accumulation of these metabolites, especially sorbitol, leads to an increase in intracellular fluids, followed by complex biochemical changes including decreased activity of the sodium-potassium adenosine triphosphatase pump (Na^+,K^+ ATPase), depletion of myo-inositol, increased oxidative stress, and altered PKC activity content (53,81). This chain of events is particularly important for the pathogenesis of diabetic cataract and peripheral neuropathy, but it is believed to contribute to the development of nephropathy as well (53). Evidence for this conclusion comes primarily from studies of diabetic rodents treated with pharmacologic inhibitors of aldose reductase (82–86). Similar studies indicate that activation of the polyol pathway may also play a role in atherogenesis by promoting intimal thickening and proliferation of smooth muscle cells (87,88). On this basis, it has been hypothesized that DNA sequence differences in the genes encoding for components of this pathway might influence susceptibility to late diabetic complications. This hypothesis has been intensively investigated for diabetic nephropathy but not for CAD.

A key regulator of this pathway is aldose reductase (*AKR1B1*, EC 1.1.1.21), a monomeric, reduced nicotinamide adenine dinucleotide phosphate (NADPH)-dependent cytosolic enzyme that catalyzes the reduction of a broad range of carbonyl-containing compounds to their respective alcohols. The human *AKR1B1* gene is located on chromosome 7q35 (89) and extends over 18 kb. Like its rat counterpart (14.1 kb), it consists of ten exons. Two rare DNA sequence differences were found in the exons of the human gene (90); one of these, located in exon 3, causes an amino acid change (Lys→Glu) in the protein. On the other hand, frequent DNA sequence differences were found in the promoter region. An $(AC)_n$ microsatellite polymorphism, located 2.1 kb upstream of *AKR1B1*, was associated with early-onset retinopathy among Chinese patients with type 2 diabetes residing in Hong Kong (91), and a number of studies have sought to determine whether this polymorphism may be a marker for risk of development of diabetic nephropathy as well. Studies in Caucasian (92) and Japanese (93,94) patients with type 2 diabetes have so far not detected an association of this polymorphism with diabetic nephropathy, and studies involving type 1 diabetics have produced inconsistent results (90,95–97). The initial report by Heesom et al. (95) described a strong protective effect of the Z+2 allele of the $(AC)_n$ microsatellite marker against the development of nephropathy in British Caucasians with type 1 diabetes. A later study of Caucasians with type 1 diabetes in the United Kingdom did not confirm this result (97). More recently, this issue was reexamined in a smaller study of Caucasians with type 1 diabetes in Australia with negative findings (98).

In the United States, Moczulski et al. (90) employed both a case-control study and the TDT study design for their investigation of nephropathy in Caucasians with type 1 diabetes (Table 7-3). The results of the case-control study indicated that carriers of the Z−2 allele have a slight but significant increase in risk of diabetic nephropathy (OR = 1.7, 95% CI, 1.1–2.5). In addition, an SNP (C−106T) located in the promoter region of *AKR1B1* was examined and was likewise found to be associated with diabetic nephropathy (90). Although subsequent TDT analyses were consistent with the results obtained in the case-control study, the difference in the transmission of the risk alleles was not

TABLE 7-3. *Frequencies of* AKR1B1 *alleles according to nephropathy status in 414 type 1 diabetic patients from the Joslin Clinic*

Allele	DN − n (%)	DN + n (%)
5′-ALR2		
Z+8	3 (0.8)	3 (0.7)
Z+6	5 (1.3)	7 (1.6)
Z+4	25 (6.5)	18 (4.1)
Z+2	71 (18.4)	75 (16.9)
Z	155 (40.1)	158 (35.7)[a]
Z−2	111 (28.8)	168 (38.0)
Z−4	14 (3.6)	10 (2.3)
Z−6	2 (0.5)	3 (0.7)
C-106T		
C	259 (67.1)	260 (58.8)
T	127 (32.9)	182 (41.2)[b]

DN, diabetic nephropathy.
[a]$p = .005$ for the comparison of Z−2 and all others combined.
[b]$p = .001$ for the comparison of the C and T alleles.
Adapted from Moczulski DK, Scott L, Antonellis A, et al. Aldose reductase gene polymorphisms and susceptibility to diabetic nephropathy in type 1 diabetes mellitus. *Diabet Med* 2000;17:111–118.

statistically significant. A caveat in interpreting this negative TDT result is the reduced power of the TDT relative to the case-control study (99).

Genes Modulating Tissue-specific Damage

Research also has been very active on downstream mediators and modulators of glucose-induced tissue damage. Genes coding for proteins involved in the reactivity of vascular cells to insults, in the regulation of renal hemodynamics, and in the insulin resistance syndrome (including hypertension and dyslipidemia) have been singled out for investigation.

Endothelial Nitric Oxide Synthase

Nitric oxide (NO) plays a pivotal role in the regulation of vessel function, both in the macrovascular circulation and in the microvasculature. Initially termed endothelium-derived relaxing factor (EDRF), NO is enzymatically generated in endothelial cells from the guanidine-nitrogen terminal of the amino acid L-arginine (100). Besides promoting vasodilation, NO has profound effects on many cell types, inhibiting platelet and leukocyte adherence to the endothelium,

promoting endothelial and preventing smooth-muscle cell migration and proliferation, influencing extracellular matrix synthesis and degradation, and regulating gene expression (101). These actions are mediated through the activation of guanylate cyclase, which leads to an increase in cyclic guanosine monophosphate (cGMP) within platelets and smooth muscle cells (102). Long-term blockade of whole-body nitric oxide synthase (NOS) leads to proinflammatory changes in the vessels, with upregulation of cellular adhesion molecules and inflammatory cell infiltration (103). Thus, NO has profound vasoprotective effects that play a crucial role in the vascular remodeling processes aimed at maintaining vascular patency.

Both type 1 and type 2 diabetes are characterized by endothelial dysfunction and decreased bioavailability of NO secondary to decreased NO production or inactivation by free radicals, or both (104,105). One important mechanism contributing to the latter process is the increased generation of reactive oxygen species that is produced by the boost in glucose oxidative metabolism caused by the increased availability of intracellular glucose in insulin-independent tissues exposed to hyperglycemia (52). Another factor is the increased formation of AGEs, which are capable of quenching and therefore interfering with the action of NO (106). Decreased NO bioavailability also appears to be an intrinsic feature of insulin resistance, which is characteristic of individuals with type 2 diabetes (105,107).

Because of its prominent role in NO production, the endothelial NOS (eNOS) gene (*NOS3*) has been considered a candidate susceptibility gene for nephropathy and premature CAD in diabetes. This gene comprises 26 exons and, coincidentally, is located near the gene for aldose reductase on human chromosome 7q35 (108). This chromosomal region has been identified in genome scans as one that possibly contains a susceptibility gene for nephropathy in patients with type 2 diabetes, among both Pima Indians (43) and Caucasians (46).

Several polymorphisms have been identified in the *NOS3* gene (Fig. 7-2). A substitution in exon 7 (c.894G→T) has been studied in patients with type 1 diabetes and nephropathy (109) and in

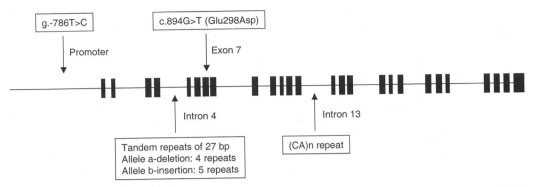

FIG. 7-2. Location of polymorphisms in the endothelial nitric oxide synthase gene (*NOS3*). The 26 exons of the *NOS3* gene are indicated by black boxes. Polymorphisms that have been investigated for association with diabetic complications are indicated by the arrows. (Adapted from Zanchi A, Moczulski DK, Hanna LS, et al. Risk of advanced diabetic nephropathy in type 1 diabetes is associated with endothelial nitric oxide synthase gene polymorphism. *Kidney Int* 2000;57:405–413.)

patients with type 2 diabetes and microalbuminuria (110); no association was found in either study. However, the former study demonstrated significant differences in allele distributions of two other intragenic polymorphisms, a substitution (g.−786C →T) in the promoter and a variable repeat (of 27 bp) in intron 4 having two alleles, one ("a-deletion") characterized by four repeats, the other ("b-insertion") by five (Fig. 7-2). The C allele at −786 and the a-deletion allele were more frequently found in patients with advanced nephropathy than in patients with proteinuria or control subjects free of diabetic nephropathy. Homozygotes for −786C (OR = 2.8, 95% CI, 1.4–5.6) and carriers of the a-deletion (OR = 2.3, 95% CI, 1.4–4.0) were more than twice as likely to develop advanced diabetic nephropathy (109). In support of these findings, TDT analyses of transmission of the a-deletion risk allele from heterozygous parents showed significant excess transmission to offspring with advanced diabetic nephropathy (65%, *p* = .03), as well as diminished transmission to offspring with normoalbuminuria that was almost significant (36%, *p* = .06) (109). The haplotypes defined by these two polymorphisms were determined, and the transmission of haplotypes from heterozygous parents was examined. Transmission of the risk haplotype (−786C/a-deletion) was significantly increased to offspring with advanced diabetic nephropathy (74%, *p* = .004), whereas transmis-

sion of the −786T/b-insertion haplotype was significantly increased to offspring with normoalbuminuria (63%, *p* = .04). At present, the molecular mechanism underlying the associations of these haplotypes with the risk of nephropathy is not clear, but difference in eNOS expression and NO production affecting glomerular function or structure might be involved. Indeed, carriers of the a-deletion allele were found to have 20% lower plasma levels of NO metabolites than noncarriers (111), and decreased renal NO production accelerated the progression of diabetic nephropathy in a rat model, presumably through enhanced vascular tone, stronger angiotensin II effects, and increased accumulation of extracellular matrix (112). It is not known at this time whether the intron 4 and −786 polymorphisms are themselves responsible for decreased eNOS expression or whether they are mere markers in linkage disequilibrium with an as yet undiscovered functional variant.

The intron 4 a-deletion allele has been also implicated in the development of CAD. In a cross-sectional study of 549 cases and 153 controls from the general population, Wang et al. (113) observed a significant interaction between the a-deletion and smoking in determining the risk of CAD. Among current or past smokers, a-deletion homozygotes (a/a) had a 1.8-fold increased risk of myocardial infarction, compared with carriers of other genotypes (113). However, this effect has not been unequivocally confirmed in subsequent studies (114,115). In the diabetic population, a/a homozygotes do not appear to be at increased risk for premature CAD, but they have elevated levels of systolic blood pressure ($p = .035$) and mean arterial blood pressure ($p = .04$) (116). Association with blood pressure and coronary vasospasm has also been reported for the -786 polymorphism (117,118).

In other studies, the association with CAD concerns the c.894G→T polymorphism, which causes the substitution of glutamate with aspartate at residue 298 in the heme-binding site of eNOS. The most convincing evidence for a role of this polymorphism has come from the Caucasian populations of the Cambridge Heart Antioxidant Studies (CHAOS) 1 and 2, in which Asp/Asp homozygosis was associated with a 4.2-fold greater risk of angiographic CAD and a 2.5-fold greater risk of myocardial infarction, compared with other genotypes (119). However, studies from Finland failed to confirm these finding among diabetic patients (116).

Renin-Angiotensin System

The genes coding for components of the renin-angiotensin system (RAS) have drawn special attention due to the central role that this system plays in the regulation of blood pressure, vascular cell functions, and renal hemodynamics (120). The RAS consists of four components—renin, angiotensinogen, angiotensin I-converting enzyme (ACE), and angiotensin receptor—which sequentially interact to produce strong vasoconstriction of the systemic vasculature (121). In addition to the action on systemic blood pressure, the system has several intrarenal actions that may act as powerful cofactors in the development of glomerular alterations. These effects include both alterations of renal hemodynamics (e.g., increased intraglomerular pressure) and direct stimulation of mesangial cell proliferation and matrix production (121). Similar effects are produced on the arterial wall, where angiotensin II stimulates smooth muscle cell proliferation and promotes inflammation (122). Genetic variability in angiotensin II generation or action has been hypothesized to contribute to variability in

susceptibility to diabetic nephropathy and CAD, and support has been provided by clinical studies showing that inhibition of angiotensin II generation or action retards the progression of renal lesions and atherosclerosis (123).

Numerous studies have sought to determine whether polymorphisms in genes encoding components of RAS are associated with renal or cardiovascular complications. The contradictory results of these studies have been extensively reviewed (14,120). Much of the controversy concerns two polymorphisms: an insertion/deletion (I/D) in intron 16 of the ACE gene and a methionine-to-threonine substitution at codon 235 of the angiotensinogen gene. The D allele of the ACE I/D polymorphism was initially found to be associated with increased ACE serum levels, increased risk of diabetic nephropathy, and increased risk of myocardial infarction both in the general population and in diabetic individuals (124–127). However, subsequent studies have not confirmed these findings (128–131). Especially striking was the lack of association between ACE genotype and ischemic heart disease among 1,250 incident cases and 2,340 controls from the Physicians' Health Study (131). Similarly, angiotensinogen allele 235T has been found to be associated with hypertension, diabetic nephropathy, or CAD in some studies but not in others (132–136). These conflicting results indicate that polymorphisms in these genes are associated with minor effects on the development of diabetic nephropathy or CAD.

Homocysteine and Methylenetetrahydrofolate Reductase

A large body of evidence indicates that hyperhomocysteinemia is a significant predictor of CVD, independent of other known risk factors (137–140), because of the toxic effects of this amino acid on the endothelium, which lead to enhanced auto-oxidation of LDL and accelerated thrombosis (141). Levels of circulating homocysteine are the result of a balance between its synthesis by demethylation of dietary methionine and its removal by *trans*-sulphuration to cystathionine or remethylation to methionine (Fig. 7-3). A common cause of

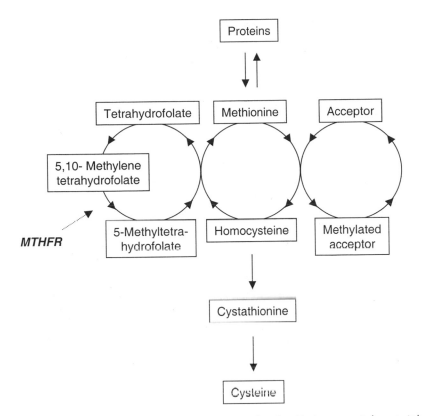

FIG. 7-3. Schematic diagram of the biochemical pathways involved in homocysteine metabolism. Homocysteine originates from the demethylation of methionine. Its removal by remethylation requires the availability of 5-methyltetrahydrofolate, which is generated from 5,10-methylenetetrahydrofolate by the enzyme methylenetetrahydrofolate reductase (MTHFR). Impaired MTHFR activity or tetrahydrofolate deficiency, or both, predispose to increased homocysteine levels.

hyperhomocysteinemia is reduced activity of the enzyme 5,10-methylenetetrahydrofolate reductase (MTHFR), which is necessary to generate 5-methyltetrahydrofolate, the methyl donor used for homocysteine remethylation to methionine (142,143). This enzymatic defect is caused by a common alanine-to-valine substitution at codon 222 of the MTHFR gene, with Val/Val homozygotes having 30% of the MTHFR activity of Ala/Ala homozygotes (144). A large series of studies have examined whether this variant is associated with an increased risk of CAD in the general population. The results have been inconsistent, possibly because of a strong gene-environment interaction that makes the effect of the MTHFR polymorphism especially evident in individuals with low folate intake (145,146). A recent metaanalysis from 40 studies involving a total of 11,162 cases and 12,758 controls indicated that the Ala222Val polymorphism is indeed a significant determinant of CAD in the general population, but its effect is rather small (OR = 1.16, 95% CI, 1.05–1.28) (145).

Hyperhomocysteinemia is a significant risk factor for CAD also when it is accompanied by diabetes (147). In fact, part of the increased cardiovascular risk observed in type 2 diabetes may be related to an association between insulin resistance and hyperhomocysteinemia (148). This effect on CAD seems to be independent of the Ala222Val polymorphism. In a study of 354 type 1 and 392 type 2 diabetic patients from Australia, homocysteine levels were significantly related to hard end points of CAD and stroke

($p < .01$), whereas no such association was observed for the MTHFR polymorphism (149). An association between the valine allele and diabetic nephropathy was reported in a small study of Japanese subjects with type 2 diabetes (150), but this has not been confirmed in larger populations from Ireland and the United States (151,152). In the latter study, T allele homozygosis was associated with a higher mortality rate among patients with diabetic nephropathy (3.9/100 person-years in Val/Val homozygotes, 2.1/100 in Ala/Val heterozygotes, and 2.6/100 in Ala/Ala homozygotes), but this finding did not reach significance ($p < .1$) (152).

Genes Involved in Insulin Resistance

Data in the literature suggest that insulin resistance may be a common denominator of renal and cardiovascular complications of diabetes. Insulin resistance and other correlates, such as increased body mass index, hypertension, and dyslipidemia, are well known cardiovascular risk factors in both diabetic and nondiabetic individuals (153). At the same time, insulin resistance is a characteristic feature of diabetic patients with microalbuminuria, as well as their nondiabetic, first-degree relatives (154–156). Furthermore, hyperinsulinemia, which is the hallmark of insulin resistance, has been reported to increase vascular permeability to albumin—a recognized feature of diabetic patients with microalbuminuria (157). Therefore, genetic factors causing insulin resistance and hyperinsulinemia may be responsible for increased susceptibility to both nephropathy and CAD in diabetes.

One gene involved in insulin resistance that has drawn much interest is the ectonucleotide pyrophosphatase/phosphodiesterase gene (*ENPP1*), also known as PC-1 (158). Discovered as a surface marker of plasma cells (158), PC-1 was subsequently found to inhibit insulin receptor tyrosine kinase activity in various cells and to cause insulin resistance (159–163). These effects appear to be mediated by a direct interaction with the insulin receptor α-unit (163). The gene encoding for ENPP1 has 25 exons and is located on chromosome 6q22-23 (164). A polymorphism causing an amino acid change from lysine to glutamine has been described at codon 121 (K121Q)

in the second somatomedin-B-like domain of ENPP1, where it may interfere with protein-protein interactions (165). *In vitro* studies have shown that the Q variant interacts with the insulin receptor and reduces its autophosphorylation more strongly than does the K allele (165). Similarly impaired by the Q allele are downstream steps of the insulin signaling cascade, such as phosphorylation of insulin receptor substrate-1, activation of phosphatidylinositol-3-kinase (PI3 kinase) activity, and glycogen synthesis (166). Consistent with these findings, human studies demonstrated that Sicilian carriers of the Q variant have lower sensitivity than do noncarriers (165). Similar results were obtained in studies of Finns and Swedes, but not of Danes (167,168).

A small follow-up study of patients with type 1 diabetes and proteinuria found that renal function declines more rapidly in carriers of the Q allele than in noncarriers (169). During 6.5 years of follow-up, the decline of the glomerular filtration rate was 7.2 mL/min per year in Q allele carriers (QQ and KQ genotypes, $n = 22$), compared with 3.7 mL/min per year in subjects with the KK genotype ($n = 22$). These findings were confirmed by Canani et al. (170) in a large cross-sectional study including 659 patients with type 1 diabetes: 307 with normal albumin excretion despite diabetes duration longer than 15 years, 200 with persistent proteinuria, and 152 with ESRD. Allele Q was significantly more common among individuals with proteinuria or ESRD (31.5% and 32.2%, respectively) than among normoalbuminuric control subjects (21.5%, $p = .01$). After stratification by duration of diabetes, the risk of early-onset ESRD for Q carriers was 2.3 times that of noncarriers (95% CI, 1.2–4.6). Similar findings were obtained in a family-based study (170). These data suggest a model by which the Q variant accelerates the natural history of diabetic nephropathy (earlier onset and faster progression through each stage), so that the association is strongest in patients with the earliest onset of ESRD. The Q allele may accelerate renal damage by causing insulin resistance and hyperinsulinemia, which may in turn stimulate renal sodium reabsorption, volume expansion, enhanced sympathetic adrenergic activity, and upregulation of the angiotensin II type 1 receptor, leading to impaired peripheral vasodilation (171). Volume overload and impaired vasodilation may predispose to hypertension and a decrease in the nocturnal dipping of blood pressure (171,172)—phenotypes that are characteristic of diabetic nephropathy.

Apolipoprotein E

In addition to their well-known effect on cardiovascular risk, lipid abnormalities also have an impact on the progression of diabetic nephropathy (173,174). Apolipoprotein E (APOE) is a 299-amino-acid glycoprotein that plays an important role in lipid metabolism. It has three common isoforms (E2, E3, and E4) encoded by three alleles (ϵ2, ϵ3, and ϵ4) in exon 4 of the APOE gene (175). Several case-control studies have examined the association between this polymorphism and diabetic nephropathy in type 1 and type 2 diabetes, but the findings were inconclusive (176–183). To clarify the association, Araki et al. (184) conducted a large case-control study, the positive results of which were examined further in a TDT family study.

In the case-control study, allele frequencies of the APOE polymorphisms in exon 4 were significantly different in the two groups (Table 7-4), with the ϵ2 allele being more frequent in patients

with advanced diabetic nephropathy than in normoalbuminuric controls with at least 15 years duration of type 1 diabetes. Genotype frequencies were also significantly different in the two groups, with those containing the ϵ2 allele being more frequent in cases (18%) than in controls (6.5%). Carriers of the ϵ2 allele had an odds ratio of 3.1 (95% CI, 1.6–5.9) for diabetic nephropathy in comparison with noncarriers. This value is very similar to the previous finding (OR = 4.3, 95% CI, 2.3–8.2) obtained in a large case-control study reported by Chowdhury et al. (176).

To be certain that the association of diabetic nephropathy with the ϵ2 allele of APOE in the case-control study was not a spurious finding due to unrecognized population stratification, the association was examined further in a TDT study. As expected for a risk allele, the ϵ2 allele was preferentially transmitted to offspring with diabetic nephropathy ($p = .03$) and was transmitted less than the expected 50% of the time to offspring without diabetic nephropathy. With the available number of control families, the low transmission of the ϵ2 allele to offspring without nephropathy was not significantly different from the null expectation of 50%, but it was significantly different from the transmission of the ϵ2 allele to offspring with diabetic nephropathy (heterogeneity test, $p = .02$). This symmetrically distorted pattern of transmission strongly supports the association of the ϵ2 allele of APOE with increased risk of diabetic nephropathy.

To explore the possibility that the association with the ϵ2 allele might be caused by linkage disequilibrium with another DNA sequence difference in the same region, Araki et al. (184) examined the distribution of four additional SNPs flanking APOE. The APOE ϵ2 allele was in significant linkage disequilibrium with all of them. However, the allele frequencies of these SNPs were similar in cases and controls, and the alleles were equally transmitted or not transmitted from heterozygous parents to offspring with or without diabetic nephropathy.

In conclusion, the case-control and family-based study provide strong evidence that the ϵ2 isoform of APOE, by itself, increases the risk of diabetic nephropathy. However, the mechanisms

TABLE 7-4. *Frequencies of apolipoprotein E (APOE) genotypes and alleles according to nephropathy status in 419 individuals with type 1 diabetes from the Joslin Clinic*

Genotype or allele	DN − n (%)	DN + n (%)
Genotypes[a]		
ϵ2/ϵ2	0 (0.0)	2 (1.0)
ϵ2/ϵ3	12 (6.0)	32 (14.0)
ϵ2/ϵ4	1 (0.5)	6 (3.0)
ϵ3/ϵ3	127 (65.0)	135 (61.0)
ϵ3/ϵ4	55 (28.0)	41 (18.0)
ϵ4/ϵ4	1 (0.5)	7 (3.0)
Alleles[b]		
ϵ2	13 (3.0)	42 (9.0)
ϵ3	321 (82.0)	343 (77.0)
ϵ4	58 (15.0)	61 (14.0)

DN, diabetic nephropathy.
[a]$p < .001$.
[b]$p = .002$.
Adapted from Araki S, Moczulski DK, Hanna L, et al. APOE polymorphisms and the development of diabetic nephropathy in type 1 diabetes. *Diabetes* 2000; 49:2190–2195.

through which this isoform causes diabetic nephropathy remain to be established (184).

CONCLUSION

A large body of evidence indicates that susceptibility to late diabetic complications is genetically determined. This evidence, which is especially strong for nephropathy and premature CAD, is derived from several family studies demonstrating an increased risk of these two complications in relatives of diabetic patients who have developed nephropathy or CAD, compared with relatives of probands who have not. The genes involved in susceptibility to these two diabetic complications may in part overlap. Interesting leads concerning the identities of these genes have come from genome-wide linkage studies of affected or discordant sib-pairs. Linkage has been detected on chromosomes 3q, 7q, 9q, and 20p for diabetic nephropathy and on 2q, 3q, and Xq for CAD. Positional cloning efforts are in progress to pinpoint the genes in these regions that affect the risk of complications. Equally active has been the investigation of candidate genes in association studies involving unrelated individuals. Findings have been far from consistent and are even conflicting in some cases. Although the cause of these discrepancies cannot be precisely determined, it is conceivable that the "detectability" of the contributions of these genes may depend on many additional factors, such as study design, ethnicity of the study population, or the modulating effect of various environmental conditions (e.g. tobacco smoking, glycemic control, hypertension control).

An additional challenge of association studies is the interpretation of positive findings. Association with nephropathy or CAD may be due to direct effects of polymorphisms on the expression or function of genes or gene products (e.g., amino acid change, frameshift mutation, premature termination), but may also result from linkage disequilibrium with as yet unidentified causative polymorphisms. Therefore, although association between a polymorphism and diabetic nephropathy or CAD may be demonstrated, confirmation that the polymorphism is actually the cause of genetic susceptibility can be ob-

tained only from functional *in vitro* and *in vivo* studies evaluating the impact of the polymorphism on the pathogenesis of these complications. Despite these challenges, it is expected that new developments such as the completion of the human genome sequence, improved understanding of genetic variation, and the availability of high-throughput technologies will eventually lead to the unambiguous identification of the genes involved in the etiology of diabetic nephropathy and premature CAD. Completion of this task holds the promise of opening new avenues for the prevention and treatment of these severe complications of diabetes.

ACKNOWLEDGMENTS

The authors' work described in this chapter was supported by National Institutes of Health grant DK58549 (A.S.K.) and by research grants from the American Diabetes Association and the American Heart Association (A.D.).

REFERENCES

1. Andersen AR, Christiansen JS, Andersen JK, et al. Diabetic nephropathy in type 1 (insulin-dependent) diabetes: an epidemiologic study. *Diabetologia* 1983; 25:496–501.
2. Krolewski AS, Warram JH, Christlieb AR, et al. The changing natural history of nephropathy in type 1 diabetes. *Am J Med* 1985;78:785–794.
3. Krolewski AS, Kosinski EJ, Warram JH, et al. Magnitude and determinants of coronary artery disease in juvenile-onset insulin-dependent diabetes mellitus. *Am J Cardiol* 1987;59:750–755.
4. Borch-Johnsen K, Kreiner S. Proteinuria: value as a predictor of cardiovascular mortality in insulin-dependent diabetes. *BMJ* 1987;294:1651–1654.
5. Valmadrid CT, Klein R, Moss SE, et al. The risk of cardiovascular disease mortality associated with microalbuminuria and gross proteinuria in persons with older-onset diabetes mellitus. *Arch Intern Med* 2000;160:1093–1100.
6. Stamler J, Vaccaro O, Neaton JD, et al. Diabetes, other risk factors, and 12-yr cardiovascular mortality for men screened in the Multiple Risk Factor Intervention Trial. *Diabetes Care* 1993;16:434–444.
7. Krolewski AS, Warram JH. Epidemiology of late complications of diabetes. In: Kahn CR, Weir G, eds. *Joslin's diabetes mellitus,* 13th ed. Philadelphia: Lea & Febiger, 1994.
8. Alaveras AE, Thomas SM, Sagriotis A, et al. Promoters of progression of diabetic nephropathy: the relative roles of blood glucose and blood pressure control. *Nephrol Dial Transplant* 1997;12[Suppl 2]:71–74.

9. Warram JH, Scott LJ, Hanna LS, et al. Progression of microalbuminuria to proteinuria in type 1 diabetes: nonlinear relationship with hyperglycemia. *Diabetes* 2000;49:94–100.

10. The Diabetes Control and Complications Trial Research Group. The effect of intensive treatment of diabetes on the development and progression of long-term complications in insulin-dependent diabetes mellitus. *N Engl J Med* 1993;329:977–986.

11. Haider A, Oh P, Peloso PM. An evidence-based review of ACE inhibitors in incipient diabetic nephropathy. *Can J Clin Pharmacol* 2000;7:115–119.

12. Krolewski AS, Warram JH, Rand LI, et al. Risk of proliferative diabetic retinopathy in juvenile-onset type I diabetes: a 40-year follow up study. *Diabetes Care* 1986;9:443–452.

13. Krolewski AS, Warram JH, Rand LI, et al. Epidemiologic approach to the etiology of diabetes mellitus and its complications. *N Engl J Med* 1987;317:1390–1398.

14. Krolewski AS. Genetics of diabetic nephropathy: evidence for major and minor gene effects [Clinical Conference]. *Kidney Int* 1999;55:1582–1596.

15. Wagenknecht LE, Bowden DW, Carr JJ, et al. Familial aggregation of coronary artery calcium in families with type 2 diabetes. *Diabetes* 2001;50:861–866.

16. Seaquist ER, Goetz FC, Rich S, et al. Familial clustering of diabetic kidney disease: evidence for genetic susceptibility to diabetic nephropathy. *N Engl J Med* 1989;320:1161–1165.

17. Borch-Johnsen K, Norgaard K, Hommel E, et al. Is diabetic nephropathy an inherited complication? *Kidney Int* 1992;41:719–722.

18. Quinn M, Angelico MC, Warram JH, et al. Familial factors determine the development of diabetic nephropathy in patients with IDDM. *Diabetologia* 1996;39:940–945.

19. Faronato PP, Maioli M, Tonolo G, et al. Clustering of albumin excretion rate abnormalities in Caucasian patients with NIDDM: the Italian NIDDM Nephropathy Study Group. *Diabetologia* 1997;40:816–823.

20. Cañani LH, Gerchman F, Gross JL. Familial clustering of diabetic nephropathy in Brazilian type 2 diabetic patients. *Diabetes* 1999;48:909–913.

21. Pettitt DJ, Saad MF, Bennett PH, et al. Familial predisposition to renal disease in two generations of Pima Indians with type 2 (non-insulin-dependent) diabetes mellitus. *Diabetologia* 1990;33:438–443.

22. Freedman BI, Tuttle AB, Spray BJ. Familial predisposition to nephropathy in African-Americans with non-insulin-dependent diabetes mellitus. *Am J Kidney Dis* 1995;25:710–713.

23. The Diabetes Control and Complications Trial Research Group. Diabetes: clustering of long-term complications in families with diabetes in the Diabetes Control and Complications Trial. *Diabetes* 1997;46:1829–1839.

24. Fogarty DG, Rich SS, Hanna L, et al. Urinary albumin excretion in families with type 2 diabetes is heritable and genetically correlated to blood pressure. *Kidney Int* 2000;57:250–257.

25. Fagerudd JA, Tarnow L, Jacobsen P, et al. Predisposition to essential hypertension and development of diabetic nephropathy in IDDM patients. *Diabetes* 1998;47:439–444.

26. Viberti GC, Keen H, Wiseman MJ. Raised arterial pressure in parents of proteinuric insulin dependent diabetics. *BMJ* 1987;295:515–517.

27. Krolewski AS, Canessa M, Warram JH, et al. Predisposition to hypertension and susceptibility to renal disease in insulin-dependent diabetes mellitus. *N Engl J Med* 1988;318:140–145.

28. Fogarty DG, Hanna LS, Wantman M, et al. Segregation analysis of urinary albumin excretion in families with type 2 diabetes. *Diabetes* 2000;49:1057–1063.

29. Imperatore G, Knowler WC, Pettitt DJ, et al. Segregation analysis of diabetic nephropathy in Pima Indians. *Diabetes* 2000;49:1049–1056.

30. Lusis AJ, et al. Genetics of atherosclerosis. In: Topol EJ, ed. *Textbook of cardiovascular medicine*. Philadelphia: Lippincott-Raven, 1998.

31. Slack J, Evans KA. The increased risk of death from ischemic heart disease in first degree relatives of 121 men and 96 women with ischemic heart disease. *J Med Genet* 1966;3:239–257.

32. Jorde LB, Williams RR. Relationship between family history of coronary artery disease and coronary risk variables. *Am J Cardiol* 1988;62:708–713.

33. Marenberg M, Risch N, Berkman LF, et al. Genetic susceptibility to death from coronary artery disease in a study of twins. *N Engl J Med* 1994;330:1041–1046.

34. Arad Y, Spadaro LA, Goodman K, et al. Predictive value of electron beam computed tomography of the coronary arteries: 19-month follow-up of 1173 asymptomatic subjects. *Circulation* 1996;93:1951–1953.

35. Wong ND, Hsu JC, Detrano RC, et al. Coronary artery calcium evaluation by electron beam computed tomography and its relation to new cardiovascular events. *Am J Cardiol* 2000;86:495–498.

36. Lange LA, Bowden DW, Langefeld CD, et al. Heritability of carotid artery intima-medial thickness in type 2 diabetes. *Stroke* 2002;33:1876–1881.

37. Earle K, Walker J, Hill C, et al. Familial clustering of cardiovascular disease in patients with insulin-dependent diabetes and nephropathy. *N Engl J Med* 1992;326:673–677.

38. Norgaard K, Mathiesen ER, Hommel E, et al. Lack of familial predisposition to cardiovascular disease in type 1 (insulin-dependent) diabetic patients with nephropathy. *Diabetologia* 1991;34:370–372.

39. Morton NE. Sequential tests for the detection of linkage. *Am J Hum Genet* 1955;7:277–318.

40. Dib C, Faure S, Fizames C, et al. A comprehensive genetic map of the human genome based on 5,264 microsatellites. *Nature* 1996;380:152–154.

41. Blackwelder WC, Elston RC. A comparison of sib-pair linkage tests for disease susceptibility loci. *Genet Epidemiol* 1995;2:85–97.

42. Rogus JJ, Krolewski AS. Using discordant sib pairs to map loci for qualitative traits with high sibling recurrence risk. *Am J Hum Genet* 1996;59:1376–1381.

43. Imperatore G, Hanson RL, Pettitt DJ, et al. Sib-pair linkage analysis for susceptibility genes for microvascular complications among Pima Indians with type 2 diabetes. *Diabetes* 1998;47:821–830.

44. Hanson RL, Ehm MG, Pettitt DJ, et al. An autosomal genomic scan for loci linked to type 2 diabetes mellitus and body-mass index in Pima Indians. *Am J Hum Genet* 1998;63:1130–1138.

45. Moczulski DK, Rogus JJ, Antonellis A, et al. Major susceptibility locus for nephropathy in type 1 diabetes on chromosome 3q: results of novel discordant sib-pair analysis. *Diabetes* 1998;47:1164–1169.

46. Fogarty DG, Moczulski DK, Makita Y, et al. Evidence for a susceptibility locus for diabetic nephropathy (DN) on chromosome 7q in Caucasian families with type 2 diabetes. *Diabetes* 1999;48[Suppl 1]:A47(abst).

47. Harrap SB, Zammit KS, Wong ZY, et al. Genome-wide linkage analysis of the acute coronary syndrome suggests a locus on chromosome 2. *Arterioscler Thromb Vasc Biol* 2002;22:874–878.

48. Pajukanta P, Cargill M, Viitanen L, et al. Two loci on chromosomes 2 and X for premature coronary heart disease identified in early- and late-settlement populations of Finland. *Am J Hum Genet* 2000;67:1481–1493.

49. Lange LA, Lange EM, Bielak LF, et al. Autosomal genome-wide scan for coronary artery calcification loci in sibships at high risk for hypertension. *Arterioscler Thromb Vasc Biol* 2002;22:418–423.

50. Spielman RS, McGinnis RE, Ewens WJ. Transmission test for linkage disequilibrium: the insulin gene region and insulin-dependent diabetes mellitus (IDDM). *Am J Hum Genet* 1993;52:506–516.

51. Brownlee M. Biochemistry and molecular cell biology of diabetic complications. *Nature* 2001;414:813–820.

52. Nishikawa T, Edelstein D, Du XL, et al. Normalizing mitochondrial superoxide production blocks three pathways of hyperglycaemic damage. *Nature* 2000;404:787–790.

53. Kinoshita JH, Nishimura C. The involvement of aldose reductase in diabetic complications. *Diabetes Metab Rev* 1988;4:323–337.

54. Thorpe SR, Baynes JW. Role of the Maillard reaction in diabetes mellitus and diseases of aging. *Drugs Aging* 1996;9:69–77.

55. Koya D, King GL. Protein kinase C activation and the development of diabetic complications. *Diabetes* 1998;47:859–866.

56. Kolm-Litty V, Sauer U, Nerlich A, et al. High glucose-induced transforming growth factor beta1 production is mediated by the hexosamine pathway in porcine glomerular mesangial cells. *J Clin Invest* 1998;101:160–169.

57. Steinberg D. Low density lipoprotein oxidation and its pathobiological significance. *J Biol Chem* 1997;272:20963–20966.

58. Krieger M, Acton S, Ashkenas J, et al. Molecular flypaper, host defense, and atherosclerosis: structure, binding properties, and functions of macrophage scavenger receptors. *J Biol Chem* 1993;268:4569–4572.

59. Tsai EC, Hirsch IB, Brunzell JD, et al. Reduced plasma peroxyl radical trapping capacity and increased susceptibility of LDL to oxidation in poorly controlled IDDM. *Diabetes* 1994;43:1010–1014.

60. Mackness MI, Mackness B, Durrington PN, et al. Paraoxonase: biochemistry, genetics and relationship to plasma lipoproteins. *Curr Opin Lipidol* 1996;7:69–76.

61. Heinecke JW, Lusis AJ. Paraoxonase-gene polymorphisms associated with coronary heart disease: support for the oxidative damage hypothesis? *Am J Hum Genet* 1998;62:20–24.

62. Mackness MI, Arrol S, Durrington PN. Paraoxonase prevents accumulation of lipoperoxides in low-density lipoprotein. *FEBS Lett* 1991;286:152–154.

63. Watson AD, Berliner JA, Hama SY, et al. Protective effect of high density lipoprotein associated paraoxonase: inhibition of the biological activity of minimally oxidized low density lipoprotein. *J Clin Invest* 1995;96:2882–2891.

64. Humbert R, Adler DA, Disteche CM, et al. The molecular basis of the human serum paraoxonase activity polymorphism. *Nat Genet* 1993;3:73–76.

65. Garin MC, James RW, Dussoix P, et al. Paraoxonase polymorphism Met-Leu54 is associated with modified serum concentrations of the enzyme: a possible link between the paraoxonase gene and increased risk of cardiovascular disease in diabetes. *J Clin Invest* 1997;99:62–66.

66. Ruiz J, Blanche H, James RW, et al. Gln-Arg192 polymorphism of paraoxonase and coronary heart disease in type 2 diabetes. *Lancet* 1995;346:869–872.

67. Odawara M, Sasaki K, Tachi Y, et al. Endothelial nitric oxide synthase gene polymorphism and coronary heart disease in Japanese NIDDM. *Diabetologia* 1998;41:365–366.

68. Pfohl M, Koch M, Enderle MD, et al. Paraoxonase 192 Gln/Arg gene polymorphism, coronary artery disease, and myocardial infarction in type 2 diabetes. *Diabetes* 1999;48:623–627.

69. Antikainen M, Murtomaki S, Syvanne M, et al. The Gln-Arg191 polymorphism of the human paraoxonase gene (HUMPONA) is not associated with the risk of coronary artery disease in Finns. *J Clin Invest* 1996;98:883–885.

70. Herrmann SM, Blanc H, Poirier O, et al. The Gln/Arg polymorphism of human paraoxonase (PON 192) is not related to myocardial infarction in the ECTIM study. *Atherosclerosis* 1996;126:299–303.

71. Gardemann A, Philipp M, Hess K, et al. The paraoxonase Leu-Met54 and Gln-Arg191 gene polymorphisms are not associated with the risk of coronary heart disease. *Atherosclerosis* 2000;152:421–431.

72. Cao H, Girard-Globa A, Berthezene F, et al. Paraoxonase protection of LDL against peroxidation is independent of its esterase activity towards paraoxon and is unaffected by the Q→R genetic polymorphism. *J Lipid Res* 1999;40:133–139.

73. Mackness B, Mackness MI, Arrol S, et al. Effect of the human serum paraoxonase 55 and 192 genetic polymorphisms on the protection by high density lipoprotein against low density lipoprotein oxidative modification. *FEBS Lett* 1998;423:57–60.

74. James RW, Leviev I, Ruiz J, et al. Promoter polymorphism T(−107)C of the paraoxonase PON1 gene is a risk factor for coronary heart disease in type 2 diabetic patients. *Diabetes* 2000;49:1390–1393.

75. Brophy VH, Jampsa RL, Clendenning JB, et al. Effects of 5′ regulatory-region polymorphisms on paraoxonase-gene (PON1) expression. *Am J Hum Genet* 2001;68:1428–1436.

76. Sanghera DK, Aston CE, Saha N, et al. DNA polymorphisms in two paraoxonase genes (PON1 and PON2) are associated with the risk of coronary heart disease. *Am J Hum Genet* 1998;62:36–44.

77. Jenkins AJ, Klein RL, Zheng D, et al. Paraoxonase genotype (192 Gln-Arg) and serum

paraoxonase-arylesterase activity: relationship with type 1 diabetes and nephropathy. *Diabetes* 2000;49 [Suppl. 1]:A157(abst).

78. Araki S, Makita Y, Canani L, et al. Polymorphisms of human paraoxonase 1 gene (PON1) and susceptibility to diabetic nephropathy in type I diabetes mellitus. *Diabetologia* 2001;43:1540–1543.

79. Pinizzotto M, Castillo E, Fiaux M, et al. Paraoxonase2 polymorphisms are associated with nephropathy in type 2 diabetes. *Diabetologia* 2001;44:104–107.

80. Canani LH, Araki S, Warram JH, et al. Comment to: Pinizzotto M, Castillo E, Fiaux M, et al. Paraoxonase 2 polymorphisms are associated with diabetic nephropathy in type 2 diabetes. *Diabetologia* 2001;44:1062–1064.

81. Greene DA, Lattimer SA, Sima AA. Sorbitol, phosphoinositides, and sodium-potassium-ATPase in the pathogenesis of diabetic complications. *N Engl J Med* 1987;316:599–606.

82. Beyer-Mears A, Mistry K, Diecke FP, et al. Zopolrestat prevention of proteinuria, albuminuria and cataractogenesis in diabetes mellitus. *Pharmacology* 1996;52:292–302.

83. McCaleb ML, McKean ML, Hohman TC, et al. Intervention with the aldose reductase inhibitor, tolrestat, in renal and retinal lesions of streptozotocin-diabetic rats. *Diabetologia* 1991;34:695–701.

84. Mauer SM, Steffes MW, Azar S, et al. Effects of sorbinil on glomerular structure and function in long-term diabetic rats. *Diabetes* 1989;38:839–846.

85. Craven PA, DeRubertis FR. Sorbinil suppresses glomerular prostaglandin production in the streptozotocin diabetic rat. *Metabolism* 1989;38:649–654.

86. Chang WP, Dimitriadis E, Allen T, et al. The effect of aldose reductase inhibitors on glomerular prostaglandin production and urinary albumin excretion in experimental diabetes mellitus. *Diabetologia* 1991;34:225–231.

87. Ramana KV, Chandra D, Srivastava S, et al. Aldose reductase mediates mitogenic signaling in vascular smooth muscle cells. *J Biol Chem* 2002;277:32063–32070.

88. Kasuya Y, Ito M, Nakamura J, et al. An aldose reductase inhibitor prevents the intimal thickening in coronary arteries of galactose-fed beagle dogs. *Diabetologia* 1999;42:1404–1409.

89. Graham A, Heath P, Morten JE, et al. The human aldose reductase gene maps to chromosome region 7q35. *Hum Genet* 1991;86:509–514.

90. Moczulski DK, Scott L, Antonellis A, et al. Aldose reductase gene polymorphisms and susceptibility to diabetic nephropathy in type 1 diabetes mellitus. *Diabet Med* 2000;17:111–118.

91. Ko BC, Lam KS, Wat NM, et al. An (A-C)n dinucleotide repeat polymorphic marker at the 5' end of the aldose reductase gene is associated with early-onset diabetic retinopathy in NIDDM patients. *Diabetes* 1995;44:727–732.

92. Moczulski DK, Burak W, Doria A, et al. The role of aldose reductase gene in the susceptibility to diabetic nephropathy in type II (non-insulin-dependent) diabetes mellitus. *Diabetologia* 1999;42:94–97.

93. Maeda S, Haneda M, Yasuda H, et al. Diabetic nephropathy is not associated with the dinucleotide re-

peat polymorphism upstream of the aldose reductase (ALR2) gene but with erythrocyte aldose reductase content in Japanese subjects with type 2 diabetes. *Diabetes* 1999;48:420–422.

94. Ichikawa F, Yamada K, Ishiyama-Shigemoto S, et al. Association of an (A-C)n dinucleotide repeat polymorphic marker at the 5'-region of the aldose reductase gene with retinopathy but not with nephropathy or neuropathy in Japanese patients with type 2 diabetes mellitus. *Diabet Med* 1999;16:744–748.

95. Heesom AE, Hibberd ML, Millward A, et al. Polymorphism in the 5'-end of the aldose reductase gene is strongly associated with the development of diabetic nephropathy in type 1 diabetes. *Diabetes* 1997;46:287–291.

96. Shah VO, Scavini M, Nikolic J, et al. Z-2 microsatellite allele is linked to increased expression of the aldose reductase gene in diabetic nephropathy. *J Clin Endocrinol Metab* 1998;83:2886–2891.

97. Dyer PH, Chowdhury TA, Dronsfield MJ, et al. The 5'-end polymorphism of the aldose reductase gene is not associated with diabetic nephropathy in Caucasian type 1 diabetic patients [Letter]. *Diabetologia* 1999;42:1030–1031.

98. Ng DP, Conn J, Chung SS, et al. Aldose reductase (AC)n microsatellite polymorphism and diabetic microvascular complications in Caucasian type 1 diabetes mellitus. *Diabetes Res Clin Pract* 2001;52:21–27.

99. Morton NE, Collins A. Tests and estimates of allelic association in complex inheritance. *Proc Natl Acad Sci U S A* 1998;95:11389–11393.

100. Harrison DG. Cellular and molecular mechanisms of endothelial cell dysfunction. *J Clin Invest* 1997;100:2153–2157.

101. Rudic RD, Sessa WC. Nitric oxide in endothelial dysfunction and vascular remodeling: clinical correlates and experimental links. *Am J Hum Genet* 1999;64:673–677.

102. Moncada S, Higgs A. The L-arginine-nitric oxide pathway. *N Engl J Med* 1993;329:2002–2012.

103. Luvara G, Pueyo ME, Philippe M, et al. Chronic blockade of NO synthase activity induces a proinflammatory phenotype in the arterial wall: prevention by angiotensin II antagonism. *Arterioscler Thromb Vasc Biol* 1998;18:1408–1416.

104. Lekakis J, Papamichael C, Anastasiou H, et al. Endothelial dysfunction of conduit arteries in insulin-dependent diabetes mellitus without microalbuminuria. *Cardiovasc Res* 1997;34:164–168.

105. Caballero AE, Arora S, Saouaf R, et al. Microvascular and macrovascular reactivity is reduced in subjects at risk for type 2 diabetes. *Diabetes* 1999;48:1856–1862.

106. Bucala R, Tracey KJ, Cerami A. Advanced glycosylation products quench nitric oxide and mediate defective endothelium-dependent vasodilatation in experimental diabetes. *J Clin Invest* 1991;87:432–438.

107. Reusch JE. Current concepts in insulin resistance, type 2 diabetes mellitus, and the metabolic syndrome. *Am J Cardiol* 2002;90:19G–26G.

108. Marsden PA, Heng HH, Scherer SW, et al. Structure and chromosomal localization of the human constitutive endothelial nitric oxide synthase gene. *J Biol Chem* 1993;268:17478–17488.

109. Zanchi A, Moczulski DK, Hanna LS, et al. Risk of advanced diabetic nephropathy in type 1 diabetes is associated with endothelial nitric oxide synthase gene polymorphism. *Kidney Int* 2000;57:405–413.

110. Cai H, Wang X, Colagiuri S, et al. A common Glu298→Asp (894G→T) mutation at exon 7 of the endothelial nitric oxide synthase gene and vascular complications in type 2 diabetes [Letter]. *Diabetes Care* 1998;21:2195–2196.

111. Tsukada T, Yokoyama K, Arai T, et al. Evidence of association of the ecNOS gene polymorphism with plasma NO metabolite levels in humans. *Biochem Biophys Res Commun* 1998;245:190–193.

112. Shultz PJ, Schorer AE, Raij L. Effects of endothelium-derived relaxing factor and nitric oxide on rat mesangial cells. *Am J Physiol* 1990;258:F162–F167.

113. Wang XL, Sim AS, Badenhop RF, et al. A smoking-dependent risk of coronary artery disease associated with a polymorphism of the endothelial nitric oxide synthase gene. *Nat Med* 1996;2:41–45.

114. Ukkola O, Erkkila PH, Savolainen MJ, et al. Lack of association between polymorphisms of catalase, copper-zinc superoxide dismutase (SOD), extracellular SOD and endothelial nitric oxide synthase genes and macroangiopathy in patients with type 2 diabetes mellitus. *J Intern Med* 2001;249:451–459.

115. Sigusch HH, Surber R, Lehmann MH, et al. Lack of association between 27-bp repeat polymorphism in intron 4 of the endothelial nitric oxide synthase gene and the risk of coronary artery disease. *Scand J Clin Lab Invest* 2000;60:229–235.

116. Pulkkinen A, Viitanen L, Kareinen A, et al. Intron 4 polymorphism of the endothelial nitric oxide synthase gene is associated with elevated blood pressure in type 2 diabetic patients with coronary heart disease. *J Mol Med* 2000;78:372–379.

117. Miyamoto Y, Saito Y, Kajiyama N, et al. Endothelial nitric oxide synthase gene is positively associated with essential hypertension. *Hypertension* 1998;32:3–8.

118. Nakayama M, Yasue H, Yoshimura M, et al. T-786→C mutation in the 5′-flanking region of the endothelial nitric oxide synthase gene is associated with coronary spasm. *Circulation* 1999;99:2864–2870.

119. Hingorani AD, Liang CF, Fatibene J, et al. A common variant of the endothelial nitric oxide synthase (Glu298→Asp) is a major risk factor for coronary artery disease in the UK. *Circulation* 1999;100:1515–1520.

120. Doria A, Warram JH, Krolewski AS. Genetic susceptibility to nephropathy in IDDM: from epidemiology to molecular genetics. *Diabetes Met Rev* 1995;11:287–314.

121. Ballerman BJ, Zeidel ML, Gunning ME, et al. Vasoactive peptides and the kidney. In: Brenner BM, Rector FC, eds. *The kidney,* 4th ed. Philadelphia: WB Saunders, 1991:510–583.

122. Strawn WB, Ferrario CM. Mechanisms linking angiotensin II and atherogenesis. *Curr Opin Lipidol* 2002;13:505–512.

123. Lewis EJ, Hunsicker LG, Bain RP, et al. The effect of angiotensin-converting enzyme inhibition on diabetic nephropathy. *N Engl J Med* 1993;329:1456–1462.

124. Rigat B, Hubert C, Alhenc-Gelas F, et al. An insertion/deletion polymorphism in the angiotensin-I converting enzyme gene accounting for half the variance of serum enzyme levels. *J Clin Invest* 1990;86:1343–1346.

125. Cambien F, Poirier O, Lecerf L, et al. Deletion polymorphism in the gene for angiotensin-converting enzyme is a potent risk factor for myocardial infarction. *Nature* 1992;359:641–644.

126. Marre M, Bernadet P, Gallois Y, et al. Relationship between angiotensin I converting enzyme gene polymorphism, plasma levels and diabetic retinal and renal complications. *Diabetes* 1994;43:384–388.

127. Ruiz J, Blanche H, Cohen N, et al. Insertion/deletion polymorphism of the angiotensin-converting enzyme gene is strongly associated with coronary heart disease in non-insulin-dependent diabetes mellitus. *Proc Natl Acad Sci U S A* 1994;91:3662–3665.

128. Doria A, Warram JH, Krolewski AS. Genetic predisposition to diabetic nephropathy: evidence for a role of the angiotensin I-converting enzyme gene. *Diabetes* 1994;43:690–695.

129. Tarnow L, Cambien F, Rossing P, et al. Lack of relationship between an insertion/deletion polymorphism in the angiotensin I-converting enzyme gene and diabetic nephropathy and proliferative retinopathy in IDDM patients. *Diabetes* 1995;44:489–494.

130. Schmidt S, Schone N, Ritz E, and the Diabetic Nephropathy Study Group. Association of ACE gene polymorphism and diabetic nephropathy. *Kidney Int* 1995;47:1176–1181.

131. Lindpaintner K, Pfeffer MA, Kreutz R, et al. A prospective evaluation of an angiotensin-converting-enzyme gene polymorphism and the risk of ischemic heart disease. *N Engl J Med* 1995;332:706–711.

132. Jeunemaitre X, Soubrier F, Kotelevtsev YV, et al. Molecular basis of human hypertension: role of angiotensinogen. *Cell* 1992;71:169–180.

133. Caulfield M, Lavender P, Newell-Price J, et al. Linkage of the angiotensinogen gene locus to essential hypertension in African Caribbeans. *J Clin Invest* 1995;96:687–692.

134. Doria A, Onuma T, Gearin G, et al. Angiotensinogen polymorphism M235T, hypertension, and nephropathy in insulin-dependent diabetes. *Hypertension* 1996;27:1134–1139.

135. Tarnow L, Cambien F, Rossing P, et al. Angiotensinogen gene polymorphism in IDDM patients with diabetic nephropathy. *Diabetes* 1996;45:367–369.

136. Fogarty DG, Harron JC, Hughes AE, et al. A molecular variant of angiotensinogen is associated with diabetic nephropathy in IDDM. *Diabetes* 1996;45:1204–1208.

137. Boers GH, Smals AG, Trijbels FJ, et al. Heterozygosity for homocystinuria in premature peripheral and cerebral occlusive arterial disease. *N Engl J Med* 1985;313:709–715.

138. Genest JJ Jr, McNamara JR, Salem DN, et al. Plasma homocyst(e)ine levels in men with premature coronary artery disease. *J Am Coll Cardiol* 1990;16:1114–1119.

139. Clarke R, Daly L, Robinson K, et al. Hyperhomocysteinemia: an independent risk factor for vascular disease. *N Engl J Med* 1991;324:1149–1155.

140. Stampfer MJ, Malinow MR, Willett WC, et al. A prospective study of plasma homocyst(e)ine and risk of myocardial infarction in US physicians. *JAMA* 1992;268:877–881.

141. Harker LA, Ross R, Slichter SJ, et al. Homocysteine induced arteriosclerosis: the role of endothelial cell injury and platelet response in its genesis. *J Clin Invest* 1976;58:731–741.

142. Kang SS, Wong PW, Susmano A, et al. Thermolabile methylenetetrahydrofolate reductase: an inherited risk factor for coronary artery disease. *Am J Hum Genet* 1991;48:536–545.

143. Engbersen AM, Franken DG, Boers GH, et al. Thermolabile 5,10-methylenetetrahydrofolate reductase as a cause of mild hyperhomocysteinemia. *Am J Hum Genet* 1995;56:142–150.

144. Frosst P, Blom HJ, Milos R, et al. A candidate genetic risk factor for vascular disease: a common mutation in methylenetetrahydrofolate reductase. *Nat Genet* 1995;10:111–113.

145. Klerk M, Verhoef P, Clarke R, et al. MTHFR 677C→T polymorphism and risk of coronary heart disease: a meta-analysis. *JAMA* 2002;288:2023–2031.

146. Girelli D, Friso S, Trabetti E, et al. Methylenetetrahydrofolate reductase C677T mutation, plasma homocysteine, and folate in subjects from northern Italy with or without angiographically documented severe coronary atherosclerotic disease: evidence for an important genetic-environmental interaction. *Blood* 1998;91:4158–4163.

147. Hoogeveen EK, Kostense PJ, Beks PJ, et al. Hyperhomocysteinemia is associated with an increased risk of cardiovascular disease, especially in non-insulin-dependent diabetes mellitus: a population-based study. *Arterioscler Thromb Vasc Biol* 1998;18:133–138.

148. Meigs JB, Jacques PF, Selhub J, et al. Fasting plasma homocysteine levels in the insulin resistance syndrome: the Framingham offspring study. *Diabetes Care* 2001;24:1403–1410.

149. Kaye JM, Stanton KG, McCann VJ, et al. Homocysteine, folate, methylene tetrahydrofolate reductase genotype and vascular morbidity in diabetic subjects. *Clin Sci* 2002;102:631–637.

150. Neugebauer S, Baba T, Watanabe T. Methylenetetrahydrofolate reductase gene polymorphism as a risk factor for diabetic nephropathy in NIDDM patients. *Lancet* 1998;352:454.

151. Smyth JS, Savage DA, Maxwell AP. MTHFR gene polymorphism and diabetic nephropathy in type 1 diabetes. *Lancet* 1999;353:1156–1157.

152. Makita Y, Moczulski DK, Bochenski J, et al. Methylenetetrahydrofolate reductase (MTHFR) gene polymorphism and susceptibility to diabetic nephropathy in type 1 diabetes. *Am J Kidney Dis* 2003;41:1189–1194.

153. Reaven GM. Role of insulin resistance in human disease. *Diabetes* 1988;37:1595–1607.

154. Yip J, Mattock MB, Morocutti A, et al. Insulin resistance in insulin-dependent diabetic patients with microalbuminuria. *Lancet* 1993;342:883–887.

155. Yip J, Mattock M, Sethi M, et al. Insulin resistance in family members of insulin-dependent diabetic patients with microalbuminuria. *Lancet* 1993;341:369–370.

156. Groop L, Ekstrand A, Forsblom C, et al. Insulin resistance, hypertension and microalbuminuria in patients with type 2 (non-insulin-dependent) diabetes mellitus. *Diabetologia* 1993;36:642–647.

157. Nestler JE, Barlascini CO, Tetrault GA, et al. Increased transcapillary escape rate of albumin in nondiabetic men in response to hyperinsulinemia. *Diabetes* 1990;39:1212–1217.

158. Goding JW, Howard MC. Ecto-enzymes of lymphoid cells. *Immunol Rev* 1998;161:5–10.

159. Maddux BA, Sbraccia P, Kumakura S, et al. Membrane glycoprotein PC-1 and insulin resistance in non-insulin-dependent diabetes mellitus. *Nature* 1995;373:448–451.

160. Kumakura S, Maddux BA, Sung CK. Overexpression of membrane glycoprotein PC-1 can influence insulin action at a post-receptor site. *J Cell Biochem* 1998;68:366–377.

161. Maddux BA, Goldfine ID. Membrane glycoprotein PC-1 inhibition of insulin receptor function occurs via direct interaction with the receptor alpha-subunit. *Diabetes* 2000;49:13–19.

162. Frittitta L, Youngren J, Vigneri R, et al. PC-1 content in skeletal muscle of non-obese, non-diabetic subjects: relationship to insulin receptor tyrosine kinase and whole body insulin sensitivity. *Diabetologia* 1996;39:1190–1195.

163. Frittitta L, Youngren JF, Sbraccia P, et al. Increased adipose tissue PC-1 protein content, but not tumour necrosis factor-alpha gene expression, is associated with a reduction of both whole body insulin sensitivity and insulin receptor tyrosine kinase activity. *Diabetologia* 1997;40:282–289.

164. Buckley MF, Loveland KA, McKinstry WJ, et al. Plasma cell membrane glycoprotein PC-1: cDNA cloning of the human molecule, amino acid sequence, and chromosomal location. *J Biol Chem* 1990;265:17506–17511.

165. Pizzuti A, Frittitta L, Argiolas A, et al. A polymorphism (K121Q) of the human glycoprotein PC-1 gene coding region is strongly associated with insulin resistance. *Diabetes* 1999;48:1881–1884.

166. Costanzo BV, Trischitta V, Di Paola R, et al. The Q allele variant (GLN121) of membrane glycoprotein PC-1 interacts with the insulin receptor and inhibits insulin signaling more effectively than the common K allele variant (LYS121). *Diabetes* 2001;50:831–836.

167. Gu HF, Almgren P, Lindholm E, et al. Association between the human glycoprotein PC-1 gene and elevated glucose and insulin levels in a paired-sibling analysis. *Diabetes* 2000;49:1601–1603.

168. Rasmussen SK, Urhammer SA, Pizzuti A, et al. The K121Q variant of the human PC-1 gene is not associated with insulin resistance or type 2 diabetes among Danish Caucasians. *Diabetes* 2000;49:1608–1611.

169. De Cosmo S, Argiolas A, Miscio G, et al. A PC-1 amino acid variant (K121Q) is associated with faster progression of renal disease in patients with type 1 diabetes and albuminuria. *Diabetes* 2000;49:521–524.

170. Canani LH, Ng DP, Smiles AM, et al. Polymorphism in ecto-nucleotide pyrophosphatase/phospodiesterase 1 gene *(ENPP1/PC-1)* and early development of advanced diabetic nephropathy in type 1 diabetes mellitus. *Diabetes* 2002;51:1188–1193.

171. Abate N. Obesity and cardiovascular disease: pathogenetic role of the metabolic syndrome and therapeutic

implications. *J Diabetes Complications* 2000;14:154–174.

172. McFarlane SI, Banerji M, Sowers JR. Insulin resistance and cardiovascular disease. *J Clin Endocrinol Metab* 2001;86:713–718.

173. Watts GF, Powrie JK, O'Brien SF, et al. Apolipoprotein B independently predicts progression of very-low-level albuminuria in insulin-dependent diabetes mellitus. *Metabolism* 1996;45:1101–1107.

174. Krolewski AS, Warram JH, Christlieb AR. Hypercholesterolemia: a determinant of renal function loss and deaths in IDDM patients with nephropathy. *Kidney Int* 1994;45[Suppl]:S125–S131.

175. Mahley RW. Apolipoprotein E: cholesterol transport protein with expanding role in cell biology. *Science* 1988;240:622–630.

176. Chowdhury TA, Dyer PH, Kumar S, et al. Association of apolipoprotein epsilon2 allele with diabetic nephropathy in Caucasian subjects with IDDM. *Diabetes* 1998;47:278–280.

177. Hadjadj S, Gallois Y, Simard G, et al. Lack of relationship in long-term type 1 diabetic patients between diabetic nephropathy and polymorphisms in apolipoprotein varepsilon, lipoprotein lipase and cholesteryl ester transfer protein. *Nephrol Dial Transplant* 2000;15:1971–1976.

178. Tarnow L, Stehouwer CD, Emeis JJ, et al. Plasminogen activator inhibitor-1 and apolipoprotein E gene polymorphisms and diabetic angiopathy. *Nephrol Dial Transplant* 2000;15:625–630.

179. Eto M, Horita K, Morikawa A, et al. Increased frequency of apolipoprotein epsilon 2 allele in non-insulin dependent diabetic (NIDDM) patients with nephropathy. *Clin Genet* 1995;48:288–292.

180. Kimura H, Suzuki Y, Gejyo F, et al. Apolipoprotein E4 reduces risk of diabetic nephropathy in patients with NIDDM. *Am J Kidney Dis* 1998;31:666–673.

181. Ukkola O, Kervinen K, Salmela PI, et al. Apolipoprotein E phenotype is related to macro- and microangiopathy in patients with non-insulin-dependent diabetes mellitus. *Atherosclerosis* 1993;101:9–15.

182. Boizel R, Benhamou PY, Corticelli P, et al. ApoE polymorphism and albuminuria in diabetes mellitus: a role for LDL in the development of nephropathy in NIDDM. *Nephrol Dial Transplant* 1998;13:72–75.

183. Vauhkonen I, Niskanen L, Ryynanen M, et al. Divergent association of apolipoprotein E polymorphism with vascular disease in patients with NIDDM and control subjects. *Diabet Med* 1997;14:748–756.

184. Araki S, Moczulski DK, Hanna L, et al. APOE polymorphisms and the development of diabetic nephropathy in type 1 diabetes. *Diabetes* 2000;49:2190–2195.

Diabetes and Cardiovascular Disease
edited by Steven P. Marso and David M. Stern
Lippincott Williams & Wilkins, Philadelphia © 2004

8

Diabetic Retinopathy and Vascular Endothelial Growth Factor

Hans-Peter Hammes and Georg Breier

Professor, Head, Fifth Medical Department, Medical School of Mannheim, University Hospital Mannheim, Mannheim, Germany; Department of Molecular Cell Biology, Max-Planck-Institute für Physiologische und Klinische Forschung, Bad Nauheim, Germany

Diabetic retinopathy is the most prevalent of all microvascular complications in diabetes, and it affects the majority of patients with both insulin-dependent (type 1) and non-insulin-dependent (type 2) diabetes mellitus. It is still the leading cause of blindness in adults despite the proven efficacy of screening programs and the favorable cost/benefit ratios of interventions. Medical treatment comprises the best feasible control of blood glucose and of blood pressure, in combination with cessation of smoking. Highly effective ophthalmologic treatment is available by laser photocoagulation, provided that routine schedules of screening for retinopathy are kept, in particular because retinopathy, even at the advanced stages, can sometimes not produce any symptoms.

NATURAL HISTORY OF DIABETIC RETINOPATHY

Retinopathy is the most prevalent microvascular complication in patients with diabetes mellitus in general, and it is the leading cause of blindness in adults (1–4). In the United States, there are an estimated 1 million patients with sight-threatening affliction of the eye due to diabetes, either proliferative diabetic retinopathy (PDR) or clinically significant macular edema (5). In Germany, the incidence of new cases of blindness due to diabetes is estimated to be 10,000 per year, and the incidence of new cases of diabetic retinopathy is

56,000 per year (6). The relative risk of blindness from diabetes is extremely high in young patients due to the absence of other blinding diseases in this group (7). The average risk of blindness in all diabetic patients is 11.6, and this figure decreases significantly with increasing age due to progression of other blinding diseases over time.

Retinopathy before puberty is a rare event, and the prepuberal status has been found to be protective against advanced stages of retinopathy. However, case reports indicate that mild retinopathy may become present after a short duration of diabetes, even before puberty (8). The shortest interval reported between onset of diabetes and onset of retinopathy is 8 months (9).

Previous data from the United States showed that patients with diabetes onset before 30 years of age had no detectable retinopathy at onset, and that the prevalence of retinopathy in this group was 20% to 25% after 5 years of disease duration (2). However, new data from the Diabetes Complications and Control Trial (DCCT) cohort, using more sophisticated techniques to detect very early retinal lesions, showed that the incidence of retinopathy in type 1 diabetes is unexpectedly high. Specifically, when 7-field-stereo fundus photography and fluorescence angiography were used to assess retinopathy during the recruiting phase of the DCCT, 44.4% of 1,613 patients with diabetes duration of less than 5 years were found to have signs of retinopathy in the photographs, and an additional 19.8% had signs of retinopathy in their fluorescein angiograms. Furthermore, another 12.9% of those with less than 5 years of diabetes developed retinopathy during their follow-up before reaching the 5-year mark. Therefore, 67.1% of patients with type 1 diabetes develop at least mild retinopathy during the first 5 years of diabetes (10).

In patients with longer disease duration, data exist from cohorts with considerable differences in glycemia. Patients in the Wisconsin study (2) had a mean hemoglobin (Hb) A_1 value of 12.5% $\pm$ 2.6% (corresponding to an HbA_{1C} level of approximately 10.5%), and 95% had developed retinopathy after 15 to 20 years of diabetes. Corresponding data from a European multicenter study (EURODIAB) showed a prevalence of 82% after 20 years of diabetes (1). Patients in this study had a mean HbA_{1C} of 6.7% $\pm$ 1.9%. PDR was present in 50% of the Wisconsin cohort after 20 years, and in 37% after 30 years in the European multicenter study. A small but relevant proportion of patients (5% to 7%) may develop advanced lesions after only 8 years of type 1 diabetes, and some 20% remain relatively unaffected despite disease duration of 40 years or longer (11).

It has always been acknowledged that patients with type 2 diabetes may have asymptomatic hyperglycemia for years before the diagnosis is made, as well as a variably long preperiod of impaired glucose tolerance (12). Therefore, it is not surprising that a major proportion of patients have retinopathy at the time of diagnosis (3). Depending on the sensitivity of the method used (direct ophthalmoscopy, fundus photography, stereo fundus photography with centralized grading, fluorescein angiography), an increasing proportion of affected patients may be identified. In the United Kingdom Prospective Diabetes Study (UKPDS), 36% of patients had at least microaneurysms at the time of diagnosis (13). An interesting question is when the process of vascular damage in the eye starts. It was previously noted that retinopathy can be present for as long as 5 years before the diagnosis is made. Linear extrapolation of data from patients in the conventional group of the UKPDS showed that microaneurysms could have been present for

as long as 14 years (95% confidence interval, 9–23 years) before diagnosis. At diagnosis, 37.5% of this group had at least one microaneurysm in one eye, and 69.2% of the group had retinopathy 12 years later (14).

Older data are not instructive as to the outcome of patients who have type 2 diabetes with and without retinopathy at the time of diagnosis. Recent information from the UKPDS determined the risk of the need for photocoagulation in these type 2 diabetics. Of those who had no retinopathy at diagnosis, 3.9% required photocoagulation at some time during the next 9 years. Of those with only microaneurysms in one eye at entry, 6.6% had photocoagulation within the subsequent 9 years. Among patients with more severe retinopathy, the risk increased to 72.4%. Most patients underwent photocoagulation for diabetic maculopathy (77.4%); preproliferative or proliferative retinopathy was treated by laser in 17.4%, confirming state-of-the-art knowledge (15).

Patients of different ethnic origins do not consistently vary in their propensity to develop diabetic retinopathy. American Indians appear to have a higher risk of retinopathy than do Europeans or Asians (16), and the risk of diabetic retinopathy among Mexican-Americans is twice as high as that among non-Hispanic white patients (17). The higher risk among South African black patients with diabetes is possibly due to comparably higher average glucose values, but a genetic influence cannot be excluded (18).

Patients with rare forms of diabetes, such as maturity-onset diabetes of youth 3 (MODY3), have the same incidence of retinopathy as do patients with type 2 diabetes (19), and those with late-onset diabetes of the adult (LODA) have the same prevalence as in type 2 diabetics (20).

CLINICAL COURSE OF DIABETIC RETINOPATHY

Conceptually, diabetic retinopathy consists of an early, nonproliferative stage and an advanced, proliferative stage. As discussed later, the term "nonproliferative diabetic retinopathy" is misleading, because there is already significant evidence for the formation of new blood vessels during the nonproliferative period of retinopathy, although not growing beyond the retina. A separate, sometimes concomitant specific condition is diabetic maculopathy, which reflects an increase in retinal permeability around the macula. The clinical stages of diabetic retinopathy are given in Table 8-1, and fundus photographs are shown in Figures 8-1 and 8-2.

The two most characteristic features of incipient diabetic retinopathy are increased vascular permeability and progressive vascular occlusion (21). In the normal retina, capillaries consist of three elementary structures: endothelial cells, basement membrane tubes, and intramural pericytes which are located within the basement

TABLE 8-1. *Stages of diabetic retinopathy*

Nonproliferative diabetic retinopathy
Mild: Microaneurysm, retinal hemorrhage in fundus (see Fig. 8-1)
Moderate: Positive venous beading, IRMAs present
Severe: 4-2-1 rule
Microaneurysms + retinal hemorrhages in *4 quadrants*
Venous beading in *2 (or more) quadrants*
IRMAs in *1 (or more) quadrant(s)*
Proliferative diabetic retinopathy
Neovascularization from the disc
Neovascularization elsewhere
Preretinal/vitreous hemorrhage
Retinal detachment

IRMAs, intraretinal microvascular abnormalities.

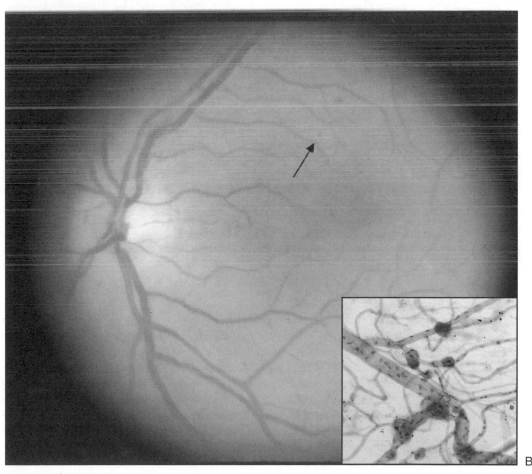

A   B

FIG. 8-1. Fundus photography of a patient with mild nonproliferative diabetic retinopathy; the arrow points to a microaneurysm. *Inset:* Retinal digest preparation of a diabetic patient; note the presence of a microaneurysm. Original magnification, ×200.

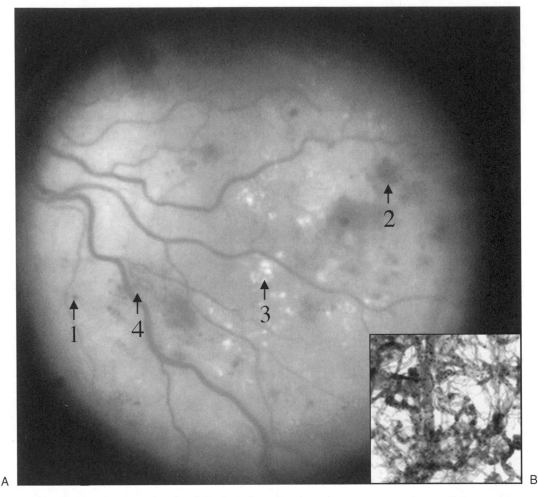

FIG. 8-2. Fundus photography of a diabetic patient showing microaneurysms *(arrow 1)*, hemorrhages *(arrow 2)*, hard exudates *(arrow 3)*, and an intraretinal microvascular abnormality (IRMA) *(arrow 4)*. *Inset:* Retinal digest preparation of a diabetic patient showing an IRMA.

membrane. The time course of hyperglycemic capillary damage has been studied in diabetic animal models (22,23). The first appreciable indication of diabetic vascular damage is the loss of intramural pericytes. Subsequently, endothelial cells disappear focally, leaving completely acellular capillaries behind, or they tend to proliferate in other areas of the capillary network. Acellular capillaries are the most significant lesions in the diabetic retina, because they (a) represent the phenotype of hyperglycemia-induced vascular cell damage, which is a general feature of diabetic complications, and (b) are the likely harbinger of all subsequent lesions in the retina.

Earlier clinicopathologic studies in human retinas demonstrated not only that acellular capillaries are no longer perfused but also that the microaneurysms which are the earliest clinically detectable signs of diabetic retinopathy tend to cluster around areas of focal capillary dropout (24–26). Microaneurysms are often locations of increased vascular permeability, and they undergo a process of involution that explains the apparent improvement in retinopathy that may be seen during follow-up examinations (25,26). Focal hard exudates and dot-blot hemorrhages are direct indicators of a breakdown of the blood-retinal barrier. As nonperfused areas

TABLE 8-2. *Risk of development of proliferative diabetic retinopathy levels requiring photocoagulation*

Retinopathy	Chance in 1 yr (%)	Chance in 5 yr (%)
Nonproliferative diabetic retinopathy		
Mild	1	16
Moderate	3–8	27–39
Severe to very severe	15–45	56–71
Proliferative diabetic retinopathy		
Early	22–46	64–75

From, Early Treatment Diabetic Retinopathy Study Research Group *Arch Ophtalmol* 1985;103:1796–1806.

become more extended due to progressive capillary occlusions, more areas may respond with intravascular endothelial proliferations, leading to hypercellular vessels (not necessarily capillaries), and with the formation of new intraretinal blood vessels resulting from sprouting angiogenesis and from vascular remodeling. Later, the formation of venous beading indicates progressive retinal ischemia, representing the extension of the response to ischemic injury to the veins. With increasing diabetes duration, and even more nonperfused retinal areas, the retina responds with the formation of new blood vessels that penetrate through the inner limiting membrane in the vitreous body. The number of newly formed vessels often correlates with the extent of nonperfusion in the retina. These neovascularizations tend to spread within the preretinal vitreous and are prone to rhexis and preretinal bleeding. Preretinal proliferations are often accompanied by increased activity of matrix-producing cells such as fibroblasts and inflammatory cells. Both tractive forces due to the tendency of new membranes to shrink and the fragility of the newly formed vessels explain the high risk of vitreous hemorrhages in patients with PDR. The chances of developing high-risk PDR within defined periods have been summarized and are given in Table 8-2.

EARLY VASCULAR CHANGES IN HUMANS

Important insight into the cellular changes that underlie diabetic retinopathy that is eventually detectable by funduscopy dates back to the early 1960s. Kuwabara and Cogan developed a method that allowed direct inspection of affected retina liberated from neuroglial tissues by means of their differential susceptibility to trypsin digestion (27). As a result of their work and that of others presented later, pericyte loss was identified as one of the earliest changes in the diabetic retina (28). Pericytes and endothelial cells are the two cell types of the retinal capillary, and they are normally distributed in a 1:1 ratio within the capillaries. Pericytes provide vascular stability and control endothelial cell proliferation (29). Pericyte recruitment to the retinal capillary marks the transition of growing to a mature vessel, characterized by longevity of the vasculature and a low replication rate of endothelial cells (30). Neither the precise reason nor the mechanisms involved are exactly defined at present.

Microaneurysms are found predominantly around areas of occluded capillaries, suggesting that microaneurysms are a first, abortive attempt of neovascularization resulting from focal retinal ischemia (26). Of note, occluded capillaries do not contain blood cells, indicating true occlusion rather than obstruction by cellular debris or white blood cells. These capillaries may be invaded by processes of glial cells, but reperfusion has also been reported, either through recanalization during early stages of retinopathy or by vascular remodeling involving intraretinal neovascularization when retinopathy is more advanced (31).

EARLY RETINAL LESIONS: INSIGHT FROM ANIMAL MODELS

Despite a large dispute about the helpfulness and relevance of diabetic animal models for human diabetic retinopathy, some insight into early processes has come from studies of rats with spontaneous or chemically induced diabetes.

In streptozotocin-diabetic rats, the earliest discernible morphologic sign of hyperglycemic damage is the loss of pericytes. It starts at between 4 and 8 weeks of diabetes, and most likely persists over the entire hyperglycemic period, although with decreasing magnitude over time (23) (Hammes et al., unpublished observations). Concomitantly, there is a steady increase in the number of endothelial cells per capillary area unit, indicating random distribution of endothelial cell proliferation. This change becomes significant after 4 to 5 months of hyperglycemia. In parallel with the increasing endothelial cell numbers, acellular occluded capillaries occur, starting with a unilateral focal obstruction in the vicinity of capillaries that still contain cells. This phenotype favors the idea that capillary occlusion in the diabetic retina is the result of both endothelial cell damage (and loss) and extraluminal factors. Although *in vivo* experiments suggest that intraluminal obstruction may occur through cellular components, acellular capillaries in retinal digest preparations of diabetic rats typically are devoid of cellular debris or blood cells (32,33) (Fig. 8-3). Acellular capillaries are also present in nondiabetic animals, but they are more numerous in diabetic animals, and they become more frequent after 3 to 4 months of diabetes (Fig. 8-4).

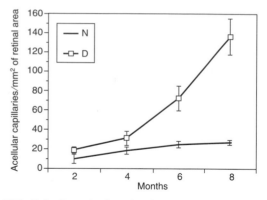

FIG. 8-4. Quantitative development of acellular capillaries in diabetic rats.

Microaneurysms resembling very early lesions in human retinas (i.e., unilateral outpouchings of the capillary) are occasionally found in diabetic rodents, appearing after 5 to 6 months of hyperglycemia (34).

Basement membrane thickening is a later event in diabetic rodents, although the transcription of basement membrane components starts after about 2 months of diabetes (35).

PATHOBIOCHEMISTRY

Chronic hyperglycemia, which characterizes all forms of diabetes, is the main causal factor of retinal damage in diabetes. Notably, all diabetes types are prone to the development of specific retinal pathology. The typical features of hyperglycemia-induced disease in the retina (i.e., abnormalities of blood flow and increased vascular permeability) are also found in other microvascular tissues, underlining the general character of the disease. With disease progression, abnormalities of the matrix occur that contribute to irreversible vascular leakage. One characteristic in diabetic retinal capillaries is cell loss. When pericytes are lost and acellular capillaries form, endothelial cells are also lost. One possible reason may be programmed cell death, which in turn can be the result of decreased production of trophic/survival factors (36,37). The link between hyperglycemia and the tissue changes leading to ischemia and hypoxia-induced

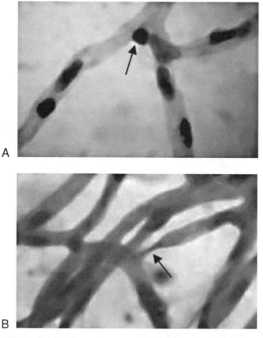

FIG. 8-3. Retinal digest preparation of rat retina. **A:** Normal retina; the arrow indicates a pericyte. **B:** Retina of a rat with diabetes of 5 months' duration, showing unilateral occlusion of a retinal capillary. Original magnification, ×400.

neovascularization is based on biochemical pathway alterations that originally were thought to work independently and with varying priorities in different target tissues of diabetic complications. It was thought for many years that chronic hyperglycemia causes retinopathy and other tissue-specific microangiopathies by four independent pathways: increased polyol pathway flux, increased formation of advanced glycation end products (AGEs), activation of protein kinase C (PKC) isoforms, and increased hexosamine pathway flux (38–41). With the identification of a common underlying hyperglycemia-driven biochemical cellular abnormality—increased mitochondrial production of reactive oxygen species—a new concept has been identified (42,43). The aspects of this new concept with relevance for the retina are summarized here.

Aldose-Reductase Pathway

The cytosolic enzyme aldose reductase (EC1.1.1.21) reduces glucose to sorbitol. Reduced nicotinamide adenine dinucleotide phosphate (NADPH) is the cofactor of this reaction and also of the regeneration of glutathione by the enzyme glutathione reductase. Because of the low affinity of glucose for aldose reductase, the pathway contributes only little to glucose metabolism under normoglycemic conditions. However, when much more glucose enters the cell in hyperglycemia, the flux through the pathway is increased, consuming NADPH and producing reduced nicotinamide adenine dinucleotide (NADH) and fructose. The cellular consequences of these alterations were thought to involve (a) osmotic stress due to intracellular sorbitol; (b) decreased activity of the sodium-potassium adenosine triphosphatase pump (Na^+,K^+-ATPase); (c) increased ratio of NADH to its oxidized form NAD^+, or reductive stress; and (d) reduction of cytosolic NADPH (exacerbation of intracellular oxidative stress).

The relative contribution of this pathway to the pathogenesis of diabetic retinopathy was tested with the use of pharmacologic inhibitors. In contrast to other complications in diabetes (e.g., neu-

ropathy), aldose reductase inhibition produced inconsistent data in animal models (44,45) and failed in human trials (46).

Protein Kinase C Activation

Excess intracellular glucose can result in the activation of some members of the PKC family by *de novo* synthesis of the lipid second messenger, diacylglycerol (DAG), which is produced by the glycolytic intermediate dihydroxyacetone phosphate through reduction and acylation steps. DAG activates primarily PKC-β and -δ, but it also specifically activates PKC-α and -ϵ in the retina. The consequences of PKC activation are manifold, the most important for the retina being changes in blood flow and vascular permeability to vasoactive molecules such as endothelial nitric oxide synthase (eNOS), endothelin-1 (ET-1), and vascular endothelial growth factor (VEGF) (47–49). Mice with transgenic overexpression of PKC-β developed more neovascularizations than did wild-type mice in a model of hypoxia-induced proliferative retinopathy, whereas mice with a genetic ablation of the gene developed fewer proliferations (50). With the use of PKC-β inhibitors, it was demonstrated that hyperglycemia-induced PKC activation can be inhibited dose-dependently, and that a decrease of blood flow through the retina of hyperglycemic animals could be normalized (51). With the same oral inhibitor of PKC, laser-induced retinal neovascularizations were also reduced, indicating that PKC activation is a possible therapeutic target in diabetic patients with various levels of retinopathy (52).

Increased Intracellular Formation of Advanced Glycation End Products

AGEs have been found in a variety of diabetic tissues, including the retina, where they are found in vascular and neuroglial areas, depending on the type of AGE investigated and the duration of disease (53,54).

The conventional concept holds that AGEs are formed from glucose by a nonenzymatic reaction with extracellular proteins. However, it has become clear recently that the reaction of glycolytic intermediates with proteins contributes to the process of intracellular AGE formation, and that this process occurs at a much higher level than previously thought (55,56). Intracellular AGE can be formed by three independent mechanisms: (a) intracellular auto-oxidation of glucose, (b) decomposition of Amadori products to 3-deoxyglucosone (3-DG), and (c) fragmentation of glyceraldehyde-3-phosphate and dihydroxyacetone phosphate to methylglyoxal (57,58). Another result of the biochemical reactions in diabetic tissues is the glycoxidation product $N\epsilon$-(carboxymethyl)lysine (CML), which is formed through oxidative cleavage of the carbohydrate moiety of an Amadori product together with erythronic acid (59). CML is found in the nondiabetic retina, but it increases in vascular and neuroglial elements of the retina in diabetes. AGEs of the 3-DG type are present only in vascular structures during the onset of retinopathy. Both CML and 3-DG-type AGEs are found throughout the entire retina in cases of advanced retinopathy in humans (54). AGEs and their intracellular precursors affect diabetic target tissues by three types of interactions: (a) they modify protein function; (b) they interact with cellular receptors on a variety of cells, including macrophages; and (c) they interfere with long-lived matrix molecules and with matrix receptors.

One important receptor system involved in the interaction of AGEs with cells is the receptor

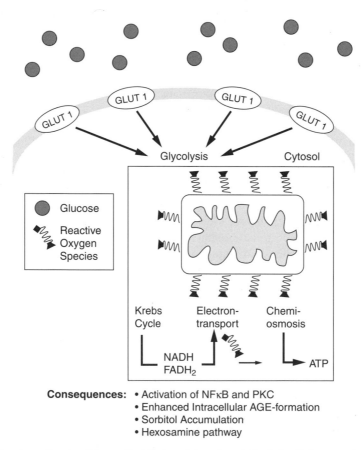

FIG. 8-5. Unifying hypothesis of the pathobiochemistry of endothelial cell damage in diabetes (modified from David Stern). Increased flux through glycolysis and the tricarboxylic acid (TCA) cycle results in mitochondrial production of reactive oxygen species, with subsequent activation of the aldose reductase and hexosamine pathways, activation of protein kinase C, and increased formation of advanced glycation end products.

for AGEs, termed RAGE. Its role in the pathogenesis of diabetic complications is outlined in Chapter 6.

Inhibitor studies in animals and humans have been performed with various unrelated AGE inhibitors. These studies yielded functional and structural ameliorations of features of diabetic retinopathy, such as pericyte loss, microaneurysms, and the formation of acellular capillaries (53,60).

The Unifying Concept

Recently, an innovative concept has been proposed to link the seemingly unrelated pathobiochemical processes and hexosamine pathway activation with hyperglycemia-induced microangiopathy (42). This concept is based on the finding that cells that are exposed to high ambient glucose, such as endothelial cells, have an increased flux through glycolysis and through the tricarboxylic acid (TCA) cycle. This generates electron donors, which cause a high electrochemical potential difference across the inner mitochondrial membrane, prolonging the half-life of superoxide-generating mediators such as coenzyme Q. The result is an increased production of superoxide by the mitochondrial electron transport chain. There is a major reduction in the activity of the glycolytic enzyme system, glyceraldehyde-3-phosphate dehydrogenase (GA3PDH), with an upstream accumulation of glycolytic metabolites such as sorbitol. Methylglyoxal, as one important intracellular AGE, may also accumulate in response to mitochondrial overproduction of reactive oxygen species (ROS), reflecting increased triose phosphate levels as a result of inhibited glycolysis on the level of GA3PDH. The same also applies to the PKC pathway, because its booster, DAG, is increasingly formed by the glycolytic intermediate dihydroxyacetone phosphate. Figure 8-5 summarizes this new concept.

Preliminary experimental support for this new hypothesis comes from studies in mice with genetic modulation of the superoxide detoxification system, but data with relevance for the retina are lacking.

EVIDENCE FOR OXIDATIVE STRESS IN THE RETINA

The *in vivo* relevance of the concept of increased ROS production for the retina, and for the pathogenesis of diabetic retinopathy in general, can be underpinned by evidence that there is oxidative stress in the diabetic retina. Because ROS have an ultrashort half-life, direct measurements of ROS in the retina are difficult. However, information from indirect measures, such as oxidation of cellular components or indicators of ROS modification of plasma constituents, have been reported.

One indicator of oxidative stress in the diabetic retina is the glycoxidation product CML. As mentioned previously, this product is increasingly formed by the oxidative fragmentation of glucose moieties in Amadori products (61). CML, however, is also a degradation product of lipid peroxidation. The presence of CML in the normal retina has been related to the high concentration of easily oxidizable membrane components of the photoreceptor layer and to the high consumption of molecular oxygen in the retina. In the normal retina, CML is found in neuroglial cells and in the photoreceptor layer. In diabetes, CML is primarily found in the inner (vascularized) parts of the retina. CML is a ligand of RAGE. RAGE colocalizes with Müller cells in the retina, and it is upregulated in the diabetic retina (54,62). The result of RAGE activation is increased oxidative stress through the generation of ROS (63). This may represent a vicious cycle, in which both the ligand and the receptor lead to perpetuated ROS formation in the retina.

Further indication of an increase in oxidative stress in the diabetic retina comes from experiments measuring estimates of lipid peroxide, such as thiobarbituric acid substances (TBARS). Kern et al. (64) measured this parameter in retinas of rats diabetic for 12 months and found a doubling of the level compared with nondiabetic controls. Confirming the hypothesis that hyperglycemia mediates induction of ROS production, and subsequently activation of PKC, the enzyme not only was activated in the retina but was inhibited to near-normal levels by a mixture of multiple antioxidants with various modes of action (64).

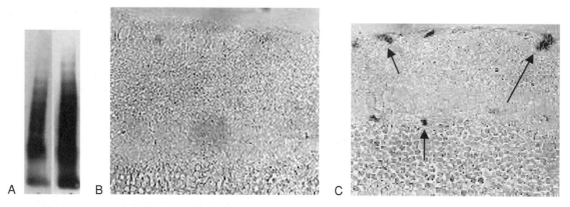

FIG. 8-6. Evidence for oxidative stress in the diabetic retina. **A:** Comparison of a normal rat retina *(left lane)* and a 6-month diabetic rat retina *(right lane)*. Protein extracts were subjected to electrophoresis and blotted against reagents detecting oxidatively modified proteins. Note that the amount of modified proteins is much higher in the diabetic retina. **B:** Nitrotyrosine immunohistology of a nondiabetic retina. **C:** Positive labeling of vascular structures with nitrotyrosine, indicating oxidative stress in diabetic retinal vessels *(arrows)*.

Another candidate indicator for oxidative stress in the diabetic retina is heme oxygenase-1 (HO-1), also known as heat shock protein-32, which is a regulatory enzyme in the heme degradation pathway. The general stimulus for HO-1 induction is increased oxidative stress in the retina. In rats that were diabetic for 6 months, HO-1 was upregulated in a pattern colocalizing with the presence of Müller cells (34).

Researchers using a method that identifies oxidatively modified proteins by an immunoblot technique found that retinas from 6 months diabetic rats yielded higher levels of carbonyl-stress modified proteins than did retinas of age-matched control rats (Fig. 8-6).

A third marker for the presence of superoxide within the retina is nitrotyrosine. In the presence of superoxide, nitric oxide nitrates proteins via heterolytic cleavage of peroxynitrite. The resultant, nitrotyrosine, is detectable by immunohistochemical methods, and it is mainly found in the vascular parts of experimentally diabetic retinas.

THE BIOLOGY OF VASCULAR ENDOTHELIAL GROWTH FACTOR

VEGF was originally discovered as the first endothelial-cell-specific angiogenic growth fac-

tor and vascular permeability factor (65,66). Research revealed that VEGF (then called VEGF-A) is a true pluripotent cytokine that stimulates various biologic responses in endothelial cells, including proliferation, migration, survival, permeability, fenestration, and tissue factor production (67,68). Several VEGF isoforms are generated by alternative splicing of a single VEGF messenger RNA (69). These isoforms form homodimeric proteins which differ in their ability to bind to heparin. This physical property allows the formation of VEGF-protein gradients in tissues, for example in the developing brain (70). VEGF is the founding member of a family of growth factors with functions in angiogenesis and lymphangiogenesis (71). However, although certain relatives of VEGF, in particular placenta growth factor, play a role in postnatal angiogenesis, VEGF is still the most universal regulator of physiologic and pathologic angiogenesis.

In the normal organism, VEGF acts primarily on the vascular system, because the high-affinity VEGF receptors, VEGFR-1 (known as flt-1) and VEGFR-2 (known as flk-1 in the mouse, KDR in humans) are expressed predominantly by vascular endothelial cells (72). All known VEGF isoforms are capable of binding VEGFR-1 and VEGFR-2. Neuropilin-1 (nrp-1), a neuronal receptor involved in axonal guidance during development, has been identified as an isoform-specific receptor for the 165-amino-acid VEGF isoform (73). Nrp-1 is expressed by both endothelial cells and neurons, which suggests that VEGF also has a function in the nervous system. This hypothesis is supported by the observation that certain neurons in the brain and in the retina also express flk-1 (74). Therefore, the VEGF/flk-1/nrp-1 system represents a molecular link between the vascular system and the nervous system.

Gene targeting experiments have shown that VEGF is essential for early-stage vascular development (75,76). VEGF-deficient mouse embryos die at midgestation as a consequence of severe malformations of the primitive cardiovascular system: although the heart is beating initially, a functional circulation does not form because large blood vessels, in particular the dorsal aorta and the vitelline vessels of the yolk sac, fail to form properly. Conditional inactivation of VEGF, either by pharmacologic inhibition or by genetic techniques, has demonstrated that VEGF is also required for angiogenesis in the corpus luteum (77), in developing long bones (78), and in the developing brain (Raab and Breier, data in preparation). Moreover, indirect evidence suggests that VEGF secreted by astrocytes guides capillary growth in the postnatal retina (79). Taken together, the available knowledge suggests that VEGF regulates blood vessel formation in all organs and throughout development. VEGF is also an important survival factor for newly formed blood vessels, as is demonstrated in the developing retina (80), whereas mature vessels no longer require VEGF for their survival (81). The survival activity of VEGF is dependent on vascular endothelial cadherin (VE-cadherin), a Ca^{2+}-dependent cell adhesion molecule that is localized in the so-called adherens junctions of endothelial cells (82).

Local or systemic hypoxia leads to a strong upregulation of VEGF expression. This remarkable property was originally discovered by analyses of VEGF expression in tumors. Cells adjacent to necrotic areas are hypoxic and express large amounts of VEGF (83–85). It was therefore suggested that VEGF upregulation in perinecrotic tumor areas stimulates the growth of new blood vessels in order to nourish the growing tumor. However, another important function of

VEGF inside the tumor is to prevent endothelial cell apoptosis and vessel regression (30). In the meanwhile, it is well established that VEGF upregulation in hypoxic tissue is a universal mechanism that stimulates the compensatory growth of blood vessels in physiologic and pathologic situations. VEGF upregulation is mediated primarily by hypoxia-inducible factor-1 (HIF-1), a central regulator of the cellular responses to hypoxia (86). HIF-1 is a heterodimeric transcription factor whose α-subunit is rapidly degraded in normoxic cells but becomes stabilized under hypoxia. Recent evidence suggests that enzymes that modify the HIF-1α subunit, so-called prolyl hydroxylases, regulate HIF-1 stability (87). Because the activity of prolyl hydroxylases is regulated by oxygen, they may serve as the long-sought oxygen sensors in cells.

VEGF cooperates with various other factors during angiogenesis and vascular morphogenesis. A second family of vascular cytokines of central importance for vascular growth and development are the angiopoietins (88). Angiopoietin-1 cooperates with VEGF to induce vascular sprouting and is required for the remodeling of the primitive vasculature into the network of small and large vessels known as the vascular tree. In the adult organism, angiopoietin-1 stabilizes blood vessels and renders them resistant to vascular leakage. Angiopoietin-2 serves as an antagonist of angiopoietin-1 activity. Angiopoietin-2 expression is strictly regulated and occurs at sites of vascular remodeling, for example in host vessels that are activated by adjacent tumors. It has been proposed that the outcome of angiopoietin-2-expressing endothelial cells depends on VEGF levels in local tissue: in the presence of high VEGF levels, endothelial cells proliferate and angiogenesis occurs, whereas low VEGF levels cause endothelial cell apoptosis, because survival activity is missing (89).

Vascular Endothelial Growth Factor and the Diabetic Retina

As outlined previously, the natural history of diabetic retinopathy is progressive vessel dropout and increased vascular permeability. The link between vascular regression and responsive neovascularizations was made more than 50 years ago, when Michaelson hypothesized that factors secreted by the hypoxic retina stimulate vessel growth (90). After an extensive search, VEGF was identified as the factor that best matches the criteria of Michaelson's hypothesis.

Vascular Endothelial Growth Factor in Ischemic Retinopathy

VEGF is present at low levels in the normal retina. Several cells in the eye are able to constantly produce VEGF, including endothelial cells, pericytes, Müller cells, and ganglion cells (91–94). Local VEGF production in the vasculature is associated with a fenestrated capillary phenotype, such as in the glomerulus of the kidney or in the choroid (95). In the inner retina, the local production of VEGF in the retina may have different functions (discussed later).

VEGF is upregulated severalfold in the vitreous and aqueous humors of patients with active ocular neovascularization, regardless of the cause of retinopathy (96). Several animal models of hypoxia-induced proliferative retinopathy exhibit high retinal VEGF levels (97–99). Many studies have confirmed and extended these findings, indicating that retinal diseases involving ischemia of a certain degree are also associated with hypoxia-induced VEGF upregulation.

VEGF is also a permeability-enhancing factor within the eye, a function that possibly contributes to the pathogenesis of macula edema (100). Intravitreal injection of VEGF into the eyes of rodents and primates mimics some early features of nonproliferative diabetic retinopathy, such as increased vascular permeability and microaneurysm formation (Fig. 8-1) (101). It is therefore possible that VEGF may be responsible for some of the changes observed during the earliest stages of retinopathy.

However, from retinal digest preparations of diabetic rats, it is known that a focal increase in the number of endothelial cells and an increase in the deposition of periodic acid-Schiff (PAS)-positive material occurs within the vessel wall, which suggests increased vascular permeability and proliferative activity of the retina in the absence of occlusive vascular changes. The expression of VEGF was therefore studied

in these models, which do not develop proliferative retinal changes, and it was found that VEGF is upregulated in association with its receptors flt-1 (VEGFR-1) and flk-1 (VEGFR-2) (37). Two important questions arise from this and concomitant studies (102–106): (a) What is the stimulus for VEGF upregulation? and (b) What is the reason for VEGF to be upregulated? With the available data, it appears that VEGF is induced by hyperglycemia-induced ROS production (107). Other likely inducers during the early course of retinopathy, in which ischemia due to capillary dropout may not yet be a significant contributor, are AGEs (108–110), which are also known to induce intraocular VEGF production, and ROS (111). Regarding the second question, it appears more difficult to find a definitive answer. VEGF, among other growth, may promote endothelial resistance to oxidative stress (112). As mentioned earlier, VEGF is also a survival factor for endothelial cells (80). Chronic hyperglycemia induces a comprehensible stress not only for vascular endothelial cells in the diabetic retina. An imbalance between survival factor demand and provision can induce programmed cell death (113). In fact, apoptosis has been observed in both vascular and neuroglial structures in diabetic retinas, and it can be reduced either by the application of growth factors or by inhibitors of oxidative stress (114,115). The upregulation of VEGF in the early diabetic retina may represent a stress-induced cell response.

Treatment of Vascular Endothelial Growth Factor-Induced Pathologies in the Eye

If VEGF is the problem, VEGF inhibition should be the solution. Therefore, several approaches were chosen in different experimental models to verify the possibility of VEGF inhibition as a therapeutic option.

Three mechanisms of VEGF antagonism have been applied to experimental eyes, for proof of the principle that VEGF is the major factor involved in retinal neovascularization and to establish novel therapies. Chimeric proteins or neutralizing antibodies that trap VEGF reduced experimental retinopathy by up to 77%, and antisense oligonucleotides that inhibit the transcription of VEGF were effective, albeit less strong (116,117).

Interference with the intracellular transduction cascade of the VEGF receptor has also been proposed. Because PKC is downstream VEGF signaling, PKC inhibitors were tested and proved effective in certain aspects of VEGF-associated pathologies, such as increased permeability, retinal blood flow, and proliferative retinopathy (51,52).

TREATMENT OF DIABETIC RETINOPATHY: CURRENT STANDARDS

Blood Glucose Control

There is no doubt that good glycemic control helps prevent the onset and delays the progression of retinopathy. Two large clinical studies have provided evidence that intensive care, both in type 1 and in type 2 diabetes, results in a beneficial outcome with regard to onset, progression to higher levels, and progression to vision-threatening retinopathy.

The results of the DCCT have been detailed many times, and there is no need to repeat them. With regard to prevention and treatment of diabetic retinopathy, the results of the study are summarized in Table 8-3. The main findings were that improved glucose control in patients with retinopathy at baseline (i.e., group average reduction of HbA_1 from 9.1% to 7.2% over a mean of 6.5 years) resulted in a 76% reduction in the development of retinopathy. If glucose control was implemented when retinopathy was already

present, the effect occurred in a delayed fashion and was overall less pronounced.

There is a level of retinopathy that represents a "point of no return," beyond which improved control may no longer be effective. This suggests that implementation of the DCCT findings in every patient with type 1 diabetes should be performed as quickly as possible (118). Interestingly, good glycemic control has an "afterburner" effect. The risk reduction achieved by good glycemic control persisted in patients of the former "intensified" treatment group compared with the former "conventional" group of the DCCT, although glycemic levels became comparable over time after the ending of the DCCT. This Epidemiology of Diabetes Interventions and Complications (EDIC) follow-up study showed benefits for retinal outcome in 52% to 75% of subjects regarding the development of severe nonproliferative retinopathy, PDR, clinically significant macular edema, and need for laser treatment (119). The risks of intensive glucose control have also been studied; they are increased frequency of hypoglycemia and weight gain.

The corresponding study in type 2 diabetes is the UKPDS, the results of which have been published and are available as a slide set from the UKPDS web site (http://www.dtu.ox.ac.uk/index.html?maindoc=/ukpds/). This large, multicenter study showed that a reduction of glycated hemoglobin from 7.9% to 7.0% over 9 years reduced the combined risk of vitreous hemorrhage, need for photocoagulation, and renal failure by 25%, regardless of whether insulin or oral hypoglycemic agents were used to achieve the aim (13,120).

The level of glycemia was determined with HbA_{1C} as the standard for assessment of the quality of control. Several guidelines have implemented thresholds for glycated hemoglobin, above which the diabetologist should be consulted for further action.

TABLE 8-3. *Important questions answered by the Diabetes Control and Complications Trial*

Can complete prevention of any retinopathy be obtained by good glycemic control (permanent HbA1c below 7%)?	No (but 27% risk reduction)
Can developing retinopathy be prevented by good glycemic control?	Yes, 76% risk reduction
Can retinopathy progression be prevented?	Yes, 63% risk reduction
Can the need for laser coagulation be prevented?	Yes, 52% risk reduction

Blood Pressure Control

Both type 1 and type 2 diabetic patients are often affected by arterial hypertension, even in the absence of diabetic nephropathy. In type 1 diabetic patients, the prevalence varies between

10% and 40%, and in type 2 diabetics it is approximately 70% (121,122). Men appear to have a higher risk, as in nondiabetic patients; further risk factors are those that can lead to overt nephropathy, such as diabetes duration and glycated hemoglobin. With nephropathy appearing, the prevalence of hypertension approaches 100%.

Treatment of hypertension in type 2 diabetes often requires more than one agent. However, if effective blood pressure lowering is achieved, the benefit for the eye may be pronounced. In the UKPDS, 1,148 patients were randomly assigned to receive or not receive intensive blood pressure control. In a follow-up period of more than 8 years, there was a reduction in risks of up to 47% for several relevant parameters, such as risk of progression of retinopathy or moderate visual acuity loss, regardless of the drug used (angiotensin-converting-enzyme inhibitor versus β-blocker) and independent from the degree of glucose control (123).

In type 1 diabetic patients, the issue is less well documented. One study (EUCLID) tested the effect of low-dose lisinopril on the incidence and progression of retinopathy in type 1 diabetic patients who were mostly normoalbuminuric and normotensive. Although no effect was observed on the prevention of diabetic retinopathy, a 50% reduction of retinopathy progression and an 80% reduction of progression to proliferative retinopathy were reported (124).

Ophthalmologic Treatment: Current Standard

Evidence-based medicine has produced a clear treatment regimen for advanced eye disease in diabetes. Retinal laser photocoagulation is established as the therapy for PDR and for clinically significant macular edema. Expert ophthalmologic summaries and periodic clinical recommendations are available and need no further extension (5,125–128). In brief, PDR is treated by panretinal laser photocoagulation because of the well-established benefit of this procedure with regard to the prevention of severe visual loss, which was demonstrated in a large clinical trial (fewer than 5 instances of visual loss in 200 treated subjects) (129,130). Those eyes with high-risk characteristics (neovascularization from the disc or vitreous hemorrhages with persisting retinal neovascularization) profited most. However, because there are side effects of laser treatment, such as modest loss of visual acuity or contraction of the visual field, only eyes approaching high-risk characteristics are primarily treated.

It is also evidence that patients with macular edema benefit from laser therapy (131,132). It is unclear at present how laser treatment exerts its effect on the retina. Angiogenesis (the formation of new blood vessels from preexisting vessels) is the product of the imbalance between proangiogenic and antiangiogenic stimuli (133). Therefore, it was hypothesized that the method works either by reducing proangiogenic or by increasing antiangiogenic factors (134). Moreover, the net amount of oxygen-consuming tissue is reduced, which can further contribute to the beneficial effect of laser treatment.

REFERENCES

1. Microvascular and acute complications in IDDM patients: the EURODIAB IDDM Complications Study. *Diabetologia* 1994;37:278–285.
2. Klein R, Klein BE, Moss SE, et al. The Wisconsin epidemiologic study of diabetic retinopathy: II. Prevalence and risk of diabetic retinopathy when age at diagnosis is less than 30 years. *Arch Ophthalmol* 1984;102:520–526.
3. Klein R, Klein BE, Moss SE, et al. The Wisconsin epidemiologic study of diabetic retinopathy: III. Prevalence and risk of diabetic retinopathy when age at diagnosis is 30 or more years. *Arch Ophthalmol* 1984;102:527–532.
4. Thylefors B, Negrel AD, Pararajasegaram R, et al. Global data on blindness. *Bull World Health Organ* 1995;73:115–121.
5. Aiello LP, Gardner TW, King GL, et al. Diabetic retinopathy. *Diabetes Care* 1998;21:143–156.
6. Trautner C, Haastert B, Giani G, et al. Incidence of blindness in southern Germany between 1990 and 1998. *Diabetologia* 2001;44:147–150.
7. Trautner C, Icks A, Haastert B, et al. Incidence of blindness in relation to diabetes: a population-based study. *Diabetes Care* 1997;20:1147–1153.
8. Danne T, Kordonouri O, Hovener G, et al. Diabetic angiopathy in children. *Diabet Med* 1997;14:1012–1025.
9. Kernell A, Dedorsson I, Johansson B, et al. Prevalence of diabetic retinopathy in children and adolescents with IDDM: a population-based multicentre study. *Diabetologia* 1997;40:307–310.

10. Malone JI, Morrison AD, Pavan PR, et al. Prevalence and significance of retinopathy in subjects with type 1 diabetes of less than 5 years' duration screened for the Diabetes Control and Complications Trial. *Diabetes Care* 2001;24:522–526.

11. Deckert T, Poulsen JE, Larsen M. Prognosis of diabetics with diabetes onset before the age of thirty-one: II. Factors influencing the prognosis. *Diabetologia* 1978;14:371–377.

12. Harris MI, Klein R, Welborn TA, et al. Onset of NIDDM occurs at least 4–7 yr before clinical diagnosis. *Diabetes Care* 1992;15:815–819.

13. United Kingdom Prospective Diabetes Study Group. Intensive blood-glucose control with sulphonylureas or insulin compared with conventional treatment and risk of complications in patients with type 2 diabetes (UKPDS 33). *Lancet* 1998;352:837–853.

14. Holman RR, Manley SE, Neil AA, et al. Retinopathy in type 2 diabetes: when does the clock start ticking? *Diabetes* 2002;51[Suppl. 2]:A64.

15. Kohner EM, Stratton IM, Aldington SJ, et al. Relationship between the severity of retinopathy and progression to photocoagulation in patients with type 2 diabetes mellitus in the UKPDS (UKPDS 52). *Diabet Med* 2001;18:178–184.

16. Lee ET, Lu M, Bennett PH, et al. Vascular disease in younger-onset diabetes: comparison of European, Asian and American Indian cohorts of the WHO Multinational Study of Vascular Disease in Diabetes. *Diabetologia* 2001;44[Suppl 2]:S78–S81.

17. Harris MI, Klein R, Cowie CC, et al. Is the risk of diabetic retinopathy greater in non-Hispanic blacks and Mexican Americans than in non-Hispanic whites with type 2 diabetes? A U.S. population study. *Diabetes Care* 1998;21:1230–1235.

18. Sobngwi E, Mauvais-Jarvis F, Vexiau P, et al. Diabetes in Africans: part 1. Epidemiology and clinical specificities. *Diabetes Metab* 2001;27:628–634.

19. Isomaa B, Henricsson M, Lehto M, et al. Chronic diabetic complications in patients with MODY3 diabetes. *Diabetologia* 1998;41:467–473.

20. Isomaa B, Almgren P, Henricsson M, et al. Chronic complications in patients with slowly progressing autoimmune type 1 diabetes (LADA). *Diabetes Care* 1999;22:1347–1353.

21. Ashton N. Pathogenesis of diabetic retinopathy. In: Little HL, Jack RL, Patz AP, et al., eds. *Diabetic retinopathy*. New York: Thieme-Stratton, 1983:85–106.

22. Engerman RL. Animal models of diabetic retinopathy. *Trans Am Acad Ophthalmol Otolaryngol* 1976;81:OP710–OP715.

23. Buscher C, Weis A, Wohrle M, et al. Islet transplantation in experimental diabetes of the rat: XII. Effect on diabetic retinopathy: morphological findings and morphometrical evaluation. *Horm Metab Res* 1989;21:227–231.

24. Kohner EM, Henkind P. Correlation of fluorescein angiogram and retinal digest in diabetic retinopathy. *Am J Ophthalmol* 1970;69:403–414.

25. De Venecia G, Davis M, Engerman R. Clinicopathologic correlations in diabetic retinopathy: I. Histology and fluorescein angiography of microaneurysms. *Arch Ophthalmol* 1976;94:1766–1773.

26. Bresnick GH, Davis MD, Myers FL, et al. Clinicopathologic correlations in diabetic retinopathy: II. Clinical and histologic appearances of retinal capillary microaneurysms. *Arch Ophthalmol* 1977;95:1215–1220.

27. Kuwabara T, Cogan DG. Studies of retinal vascular pattern: I. Normal architecture. *Arch Ophthalmol* 1960;64:904–911.

28. Cogan DG, Toussaint D, Kuwabara T. Retinal vascular pattern: IV. Diabetic retinopathy. *Arch Ophthalmol* 1961;66:366–378.

29. Hirschi KK, D'Amore PA. Pericytes in the microvasculature. *Cardiovasc Res* 1996;32:687–698.

30. Benjamin LE, Hemo I, Keshet E. A plasticity window for blood vessel remodelling is defined by pericyte coverage of the preformed endothelial network and is regulated by PDGF-B and VEGF. *Development* 1998;125:1591–1598.

31. Takahashi K, Kishi S, Muraoka K, et al. Reperfusion of occluded capillary beds in diabetic retinopathy. *Am J Ophthalmol* 1998;126:791–797.

32. Schroder S, Palinski W, Schmid-Schonbein GW. Activated monocytes and granulocytes, capillary nonperfusion, and neovascularization in diabetic retinopathy. *Am J Pathol* 1991;139:81–100.

33. Miyamoto K, Hiroshiba N, Tsujikawa A, et al. In vivo demonstration of increased leukocyte entrapment in retinal microcirculation of diabetic rats. *Invest Ophthalmol Vis Sci* 1998;39:2190–2194.

34. Hammes HP, Bartmann A, Engel L, et al. Antioxidant treatment of experimental diabetic retinopathy in rats with nicanartine. *Diabetologia* 1997;40:629–634.

35. Nishikawa T, Giardino I, Edelstein D, et al. Changes in diabetic retinal matrix protein mRNA levels in a common transgenic mouse strain. *Curr Eye Res* 2000;21:581–587.

36. Mizutani M, Kern TS, Lorenzi M. Accelerated death of retinal microvascular cells in human and experimental diabetic retinopathy. *J Clin Invest* 1996;97:2883–2890.

37. Hammes HP, Lin J, Bretzel RG, et al. Upregulation of the vascular endothelial growth factor/vascular endothelial growth factor receptor system in experimental background diabetic retinopathy of the rat. *Diabetes* 1998;47:401–406.

38. Lee AY, Chung SK, Chung SS. Demonstration that polyol accumulation is responsible for diabetic cataract by the use of transgenic mice expressing the aldose reductase gene in the lens. *Proc Natl Acad Sci U S A* 1995;92:2780–2784.

39. Brownlee M. Advanced protein glycosylation in diabetes and aging. *Annu Rev Med* 1995;46:223–234.

40. Koya D, King GL. Protein kinase C activation and the development of diabetic complications. *Diabetes* 1998;47:859–866.

41. Kolm-Litty V, Sauer U, Nerlich A, et al. High glucose-induced transforming growth factor beta1 production is mediated by the hexosamine pathway in porcine glomerular mesangial cells. *J Clin Invest* 1998;101:160–169.

42. Nishikawa T, Edelstein D, Du XL, et al. Normalizing mitochondrial superoxide production blocks three pathways of hyperglycaemic damage. *Nature* 2000;404:787–790.

43. Brownlee M. Biochemistry and molecular cell biology of diabetic complications. *Nature* 2001;414:813–820.

44. Engerman RL, Kern TS. Aldose reductase inhibition fails to prevent retinopathy in diabetic and galactosemic dogs. *Diabetes* 1993;42:820–825.

45. Robison WG Jr, Laver NM, Jacot JL, et al. Sorbinil prevention of diabetic-like retinopathy in the galactose-fed rat model. *Invest Ophthalmol Vis Sci* 1995;36:2368–2380.

46. Sorbinil Retinopathy Trial Research Group. A randomized trial of sorbinil, an aldose reductase inhibitor, in diabetic retinopathy. *Arch Ophthalmol* 1990;108:1234–1244.

47. Kowluru RA, Engerman RL, Kern TS. Abnormalities of retinal metabolism in diabetes or experimental galactosemia: VIII. Prevention by aminoguanidine. *Curr Eye Res* 2000;21:814–819.

48. Park JY, Takahara N, Gabriele A, et al. Induction of endothelin-1 expression by glucose: an effect of protein kinase C activation. *Diabetes* 2000;49:1239–1248.

49. Xia P, Aiello LP, Ishii H, et al. Characterization of vascular endothelial growth factor's effect on the activation of protein kinase C, its isoforms, and endothelial cell growth. *J Clin Invest* 1996;98:2018–2026.

50. Suzuma K, Takahara N, Suzuma I, et al. Characterization of protein kinase C beta isoform's action on retinoblastoma protein phosphorylation, vascular endothelial growth factor-induced endothelial cell proliferation, and retinal neovascularization. *Proc Natl Acad Sci U S A* 2002;99:721–726.

51. Ishii H, Jirousek MR, Koya D, et al. Amelioration of vascular dysfunctions in diabetic rats by an oral PKC beta inhibitor. *Science* 1996;272:728–731.

52. Danis RP, Bingaman DP, Jirousek M, et al. Inhibition of intraocular neovascularization caused by retinal ischemia in pigs by PKCbeta inhibition with LY333531. *Invest Ophthalmol Vis Sci* 1998;39:171–179.

53. Hammes HP, Martin S, Federlin K, et al. Aminoguanidine treatment inhibits the development of experimental diabetic retinopathy. *Proc Natl Acad Sci U S A* 1991;88:11555–11558.

54. Hammes HP, Alt A, Niwa T, et al. Differential accumulation of advanced glycation end products in the course of diabetic retinopathy. *Diabetologia* 1999;42:728–736.

55. Giardino I, Edelstein D, Brownlee M. BCL-2 expression or antioxidants prevent hyperglycemia-induced formation of intracellular advanced glycation endproducts in bovine endothelial cells. *J Clin Invest* 1996;97:1422–1428.

56. Shinohara M, Thornalley PJ, Giardino I, et al. Overexpression of glyoxalase-I in bovine endothelial cells inhibits intracellular advanced glycation endproduct formation and prevents hyperglycemia-induced increases in macromolecular endocytosis. *J Clin Invest* 1998;101:1142–1147.

57. Wells-Knecht KJ, Zyzak DV, Litchfield JE, et al. Mechanism of autoxidative glycosylation: identification of glyoxal and arabinose as intermediates in the autoxidative modification of proteins by glucose. *Biochemistry* 1995;34:3702–3709.

58. Thornalley PJ. The glyoxalase system: new developments towards functional characterization of a metabolic pathway fundamental to biological life. *Biochem J* 1990;269:1–11.

59. Fu MX, Requena JR, Jenkins AJ, et al. The advanced glycation end product, N-epsilon-(carbox-ymethyl)lysine, is a product of both lipid peroxidation and glycoxidation reactions. *J Biol Chem* 1996;271:9982–9986.

60. Kern TS, Engerman RL. Pharmacological inhibition of diabetic retinopathy: aminoguanidine and aspirin. *Diabetes* 2001;50:1636–1642.

61. Hammes HP, Brownlee M, Lin J, et al. Diabetic retinopathy risk correlates with intracellular concentrations of the glycoxidation product N-epsilon-(carboxymethyl) lysine independently of glycohaemoglobin concentrations. *Diabetologia* 1999;42:603–607.

62. Soulis T, Thallas V, Youssef S, et al. Advanced glycation end products and their receptors co-localise in rat organs susceptible to diabetic microvascular injury. *Diabetologia* 1997;40:619–628.

63. Kislinger T, Fu C, Huber B, et al. Nε-(carboxymethyl)lysine adducts of proteins are ligands for receptor for advanced glycation end products that activate cell signaling pathways and modulate gene expression. *J Biol Chem* 1999;274:31740–31749.

64. Kowluru RA, Tang J, Kern TS. Abnormalities of retinal metabolism in diabetes and experimental galactosemia: VII. Effect of long-term administration of antioxidants on the development of retinopathy. *Diabetes* 2001;50:1938–1942.

65. Connolly DT, Olander JV, Heuvelman D, et al. Human vascular permeability factor: isolation from U937 cells. *J Biol Chem* 1989;264:20017–20024.

66. Leung DW, Cachianes G, Kuang WJ, et al. Vascular endothelial growth factor is a secreted angiogenic mitogen. *Science* 1989;246:1306–1309.

67. Clauss M, Gerlach M, Gerlach H, et al. Vascular permeability factor: a tumor-derived polypeptide that induces endothelial cell and monocyte procoagulant activity, and promotes monocyte migration. *J Exp Med* 1990;172:1535–1545.

68. Ferrara N. Vascular endothelial growth factor and the regulation of angiogenesis. *Recent Prog Horm Res* 2000;55:15–35; discussion 35–36.

69. Ferrara N, Houck KA, Jakeman LB, et al. The vascular endothelial growth factor family of polypeptides. *J Cell Biochem* 1991;47:211–218.

70. Breier G, Albrecht U, Sterrer S, et al. Expression of vascular endothelial growth factor during embryonic angiogenesis and endothelial cell differentiation. *Development* 1992;114:521–532.

71. Veikkola T, Alitalo K. VEGFs, receptors and angiogenesis. *Semin Cancer Biol* 1999;9:211–220.

72. Breier G. Functions of the VEGF/VEGF receptor system in the vascular system. *Semin Thromb Hemost* 2000;26:553-559.

73. Neufeld G, Cohen T, Gengrinovitch S, et al. Vascular endothelial growth factor (VEGF) and its receptors. *FASEB J* 1999;13:9–22.

74. Sondell M, Sundler F, Kanje M. Vascular endothelial growth factor is a neurotrophic factor which stimulates axonal outgrowth through the flk-1 receptor. *Eur J Neurosci* 2000;12:4243–4254.

75. Carmeliet P, Ferreira V, Breier G, et al. Abnormal blood vessel development and lethality in embryos lacking a single VEGF allele. *Nature* 1996;380:435–439.

76. Ferrara N, Carver-Moore K, Chen H, et al. Heterozygous embryonic lethality induced by targeted inactivation of the VEGF gene. *Nature* 1996;380:439–442.

77. Ferrara N, Chen H, Davis-Smyth T, et al. Vascular endothelial growth factor is essential for corpus luteum angiogenesis. *Nat Med* 1998;4:336–340.

78. Gerber HP, Vu TH, Ryan AM, et al. VEGF couples hypertrophic cartilage remodeling, ossification and angiogenesis during endochondral bone formation. *Nat Med* 1999;5:623–628.

79. Stone J, Itin A, Alon T, et al. Development of retinal vasculature is mediated by hypoxia-induced vascular endothelial growth factor (VEGF) expression by neuroglia. *J Neurosci* 1995;15:4738–4747.

80. Alon T, Hemo I, Itin A, et al. Vascular endothelial growth factor acts as a survival factor for newly formed retinal vessels and has implications for retinopathy of prematurity. *Nat Med* 1995;1:1024–1028.

81. Gerber HP, Hillan KJ, Ryan AM, et al. VEGF is required for growth and survival in neonatal mice. *Development* 1999;126:1149–1159.

82. Carmeliet P, Lampugnani MG, Moons L, et al. Targeted deficiency or cytosolic truncation of the VE-cadherin gene in mice impairs VEGF-mediated endothelial survival and angiogenesis. *Cell* 1999;98:147–157.

83. Plate KH, Breier G, Weich HA, et al. Vascular endothelial growth factor is a potential tumour angiogenesis factor in human gliomas in vivo. *Nature* 1992;359:845–848.

84. Shweiki D, Itin A, Soffer D, et al. Vascular endothelial growth factor induced by hypoxia may mediate hypoxia-initiated angiogenesis. *Nature* 1992;359:843–845.

85. Damert A, Machein M, Breier G, et al. Up-regulation of vascular endothelial growth factor expression in a rat glioma is conferred by two distinct hypoxia-driven mechanisms. *Cancer Res* 1997;57:3860–3864.

86. Ratcliffe PJ, O'Rourke JF, Maxwell PH, et al. Oxygen sensing, hypoxia-inducible factor-1 and the regulation of mammalian gene expression. *J Exp Biol* 1998;201:1153–1162.

87. Mole DR, Pugh CW, Ratcliffe PJ, et al. Regulation of the HIF pathway: enzymatic hydroxylation of a conserved prolyl residue in hypoxia-inducible factor alpha subunits governs capture by the pVIIL E3 ubiquitin ligase complex. *Adv Enzyme Regul* 2002;42:333–347.

88. Davis S, Yancopoulos GD. The angiopoietins: yin and yang in angiogenesis. *Curr Top Microbiol Immunol* 1999;237:173–185.

89. Holash J, Maisonpierre PC, Compton D, et al. Vessel cooption, regression, and growth in tumors mediated by angiopoietins and VEGF. *Science* 1999;284:1994–1998.

90. Michaelson IC. The mode of development of the vascular system of the retina, with some observations on its significance for certain retinal diseases. *Trans Ophthalmol Soc UK* 1948;68:137–180.

91. Eichler W, Kuhrt H, Hoffmann S, et al. VEGF release by retinal glia depends on both oxygen and glucose supply. *Neuroreport* 2000;11:3533–3537.

92. Yi X, Mai LC, Uyama M, et al. Time-course expression of vascular endothelial growth factor as related to the development of the retinochoroidal vasculature in rats. *Exp Brain Res* 1998;118:155–160.

93. Yamagishi S, Amano S, Inagaki Y, et al. Advanced glycation end products-induced apoptosis and overexpression of vascular endothelial growth factor in bovine retinal pericytes. *Biochem Biophys Res Commun* 2002;290:973–978.

94. Nomura M, Yamagishi S, Harada S, et al. Possible participation of autocrine and paracrine vascular endothelial growth factors in hypoxia-induced proliferation of endothelial cells and pericytes. *J Biol Chem* 1995;270:28316–28324.

95. Esser S, Wolburg K, Wolburg H, et al. Vascular endothelial growth factor induces endothelial fenestrations in vitro. *J Cell Biol* 1998;140:947–959.

96. Aiello LP, Avery RL, Arrigg PG, et al. Vascular endothelial growth factor in ocular fluid of patients with diabetic retinopathy and other retinal disorders. *N Engl J Med* 1994;331:1480–1487.

97. Pierce EA, Avery RL, Foley ED, et al. Vascular endothelial growth factor/vascular permeability factor expression in a mouse model of retinal neovascularization. *Proc Natl Acad Sci U S A* 1995;92:905–909.

98. Robbins SG, Conaway JR, Ford BL, et al. Detection of vascular endothelial growth factor (VEGF) protein in vascular and non-vascular cells of the normal and oxygen-injured rat retina. *Growth Factors* 1997;14:229–241.

99. Miller JW, Adamis AP, Shima DT, et al. Vascular endothelial growth factor/vascular permeability factor is temporally and spatially correlated with ocular angiogenesis in a primate model. *Am J Pathol* 1994;145:574–584.

100. Murata T, Ishibashi T, Khalil A, et al. Vascular endothelial growth factor plays a role in hyperpermeability of diabetic retinal vessels. *Ophthalmic Res* 1995;27:48–52.

101. Tolentino MJ, Miller JW, Gragoudas ES, et al. Intravitreous injections of vascular endothelial growth factor produce retinal ischemia and microangiopathy in an adult primate. *Ophthalmology* 1996;103:1820–1828.

102. Ellis EA, Guberski DL, Somogyi-Mann M, et al. Increased H2O2, vascular endothelial growth factor and receptors in the retina of the BBZ/Wor diabetic rat. *Free Radic Biol Med* 2000;28:91–101.

103. Segawa Y, Shirao Y, Yamagishi S, et al. Upregulation of retinal vascular endothelial growth factor mRNAs in spontaneously diabetic rats without ophthalmoscopic retinopathy: a possible participation of advanced glycation end products in the development of the early phase of diabetic retinopathy. *Ophthalmic Res* 1998;30:333–339.

104. Gilbert RE, Vranes D, Berka JL, et al. Vascular endothelial growth factor and its receptors in control and diabetic rat eyes. *Lab Invest* 1998;78:1017–1027.

105. Sone H, Kawakami Y, Okuda Y, et al. Ocular vascular endothelial growth factor levels in diabetic rats are elevated before observable retinal proliferative changes. *Diabetologia* 1997;40:726–730.

106. Murata T, Nakagawa K, Khalil A, et al. The relation between expression of vascular endothelial growth factor and breakdown of the blood-retinal barrier in diabetic rat retinas. *Lab Invest* 1996;74:819–825.

107. Chandel NS, Maltepe E, Goldwasser E, et al. Mitochondrial reactive oxygen species trigger hypoxia-induced transcription. *Proc Natl Acad Sci U S A* 1998;95:11715–11720.

108. Okamoto T, Tanaka S, Stan AC, et al. Advanced gly-cation end products induce angiogenesis in vivo. *Microvasc Res* 2002;63:186–195.

109. Treins C, Giorgetti-Peraldi S, Murdaca J, et al. Regulation of vascular endothelial growth factor expression by advanced glycation end products. *J Biol Chem* 2001;276:43836–43841.

110. Lu M, Kuroki M, Amano S, et al. Advanced glycation end products increase retinal vascular endothelial growth factor expression. *J Clin Invest* 1998;101:1219–1224.

111. Kuroki M, Voest EE, Amano S, et al. Reactive oxygen intermediates increase vascular endothelial growth factor expression in vitro and in vivo. *J Clin Invest* 1996;98:1667–1675.

112. Yang W, de Bono DP. A new role for vascular endothelial growth factor and fibroblast growth factors: increasing endothelial resistance to oxidative stress. *FEBS Lett* 1997;403:139–142.

113. Carmeliet P. Mechanisms of angiogenesis and arteriogenesis. *Nat Med* 2000;6:389–395.

114. Hammes HP, Federoff HJ, Brownlee M. Nerve growth factor prevents both neuroretinal programmed cell death and capillary pathology in experimental diabetes. *Mol Med* 1995;1:527–534.

115. Giardino I, Fard AK, Hatchell DL, et al. Aminoguanidine inhibits reactive oxygen species formation, lipid peroxidation, and oxidant-induced apoptosis. *Diabetes* 1998;47:1114–1120.

116. Aiello LP, Pierce EA, Foley ED, et al. Suppression of retinal neovascularization in vivo by inhibition of vascular endothelial growth factor (VEGF) using soluble VEGF-receptor chimeric proteins. *Proc Natl Acad Sci U S A* 1995;92:10457–10461.

117. Robinson GS, Pierce EA, Rook SL, et al. Oligodeoxynucleotides inhibit retinal neovascularization in a murine model of proliferative retinopathy. *Proc Natl Acad Sci U S A* 1996;93:4851–4856.

118. Diabetes Control and Complications Trial Research Group. Progression of retinopathy with intensive versus conventional treatment in the Diabetes Control and Complications Trial. *Ophthalmology* 1995;102:647–661.

119. The Diabetes Control and Complications Trial/Epidemiology of Diabetes Interventions and Complications Research Group. Retinopathy and nephropathy in patients with type 1 diabetes four years after a trial of intensive therapy. *N Engl J Med* 2000;342:381–389.

120. United Kingdom Prospective Diabetes Study Group. Effect of intensive blood-glucose control with metformin on complications in overweight patients with type 2 diabetes (UKPDS 34). *Lancet* 1998;352:854–865.

121. Collado-Mesa F, Colhoun HM, Stevens LK, et al. Prevalence and management of hypertension in type 1 diabetes mellitus in Europe: the EURODIAB IDDM Complications Study. *Diabet Med* 1999;16:41–48.

122. Ritz E, Keller C, Bergis KH. Nephropathy of type II diabetes mellitus. *Nephrol Dial Transplant* 1996;11[Suppl 9]:38–44.

123. United Kingdom Prospective Diabetes Study Group. Efficacy of atenolol and captopril in reducing risk of macrovascular and microvascular complications in type 2 diabetes: UKPDS 39. *BMJ* 1998;317:713–720.

124. Chaturvedi N, Sjolie AK, Stephenson JM, et al. Effect of lisinopril on progression of retinopathy in normotensive people with type 1 diabetes. The EUCLID Study Group. EURODIAB Controlled Trial of Lisinopril in Insulin-Dependent Diabetes Mellitus. *Lancet* 1998;351:28–31.

125. Kohner EM. Diabetic retinopathy. *BMJ* 1993;307:1195–1199.

126. Ferris FL 3rd, Davis MD, Aiello LM. Treatment of diabetic retinopathy. *N Engl J Med* 1999;341:667–678.

127. Klein R, Klein BE. Diabetic eye disease. *Lancet* 1997;350:197–204.

128. Association AD. Diabetic retinopathy. *Diabetes Care* 2002;25:S90–S93.

129. The Diabetic Retinopathy Study Research Group. Indications for photocoagulation treatment of diabetic retinopathy: Diabetic Retinopathy Study Report no.14. *Int Ophthalmol Clin* 1987;27:239–253.

130. The Diabetic Retinopathy Study Research Group. Photocoagulation treatment of proliferative diabetic retinopathy: clinical application of Diabetic Retinopathy Study (DRS) findings. DRS Report no. 8. *Ophthalmology* 1981;88:583–600.

131. Early Treatment Diabetic Retinopathy Study Research Group. Early photocoagulation for diabetic retinopathy. ETDRS Report no. 9. *Ophthalmology* 1991;98:766–785.

132. Early Treatment Diabetic Retinopathy Study Research Group. Photocoagulation for diabetic macular edema. Early Treatment Diabetic Retinopathy Study report no.1. *Arch Ophthalmol* 1985;103:1796–1806.

133. Folkman J, D'Amore PA. Blood vessel formation: what is its molecular basis? *Cell* 1996;87:1153–1155.

134. Spranger J, Hammes HP, Preissner KT, et al. Release of the angiogenesis inhibitor angiostatin in patients with proliferative diabetic retinopathy: association with retinal photocoagulation. *Diabetologia* 2000;43:1404–1407.

PART II

Clinical Topics

Diabetes and Cardiovascular Disease
edited by Steven P. Marso and David M. Stern
Lippincott Williams & Wilkins, Philadelphia © 2004

9

Epidemiology of Diabetes Mellitus and Cardiovascular Disease

Sunil V. Rao and Darren K. McGuire

Cardiology Fellow, Duke University Medical Center, Duke Clinical Research Institute, Durham, North Carolina; Assistant Professor, Department of Internal Medicine, University of Texas–Southwestern Medical Center, Director, Outpatient Cardiology Services, Parkland Hospital and Health System, Dallas, Texas

The incidence and prevalence of diabetes mellitus worldwide is increasing, due almost exclusively to an increase in non-insulin-dependent (type 2) diabetes mellitus, which represents more than 90% of all cases of diabetes (1–3). The concomitant increase in the risk factors for glucose intolerance among individuals (obesity, sedentary lifestyle) in developed and developing countries around the world suggests that diabetes will be a significant strain on health care resources for the foreseeable future. Given that the leading cause of morbidity and mortality for patients with diabetes is atherosclerotic vascular disease, knowledge of the epidemiology of diabetes and its associated cardiovascular complications is essential for targeting interventions designed to improve health outcomes in this high-risk population. This chapter reviews the epidemiology of diabetes, with specific focus on the incidence and prevalence of type 2 diabetes and diabetes-related cardiovascular disease.

GLOBAL BURDEN OF DIABETES MELLITUS

Presently, there is a global pandemic of type 2 diabetes mellitus and its clinical sequelae. The World Health Organization (WHO) estimates that there will be 300 million people with diabetes worldwide by the year 2025 (2), which is more than twice the estimated prevalence reported in 1995. These figures are most likely a gross underestimation of the problem, given that as many as half of affected patients remain undiagnosed (4–6), especially in light of the recently modified diagnostic criteria for type 2 diabetes mellitus (7,8). The American Diabetes Association (ADA) criterion requires merely a fasting plasma glucose (FPG) concentration of 126 mg/dL (7.0 mmol/L), whereas the WHO 1999 criteria define diabetes as being present when there is either an FPG level of 126 mg/dL (7.0 mmol/L) or a 2-hour postload glucose level of 200 mg/dL (11.1 mmol/L). These diagnostic criteria are depicted in Table 9-1.

The choice of diagnostic criteria has implications for the reported incidence of diabetes mellitus. The Hoorn Study recently evaluated the various diagnostic criteria with respect to the cumulative incidence of type 2 diabetes mellitus among an exclusively white, elderly Danish population (9). With the ADA criteria, the 6-year cumulative incidence of type 2 diabetes mellitus was 3.7% for persons with normal glucose tolerance at baseline (FPG <126 mg/dL, 2-hour postload glucose level <140 mg/dL) and 32.4% for those with impaired glucose tolerance (IGT) at baseline (FPG <126 mg/dL, postload level 140 to 200 mg/dL). Using the WHO 1999 criteria, the 6-year cumulative incidence of type 2 diabetes mellitus was 4.5% among persons with normal basal glucose levels, 33.0% among those

TABLE 9-1. *The WHO and ADA diagnostic criteria*

1985 WHO	1999 WHO	1997 ADA
FPG = 7.8 mmol/L *or* 2-hr post load plasma glucose = 11.1 mmol/L	FPG = 7.0 mmol/L *or* 2-hr post load plasma glucose = 11.1 mmol/L	FPG = 7.0 mmol/L (126 mg/dL)

ADA, American Diabetes Association; FPG, fasting plasma glucose concentration; WHO, World Health Organization.

with impaired fasting glucose (IFG; 110 to 126 mg/dL) and normal glucose tolerance (postload level <140 mg/dL), and 64.5% among persons with both IFG and IGT (140 to 200 mg/dL). The overall 6-year incidence of type 2 diabetes mellitus in the Hoorn Study was 9.9% using the WHO 1999 criteria and 8.3% according to the ADA diagnostic criterion. Clearly, the annualized risk of type 2 diabetes is dependent on the basal metabolic state.

United States

The second National Health and Nutrition Survey (NHANES II) examined the prevalence of physician-diagnosed and undiagnosed diabetes among Americans age 20 to 74 years (10). Using a combination of self-reported diabetes and the results of randomly administered oral glucose tolerance tests (OGTTs), its results suggested a prevalence of diabetes approximating 6.6% of the U. S. population age 20 to 74 years, with almost equal proportions of diagnosed and undiagnosed diabetes. The rates were equal by gender, increased with increasing age, and were higher among black Americans. By the time NHANES III was reported in 1998, the prevalence had increased to 7.8% of adults older than 20 years of age (11). Between 1980 and 1996, the estimated number of diagnosed cases of diabetes in the United States increased by more than 33%, from fewer than 6 million to more than 8 million individuals (Fig. 9-1) (7,8). The majority of the increase reflects the continually increasing prevalence of type 2 diabetes. Presently, approximately 625,000 new cases of type 2 diabetes are diagnosed each year in the United States (12). The Centers for Disease Control and Prevention,

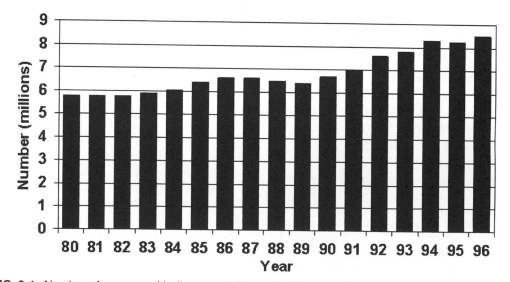

FIG. 9-1. Number of persons with diagnosed diabetes in the United States between 1980 and 1996. (From Centers for Disease Control and Prevention, Diabetes Surveillance, 1999 [110].)

using data from NHANES III to model diabetes prevalence, has estimated that 8.6% of U. S. adults had diabetes in the year 2002 (13).

Diabetes is a major contributor to morbidity and mortality and usurps a substantial proportion of health care resources. Data extrapolated from the National Hospital Discharge Survey and the National Hospital Ambulatory Care Survey indicate that, in 1996 (14,15), diabetes accounted for 503,000 primary discharge diagnoses and 1.2 million emergency room visits in the United States. Ramsey et al. (16) surveyed the claims database from a Fortune 500 company with more than 100,000 employees and found that the mean annual per capita cost for employees with diabetes was twice as high as for those without diabetes ($7,778.00 versus $3,367.00). In addition, Yassin et al. (17) found that people with diabetes were three times as likely as those without diabetes to stop working outside the home, with an annual estimated cost of disability of $9.3 billion.

Overall, diabetes is the seventh leading reported cause of death in the United States. Data from NHANES I showed that the age-adjusted risk of death for Americans age 25 to 44 years with diabetes was 3.6 times higher than for adults of the same age group without diabetes (18). Using data abstracted from death certificates to estimate disease-specific mortality, this study found that heart disease was listed in 69.5% of death certificates of people with diabetes. That is probably an underestimation of the true mortality rate attributable to heart disease among diabetics, because this comorbidity is rarely listed on death certificates (3,19).

Worldwide

Although type 2 diabetes has historically been a public health problem principally in developed countries, due to its close association with the "Western" lifestyle (2), the greatest anticipated threat of diabetes over the next several decades is in developing countries. Modernization has resulted in increased rates of diabetes, primarily as a result of decreasing physical activity, increasing prevalence of obesity, and increasing consumption of high-caloric diets in these nations

(20). In addition, increases in life expectancy will most likely translate into an increasing prevalence of diabetes in developing countries.

By the year 2025, the worldwide prevalence of diabetes is expected to increase by 35%, with 5.4% of the entire world's population expected to be affected by diabetes (2). The largest increase is expected in the developing world, and more than 75% of all people with diabetes will be residents of developing countries. China will be a country burdened with a marked increase in the prevalence of type 2 diabetes in the near future. As evidence, Pan et al. (21) examined 224,251 people in a study of 19 Chinese provinces and found that the prevalence of diabetes had tripled when compared with epidemiologic data collected 10 years earlier. Seventy percent of the cases were newly diagnosed. Compared with nondiabetic persons, subjects with diabetes as a group were older, had a higher income, had a family history of diabetes, had a higher mean body mass index (BMI), and had a higher waist-to-hip ratio (WHR). Multivariable regression showed that age, BMI, WHR, family history, hypertension, physical inactivity, and higher annual income were independent risk factors for diabetes in this Chinese study. Over the next two decades, China is expected to see an increase from 16 million to 38 million diabetics, which represents a 134% increase (2).

Ko et al. (22) assessed the prevalence of undiagnosed diabetes among Chinese inhabitants of Hong Kong. Among asymptomatic subjects, the age-standardized prevalence of undiagnosed diabetes was 2.8%; the age-standardized prevalence of IFG was 7.3%. These data reflected a doubling of the prevalence over a 7-year period. Tan et al. (23) examined the population of Singapore in the 1992 Singapore National Health Survey and found that the age-standardized prevalence of diabetes had increased twofold, to 8.4%, between 1984 and 1992. Among the three major ethnic groups in Singapore at the time, the prevalence was 7.8% in the Chinese group, 10.1% in Malays, and 12.2% in Asian Indians. The prevalence of IGT in these groups was 16.7%, 14.0%, and 13.1%, respectively.

The country with the highest number of people with diabetes is India (2). In 1995, there were an estimated 19.4 million people with diabetes in India. This number is expected to increase to more than 57 million by the year 2025. There appears to be regional variation in the prevalence of diabetes on the Indian subcontinent. For example, Misra et al. (24) examined the prevalence of diabetes, obesity, and dyslipidemia among the urban poor in northern India and found that 10.3% of the study population had diabetes. In contrast, Asha Bai et al. (25) surveyed 26,066 adults in Chennai (southern India) and found that only 779 (3.0%) had diagnosed diabetes. In an attempt to more accurately estimate the national prevalence of diabetes and IFG in India, Ramachandran et al. (26) performed OGTTs on 11,216 adults in six major cities across India. The age-standardized prevalence of diabetes was 12.1%, and that of IGT was 14.0%. As expected, age, BMI, WHR, family history, income, and sedentary lifestyle were all independently associated with diabetes. These data reinforce the contribution of risk factors associated with modernization to the development of glucose intolerance. The rising incomes of the inhabitants of developing countries have led to greater availability of calorie-dense foods, lower levels of physical activity, higher rates of obesity, and increased prevalence of hyperinsulinemia and diabetes among those with higher socioeconomic status (27). Obesity, defined according to BMI, was prevalent in 15.6% of women and 13.3% of men; however, if the percentage of body fat is used to define obesity, the prevalence among women increased to 40.2%. This geographic variation in diabetes prevalence is reinforced by data from the Indian Council of Medical Research, which indicate that the prevalence of diabetes is higher in urban areas than in rural areas (28).

SPECIAL POPULATIONS AT RISK FOR DIABETES

Elderly

The world's population is aging. Increased life expectancy has led to an increase in the number of people older than 65 years of age in both the developed and the developing world (29). By the year 2020, 12.9% of the world's population is expected to be older than age 60, compared with 9.9% in the year 2000 (30). The elderly are disproportionately affected by diabetes (2,3,10,31), and the prevalence of diabetes increases with age until age 75 years (Fig. 9-2). The aging of the global population is expected to account for at least half of the projected increase in the prevalence of diabetes over the coming years, due to the high incidence of diabetes among the elderly population (12).

In NHANES III, the prevalence of diagnosed and undiagnosed diabetes was 1.6% in men age 20 to 39 years, rising to 21.1% in men older than 75 years of age (11). Estimates from the National Health Interview Survey (NHIS) showed that the prevalence of diabetes among Americans older than 75 years in 1993 was 10.1%, compared with 1.3% among those age 18 to 44 years (32). Similarly, in the Framingham Study, glucose intolerance or diabetes was present in 30% to 40% of study subjects older than 65 years of age (31). However, after adjustment for age in the NHANES III study, the prevalence of diabetes still increased by 19% between 1980 and 1996. Therefore, the observed increase in diagnosed cases cannot be attributed solely to the aging of the population (11).

Ethnic Groups

The rising incidence and prevalence of diabetes have been especially evident among certain ethnic groups, including African-Americans, Hispanics, Asians, Native Americans, and Asian Indians, among others. For example, more than 35% of the increased incidence of newly diagnosed diabetes in the United States over the coming 50 years is expected to be accounted for by the increasing proportion of minority group members in the population (33). The ethnic association with diabetes risk most likely results from a complex interaction between genetic predisposition and environmental influences that results in a clustering of risk factors for diabetes in these populations.

The African-American population in the United States is at especially great risk for development of type 2 diabetes. In NHANES III, diabetes was more common among non-Hispanic blacks than among non-Hispanic whites; the

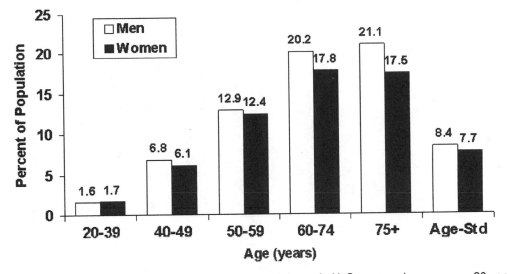

FIG. 9-2. Prevalence of diagnosed and undiagnosed diabetes in U. S. men and women age 20 years or older, based on the second National Health and Nutrition Survey (NHANES II). (Adapted from Harris MI, et al. Prevalence of diabetes, impaired fasting glucose, and impaired glucose tolerance in U.S. adults. The Third National Health and Nutrition Examination Survey, 1988–1994. *Diabetes Care* 1998;21:518–524.)

ratio of the age and sex-standardized prevalence among blacks versus whites was 1.6 (11). Data from the NHIS indicate that the prevalence of diabetes is higher in blacks compared with whites at all ages (12). For example, 19.3% of adult blacks between the ages of 20 and 44 years have diabetes, compared with 12.0% of age-matched whites (10). Furthermore, prevalence rates appear to be disproportionately greater for black women than for black men (12).

The prevalence of diabetes among Hispanics is estimated to be 25% higher than among African-Americans (34). The Hispanic Health and Nutrition Survey (HHANES), conducted between 1982 and 1984, showed that 26% of Puerto Ricans and 24% of Mexican-Americans between 45 and 74 years of age had diabetes (35). A Massachusetts survey (36) showed that the incidence was higher among Puerto Ricans (38%) than among Dominicans (35%) or non-Hispanic whites (23%) in that state. These differences were significant after multivariable adjustment. Puerto Rican ethnicity was associated with a 2.3 times higher risk for diabetes and a 3.5 times higher risk for insulin use, compared with white ethnicity.

The minority group that has been studied the most with regard to risk for type 2 diabetes is the Native American population in North America. Studies of Native American youth indicate that glucose intolerance and diabetes develop early in life. Using the National Indian Health Service database, Fagot-Campagna et al. (37) found that the prevalence of diabetes among Native American adolescents age 15 to 19 years increased 61% between 1988 and 1997, with an estimated prevalence of approximately 4.5 per 1,000 adolescents (Fig. 9-3). In 1965, the National Institutes of Health began a longitudinal cohort study evaluating the incidence and prevalence of type 2 diabetes in a population of 12,000 Pima Indians residing in the Gila River Indian Community in Central Arizona. The prevalence of diabetes among this population is the highest in the world; the disease affects more than 50% of Pima Indian adults (38). Among the explanations for this high prevalence of diabetes in Native American populations is the high prevalence of risk factors associated with diabetes, such as obesity, sedentary lifestyle, and family history. In addition, the theory of a "thrifty genotype" (a propensity to store calories more efficiently in the presence

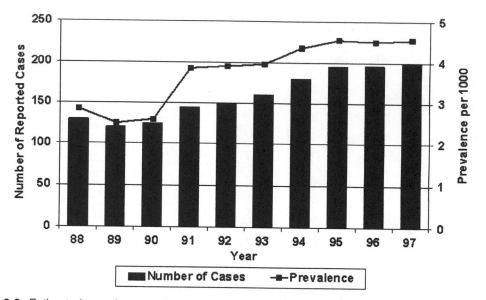

FIG. 9-3. Estimated prevalence and number of reported cases of diagnosed diabetes among Native American adolescents age 15 to 19 years in the southwestern United States between 1988 and 1997. (Adapted from Fagot-Campagna A, Burrows NR, Williamson DF. The public health epidemiology of type 2 diabetes in children and adolescents: a case study of American Indian adolescents in the Southwestern United States. *Clin Chim Acta* 1999;286:81–95.)

of scarce food supplies) has been raised in this population, suggesting that when food is plentiful, efficient calorie storage leads to accelerated obesity, hyperinsulinemia, and glucose intolerance (37). Environmental factors are quite likely to play a deterministic role. The prevalence of diabetes among the Pima Indians in Mexico is distinctly lower than among Pima Indians in Arizona (39).

The prevalence of obesity remains disproportionately elevated in these ethnic populations, a fact that probably plays a causative role in the increased rate of type 2 diabetes (11,40). Data from NHANES III indicate that 20.2% of black men in the United States are obese (41), and the rise in the incidence of obesity among African-Americans parallels the increased incidence and prevalence of diabetes. For example, in the Atherosclerosis in Communities Study (42), 50% of the increased risk for diabetes among black women was explained by modifiable risk factors such as adiposity. Other studies have confirmed the high prevalence of central obesity among Hispanics and its association with diabetes (43). There appears to be a strong associ-

ation between overweight (i.e., a BMI between 25 and 29 kg/m^2) and diabetes in Hispanics, suggesting that glucose intolerance occurs at lower levels of adiposity in Hispanics than in whites. Among Pima Indians, the prevalence of overweight and obesity is high even in children (44). In one study, the mean BMI for adult Pima Indian men age 21 to 60 years was 33; for women in the same age group, it was 35 (45).

Asians who have immigrated to Western countries also appear to have high rates of diabetes and glucose intolerance. The Japanese-American Community Diabetes Study examined the rates of diabetes among 418 second-generation Americans of 100% Japanese ancestry residing in King County, Washington (46). Subjects underwent OGTT and were classified as having normal glucose tolerance, IGT, or diabetes, based on the WHO definitions. An estimated 56% of the study population had abnormal glucose tolerance. Only 13% reported a previous diagnosis of diabetes. Extrapolation to the general population of Japanese-Americans suggested that 20% have diabetes and 36% have IGT. A follow-up study of 503 second- and third-generation

Japanese-Americans from the same area demonstrated a high prevalence of adiposity; high insulin, C peptide, and triglyceride levels; low levels of high-density lipoprotein (HDL); and high blood pressure even among subjects with IGT (47). This suggests that obesity is also a risk factor among Asian-Americans, although, as a group, they tend to have lower BMIs than do Americans of European descent (48). The higher prevalence of central adiposity may explain some of the risk for obesity-related disorders; however, the National Heart Lung and Blood Institute definitions for overweight and obesity have been shown to be effective markers of risk among Japanese-Americans (49).

Studies of Asian Indians in England have provided valuable information on diabetes among Indians who have immigrated to Western countries (50,51). The Coventry Diabetes Study examined the prevalence of diabetes among 2,130 Asian adults by administering the OGTT and found that 11.2% of Asian men and 8.9% of Asian women had diabetes, compared with 2.8% of white men and 4.3% of white women (50). Among Asians found to have diabetes, 30% did not carry a prior diagnosis. Although this study did not find significant differences in BMI between the Asian and white subjects, other studies in London have found high rates of central obesity and hyperinsulinemia among Asian Indians (51). Because there are few data on changes in prevalence among Asian-Americans over time, no comment can be made as to whether risk factors for diabetes or diabetes itself is increasing among Asians in the United States.

Individuals with the Metabolic Syndrome

Two specific groups of persons at heightened risk for development of type 2 diabetes are those with IGT and those with the metabolic syndrome. There remains no doubt that these groups are at heightened risk and that diabetes remains a preventable disease. The Diabetes Prevention Program (DPP) randomly assigned participants with increased levels of FPG (95 to 125 mg/dL) and postload plasma glucose (2 hours after 75-g oral glucose, 140 to 199 mg/dL) to one of three strategies: intensive lifestyle modification, metformin,

or usual lifestyle modification treatment (52). There was a noteworthy 58% reduction in the development of type 2 diabetes mellitus in the intensive lifestyle modification arm and a 31% reduction in the metformin arm. The annual incidence of type 2 diabetes was approximately 11% in the group receiving usual lifestyle modification treatment. According to the third National Health and Nutrition Examination Survey (53), there are an estimated 10 million people in the United States that resemble the DPP participants. The number of at-risk persons is probably greater than that defined in the DPP and will certainly increase in the near future.

Like the prevalence of type 2 diabetes, the prevalence of the metabolic syndrome also varies across ethnic background and age. The National Cholesterol Education Program-Adult Treatment Panel (NCEP-ATP III) recently defined the metabolic syndrome as shown in Table 9-2. The NHANES III report suggested that the prevalence of the metabolic syndrome, using 2000 Census data, approaches 47 million persons in the United States, almost 22% of the entire population (54). The prevalence increased from 6.7% among persons in their twenties to approximately 43% among those approaching 70 years of age. There remains a disconcerting susceptibility among certain minority groups to development of features of the metabolic syndrome. Hispanic-Americans had the greatest age-adjusted prevalence (31.9%), followed by whites (23.8%) and African-Americans (21.6%). Although the prevalence was similar among men and women overall (24.0% versus 23.4%), there was a propensity toward presence of the

TABLE 9-2. *National Cholesterol Education Program–Adult Treatment Panel III (NCEP-ATP III) diagnostic criteria for the metabolic syndrome*

Any three of the following :
 Fasting Glucose $\geq$110 mg/dL
 Triglycerides $>$150 mg/dL
 Central adiposity
  Male $>$102 cm (40 in)
  Female $>$88 cm (35 in)
 Hypertension $\geq$130/85 mm Hg
 High-density lipoprotein
  Male $<$40 mg/dL
  Female $<$50 mg/dL

metabolic syndrome among Hispanic-American women compared with men (35.6% versus 28.3%) and among African-American women compared with men (25.7% versus 16.4%). Given the increasing age prevalence of obesity, it is likely that the metabolic syndrome will become an ever more important cardiovascular risk factor.

Children

Estimates of the incidence and prevalence of diabetes among children and adolescents come from three main sources: population-based studies, clinic-based studies, and case series. Table 9-3 shows the current prevalence estimates from the three study types (55). The NHANES III study included 2,867 adolescents in the United States surveyed between 1988 and 1994 and suggested that the prevalence of all types of diabetes among 12- to 19-year-olds was 0.41%. The prevalence of glucose intolerance in the same age group was 1.76%. Thirty-one percent of the diabetes cases were considered to be type 2 diabetes, and all occurred in members of ethnic minority groups (56). Indeed, much of the data on diabetes in children comes from surveys conducted among minority groups (in particular, Native American populations in the United States and Canada). These show that the prevalence of type 2 diabetes among 15- to 19-year-olds ranges from 2.3 per 1,000 in the Canadian Cree and Manitoba Ojibwa tribes (57) to 50.9 per 1,000 in U. S. Pima Indians (58). The prevalence of childhood obesity is higher among African-American children than among white children (59), suggesting that risk factors for diabetes are present at an earlier age in minority populations.

Insulin-dependent (type 1) diabetes mellitus affects 120,000 people younger than 18 years of age in the United States. There is geographic variation in the prevalence of type 1 diabetes globally, with a prevalence of 0.7 per 100,000 in Shanghai and up to 35 per 100,000 in Finland (60). These cases represent the majority of patients affected by diabetes before the age of 19 years, but type 1 diabetes accounts for a small minority of cases of diabetes overall. Overlap among

the clinical features of type 1 and type 2 diabetes has led to some diagnostic uncertainty in the pediatric population (61). For example, the initial classification is based on the sentinel clinical presentation: patients who have recent weight loss, are of normal weight or underweight, and have ketoacidosis are considered to have type 1 diabetes. However, up to 33% of children with type 2 diabetes have ketonuria at presentation. Other features strongly associated with type 2 diabetes have been suggested to improve the diagnostic accuracy between the two clinical syndromes, including the presence of obesity or overweight, a strong family history of type 2 diabetes, acanthosis nigricans, and the polycystic ovary syndrome.

The prevalence of both type 1 and type 2 diabetes appears to be increasing among children and adolescents. The European Diabetes Study Group (EURODIAB) collaborative group studied the incidence of new cases of type 1 diabetes mellitus in Europe and Israel from 1988 to 1994 among subjects younger than 15 years of age (62). There was great variability in annual incidence across countries, ranging from 3 to 25 cases per 100,000 persons per year in Macedonia, to 40.2 cases per 100,000 per year in Finland. There was a concerning 6.3% increase in the annual incidence of type 1 diabetes among both boys and girls age 0 to 4 years. The large variability across Europe and the rapid increase in cases of type 2 diabetes mellitus probably are not related to either a difference in genetic makeup or a shift in susceptibility genes. Rather, this changing profile is best accounted for by a change in environmental factors occurring early in life.

There are few epidemiologic data on the incidence and prevalence of type 2 diabetes in children. Until recently, type 2 diabetes was believed to be a disease of adulthood. However, an alarming trend is emerging around the world as children are becoming less active and more obese, resulting in a steady increase in the prevalence of type 2 diabetes in this historically low-risk population (63). Before 1992, the diagnosis of type 2 diabetes mellitus in a child was a rare occurrence. Currently, reports suggest that type 2 diabetes accounts for 10% to 50% of all new cases of diabetes in children. This increase is quite

TABLE 9-3. *Selected current estimates of the magnitude of type 2 diabetes in North American children and adolescents in population and clinic-based studies and case series*

Study (ref. no.)	Years	Race/ethnicity	Age (yr)	Prevalence per 1000 (95% confidence interval)[a]
Population-based studies				
New Mexico (211)	1991–1992	Navajo Indians	12–19	14.1 *(0–33.5)*[b]
Arizona (64)[c]	1992–1996	Pima Indians	10–14	22.3 *(11.1–33.5)*
			15–19	50.9 *(32.2–69.6)*
Manitoba (57)	1996–1997	Cree and Ojibway Indians	4–19	11.1 *(3.4–18.8)*
			10–19	0 for boys, 36.0 for girls
NHANES III[d]	1988–1994	Whites, African, and African-Americans, all U.S.	12–19	4.1 *(0–8.6)*[b]
Clinic-based studies				
Indian Health Services (212)	1996	American Indians, all U.S.	0–14	1.3[b]
			15–19	4.5[b]
Manitoba[e]	1998	Cree and Ojibway Indians	5–14	1.0
			15–19	2.3
Clinic-based study, Cincinnati, OH (213)	1994	Whites and African-Americans	0–19	Incidence per 100,000/yr, 3.5
			10–19	7.2% of type 2 diabetes among new cases of diabetes
Cincinnati, OH (213)	1982–1994	Whites and African-Americans	0–19	16[e (in 1994)]
			10–19	33[e (in 1994)]
Charleston, SC (214)	1997	African-Americans	10–19	46
Little Rock, AR (215)	1988–1995	Whites, Hispanics, and African-Americans	0–19	U
San Diego, CA (216)	1993–1994	Whites, Hispanics, African- and Asian-Americans	0–16	8[e]
San Antonio, TX (217)	1990–1997	Whites, Hispanics	U	18[e]
Ventura, CA (218)	1990–1994	Hispanics	0–17	45[e]

NHANES III, National Health and Nutrition Examination Survey III; U, unknown data.
[a]Numbers in italics are estimates.
[b]Estimates include cases of type 1 diabetes.
[c]D. Dabelea, personal communication.
[d]A. Fagot-Campagna, personal communication.
[e]H. Dean, personal communication.
Adapted from Fagot-Campagna A, et al. Type 2 diabetes among North American children and adolescents: an epidemiologic review and a public health perspective. *J Pediatr* 2000;136:664–672.

apparent among Pima Indian children and adolescents (64). There appears to be a high incidence of associated risk factors for type 2 diabetes in children, including obesity, hypertension, dyslipidemia, and physical inactivity. Additionally, gestational diabetes and low birth weight are associated with future risk of childhood type 2 diabetes mellitus. Given the emerging data with respect to childhood obesity and diabetes, a concerted effort toward early identification of at-risk children and early implementation of risk factor modification is crucial. A recent American Heart Association scientific statement regarding cardiovascular health in childhood highlighted the real need to effect change among this cohort (65). This summary document suggested that an FPG level be determined for children thought to be at increased risk for type 2 diabetes, including children who are overweight, have a family history of type 2 diabetes, are at risk because of their ethnicity, or have signs of insulin resistance. Additionally, children with these features should have their serum cholesterol level and blood pressure checked. Given the long-term implications with respect to the future risk of diabetes and development of cardiovascular disease, a multidisciplinary team approach with specific focus on lifestyle modification, risk factor management, and early detection of type 2 diabetes and associated cardiovascular risk factors is crucial.

FACTORS CONTRIBUTING TO THE PANDEMIC OF DIABETES

Modification of Diagnostic Criteria

The criteria for the diagnosis of glucose intolerance and diabetes have undergone significant changes over the past decade, resulting in increased numbers of patients meeting the clinical criteria for disease. WHO published revised diagnostic criteria for IGT and diabetes in 1985 (66), basing the diagnosis on both the FPG and OGTT results (Table 9-1). In NHANES III, the number of previously undiagnosed people meeting criteria for diabetes was 4.4% when the ADA definition (FPG, 126 mg/dL) was used and 6.4% when the WHO definition (2-hour postload plasma glucose, 200 mg/dL) was used (67). This suggests that many patients with diabetes would not have been diagnosed without the use of OGTT, a procedure seldom performed in contemporary clinical practice. In 1997, the ADA published its revised diagnostic criteria for diabetes (7), which minimized the reliance on the OGTT. According to the revised ADA diagnostic guidelines, an FPG of 126 mg/dL (7 mmol/L) or greater on two or more occasions is diagnostic of diabetes. The diagnostic sensitivity of this new FPG cutoff very closely approximates that of the OGTT. Still, concern remains as to whether the decreased emphasis on OGTT in clinical practice will result in failure to capture a significant portion of patients with diabetes (68,69). This uncertainty prompted WHO to revisit its diagnostic criteria and update the parameters by which diabetes

should be diagnosed. These new criteria, published in 1999, incorporated the ADA FPG criterion but also retained the use of the OGTT (8). Examination of the NHANES III data demonstrated that the WHO criteria identified more patients with diabetes than did the ADA criteria (67). Similarly, in a study of 5,023 Pima Indians, the ADA criteria identified fewer patients as diabetic, compared with the revised WHO criteria (70). In addition, the intermediate category of IGT based on OGTT was more predictive of later progression to diabetes at first follow-up than was the ADA classification of IFG. Therefore, the latest diagnostic criteria proposed by WHO identify more patients as diabetic and more patients as being at risk for the development of diabetes.

Aging Population

During the 20th century, the life expectancy in industrialized countries increased by more than 25 years. People older than 80 years of age are now the fastest-growing age group. Concomitant with this increase in longevity has been an improvement in the health status of those living longer. For example, in the United States, the rate of disability has declined despite the aging of the population (71). Although the increase in longevity has not been as dramatic in developing countries, 60% of the global population age 60 years and older live in developing countries, and this percentage is expected to rise throughout the 21st century (29). This has profound implications for the increase in certain chronic diseases associated with increasing age, including type 2 diabetes. The risk of type 2 diabetes increases with increasing age. For example, the prevalence of type 2 diabetes increases from approximately 6% at age 40 years to almost 20% for persons older than 75 years of age (11).

Obesity

The WHO and the National Institutes of Health define overweight as a BMI of 25 kg/m^2 or higher but less than 30 kg/m^2; obesity as a BMI of 30 kg/m^2 or higher but less than 39.9 kg/m^2; and extreme obesity as a BMI of 40 kg/m^2 or higher

(72). Among developed and developing countries, obesity, which is directly associated with the development of insulin resistance, glucose intolerance, and diabetes, has been increasing at an alarming rate (73–75). Results from NHANES III (1988–1991) demonstrate that approximately 33% of the U. S. population is obese, up from 25% observed 10 years earlier in NHANES II (1976–1980) (74).

The increased prevalence of glucose intolerance and diabetes throughout the world is inextricably linked to increases in the proportion of the population who are overweight or obese. Several longitudinal cohort studies have demonstrated the association between obesity and glucose intolerance (11,42,76,77). Data from NHANES III show that 67% of those with type 2 diabetes mellitus have a BMI that meets the criteria for overweight, and almost half have a BMI that meets the definition of obesity (72). In the Iowa Women's Health Study, women in the highest quintile of BMI had a relative risk of 29 for the development of diabetes over the 12-year follow-up period (76). Waist circumference and WHR may be even better markers of diabetes risk than either weight or BMI alone (36,78). Even among nonobese patients, abdominal distribution of fat and increased WHR are independently associated with the risk for diabetes (79,80). Although the molecular mechanisms by which obesity contributes to glucose intolerance remain elusive, they most likely involve a combination of genetic factors and mechanisms in which skeletal myocytes and central adipocytes play a deterministic role (81–83).

Decreasing Levels of Physical Activity

Leisure-time physical activity continues to decrease worldwide, resulting in an increasingly sedentary population and incrementing risk for diabetes (20). Data from the Nurses' Health Study demonstrated that even physical activity of moderate intensity and duration was associated with a decreased risk for diabetes (84). The favorable impact of physical activity on diabetes risk extends beyond issues of weight management. Physical activity is directly associated with improved glycometabolism, as demonstrated

by decreased insulin levels, increased insulin sensitivity, and a lower incidence of diabetes (85–87).

Diet

Other lifestyle factors, such as diets that are low in dietary fiber with a high glycemic load (88) and high-fat diets (89), have also been associated with the development of diabetes. An analysis of 42,504 subjects in the Physicians' Health Study found a relative risk of 1.59 for the development of diabetes with consumption of a high-fat diet (90). Similarly, in the Nurses' Health Study, increased intake of dietary cereal fiber, whole-grain foods (91), and trans-fatty acids and decreased intake of saturated fat were associated with a reduced risk for development of type 2 diabetes (92,93).

Genetic Associations

The familial occurrence of diabetes suggests a genetic predisposition to abnormalities of glucose tolerance. The fundamental differences between type 1 diabetes (beta-cell dysfunction leading to absolute insulin deficiency) and type 2 diabetes (hyperinsulinemia and insulin resistance) imply that different genes are involved in each disease process. Human leukocyte antigens (HLAs) appear to be associated with susceptibility to and development of type 1 diabetes (94). For example, many Caucasians with type 1 diabetes have HLA-DR3, HLA-DR4, or both (95). The HLA-DQβ gene is associated with susceptibility to autoimmune beta-cell destruction (96).

Similarly, type 2 diabetes appears to have strong genetic associations. Studies in twins have demonstrated that the concordance rates of type 2 diabetes in monozygotic twins range between 34% and 83% (97,98). The broad range of observed correlation suggests both a complex genetic predisposition and an interaction between environmental and genetic factors in the pathogenesis of type 2 diabetes. As evidence of the complexity of the genetic determinants, no single genetic locus has been linked definitively with type 2 diabetes despite the examination of more than 250 candidate genes (99). In specific populations, an association between certain chromosome loci and diabetic traits has been observed (91). In addition, some gene products, such as the glucagon receptor and the product of the *MAPKBIP1* gene, may contribute to the pathogenesis of type 2 diabetes (100,101). Given the complexity of the disease, newer techniques that allow for the screening of a large number of genes and genetic loci will be needed to establish clear genetic associations with diabetes (91).

EPIDEMIOLOGY OF DIABETIC CARDIOVASCULAR DISEASE

Macrovascular disease (myocardial infarction [MI], stroke, and peripheral arterial disease) accounts for the majority of morbidity and mortality associated with type 2 diabetes (102–106). For example, in the United Kingdom Prospective Diabetes Study (UKPDS), the 10-year risk for all macrovascular complications was more than four times that for microvascular complications (107). Nevertheless, a survey conducted by the ADA and the American College of Cardiology of 2,008 subjects with diabetes revealed that almost 70% of those surveyed did not believe that cardiovascular disease was a serious risk associated with diabetes (108).

Ischemic Heart Disease

The most common cause of death among patients with diabetes is ischemic heart disease (18). In the NHIS, there was a correlation between age and the prevalence of ischemic heart disease among subjects with diabetes: 3% of subjects age 18 to 44 years reported such a history, compared with 14% of those age 45 to 64 years, and 20% of those older than 65 years of age (104). There appears to be some ethnic variation in the prevalence and incidence of heart disease among persons with type 2 diabetes. For example, cardiovascular disease was reported in approximately 14% of white patients with diabetes, compared with 50% to 80% of Native Americans with diabetes (11). In the Strong Heart Study of Native American tribes in central Arizona, southwestern Oklahoma, South Dakota, and North Dakota, the incidence of coronary heart disease was twice as high as in the Atherosclerosis Risk in Communities Study, which involved mostly white subjects (109).

Some data suggest that, among the population with diabetes, women are at higher cardiovascular risk than men are. Data from NHANES I showed that mortality over a 9-year period declined for men and women without diabetes as well as for men with diabetes, but increased 23% for women with diabetes (110). Furthermore, African-American women with diabetes appear to be at higher risk than white women with diabetes (111). Similarly, analysis of data from the NHIS and the Nationwide Inpatient Sample show that the age-adjusted prevalence of major cardiovascular disease for women with diabetes is twice that for women without diabetes (112). Among Native Americans in the Strong Heart Study, however, men with diabetes had almost twice the incidence of fatal and nonfatal cardiovascular disease than did women with diabetes (109). There are a number of pathophysiologic mechanisms by which diabetes is associated with an increased susceptibility to acute ischemic events; these are reviewed elsewhere in this text.

Patients with diabetes also have worse clinical outcomes than do nondiabetic patients after acute coronary syndromes. The increased risk associated with diabetes after acute coronary syndromes has been reported among patients with ST-elevation MI (113–115) and among those with non-ST-elevation acute coronary syndromes (116,117). Likewise, the Framingham Study documented a significantly higher rate of mortality and a higher rate of reinfarction and heart failure for patients with diabetes, both acutely and in the postinfarction period, after adjusting for other factors (118).

Congestive Heart Failure

The most common cause of left ventricular systolic dysfunction with congestive heart failure (CHF) in the United States is ischemic heart disease (119). However, after adjusting for the prevalence of coronary artery disease, diabetes remains an independent predictor for CHF (120) and an independent predictor of mortality among patients with CHF (121). Glucose intolerance, even in the prediabetic setting, has been associated with CHF, suggesting that the glycometabolic state may play a pathophysiologic role (120,122–124).

Patients with diabetes develop heart failure after MI at higher rates than do patients without diabetes, independent of infarct size (125,126). The increased risk for CHF was demonstrated in the Multicenter Investigation of the Limitation of Infarct Size (MILIS) trial, in which diabetes was independently associated with CHF and decreased systolic function after MI (126). Similarly, patients with diabetes and ST-elevation MI enrolled in the Global Utilization of Streptokinase and Tissue Plasminogen Activator for Occluded Coronary Arteries I (GUSTO I) trial had twice the incidence of post-MI heart failure of patients without diabetes (115). The increased risk for CHF associated with diabetes has been demonstrated across the entire spectrum of acute coronary syndromes (116).

Cerebrovascular Disease

The constellation of metabolic and physiologic abnormalities that coexist with diabetes (e.g., hypertension, dyslipidemia) confers a high risk of stroke in this population. However, even after adjustment for these factors, diabetes remains an independent predictor for ischemic neurologic events, suggesting that additional diabetes-related factors are contributing (127). In both the Framingham Study and the Honolulu Heart Study, diabetes was associated with twice the risk of stroke after adjustment for other cardiovascular risk factors (103,127).

Peripheral Vascular Disease

A significant contributor to the morbidity associated with diabetes is peripheral arterial disease, which commonly manifests as lower-extremity ulceration or gangrene (or both) and can result in amputation. The occurrence of peripheral vascular disease among patients with diabetes is associated with a 70% to 80% higher mortality rate, compared with the absence of peripheral vascular disease (128,129). Between 1983 and 1990,

6% of hospitalizations that contained diabetes as a discharge diagnosis also listed lower-extremity ulcer (130). Data from the ADA have identified male gender, duration of diabetes greater than 10 years, poor glucose control, and the presence of cardiovascular, retinal, or renal complications as risk factors for foot ulcers. Population-based studies in the United States have shown that 10% to 17% of patients with diabetes have foot ulceration, with a greater prevalence among male patients, those treated with insulin, and those with longer duration of diabetes (131).

Because of compromised peripheral circulation, diabetes results in approximately 45% of the extremity amputations in the United States, and amputation is 15 times more common in diabetics than in patients without diabetes (132–134). Population studies indicate that the highest incidence of lower-extremity amputation occurs among Pima Indians with diabetes; the amputation rate in this population was 137 times that among Pima Indians without diabetes (135). Examination of statewide data from Texas suggested that blacks have higher amputation rates than whites (130). However, more recent data from a large health maintenance organization in northern California showed that Asian-Americans have a lower risk of amputation and that there were no apparent differences in risk between Hispanics, African-Americans, and Caucasians (136).

The pathophysiology of peripheral vascular disease in diabetes differs from that of "routine" peripheral atherosclerosis. The distal lower-extremity arterial circulation appears to be affected more often in patients with diabetes, whereas the more proximal vessels are affected more often in patients without diabetes (137) (Fig. 9-4), who have relative sparing of the pedal vessels (138). This pattern often requires a distal anastomosis at the time of vascular surgery.

The prognosis for patients with diabetes after the development of peripheral arterial disease is poor, especially if amputation is required. Outcomes are worse for diabetics than for patients who do not have diabetes or patients who have diabetes but do not require amputation (135,139). The 3-year mortality rate after lower-extremity amputation in patients with diabetes has been

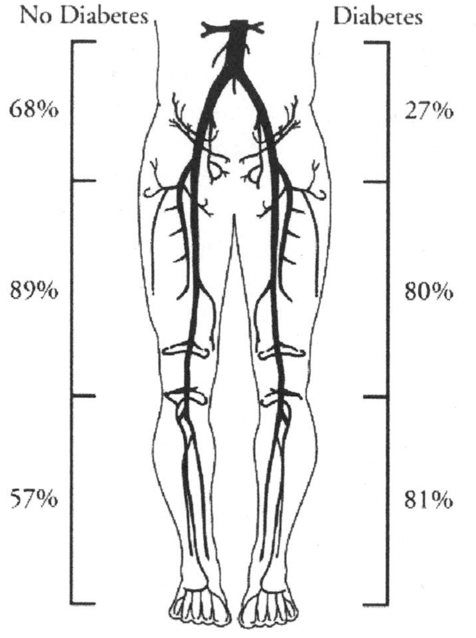

FIG. 9-4. Topographic distribution of nondiabetic peripheral arteriopathy *(left)* and diabetic peripheral arteriopathy *(right)*. (Adapted from Lanzer P. Topographic distribution of peripheral arteriopathy in non-diabetics and type 2 diabetics. *Z Kardiol* 2001;90:99–103.)

reported to be 20% to 50% (140,141), and 5-year mortality rate is 39% to 68% (135,142).

Hypertension

Hypertension affects up to 70% of patients with diabetes and accounts for 35% to 45% of cardiovascular and renal complications among the diabetic cohort (104,143). In the NHANES II study, the prevalence of hypertension, defined as a blood pressure greater than 160/95 mm Hg among individuals age 65 to 74 years, increased with decreasing glucose tolerance. Approximately 60% of subjects with diabetes, 50.7% of those with IGT, and 38.3% of those with normal glucose were affected (10). In NHANES II, with hypertension defined as blood pressure greater than 140/90 mm Hg, 71% of patients with diabetes had hypertension (143). Older patients have a higher risk for hypertension with or without diabetes (10), and, among the diabetic population, men are twice as likely as women to

have hypertension (144). Ethnic and gender differences are also present. A community-based study of 765 patients with insulin-requiring diabetes found that men were almost twice as likely as women to have hypertension (144). Age, male sex, duration of diabetes, glycemic control (defined as percentage of glycosylated hemoglobin), and proteinuria are independent predictors of hypertension (144). Pooled, unpublished data from NHANES II and HHANES showed that the prevalence of hypertension was highest in black women and lowest in Mexican-Americans. Mean systolic pressure was highest among whites in the Rancho Bernardo Diabetes Study and lowest among Dakota Indians in the Strong Heart Study, whereas diastolic pressure was highest among blacks and lowest among Mexican-Americans and whites in the San Antonio Texas Diabetes Study (145).

Dyslipidemia

The lipid profile in diabetes that is associated with increased risk of coronary artery disease consists of a low HDL concentration; a high concentration of low-density lipoprotein (LDL) with a preponderance of small, dense LDL particles; and increased apolipoprotein A-IV (146–149). Triglycerides are also often elevated, and the degree of elevation is related to the degree of glucose intolerance, with higher levels in patients who have diabetes compared with those who have IGT or normal glucose (145). In the Atherosclerosis Risk in Communities Study, African-American men and women who developed diabetes during the follow-up period had higher levels of HDL and lower levels of LDL and triglycerides, compared with their white counterparts (42). Pooling of unpublished data by the ADA from NHANES II, the Rancho Bernardo California Diabetes Study, the Japanese-American Study of Diabetes, the San Antonio Texas Heart Study, and the San Luis Valley Study showed that, among patients with diabetes, mean total cholesterol and HDL levels were higher in women compared with men (145). The highest HDL levels occurred in Japanese-American women and white women from the Rancho Bernardo study. The highest

LDL cholesterol levels were observed in white women from the NHANES II, and the lowest levels were found in Native American women. Hispanic women in the San Luis Valley study and white men in the San Antonio study had the highest levels of triglycerides.

Abnormalities of lipids in type 2 diabetes develop concomitantly with the failure of insulin activity, which leads to the release of fatty acids from adipose tissue, increased delivery of free fatty acids to the liver, and increased hepatic synthesis of very-low-density lipoproteins (VLDL) (146,150,151). This abnormal lipid profile, characterized by normal or modestly elevated LDL cholesterol, low HDL cholesterol, high triglycerides, and a preponderance of small, dense LDL particles, is associated with markedly increased cardiovascular risk among diabetic patients (148,152).

Ethnic Differences

Although macrovascular disease is the most common complication of diabetes in the overall population, Pima Indians are much more prone to develop microvascular complications, a phenomenon known as the "Pima paradox" (153). A similar disparity in the risk for diabetic complications has been reported in other ethnic groups, such as African-, Hispanic-, and Asian-Americans. Among these populations, the rate of end-stage renal disease is higher relative to whites, and the rates of macrovascular complications are relatively lower (136).

PREVENTION OF DIABETES MELLITUS

The identification of groups at high risk for diabetes has led to increasing interest in the primary prevention of diabetes and has indicated the populations to target for aggressive prevention efforts. High-risk groups include obese individuals and those with IFG, IGT, or both. For example, 16% of individuals with IGT in the Finnish Diabetes Prevention Program developed diabetes during the 3-year follow-up period (154).

Selected minority populations also exhibit excessive risk for diabetes. The Pima Indians of North America have the highest reported rates of diabetes of any ethnic population in the world, with more than 50% of adults affected (155). Among Asian-Indians, Chinese, and Creoles living on the island of Mauritius in the Indian Ocean off the coast of Madagascar, the presence of both IGT and IFG was associated with a progression rate of 40% at 5 years; the presence of either abnormality was associated with a progression rate of 20% (156). Although ethnic predisposition has been clearly documented in a number of minority groups, the majority of risk in these populations derives from the prevalence of lifestyle factors that contribute to diabetes, as discussed earlier. This implies that behavioral interventions may be effective in such populations.

Lifestyle approaches to diabetes prevention have centered on diet, weight loss, physical activity, and, in those with established diabetes, improved glycemic control (154,157–159). The Malmo feasibility study of 181 subjects with IGT examined the effect of dietary and exercise intervention and found a progression rate to diabetes of 10.2% at 6 years in the intervention group, compared with 29% in the reference group (158). This study was not randomized, but its results were replicated in the randomized Da Qing study conducted in China (160), which showed that diet and exercise therapy resulted in a 42% reduction in progression to diabetes over 5 years among 577 subjects with IGT. The Finnish Diabetes Prevention Study Group randomly assigned 522 overweight subjects with IGT to receive either dietary and exercise intervention or usual care (154). After 3 years of follow-up, there was a 58% relative risk reduction for progression to diabetes in the intervention group.

Supporting the initial feasibility studies, the DPP randomized clinical trial (52) evaluated the effect of lifestyle intervention on the prevention of diabetes in subjects with IGT. There was a remarkable 58% reduction in the risk of developing diabetes over the 3-year study period: as a result, one case of diabetes was prevented for every seven subjects treated with the intervention. Metformin, which reduces hepatic gluconeogenesis and increases insulin sensitivity, reduces insulin levels and potentially delays the onset of diabetes. Although lifestyle intervention was substantially more effective than metformin in

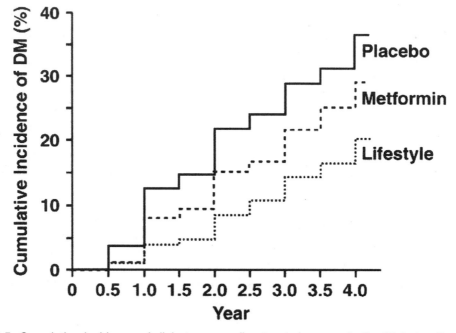

FIG. 9-5. Cumulative incidence of diabetes according to study group in the Diabetes Prevention Program. (Adapted from Knowler WC, et al. Reduction in the incidence of type 2 diabetes with lifestyle intervention or metformin. *N Engl J Med* 2002;346:393–403.)

the DPP study, metformin reduced the incidence of diabetes over 4 years by an impressive 31% (52) (Fig. 9-5). With this reduction, the number needed to treat to prevent a case of diabetes was only 13.9.

Other medications that may prevent or delay the development of diabetes include angiotensin-converting enzyme (ACE) inhibitors, α-glucosidase inhibitors, meglitinides, thiazolidinediones, and angiotensin receptor blockers (ARBs). With regard to ACE inhibitors, literature exists documenting the acute and chronic favorable effects of these drugs on insulin sensitivity, which are similar in magnitude to the effects of metformin (161–163). Although the biologic underpinnings of diabetes prevention with the administration of ACE inhibitors is unclear, captopril and ramipril were shown to decrease the risk of developing incident diabetes in subanalyses from two large-scale, randomized clinical trials (164–166). Furthermore, data from the SE-CURE study (UKPDS) support an attenuated increase in glucose levels due to treatment with

ACE inhibitors (167). The ARB losartan also seems to be associated with a decreased incidence of diabetes (168), but whether this represents a benefit of losartan or a detrimental effect on glucose metabolism is unclear given this trial design.

Acarbose is a pseudooligosaccharide that delays the absorption of glucose and reduces serum glucose concentration, insulin levels, and insulin resistance. Acarbose could theoretically reduce the toxic effects of glucose on pancreatic beta cells and prevent the onset of diabetes (169). The Study to Prevent Non-Insulin Dependent Diabetes Mellitus (STOP-NIDDM) trial randomly assigned 1,368 subjects with IGT to receive either acarbose or placebo (170). Over a mean follow-up period of 3.3 years, acarbose was associated with a statistically significant 25% reduction in relative risk for the development of diabetes.

Studies are presently underway to directly test the effects of many of these therapies on the risk of incident diabetes in prospective clinical investigations. For example, the Nateglinide and Valsartan in Impaired Glucose Tolerance Outcomes Research (NAVIGATOR) trial plans to randomly assign 7,500 patients with IGT to receive either nateglinide (a meglitinide), valsartan (an ARB), or both, to evaluate the effects of these therapies on the progression to diabetes. A similar trial that is primarily evaluating progression to diabetes, the DREAM study, plans to enroll 3,000 patients with IGT and randomly assign them factorially to ramipril versus placebo and to rosiglitazone versus placebo. Both trials will secondarily evaluate the influence of these therapies on cardiovascular outcomes.

PREVENTION OF DIABETIC CARDIOVASCULAR COMPLICATIONS

Diabetes is strongly associated with cardiovascular disease risk, which is the primary cause of morbidity and mortality among patients with diabetes, accounting for more than 80% of deaths in this population (171,172). Based on epidemiologic data, diabetes alone confers long-term cardiovascular risk similar to that observed among patients who are without diabetes but have had a prior MI (173). Once coronary artery disease develops, diabetes doubles the risk for acute coronary syndromes, and there is an additional doubling of clinical risk once these events occur (116,117,174).

Despite the prevalence of diabetes and the associated cardiovascular risk, few studies have specifically examined the effects of medical therapies and interventions in this high-risk population of patients. Most available data in this area derive from epidemiologic observations and subgroup analyses of clinical trial data.

The effect of glycemic control on cardiovascular risk has yet to be definitively established. Although epidemiologic data have clearly demonstrated a correlation between degree of glycometabolic control and clinical risk (175–178), randomized clinical trial data have suggested that the benefit of intensive glycemic control is less clear (107,179–181). The UKPDS demonstrated a beneficial effect of intensive glycemic control (107), but this effect was much more modest than expected, and the trial was not adequately powered to evaluate the effects of such a strategy specifically on cardiovascular risk. Furthermore, it appears that the strategy used for glycemic control may be more important than the degree of control achieved. A prospective, randomized substudy of the UKPDS demonstrated the superiority of metformin compared with either insulin or sulfonylureas for cardiovascular risk modification (182). In a subset of 1,700 overweight patients in UKPDS, metformin was associated with a significant reduction in cardiovascular events, compared with other glycemic treatment options (Fig. 9-6). Likewise, the Diabetes Mellitus, Insulin Glucose Infusion in Acute Myocardial Infarction (DIGAMI) study demonstrated the benefit of acute intravenous hyperinsulinemic/hyperglycemic treatment followed by chronic subcutaneous insulin therapy, compared with "usual care" among patients presenting with an acute coronary syndrome (183).

Although the role of glycemic control and the merits of various hypoglycemic strategies remain to be defined with regard to cardiovascular risk modification, several treatment strategies have been associated with marked improvement in clinical outcomes among subsets of patients with diabetes enrolled in cardiovascular randomized clinical trials in both the primary and secondary prevention settings. The details of these strategies are covered elsewhere in this text.

Briefly, antiplatelet therapy (aspirin, clopidogrel, or both) is particularly effective in the population of patients with diabetes for primary and for secondary cardiovascular risk modification (184–188). Similarly, the potent antiplatelet effects of the glycoprotein IIb/IIIa antagonists have demonstrated particular efficacy in the setting of diabetes for patients with acute coronary syndromes (189–192) and for those undergoing percutaneous coronary intervention (193). Patients with diabetes derive particular benefit from ACE inhibitors, with improvements in both macrovascular and microvascular risk (165,194–196). This benefit was demonstrated most clearly in the Heart Outcomes Prevention Evaluation (HOPE) trial (195), in which daily treatment with the ACE inhibitor, ramipril, was associated with

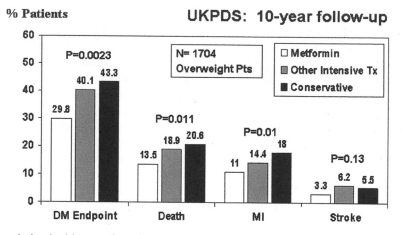

FIG. 9-6. Cumulative incidence of cardiovascular end points for various treatment strategies in patients with diabetes. (Data from United Kingdom Prospective Diabetes Study Group. Effect of intensive blood-glucose control with metformin on complications in overweight patients with type 2 diabetes [UKPDS 34]. *Lancet* 1998;352:854–865.)

a 25% relative reduction in the long-term risk of major adverse cardiovascular events among the large subset of patients with diabetes enrolled in that trial. Extending the observed benefits associated with modification of the renin-angiotensin axis among patients with diabetes, losartan (an ARB) was found to be superior to atenolol for cardiovascular risk reduction in a large-scale randomized trial (197). The effect of adding an ARB to treatment with ACE inhibitors or β-blockers remains unknown.

β-Blockers were once considered to be relatively contraindicated in patients with diabetes, due to concerns regarding adverse glycometabolic effects and worsening of dyslipidemia, as well as the masking of symptoms of hypoglycemia with β-blockade. However, β-blockers have proved to be especially effective among diabetic patients, including treatment in the primary prevention setting (196) as well as during and after acute coronary syndromes (198–200). Despite the evidence from large-scale clinical trials, physicians remain hesitant to prescribe β-blockers for diabetic patients. However, the accumulated data definitively dispel the historical concerns about use of these drugs for patients with diabetes.

Large-scale trials among diabetic patients have clearly supported aggressive treatment of dys-

lipidemia with statin therapy (201–204). Based on these data and the underlying cardiovascular risk associated with diabetes, the ATP III designated diabetes as a "coronary disease equivalent," recommending that all patients with diabetes be treated to secondary prevention lipid targets (205).

Clinical practice guidelines now recommend consideration of aspirin (or clopidogrel) and ACE inhibitors for all patients with diabetes; statins for patients with dyslipidemia, with therapeutic lipid targets for all patients with diabetes identical to the targets for the population with coronary artery disease (205); and β-blockers, ACE inhibitors, and thiazide diuretics for patients with hypertension, with aggressive blood pressure targets (206).

The complications of cardiovascular disease account for the majority of the increased morbidity and mortality associated with type 2 diabetes. Therefore, a primary goal of therapy should be improved cardiovascular clinical outcomes in these high-risk patients. Until more definitive data are available regarding the impact of current hypoglycemic strategies on important clinical outcomes, it is critical that some of the focus of therapy be directed from achievement of glycemic control to aggressive modification of cardiovascular risk.

MODIFICATION OF
CEREBROVASCULAR RISK

The most effective interventions to improve the stroke risk of patients with diabetes involve aggressive blood pressure control, antiplatelet therapy, and lipid lowering. Intensive control of glycemia has failed to demonstrate a benefit with regard to prevention of stroke (182).

Arterial hypertension, effecting up to 70% of patients with diabetes, accounts for a large proportion of the increased stroke risk among these patients. Modification of stroke risk by aggressive management of blood pressure is supported by several trials in which β-blockers, ACE inhibitors, thiazide diuretics, and ARBs were used (165,196,197,207). In the UKPDS (196), tight control of blood pressure (144/82 mm Hg compared with 154/87 mm Hg) with a primary strategy using captopril or atenolol resulted in a 44% reduction in relative risk for stroke. Subsequent statistical modeling from the UKPDS database estimated that every reduction of 10 mm Hg in blood pressure yielded a 19% decrease in stroke risk (208). Ramipril and losartan appear to decrease stroke risk beyond their effects on blood pressure (165,197).

Aspirin therapy for the prevention of stroke among patients with diabetes was evaluated in a metaanalysis of secondary prevention trials that demonstrated significant reductions in the incidence of MI, stroke, and vascular death among individuals with diabetes who had already experienced a major vascular event (184). No trials have specifically evaluated the effect of ticlopidine or clopidogrel in the prevention of stroke among patients with diabetes, but in the Clopidogrel versus Aspirin in Patients at Risk of Ischaemic Events (CAPRIE) study, which used a primary end point including stroke, clopidogrel was especially effective among the diabetic subset (187).

Few studies have specifically addressed the effect of lipid-lowering therapy on stroke risk among patients with diabetes. However, most large-scale, randomized trials of statin therapy have reported improvements in the risk of stroke for the overall population, and there is no reason to believe that patients with diabetes would not derive similar benefit (201–204). In one study that modeled the effect of treatment with simvastatin on stroke risk among patients with diabetes using data from the Scandinavian Simvastatin Survival Study, drug treatment was associated with an estimated 43% reduction in risk (209).

CONCLUSION

Diabetes is a widespread disease that, left unchecked, has serious and global public health implications extending into the foreseeable future. Review of the current literature suggests that elderly individuals and members of minority groups will be disproportionately affected, and the increasing rate of diabetes among children constitutes an emerging public health concern. Worldwide, the aging of the population and the industrialization of developing countries contribute to the increased prevalence of diabetes. The major cause of morbidity and mortality from diabetes is atherosclerotic macrovascular disease, including peripheral, cerebrovascular, and coronary artery disease. The concomitant increases in these diseases as the prevalence of diabetes continues to climb will inevitably strain health care resources. Thus far, the only interventions that have proved effective at reducing the macrovascular disease complications associated with diabetes are those that modify the coexistent risk factors, such as aberrant lifestyles, obesity, dyslipidemia, and hypertension. Disappointingly, strategies targeting improvements in glycemic metabolism have had little effect on cardiovascular risk. Therefore, the development of new strategies aimed at both primary prevention of diabetes and prevention of diabetic complications remains an important research and clinical objective.

REFERENCES

1. Eschwege E, Simon D, Balkau B. The growing burden of diabetes in the world population. *International Diabetes Federation Bulletin* 1997;42:14–19.
2. King H, Aubert RE, Herman WH. Global burden of diabetes, 1995–2025: prevalence, numerical estimates, and projections. *Diabetes Care* 1998;21:1414–1431.
3. Boyle JP, et al. Projection of diabetes burden through 2050: impact of changing demography and disease

prevalence in the U.S. *Diabetes Care* 2001;24:1936–1940.

4. Saydah SH, et al. Subclinical states of glucose intolerance and risk of death in the U.S. *Diabetes Care* 2001;24:447–453.

5. Taubert G, et al. Prevalence, predictors, and consequences of unrecognized diabetes mellitus in 3266 patients scheduled for coronary angiography. *Am Heart J* 2002 *(in press)*.

6. Norhammar A, et al. Glucose metabolism in patients with acute myocardial infarction and no previous diagnosis of diabetes mellitus: a prospective study. *Lancet* 2002;359:2140–2144.

7. The Expert Committee on the Diagnosis and Classification of Diabetes Mellitus. Report of the Expert Committee on the Diagnosis and Classification of Diabetes Mellitus. *Diabetes Care* 1997;20:1183–1197.

8. World Heath Organization. Definition, diagnosis and classification of diabetes mellitus and its complications: part 1. Report of a WHO Consultation: Diagnosis and Classification of Diabetes Mellitus. Geneva: World Health Organization, 1999.

9. de Vegt F, et al. Relation of impaired fasting and postload glucose with incident type 2 diabetes in a Dutch population: the Hoorn Study. *JAMA* 2001;285:2109–2113.

10. Harris MI, et al. Prevalence of diabetes and impaired glucose tolerance and plasma glucose levels in U.S. population aged 20–74 yr. *Diabetes* 1987;36:523–534.

11. Harris MI, et al. Prevalence of diabetes, impaired fasting glucose, and impaired glucose tolerance in U.S. adults. The Third National Health and Nutrition Examination Survey, 1988–1994. *Diabetes Care* 1998;21:518–524.

12. Kenny SJ, Aubert RE, Geiss LS. Prevalence and incidence of non-insulin-dependent diabetes. In: Harris M, ed. *Diabetes in America*. Bethesda, MD: National Institute of Diabetes and Digestive and Kidney Diseases, 1995:47–68.

13. National Center for Chronic Disease Prevention and Health Promotion, Public Health Resource National Estimates on Diabetes. Available at: http://www.cdc.gov/diabetes/pubs/estimates.htm#prev3. Accessed June 16, 2003.

14. Graves EJ. National hospital discharge survey. *Vital Health Stat 13* 1992;112:1–62.

15. McCaig LF, McLemore T. Plan and operation of the National Hospital Ambulatory Medical Survey. Series 1: programs and collection procedures. *Vital Health Stat 1* 1994;34:1–78.

16. Ramsey S, et al. Productivity and medical costs of diabetes in a large employer population. *Diabetes Care* 2002;25:23–29.

17. Yassin AS, Beckles GL, Messonnier ML. Disability and its economic impact among adults with diabetes. *J Occup Environ Med* 2002;44:136–142.

18. Gu K, Cowie CC, Harris MI. Mortality in adults with and without diabetes in a national cohort of the U.S. population, 1971–1993. *Diabetes Care* 1998;21:1138–1145.

19. Bild DE, Stevenson JM. Frequency of recording of diabetes on U.S. death certificates: analysis of the 1986 National Mortality Followback Survey. *J Clin Epidemiol* 1992;45:275–281.

20. Popkin BM, et al. Trends in diet, nutritional status, and diet-related noncommunicable diseases in China and India: the economic costs of the nutrition transition. *Nutr Rev* 2001;59:379–390.

21. Pan XR, et al. Prevalence of diabetes and its risk factors in China, 1994. National Diabetes Prevention and Control Cooperative Group. *Diabetes Care* 1997;20:1664–1669.

22. Ko GT, et al. Rapid increase in the prevalence of undiagnosed diabetes and impaired fasting glucose in asymptomatic Hong Kong Chinese. *Diabetes Care* 1999;22:1751–1752.

23. Tan CE, et al. Prevalence of diabetes and ethnic differences in cardiovascular risk factors. The 1992 Singapore National Health Survey. *Diabetes Care* 1999;22:241–247.

24. Misra A, et al. High prevalence of diabetes, obesity and dyslipidaemia in urban slum population in northern India. *Int J Obes Relat Metab Disord* 2001;25:1722–1729.

25. Asha Bai PV, et al. Prevalence of known diabetes in Chennai City. *J Assoc Physicians India* 2001;49:974–981.

26. Ramachandran A, et al. High prevalence of diabetes and impaired glucose tolerance in India: National Urban Diabetes Survey. *Diabetologia* 2001;44:1094–1101.

27. Mohan V, et al. Intra-urban differences in the prevalence of the metabolic syndrome in southern India: the Chennai Urban Population Study (CUPS No.4). *Diabet Med* 2001;18:280–287.

28. Fujimoto WY. Diabetes in Asian and Pacific Islander Americans. In: Harris M, ed. *Diabetes in America*. Bethesda, MD: National Institutes of Health, National Institute of Diabetes and Digestive and Kidney Diseases, 1995.

29. Butler RN. Population aging and health. *BMJ* 1997; 315:1082–1084.

30. Kunugi T. Women and population aging. *Asia Pac Popul J* 1989;4:75–79.

31. Wilson PW, Kannel WB. Obesity, diabetes, and risk of cardiovascular disease in the elderly. *Am J Geriatr Cardiol* 2002;11:119–123, 125.

32. National Center for Health Statistics. Current estimates from the National Health Interview Survey, 1993. *Vital Health Stat 10* 1994;190:1–221.

33. Day JC. Population projections of the U.S. by age, sex, race, and Hispanic origin 1995–2050. Washington DC: U.S. Bureau of the Census. Current Population Reports, 1996

34. Bassford TL. Health status of Hispanic elders. *Clin Geriatr Med* 1995;11:25–38.

35. Flegal KM, et al. Prevalence of diabetes in Mexican Americans, Cubans, and Puerto Ricans from the Hispanic Health and Nutrition Examination Survey, 1982–1984. *Diabetes Care* 1991;14:628–638.

36. Tucker KL, Bermudez OI, Castaneda C. Type 2 diabetes is prevalent and poorly controlled among Hispanic elders of Caribbean origin. *Am J Public Health* 2000;90:1288–1293.

37. Fagot-Campagna A, Burrows NR, Williamson DF. The public health epidemiology of type 2 diabetes in children and adolescents: a case study of American Indian adolescents in the Southwestern United States. *Clin Chim Acta* 1999;286:81–95.

38. Knowler WC, et al. Diabetes incidence and prevalence

in Pima Indians: a 19-fold greater incidence than in Rochester, Minnesota. *Am J Epidemiol* 1978;108:497–505.

39. Ravussin E. Energy metabolism in obesity. Studies in the Pima Indians. *Diabetes Care* 1993;16:232–238.

40. Harris MI. Epidemiological correlates of NIDDM in Hispanics, whites, and blacks in the U.S. population. *Diabetes Care* 1991;14:639–648.

41. Okosun IS, Prewitt TE, Cooper RS. Abdominal obesity in the United States: prevalence and attributable risk of hypertension. *J Hum Hypertens* 1999;13:425–430.

42. Brancati FL, et al. Incident type 2 diabetes mellitus in African American and white adults: the Atherosclerosis Risk in Communities Study. *JAMA* 2000;283:2253–2259.

43. Bermudez OI, Tucker KL. Total and central obesity among elderly Hispanics and the association with type 2 diabetes. *Obes Res* 2001;9:443–451.

44. Odeleye OE, et al. Fasting hyperinsulinemia is a predictor of increased body weight gain and obesity in Pima Indian children. *Diabetes* 1997;46:1341–1345.

45. Fitzgerald SJ, et al. Associations among physical activity, television watching, and obesity in adult Pima Indians. *Med Sci Sports Exerc* 1997;29:910–915.

46. Fujimoto WY, et al. Prevalence of diabetes mellitus and impaired glucose tolerance among second generation Japanese American men. *Diabetes* 1987;36:721–729.

47. Liao D, et al. Abnormal glucose tolerance and increased risk for cardiovascular disease in Japanese-Americans with normal fasting glucose. *Diabetes Care* 2001;24:39–44.

48. Whitty CJ, et al. Differences in biological risk factors for cardiovascular disease between three ethnic groups in the Whitehall II study. *Atherosclerosis* 1999;142:279–286.

49. McNeely MJ, et al. Standard definitions of overweight and central adiposity for determining diabetes risk in Japanese Americans. *Am J Clin Nutr* 2001;74:101–107.

50. Simmons D, Williams DR, Powell MJ. Prevalence of diabetes in a predominantly Asian community: preliminary findings of the Coventry diabetes study. *BMJ* 1989;298:18–21.

51. McKeigue PM, Shah B, Marmot MG. Relation of central obesity and insulin resistance with high diabetes prevalence and cardiovascular risk in South Asians. *Lancet* 1991;337:382–386.

52. Knowler WC, et al. Reduction in the incidence of type 2 diabetes with lifestyle intervention or metformin. *N Engl J Med* 2002;346:393–403.

53. Trends in the prevalence and incidence of self-reported diabetes mellitus—United States, 1980–1994. *MMWR Morb Mortal Wkly Rep* 1997;46:1014–1018.

54. Ford ES, Giles WH, Dietz WH. Prevalence of the metabolic syndrome among US adults: findings from the third National Health and Nutrition Examination Survey. *JAMA* 2002;287:356–359.

55. Fagot-Campagna A, et al. Type 2 diabetes among North American children and adolescents: an epidemiologic review and a public health perspective. *J Pediatr* 2000;136:664–672.

56. Fagot-Campagna A, et al. Diabetes, impaired fasting glucose, and elevated HbA1c in U.S. adolescents: the Third National Health and Nutrition Examination Survey. *Diabetes Care* 2001;24:834–837.

57. Dean HJ, et al. Screening for type-2 diabetes in aboriginal children in northern Canada. *Lancet* 1998;352:1523–1524.

58. Fagot-Campagna A, Knowler WC, Pettitt DJ. Type 2 diabetes in Pima Indian children: cardiovascular risk factors at diagnosis and 10 years later. *Diabetes* 1998;47[Suppl 1]:155A.

59. Dwyer JT, et al. Prevalence of marked overweight and obesity in a multiethnic pediatric population: findings from the Child and Adolescent Trial for Cardiovascular Health (CATCH) study. *J Am Diet Assoc* 2000;100:1149–1156.

60. Laporte RE, Matsushima M, Chang YF. Prevalence and incidence of insulin-dependent diabetes. In: Harris M, ed. *Diabetes in America*. Bethesda, MD: National Institutes of Health, National Institute of Diabetes and Digestive and Kidney Diseases, 1995.

61. American Diabetes Association. Type 2 diabetes in children and adolescents. *Diabetes Care* 2000;23:381–389.

62. Variation and trends in incidence of childhood diabetes in Europe. EURODIAB ACE Study Group. *Lancet* 2000;355:873–876.

63. Greger N, Edwin CM. Obesity: a pediatric epidemic. *Pediatr Ann* 2001;30:694–700.

64. Dabelea D, et al. Increasing prevalence of type II diabetes in American Indian children. *Diabetologia* 1998;41:904–910.

65. Williams CL, et al. Cardiovascular health in childhood: a statement for health professionals from the Committee on Atherosclerosis, Hypertension, and Obesity in the Young (AHOY) of the Council on Cardiovascular Disease in the Young, American Heart Association. *Circulation* 2002;106:143–160.

66. World Health Organization. Diabetes mellitus: report of a WHO Study Group. Geneva, World Health Organization, 1985.

67. Harris MI, et al. Comparison of diabetes diagnostic categories in the U.S. population according to the 1997 American Diabetes Association and 1980–1985 World Health Organization diagnostic criteria. *Diabetes Care* 1997;20:1859–1862.

68. Wahl PW, et al. Diabetes in older adults: comparison of 1997 American Diabetes Association classification of diabetes mellitus with 1985 WHO classification. *Lancet* 1998;352:1012–1015.

69. Vaccaro O, et al. Risk of diabetes in the new diagnostic category of impaired fasting glucose: a prospective analysis. *Diabetes Care* 1999;22:1490–1493.

70. Gabir MM, et al. The 1997 American Diabetes Association and 1999 World Health Organization criteria for hyperglycemia in the diagnosis and prediction of diabetes. *Diabetes Care* 2000;23:1108–1112.

71. Manton KG, Corder L, Stallard E. Chronic disability trends in elderly United States populations: 1982–1994. *Proc Natl Acad Sci U S A* 1997;94:2593–2598.

72. National Task Force on the Prevention and Treatment of Obesity. Overweight, obesity, and health risk. *Arch Intern Med* 2000;160:898–904.

73. Kuczmarski RJ, et al. Increasing prevalence of overweight among US adults: the National Health and Nutrition Examination Surveys, 1960 to 1991. *JAMA* 1994;272:205–211.

74. Flegal KM, et al. Overweight and obesity in the United

States: prevalence and trends, 1960–1994. *Int J Obes Relat Metab Disord* 1998;22:39–47.

75. James PT, et al. The worldwide obesity epidemic. *Obes Res* 2001;9[Suppl 4]:228S–233S.

76. Folsom AR, et al. Associations of general and abdominal obesity with multiple health outcomes in older women: the Iowa Women's Health Study. *Arch Intern Med* 2000;160:2117–2128.

77. Ohlson LO, et al. The influence of body fat distribution on the incidence of diabetes mellitus: 13.5 years of follow-up of the participants in the study of men born in 1913. *Diabetes* 1985;34:1055–1058.

78. Morricone L, et al. The role of central fat distribution in coronary artery disease in obesity: comparison of nondiabetic obese, diabetic obese, and normal weight subjects. *Int J Obes Relat Metab Disord* 1999;23:1129–1135.

79. Carey DG, et al. Abdominal fat and insulin resistance in normal and overweight women: direct measurements reveal a strong relationship in subjects at both low and high risk of NIDDM. *Diabetes* 1996;45:633–638.

80. Warne DK, et al. Comparison of body size measurements as predictors of NIDDM in Pima Indians. *Diabetes Care* 1995;18:435–439.

81. Kahn BB, Flier JS. Obesity and insulin resistance. *J Clin Invest* 2000;106:473–481.

82. Ryder JW, Gilbert M, Zierath JR. Skeletal muscle and insulin sensitivity: pathophysiological alterations. *Front Biosci* 2001;6:D154–D163.

83. Kraus W. Insulin resistance syndrome and cardiovascular disease: genetics and connections to skeletal muscle function. *Am Heart J* 1999;138:S413–S416.

84. Hu FB, et al. Walking compared with vigorous physical activity and risk of type 2 diabetes in women: a prospective study. *JAMA* 1999;282:1433–1439.

85. Wannamethee SG, Shaper AG, Alberti KG. Physical activity, metabolic factors, and the incidence of coronary heart disease and type 2 diabetes. *Arch Intern Med* 2000;160:2108–2116.

86. Kriska AM, et al. Association of physical activity and serum insulin concentrations in two populations at high risk for type 2 diabetes but differing by BMI. *Diabetes Care* 2001;24:1175–1180.

87. Hu FB, et al. Physical activity and television watching in relation to risk for type 2 diabetes mellitus in men. *Arch Intern Med* 2001;161:1542–1548.

88. Salmeron J, et al. Dietary fiber, glycemic load, and risk of NIDDM in men. *Diabetes Care* 1997;20:545–550.

89. Meyer KA, et al. Dietary fat and incidence of type 2 diabetes in older Iowa women. *Diabetes Care* 2001;24:1528–1535.

90. van Dam RM, et al. Dietary patterns and risk for type 2 diabetes mellitus in U.S. men. *Ann Intern Med* 2002;136:201–209.

91. van Tilburg J, et al. Defining the genetic contribution of type 2 diabetes mellitus. *J Med Genet* 2001;38:569–578.

92. Hu FB, et al. Diet, lifestyle, and the risk of type 2 diabetes mellitus in women. *N Engl J Med* 2001;345:790–797.

93. Liu S, et al. A prospective study of whole-grain intake and risk of type 2 diabetes mellitus in US women. *Am J Public Health* 2000;90:1409–1415.

94. Barbosa J, et al. The histocompatibility system in juvenile, insulin-dependent diabetic multiplex kindreds. *J Clin Invest* 1977;60:989–998.

95. Nerup J, Mandrup-Poulsen T, Molvig J. The HLA-IDDM association: implications for etiology and pathogenesis of IDDM. *Diabetes Metab Rev* 1987;3:779–802.

96. Todd JA, Bell JI, McDevitt HO. HLA-DQ beta gene contributes to susceptibility and resistance to insulin-dependent diabetes mellitus. *Nature* 1987;329:599–604.

97. Kaprio J, et al. Concordance for type 1 (insulin-dependent) and type 2 (non-insulin-dependent) diabetes mellitus in a population-based cohort of twins in Finland. *Diabetologia* 1992;35:1060–1067.

98. Japan Diabetes Society, Committee on Diabetic Twins. Diabetes mellitus in twins: a cooperative study in Japan. *Diabetes Res Clin Pract* 1988;5:271–280.

99. DeFronzo RA. Pathogenesis of type 2 diabetes: metabolic and molecular implications for identifying diabetes genes. *Diabetes Rev* 1997;5:177–269.

100. Hager J, et al. A missense mutation in the glucagon receptor gene is associated with non-insulin-dependent diabetes mellitus. *Nat Genet* 1995;9:299–304.

101. Waeber G, et al. The gene MAPK8IP1, encoding islet-brain-1, is a candidate for type 2 diabetes. *Nat Genet* 2000;24:291–295.

102. American Diabetes Association. Role of cardiovascular risk factors in prevention and treatment of macrovascular disease in diabetes. *Diabetes Care* 1989;12:573–579.

103. Kannel WB, McGee DL. Diabetes and cardiovascular disease: the Framingham study. *JAMA* 1979;241:2035–2038.

104. Wingard DL, Barrett-Connor E. Heart disease and diabetes. In: Harris M, ed. *Diabetes in America.* Bethesda, MD: National Institutes of Health, National Institute of Diabetes and Digestive and Kidney Diseases, 1995:429–456.

105. Geiss LS, Herman WH, Smith PJ. Mortality in non-insulin dependent diabetes. In: Harris M, ed. *Diabetes in America.* Bethesda, MD: National Institutes of Health, National Institute of Diabetes and Digestive and Kidney Diseases, 1995:233–255.

106. Stamler J, et al. Diabetes, other risk factors, and 12-yr cardiovascular mortality for men screened in the Multiple Risk Factor Intervention Trial. *Diabetes Care* 1993;16:434–444.

107. United Kingdom Prospective Diabetes Study Group. Intensive blood-glucose control with sulphonylureas or insulin compared with conventional treatment and risk of complications in patients with type 2 diabetes (UKPDS 33). *Lancet* 1998;352:837–853.

108. The Diabetes-Heart Disease Link: Surveying Attitudes, Knowledge, and Risk. Available at: http://www.diabetes.org/main/uedocuments/executivesummary.pdf. Accessed June 16, 2003.

109. Howard BV, et al. Rising tide of cardiovascular disease in American Indians: the Strong Heart Study. *Circulation* 1999;99:2389–2395.

110. Gu K, Cowie CC, Harris MI. Diabetes and decline in heart disease mortality in US adults. *JAMA* 1999;281:1291–1297.

111. Gillum RF, Mussolino ME, Madans JH. Diabetes mellitus, coronary heart disease incidence, and death from

all causes in African American and European American women: The NHANES I epidemiologic follow-up study. *J Clin Epidemiol* 2000;53:511–518.

112. Centers for Disease Control and Prevention. Major cardiovascular disease (CVD) during 1997–1999 and major CVD hospital discharge rates in 1997 among women with diabetes—United States. *MMWR Morb Mortal Wkly Rep* 2001;50:948–954.

113. Fibrinolytic Therapy Trialists' Collaborative Group. Indications for fibrinolytic therapy in suspected acute myocardial infarction: collaborative overview of early mortality and major morbidity results from all randomised trials of more than 1000 patients. Fibrinolytic Therapy Trialists' (FTT) Collaborative Group. *Lancet* 1994;343:311–322.

114. Granger CB, et al. Outcome of patients with diabetes mellitus and acute myocardial infarction treated with thrombolytic agents: the Thrombolysis and Angioplasty in Myocardial Infarction (TAMI) Study Group. *J Am Coll Cardiol* 1993;21:920–925.

115. Mak KH, et al. Influence of diabetes mellitus on clinical outcome in the thrombolytic era of acute myocardial infarction. GUSTO-I Investigators. Global Utilization of Streptokinase and Tissue Plasminogen Activator for Occluded Coronary Arteries. *J Am Coll Cardiol* 1997;30:171–179.

116. McGuire DK, et al. Influence of diabetes mellitus on clinical outcomes across the spectrum of acute coronary syndromes. Findings from the GUSTO-IIb study. GUSTO IIb Investigators. *Eur Heart J* 2000;21:1750–1758.

117. Malmberg K, et al. Impact of diabetes on long-term prognosis in patients with unstable angina and non-Q-wave myocardial infarction: results of the OASIS (Organization to Assess Strategies for Ischemic Syndromes) Registry. *Circulation* 2000;102:1014–1019.

118. Abbott RD, et al. The impact of diabetes on survival following myocardial infarction in men vs women: the Framingham Study. *JAMA* 1988;260:3456–3460.

119. Kannel WB, Ho K, Thom T. Changing epidemiological features of cardiac failure. *Br Heart J* 1994;72[2 Suppl]:S3–S9.

120. Kannel WB, Hjortland M, Castelli WP. Role of diabetes in congestive heart failure: the Framingham study. *Am J Cardiol* 1974;34:29–34.

121. Dries DL, et al. Prognostic impact of diabetes mellitus in patients with heart failure according to the etiology of left ventricular systolic dysfunction. *J Am Coll Cardiol* 2001;38:421–428.

122. Coutinho M, et al. The relationship between glucose and incident cardiovascular events: a metaregression analysis of published data from 20 studies of 95,783 individuals followed for 12.4 years. *Diabetes Care* 1999;22:233–240.

123. Suskin N, et al. Glucose and insulin abnormalities relate to functional capacity in patients with congestive heart failure. *Eur Heart J* 2000;21:1368–1375.

124. Norhammar A, Malmberg K. Heart failure and glucose abnormalities: an increasing combination with poor functional capacity and outcome. *Eur Heart J* 2000;21:1293–1294.

125. Jaffe AS, et al. Increased congestive heart failure after myocardial infarction of modest extent in patients with diabetes mellitus. *Am Heart J* 1984;108:31–37.

126. Stone PH, et al. The effect of diabetes mellitus on prognosis and serial left ventricular function after acute myocardial infarction: contribution of both coronary disease and diastolic left ventricular dysfunction to the adverse prognosis. The MILIS Study Group. *J Am Coll Cardiol* 1989;14:49–57.

127. Burchfiel CM, et al. Glucose intolerance and 22-year stroke incidence: the Honolulu Heart Program. *Stroke* 1994;25:951–957.

128. Kreines K, et al. The course of peripheral vascular disease in non-insulin-dependent diabetes. *Diabetes Care* 1985;8:235–243.

129. Niskanen L, et al. Medial artery calcification predicts cardiovascular mortality in patients with NIDDM. *Diabetes Care* 1994;17:1252–1256.

130. Reiber GE, Boyko EJ, Smith DG. Lower extremity foot ulcers and amputations in diabetes. In: Harris M, ed. *Diabetes in America*. Bethesda, MD: National Institutes of Health, National Institute of Diabetes and Digestive and Kidney Diseases, 1995.

131. Palumbo PJ, Melton LJ. Peripheral vascular disease and diabetes. In: Harris M, ed. *Diabetes in America*. Bethesda, MD: National Institutes of Health, National Institute of Diabetes and Digestive and Kidney Diseases, 1995.

132. Reiber GE, Pecoraro RE, Koepsell TD. Risk factors for amputation in patients with diabetes mellitus: a case-control study. *Ann Intern Med* 1992;117:97–105.

133. Most RS, Sinnock P. The epidemiology of lower extremity amputations in diabetic individuals. *Diabetes Care* 1983;6:87–91.

134. Van Gils CC, et al. Amputation prevention by vascular surgery and podiatry collaboration in high-risk diabetic and nondiabetic patients: the Operation Desert Foot experience. *Diabetes Care* 1999;22:678–683.

135. Nelson RG, et al. Lower-extremity amputations in NIDDM: 12-yr follow-up study in Pima Indians. *Diabetes Care* 1988;11:8–16.

136. Karter AJ, et al. Ethnic disparities in diabetic complications in an insured population. *JAMA* 2002;287:2519–2927.

137. Lanzer P. Topographic distribution of peripheral arteriopathy in non diabetics and type 2 diabetics. *Z Kardiol* 2001;90:99–103.

138. Kamal K, Powell RJ, Sumpio BE. The pathobiology of diabetes mellitus: implications for surgeons. *J Am Coll Surg* 1996;183:271–289.

139. Lee JS, et al. Lower-extremity amputation: incidence, risk factors, and mortality in the Oklahoma Indian Diabetes Study. *Diabetes* 1993;42:876–882.

140. Ebskov B, Josephsen P. Incidence of reamputation and death after gangrene of the lower extremity. *Prosthet Orthot Int* 1980;4:77–80.

141. Whitehouse FW, Jurgensen C, Block MA. The later life of the diabetic amputee: another look at fate of the second leg. *Diabetes* 1968;17:520–521.

142. Larsson J, et al. Long-term prognosis after healed amputation in patients with diabetes. *Clin Orthop* 1998 May;(350):149–158.

143. Geiss LS, Rolka DB, Engelgau MM. Elevated blood pressure among U.S. adults with diabetes, 1988–1994. *Am J Prev Med* 2002;22:42–48.

144. Klein R, et al. The incidence of hypertension in insulin-dependent diabetes. *Arch Intern Med* 1996;156:622–627.

145. Cowie CC, Harris MI. Physical and metabolic characteristics of persons with diabetes. In: Harris M, ed. *Diabetes in America*. Bethesda, MD: National Institutes of Health, National Institute of Diabetes and Digestive and Kidney Diseases, 1995.

146. Garg A, Grundy SM. Diabetic dyslipidemia and its therapy. *Diabetes Rev* 1997;5:425–433.

147. Turner RC, et al. Risk factors for coronary artery disease in non-insulin dependent diabetes mellitus: United Kingdom Prospective Diabetes Study (UKPDS: 23). *BMJ* 1998;316:823–828.

148. Lamarche B, et al. Small, dense low-density lipoprotein particles as a predictor of the risk of ischemic heart disease in men: prospective results from the Quebec Cardiovascular Study. *Circulation* 1997;95:69–75.

149. Verges BL, et al. Macrovascular disease is associated with increased plasma apolipoprotein A-IV levels in NIDDM. *Diabetes* 1997;46:125–132.

150. Reaven GM. Banting Lecture 1988: role of insulin resistance in human disease. *Diabetes* 1988;37:1595–1607.

151. Bierman EL. George Lyman Duff Memorial lecture: atherogenesis in diabetes. *Arterioscler Thromb* 1992;12:647–656.

152. Stampfer MJ, et al. A prospective study of triglyceride level, low-density lipoprotein particle diameter, and risk of myocardial infarction. *JAMA* 1996;276:882–888.

153. Stern MP. Cardiovascular mortality in American Indians: paradox explained? [Invited commentary]. *Am J Epidemiol* 1998;147:1009–1010.

154. Tuomilehto J, et al. Prevention of type 2 diabetes mellitus by changes in lifestyle among subjects with impaired glucose tolerance. *N Engl J Med* 2001;344:1343–1350.

155. Yale JF. Prevention of type 2 diabetes. *Int J Clin Pract Suppl* 2000 Oct;(113):35–39.

156. Shaw JE, et al. Impaired fasting glucose or impaired glucose tolerance: what best predicts future diabetes in Mauritius? *Diabetes Care* 1999;22:399–402.

157. Henry RR, Wallace P, Olefsky JM. Effects of weight loss on mechanisms of hyperglycemia in obese non-insulin-dependent diabetes mellitus. *Diabetes* 1986;35:990–998.

158. Eriksson KF, Lindgarde F. Prevention of type 2 (non-insulin-dependent) diabetes mellitus by diet and physical exercise: the 6-year Malmo feasibility study. *Diabetologia* 1991;34:891–898.

159. The Diabetes Prevention Program Research Group. The Diabetes Prevention Program: design and methods for a clinical trial in the prevention of type 2 diabetes. *Diabetes Care* 1999;22:623–634.

160. Pan XR, et al. Effects of diet and exercise in preventing NIDDM in people with impaired glucose tolerance. the Da Qing IGT and Diabetes Study. *Diabetes Care* 1997;20:537–544.

161. Henriksen EJ, et al. ACE inhibition and glucose transport in insulinresistant muscle: roles of bradykinin and nitric oxide. *Am J Physiol* 1999;277:R332–R336.

162. Velloso LA, et al. Cross-talk between the insulin and angiotensin signaling systems. *Proc Natl Acad Sci U S A* 1996;93:12490–12495.

163. Frossard M, et al. Paracrine effects of angiotensin-converting-enzyme and angiotensin-II-receptor inhibition on transcapillary glucose transport in humans. *Life Sci* 2000;66:PL147–PL154.

164. Hansson L, et al. Effect of angiotensin-converting-enzyme inhibition compared with conventional therapy on cardiovascular morbidity and mortality in hypertension: the Captopril Prevention Project (CAPPP) randomised trial. *Lancet* 1999;353:611–616.

165. Heart Outcomes Prevention Evaluation Study Investigators. Effects of ramipril on cardiovascular and microvascular outcomes in people with diabetes mellitus: results of the HOPE study and MICRO-HOPE substudy. *Lancet* 2000;355:253–259.

166. Yusuf S, et al. Ramipril and the development of diabetes. *JAMA* 2001;286:1882–1885.

167. United Kingdom Prospective Diabetes Study Group. Efficacy of atenolol and captopril in reducing risk of macrovascular and microvascular complications in type 2 diabetes (UKPDS 39). *BMJ* 1998;317:713–720.

168. Dahlof B, et al. Cardiovascular morbidity and mortality in the Losartan Intervention For Endpoint reduction in hypertension study (LIFE): a randomised trial against atenolol. *Lancet* 2002;359:995–1003.

169. Rossetti L, Giaccari A, DeFronzo RA. Glucose toxicity. *Diabetes Care* 1990;13:610–630.

170. Chiasson JL, et al. Acarbose for prevention of type 2 diabetes mellitus: the STOP-NIDDM randomised trial. *Lancet* 2002;359:2072–2077.

171. Webster MW, Scott RS. What cardiologists need to know about diabetes. *Lancet* 1997;350[Suppl 1]:SI23–SI28.

172. Savage PJ. Cardiovascular complications of diabetes mellitus: what we know and what we need to know about their prevention. *Ann Intern Med* 1996;124:123–126.

173. Haffner SM, et al. Mortality from coronary heart disease in subjects with type 2 diabetes and in nondiabetic subjects with and without prior myocardial infarction. *N Engl J Med* 1998;339:229–234.

174. Aronson D, Rayfield EJ, Chesebro JH. Mechanisms determining course and outcome of diabetic patients who have had acute myocardial infarction. *Ann Intern Med* 1997;126:296–306.

175. Gerstein HC, et al. Relationship of glucose and insulin levels to the risk of myocardial infarction: a case-control study. *J Am Coll Cardiol* 1999;33:612–619.

176. Kuusisto J, et al. NIDDM and its metabolic control predict coronary heart disease in elderly subjects. *Diabetes* 1994;43:960–967.

177. Singer DE, et al. Association of HbA1c with prevalent cardiovascular disease in the original cohort of the Framingham Heart Study. *Diabetes* 1992;41:202–208.

178. Malmberg K, et al. Glycometabolic state at admission: important risk marker of mortality in conventionally treated patients with diabetes mellitus and acute myocardial infarction: long-term results from the Diabetes and Insulin-Glucose Infusion in Acute Myocardial Infarction (DIGAMI) study. *Circulation* 1999;99:2626–2632.

179. Stern MP. The effect of glycemic control on the incidence of macrovascular complications of type 2 diabetes. *Arch Fam Med* 1998;7:155–162.

180. Meinert CL, et al. A study of the effects of hypoglycemic agents on vascular complications in patients with adult-onset diabetes: II. Mortality results. *Diabetes* 1970;19[Suppl]:789–830.

181. Abraira C, et al. Veterans Affairs Cooperative Study on Glycemic Control and Complications in Type II Diabetes (VA CSDM): results of the feasibility trial. Veterans Affairs Cooperative Study in Type II Diabetes. *Diabetes Care* 1995;18:1113–1123.

182. United Kingdom Prospective Diabetes Study Group. Effect of intensive blood-glucose control with metformin on complications in overweight patients with type 2 diabetes (UKPDS 34). *Lancet* 1998;352:854–865.

183. Malmberg K, et al. Randomized trial of insulin-glucose infusion followed by subcutaneous insulin treatment in diabetic patients with acute myocardial infarction (DIGAMI study): effects on mortality at 1 year. *J Am Coll Cardiol* 1995;26:57–65.

184. Antiplatelet Trialist's Collaboration. Collaborative overview of randomised trials of antiplatelet therapy: I. Prevention of death from myocardial infarction and stroke by prolonged antiplatelet therapy in various categories of patients. *BMJ* 1994;308:81–106.

185. Steering Committee of the Physicians' Health Study Research Group. Final report on the aspirin component of the ongoing Physicians' Health Study. *N Engl J Med* 1989;321:129–135.

186. ETDRS Investigators. Aspirin effects on mortality and morbidity in patients with diabetes mellitus: Early Treatment Diabetic Retinopathy Study report 14. *JAMA* 1992;268:1292–1300.

187. CAPRIE Steering Committee. A randomised, blinded, trial of Clopidogrel versus Aspirin in Patients at Risk of Ischaemic Events (CAPRIE). *Lancet* 1996;348:1329–1339.

188. Yusuf S, et al. Effects of clopidogrel in addition to aspirin in patients with acute coronary syndromes without ST-segment elevation. *N Engl J Med* 2001;345:494–502.

189. The PURSUIT Trial Investigators. Inhibition of platelet glycoprotein IIb/IIIa with eptifibatide in patients with acute coronary syndromes: the PURSUIT Trial Investigators. Platelet Glycoprotein IIb/IIIa in Unstable Angina: Receptor Suppression Using Integrilin Therapy. *N Engl J Med* 1998;339:436–443.

190. The Platelet Receptor Inhibition in Ischemic Syndrome Management (PRISM) Study Investigators. A comparison of aspirin plus tirofiban with aspirin plus heparin for unstable angina. *N Engl J Med* 1998;338:1498–1505.

191. The Platelet Receptor Inhibition in Ischemic Syndrome Management in Patients Limited by Unstable Angina Signs and Symptoms (PRISM-PLUS) Study Investigators. Inhibition of the platelet glycoprotein IIb/IIIa receptor with tirofiban in unstable angina and non-Q-wave myocardial infarction. *N Engl J Med* 1998;338:1488–1497.

192. Roffi M, et al. Platelet glycoprotein IIb/IIIa inhibitors reduce mortality in diabetic patients with non-ST-segment-elevation acute coronary syndromes. *Circulation* 2001;104:2767–2771.

193. Bhatt DL, et al. Abciximab reduces mortality in diabetics following percutaneous coronary intervention. *J Am Coll Cardiol* 2000;35:922–928.

194. Nesto RW, Zarich S. Acute myocardial infarction in diabetes mellitus: lessons learned from ACE inhibition. *Circulation* 1998;97:12–15.

195. Yusuf S, et al. Effects of an angiotensin-converting-enzyme inhibitor, ramipril, on cardiovascular events in high-risk patients: the Heart Outcomes Prevention Evaluation study investigators. *N Engl J Med* 2000;342:145–153.

196. United Kingdom Prospective Diabetes Study Group. Tight blood pressure control and risk of macrovascular and microvascular complications in type 2 diabetes: UKPDS 38. *BMJ* 1998;317:703–713.

197. Lindholm LH, et al. Cardiovascular morbidity and mortality in patients with diabetes in the Losartan Intervention For Endpoint reduction in hypertension study (LIFE): a randomised trial against atenolol. *Lancet* 2002;359:1004–1010.

198. Malmberg K, et al. Effects of metoprolol on mortality and late infarction in diabetics with suspected acute myocardial infarction: retrospective data from two large studies. *Eur Heart J* 1989;10:423–428.

199. Kjekshus J, et al. Diabetic patients and beta-blockers after acute myocardial infarction. *Eur Heart J* 1990;11:43–50.

200. Kendall MJ, et al. Beta-blockers and sudden cardiac death. *Ann Intern Med* 1995;123:358–367.

201. Pyorala K, et al. Cholesterol lowering with simvastatin improves prognosis of diabetic patients with coronary heart disease: a subgroup analysis of the Scandinavian Simvastatin Survival Study (4S). *Diabetes Care* 1997;20:614–620.

202. Sacks FM, et al. The effect of pravastatin on coronary events after myocardial infarction in patients with average cholesterol levels: Cholesterol and Recurrent Events Trial investigators. *N Engl J Med* 1996;335:1001–1009.

203. The Long-term Intervention with Pravastatin in Ischaemic Disease (LIPID) Study Group. Prevention of cardiovascular events and death with pravastatin in patients with coronary heart disease and a broad range of initial cholesterol levels. *N Engl J Med* 1998;339:1349–1357.

204. The Heart Protection Study Investigators. MRC/BHF Heart Protection Study of cholesterol lowering with simvastatin in 20,536 high-risk individuals: a randomised placebo-controlled trial. *Lancet* 2002;360:7–22.

205. Expert Panel on Detection, Evaluation, and Treatment of High Blood Cholesterol in Adults (Adult Treatment Panel III). Executive summary of the Third Report of the National Cholesterol Education Program (NCEP). *JAMA* 2001;285:2486–2497.

206. The Joint National Committee on Prevention, Detection, Evaluation, and Treatment of High Blood Pressure. The sixth report of the Joint National Committee on Prevention, Detection, Evaluation, and Treatment of High Blood Pressure. *Arch Intern Med* 1997;157:2413–2446.

207. Curb JD, et al. Effect of diuretic-based antihypertensive treatment on cardiovascular disease risk in older diabetic patients with isolated systolic hypertension: Systolic Hypertension in the Elderly Program Cooperative Research Group. *JAMA* 1996;276:1886–1892.

208. Adler AI, et al. Association of systolic blood pressure with macrovascular and microvascular complications of type 2 diabetes (UKPDS 36): prospective observational study. *BMJ* 2000;321:412–419.

209. Grover SA, et al. Cost-effectiveness of treating hyper-lipidemia in the presence of diabetes: who should be treated? *Circulation* 2000;102:722–727.
210. Centers for Disease Control and Prevention, Diabetes Surveillance, 1999.
211. Freedman DS, et al. Obesity, levels of lipids and glucose, and smoking among Navajo adolescents. *J Nutr* 1997;127[10 Suppl]:2120S–2127S.
212. Rios BN, Acton K, Geiss L, et al. Trends in diabetes prevalence among American Indian and Alaska Native children, adolescents and young adults, 1991–1997. 11th Annual Indian Health Service Research Conference. Albuquerque, NM: Indian Health Service, 1999;19.
213. Pinhas-Hamiel O, et al. Increased incidence of non-insulin-dependent diabetes mellitus among adolescents. *J Pediatr* 1996;128:608–615.

214. Willi SM, et al. Insulin resistance and defective glucose-insulin coupling in ketosis-prone type 2 diabetes of African-American youth. *Diabetes* 1998;47[Suppl 1]:A306.
215. Scott CR, et al. Characteristics of youth-onset noninsulin-dependent diabetes mellitus and insulin-dependent diabetes mellitus at diagnosis. *Pediatrics* 1997;100:84–91.
216. Glaser NS, Jones KL. Non-insulin dependent diabetes mellitus in Mexican-American children. *West J Med* 1998;168:11–16.
217. Hale DE, Danney DK. Non-insulin dependent diabetes in Hispanic youth (type 2Y). *Diabetes* 1998;47:A82[abstr].
218. Neufeld ND, et al. Early presentation of type 2 diabetes in Mexican-American youth. *Diabetes Care* 1998;21:80–86.

Diabetes and Cardiovascular Disease
edited by Steven P. Marso and David M. Stern
Lippincott Williams & Wilkins, Philadelphia © 2004

10

Economic Implications of Diabetes Mellitus

John D. Nachtigal and Cathryn A. Carroll

*Research Scholar, Mid America Heart Institute, Saint Luke's Hospital; Assistant Professor,
Division of Pharmacy Practice, University of Missouri–Kansas City, Kansas City, Missouri*

Diabetes mellitus produces a substantial economic burden in the United States, and it is anticipated that this burden will continue to increase over time. Current projections suggest that the number of individuals older than 20 years of age with diabetes, whether diagnosed or undiagnosed, will rise from 13.9 million in 1995 to almost 22 million in 2025 (1). If consideration is given only to patients with diagnosed diabetes, approximately 14.5 million diabetics will consume health care resources in 2025.

The estimated growth in this patient population and the resulting growth in expenditures are expected to continue increasing for the foreseeable future because of several factors. First, the U. S. population continues to age. Second, obesity, a major risk factor for diabetes, is now considered an epidemic in the country (2). The impact of the aging population will be observed primarily through an increase in both the incidence and the prevalence of non-insulin-dependent (type 2) diabetes mellitus. Third, those with diabetes consume a disproportionate amount of care compared with their nondiabetic counterparts. Rubin et al. (3) reported in 1994 that persons with diabetes constituted 4.5% of the U. S. population but accounted for 14.6% of total U. S. health care expenditures. A comparison of expenditures for diabetes relative to other disease states, as defined by Druss et al. (4), is presented in Table 10-1. Finally, no cure for diabetes appears imminent; therefore, patients, providers, payers, and policy makers should expect continued growth in expenditures for the diagnosis and treatment of this disease.

Multiple investigators using multiple methods have developed cost of illness evaluations related to diabetes. These estimates place the total annual cost of diabetes (in U. S. dollars) between $291 million and $98 billion. Pagano et al. (5) reviewed the methodologies used to derive these estimates. In 1997, approximately $98 billion was spent on direct and indirect medical costs for diabetes in the United States, with complications accounting for approximately 50% of this total cost (6). The direct medical costs of diabetes represent approximately 5% to 6% of all health care expenditures in the United States, an amount consistent with expenditures by other developed countries. Of these expenditures, Medicare and Medicaid cover 27% and 15% of total payments, respectively; employer-based insurance covers 20%; and patients pay 12% of all expenditures out of pocket (3).

In 1997, the direct medical costs of treating diabetes were estimated to be $44 billion, and the indirect costs were reported to be $54 billion (7). With respect to direct medical costs only, Basile (8) noted that hospitals are the largest cost center, consuming 39% of total direct medical costs. Hospitalizations alone were estimated to account for approximately $27.5 billion dollars per year in 1997 (7).

The large expenditures for hospital services are influenced by many factors. First, patients with diabetes are three times more likely to be hospitalized than are nondiabetic patients (9). This excess risk of hospitalizations is primarily due to complications, including hyperglycemia, hypoglycemia, and cellulitis, as well as other

TABLE 10-1. *Health costs, in 1996 dollars, among persons with one or more of five chronic conditions, 1996*

Condition	Direct per capita health costs for treatment of condition ($)	Total U.S. costs for treatment of condition ($ billion)	Percentage paid out of pocket for payments associated with condition (%)	Mean per capita health care cost per person with condition ($)	Estimated total health costs ($ billion) for persons with condition
Mood disorder	1,122	10.2	39	4,328	54.9
Diabetes	1,097	10.1	39	5,646	54.2
Heart disease	6,463	21.5	29	10,828	38.5
Hypertension	569	14.8	43	4,073	110.3
Asthma	663	5.74	38	2,779	27.7

short-term conditions such as pneumonia, urinary tract infections, and electrolyte imbalances (10). Compounding the impact of this excess risk, when diabetic patients are admitted to an institution their treatment is more resource intensive and their length of stay tends to be longer than for other patients. For example, one comparison of cardiovascular patients enrolled in the Arterial Revascularization Therapy Study (ARTS) noted that the total 1-year costs for stenting and coronary artery bypass grafting (CABG) were $12,855 and $16,585, respectively, in patients with diabetes and $10,164 and $13,082, respectively, in nondiabetics (11).

In addition to the large expenditures for hospital services, 28% of all direct medical expenditures on patients with diabetes are for outside referrals, and 9% of all medical costs are due to prescription drug use. By one estimate, people with diabetes are 1.7 times more likely to be dispensed a drug item than are people without diabetes, and a large proportion of diabetic patients' expenses for prescription medications are paid out of pocket (12). Other direct medical costs include specialty outpatient care, primary care, emergency care, and nonphysician outpatient care for services such as education.

As noted earlier, the indirect medical costs of diabetes are also significant. They are primarily expressed through absenteeism, lost productivity, disability, and mortality. Of particular importance is the economic burden resulting from losses in productivity associated with the disease. Payers, patients, and employers bear the burden of productivity losses. One estimate, by Ng et al. (13), suggested that complications of diabetes are

the single most important determinant of productivity losses. When complications and losses do occur, patients with diabetes can expect reductions in income of up to about $9,000 per year (13). The impact is felt not only by the patient but also by employers, who incur significant losses. One study estimated that the annual work-loss cost for employees with diabetes ranged from 1.7 to 2.2 times that of matched control employees (14). Patients with diabetes also were more likely to file disability claims, and the average disability absence for employees with diabetes was 41 days, compared with 22 days for the matched control group.

Even though the economic costs of diabetes in general are high, not all populations of diabetic patients are equal in their distribution of health care expenditures. Laditka et al. (15) reported that individuals with insulin-dependent (type 1) diabetes are at higher risk for long-term complications, use more physician services, and have higher costs than those with type 2 diabetes. Moreover, the economic burden of older diabetic patients is different from that of their younger counterparts. Ramsey et al. (14) reported that the incremental cost of diabetes among employees ranged from $4,671 for those age 18 to 35 years to $43,569 for those age 56 to 64 years. Younger diabetic patients are frequently hospitalized for different reasons than their senior counterparts. For example, younger patients are more likely to be hospitalized for peritonitis, followed by respiratory failure and liver disease, whereas older patients are more likely to be hospitalized for liver disease, followed by septicemia and diseases of the pulmonary circulation (16).

This section has outlined very general considerations in the economics of diabetes. The remaining sections focus on both clinical and administrative strategies that may be used to reduce the economic burden of diabetes.

CLINICAL STRATEGIES TO REDUCE THE ECONOMIC BURDEN OF DIABETES

The economic burden of diabetes, although large, can be reduced by several means. First, the economic burden can be reduced through the prevention of disease onset. Second, the impact of diabetes on payers and patients can be managed through more efficient and effective disease management. Disease management initiatives include patient education, prevention and management of the macrovascular and microvascular complications of diabetes, and appropriate management of common comorbidities of diabetes, such as hypertension and dyslipidemia.

Prevention of Disease Onset

Given that no cure for diabetes appears imminent, the next best method to control the costs of diabetes is through prevention of disease onset. This can occur through behavior modification and lifestyle changes, and the target populations for such lifestyle modification programs are numerous. According to one report by Mokhad et al. (2), the prevalence of obesity and diabetes continues to increase among U. S. adults. In addition, their analysis noted that 27% of U. S. adults did not engage in any physical activity and another 28.2% did not exercise regularly.

To evaluate the effectiveness of lifestyle changes on disease onset for patients with type 2 diabetes, a large, randomized clinical trial was begun. This study, known as the Diabetes Prevention Program, evaluated the rate of onset of type 2 diabetes in three patient groups: patients treated with metformin, patients treated with placebo, and patients enrolled in lifestyle-modification programs. The results of the study revealed that lifestyle changes were significantly more effective than metformin in reducing the incidence of diabetes in persons at high risk. The lower incidence of type 2 diabetes in the intervention group translates to the need for less direct and indirect medical expenditures, although the exact magnitudes of such reductions achieved by the Diabetes Prevention Program have not been reported.

Diabetes Education

The lack of educational awareness on the part of patients with diabetes translates into poor self-management by these patients. Hodgson et al. (17) found that only 38% of persons with diabetes performed self-monitoring of blood glucose, and a similarly low number had seen a health care professional regarding diabetes in the proceeding year. Additionally, at least two thirds of these individuals were not aware of the term hemoglobin A_{1C} (an indicator of having received diabetes education), more than 25% had not had their feet examined, and more than 20% had not had a dilated-eye examination in the preceding year.

According to some, many people are denied diabetes education. Assal (18) reported that this may be a result of either a lack of patient education programs, secondary to the scarcity of financial resources available for such programs, or inadequate educational methodologies used by health care providers. The lack of investment in patient education programs is surprising, given that the cost-benefit of education for diabetes has been reported to be $3 to $4 of savings for every $1 invested. This savings is attributed primarily to the reduction in exacerbations and complications associated with the disease. Kaplan and Davis (19) provided a comprehensive review of the literature on the costs and benefits of outpatient diabetes education programs.

Prevention and Management of Macrovascular and Microvascular Complications

As previously mentioned, diabetes predisposes those affected to numerous complications, several of them life-threatening. With these complications, diabetes is the fifth leading cause of death by disease and the seventh leading cause of death overall in the United States. However, the leading cause of death among persons with diabetes is cardiovascular disease, which accounts for 60% to 70% of all case-fatalities. The complications of diabetes can be subdivided into macrovascular and microvascular complications. Macrovascular complications include coronary artery disease (CAD), cerebral vascular disease, and peripheral vascular disease (PVD) and result in angina, myocardial infarction (MI), stroke, and claudication. Microvascular complications include nephropathy and retinopathy. Although the link between diabetes and cardiovascular mortality has been understood for some time, persons with diabetes remain unaware of this association. According to a survey conducted by the American Diabetes Association and the American College of Cardiology, 70% of 2,008 subjects with diabetes did not believe that cardiovascular disease was a serious risk associated with diabetes. In this survey, 66% of patients believed blindness to be the major complication of diabetes (20).

Although the economic burden of diabetes itself is substantial, the burden increases significantly when the cost of treating diabetes is coupled with the presence of complications. In fact, more resources are spent on treating complications than on managing the disease itself (17). Not only does diabetes predispose to numerous complications, but also treatment of those complications is significantly more expensive in the presence of diabetes (e.g., doubling or tripling the cost of CAD or cerebral vascular disease) (21). Individuals with complicated diabetes are more likely to be unemployed, to have lower income, and to receive social support than are people with uncomplicated diabetes or nondiabetics (22).

Of the various complications of diabetes, cardiovascular disease and end-stage renal disease (ESRD) are among the most costly (Fig. 10-1). Cardiovascular complications attributable to insulin resistance alone were estimated to have cost $12.5 billion in the United States in 1999 (23). The complications of diabetes are also responsible for the majority of productivity loss and

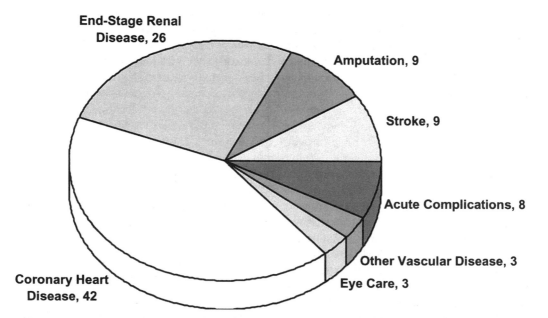

FIG. 10-1. Partitioned health care expenditures for patients with diabetes, according to complication, in an 85,000-member health maintenance organization ($283 million excess spending). (Reprinted with permission from The American Diabetes Association. Selby JV, Ray GT, Zhang D, et al. Excess costs of medical care for patients with diabetes in a managed care population. *Diabetes Care* 1997;20:1396–1402.)

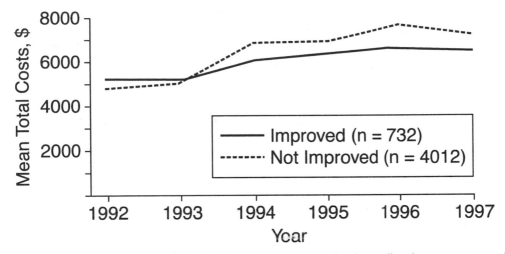

FIG. 10-2. Annual mean total health care costs among diabetic patients resulting from improvement in hemoglobin A$_{1C}$ (HbA$_{1C}$) levels. (Reprinted with permission from The American Medical Association. Wagner EH, Sandhu N, Newton KM, et al. Effect of improved glycemic control on health care costs and utilization. *JAMA* 2001;285:182–189.)

reduced quality of life seen in patients with diabetes.

Glycemic Control: An Overall Strategy to Prevent Microvascular and Macrovascular Complications

Glycemic control remains the cornerstone of diabetes treatment. Tight glycemic control leads to a significant reduction in microvascular complications for persons with either type 1 or type 2 diabetes and translates into a decreased economic burden for society (24). Poor glycemic control leads to a higher risk of diabetes-related complications. Two strategies have been evaluated with respect to clinical efficacy and are available for economic study. The intensive strategy employs an early and aggressive pharmacologic approach focused on heightened glycemic control. This strategy is associated with an early increased economic cost related to drug therapy, outpatient visits, self-testing, and case management. The adequacy of control is often assessed by measurements of glycosylated hemoglobin (HbA$_{1C}$); an HbA$_{1C}$ value of 7.0% or less is the recommended goal. The United Kingdom Prospective Diabetes Study (UKPDS) found that lowering HbA$_{1C}$ levels by as little as 1 percentage point reduces the complications of diabetes by approximately

25%, thereby reducing health care utilization and costs (Fig. 10-2) (25,26). Conversely, the work of Gilmer et al. (27) indicated that medical care charges increase by 10% or more for every 1% increase in HbA$_{1C}$.

After the finding of the UKPDS and other trials that intensive glycemic control reduces the incidence of diabetes-related complications, several studies examined the cost-effectiveness of intensive glycemic control. The UKPDS randomly assigned patients with type 2 diabetes to receive either conventional therapy or intensive glucose control with insulin, a sulfonylurea, or metformin. Although intensive therapy did increase treatment costs, the improved blood glucose control resulting from such therapy led to better outcomes and reduced the cost of complications, yielding a net incremental cost of £478 per patient per year, or £1,166 per event-free year of life (YOL) gained (25).

The Centers for Disease Control and Prevention (CDC), using a model based on the UKPDS results, found that intensive glycemic control using chlorpropamide, glipizide, or insulin resulted in an intervention cost of $12,213 (Table 10-2). However, intensive control directly reduced the incidence of nephropathy, retinopathy, and neuropathy by 11% to 27% and resulted in a 0.1915 quality-adjusted life-year (QALY)

TABLE 10-2. *Incremental cost-effectiveness by intervention*

	Cost ($)[a]				Quality-adjusted life-years (QALYs)[a]	Incremental cost-effectiveness ratio (total cost/QALY, $)
	Standard treatment	Complications	Intervention	Total		
Intensive glycemic control[b]						
Conventional glycemic control (standard treatment)	10,741	37,602	0	48,343	11.8791	
Intervention	10,785	33,271	12,213	56,270	12.0707	
Incremental	44	−4330	12,213	7,927	0.1915	41,384
Intensive hypertension control[c]						
Moderate hypertension control (standard treatment)	10,679	33,738	0	44,417	10.3990	
Intervention	11,030	28,902	3,708	43,641	10.7952	
Incremental	351	−4836	3,708	−776	0.3962	−1959
Reduction in serum cholesterol level[d]						
Standard treatment	10,353	34,819	0	45,171	11.4690	
Intervention	10,756	36,505	15,942	63,204	11.8165	
Incremental	404	1,687	15,942	18,033	0.3475	51,889

[a]Discounted at 3% annual rate. Costs are for patient's lifetime and are reported in 1997 dollars.
[b]All patients who were newly diagnosed as having type 2 diabetes.
[c]All patients who were newly diagnosed as having type 2 diabetes and hypertension.
[d]All patients who were newly diagnosed as having type 2 diabetes and above normal serum cholesterol level.
From The Centers for Disease Control Diabetes Cost-Effectiveness Group: Cost-effectiveness of intensive glycemic control, intensified hypertension control and serum cholesterol level reduction for type 2 diabetes. *JAMA* 2002;287:2542–2551, with permission from The American Medical Association.

gain. As a result, the incremental total cost of intensive treatment was reduced to $7,927, with a cost-effectiveness ratio of $41,384 per QALY gained (28). The CDC concluded that intensive glycemic control improves health outcomes, although it also increases health costs. The cost-effectiveness ratio of $41,384 per QALY is comparable to that of other commonly funded interventions, such as heart transplantation, neonatal intensive care, and dual air bags.

The Diabetes Control and Complications Trial (DCCT), like the UKPDS, analyzed the cost-effectiveness of intensive therapy, but for type 1 rather than type 2 diabetes. Conventional therapy consisted of one or two insulin injections per day, daily self-monitoring, and quarterly visits. Intensive therapy comprised three or more daily insulin injections or use of an insulin pump, self-monitoring four times per day, and monthly outpatient visits. Considering only direct medical costs (e.g., inpatient and outpatient costs, medication, equipment), intensive therapy was found to be substantially more expensive, with an annual cost almost three times that of conventional therapy for the insulin injection protocol and almost four times that of conventional therapy for the insulin pump protocol (29). The additional cost of the insulin pump protocol was essentially all due to the cost of the infusion pump and related supplies. The DCCT also found that intensive therapy, although it was more costly, reduced the incidence of retinopathy by 47% and that of nephropathy by 54%, providing intensive therapy patients with 7.7 additional years of sight, 5.8 additional years free from ESRD, and 5.6 additional years free from lower-extremity amputation, compared with conventional therapy. In terms of survival, these benefits translate to 5.1 additional YOL gained. Total incremental costs of intensive treatment were $33,476 per patient, equivalent to $28,661 per YOL gained and $19,987 per QALY gained (30). Similar to the results of the UKPDS and CDC trials, the DCCT ratios are within the generally accepted

TABLE 10-3. *Lifetime per-person costs[a] of diabetes: standard versus comprehensive care for type 2 diabetes mellitus*

Complication	Standard care ($)	Comprehensive care ($)	Difference ($)
General medical diabetes-related care	32,365	58,312	25,947
Eye disease	3,128	1,536	−1,592
Renal disease	9,437	960	−8,477
Neuropathy/amputation	4,381	1,469	−2,912
Coronary artery disease	13,458	14,414	956
Total costs	62,769	76,922	13,922
Incremental cost per quality-adjusted life-year			16,002

[a]Figures based on present value costs (3% discounted rate).
Adapted from Eastman RC, Javitt JC, Herman WH, et al. Model of complications of NIDDM: II. Analysis of the health benefits and cost-effectiveness of treating NIDDM with the goal of normoglycemia. *Diabetes Care* 1997;20:735–744; with permission from The American Diabetes Association.

range of cost-effectiveness and are similar to cost-effectiveness ratios for other widely used medical treatments.

A study by Eastman et al. (31), based on the DCCT, found that if HbA$_{1C}$ levels were decreased to and maintained at 7.2%, the cumulative incidences of blindness, ESRD, and lower-extremity amputation would be reduced by 76%, 88%, and 67%, respectively. At the same time, life expectancy would be extended by 1.4 years, resulting in an incremental cost of $16,000 per QALY (Table 10-3).

Although the UKPDS and DCCT were longer-term studies, the benefits of tight glycemic control are not limited to the long term; over a 3 year period, better glycemic control (as measured by the HbA$_{1C}$) was associated with a reduced rate of hospital admissions and reduced charges for acute complications of diabetes such as hyperglycemia, hypoglycemia, and infections (10). The economic benefits were even more marked among patients with existing long-term diabetic complications such as hypertension or CAD. Health plan studies have also concluded that cost savings from improved glucose control are attainable within just a few years after the improvement (32).

Based on the results of these studies, it is evident that intensive glycemic control reduces the incidence and cost of diabetic complications and is cost-effective. With respect to therapeutic options, pharmaceutical costs related to diabetes fluctuate between 7% and 10% of the total cost of diabetes care (33), or approximately $10 billion in the United States in 1992 (3). Common drug classes used for glycemic control include oral agents such as the sulfonylureas, metformin, the thiazolidinediones, and insulin. Annual costs of treatment have been estimated at $4,400 for sulfonylureas, $4,187 for metformin, and $7,356 for insulin (34). Glipizide, a second-generation sulfonylurea, has a well-established role as an oral antihyperglycemic agent. In a 3-year comparison with metformin and acarbose, glipizide was determined to be the least costly first-line strategy, with a per-patient cost of $4,971, compared with $5,273 for metformin and $5,311 for acarbose (35). The savings were attributed to both a lower failure rate and lower medication costs. There are not large differences in efficacy between sulfonylurea agents and metformin, but acarbose is generally recognized as less effective. The thiazolidinediones have also been found to be cost-effective in reducing HbA$_{1C}$ and achieving glycemic control, comparing favorably to the cost of insulin therapy (36).

Macrovascular Complications of Diabetes

Coronary Artery Disease

Cardiovascular disease is not only the leading cause of death and the leading source of health care expenditures in the U. S. population as a whole; it is also the leading cause of death in patients with diabetes (accounting for approximately 80% of deaths) and one of the most costly complications of diabetes. Diabetes is associated with a marked increase in the incidence of CAD, which may be as much as 76% more prevalent in patients with diabetes than in those without the disease (37). The common diabetic comorbidities, hypertension and dyslipidemia, are also risk factors for cardiovascular disease (38).

The direct cost of treating cardiovascular disease in patients with diabetes has been estimated to exceed $7.6 billion annually (39), much higher than the corresponding expenditure for nondiabetic patients. One contributing factor to this excess cost is that, in the presence of diabetes, CAD tends to be more severe and to develop at an earlier age. Moreover, the incidence of adverse events after revascularization, whether by percutaneous transluminal coronary angioplasty (PTCA) or CABG, is higher in patients with diabetes. As a result, patients with diabetes who undergo revascularization consume more hospital resources than do similar nondiabetic persons (40,41). The causes of the increased risk for CAD in diabetes are multifactorial and include dyslipidemia, hypertension, and obesity. Control of these three factors is the mainstay of CAD prevention and treatment in diabetes, as discussed elsewhere in this text. With respect to hypertension, angiotensin-converting enzyme (ACE) inhibitors have been found to delay the onset of CAD, cerebral vascular disease, and nephropathy. In addition, in patients with diabetes and CAD, low-dose aspirin therapy (75 to 325 mg/day) is recommended by the American Diabetes Association to reduce CAD and cerebral vascular disease event rates.

As mentioned previously, the management of macrovascular disease is the largest cost component of treating diabetic complications, amounting to 52% of costs, or $24,330 per patient over 30 years, as estimated by Caro et al. (42). In the acute care setting, an analysis by O'Brien et al. (43) found that acute myocardial infarctions (AMIs) in patients with diabetes led to direct medical costs of $27,630 per event, much higher than the same cost in nondiabetics, and angina cost $2,477 per event (Table 10-4). Ramsey et al. (44) estimated that the presence of dia-

TABLE 10-4. *Per-event costs of diabetes complications*

Complications	Cost ($)
Cardiovascular	
Acute myocardial infarction	27,630
Angina	2,477
Cerebrovascular	
Ischemic stroke	40,616
Transient ischemic attack	6,204
End-stage renal disease[a]	53,659
Retinopathy	
Macular edema	1,100
Proliferative diabetic retinopathy	1,044
First lower-extremity amputation	26,894
Second lower-extremity amputation	27,132

[a]Average annual Medicare payment for patient with end-stage renal disease.
Modified from O'Brien JA, Shomphe LA, Kavanagh PL, et al. Direct medical costs of complications resulting from type 2 diabetes in the U.S. *Diabetes Care* 1998;21:1122–1128. Reprinted with permission from The American Diabetes Association.

betes increases the annual cost of care for an MI by a multiple of 4.1. In regard to post-MI treatment, the Diabetes Mellitus, Insulin Glucose Infusion in Acute Myocardial Infarction (DIGAMI) trial, a European study, compared intensive insulin therapy after AMI with standard antidiabetic therapy. With intense treatment, the 1-year mortality rate was reduced from 26% to 19%; the overall mortality rate over 3 to 4 years was 33% in the insulin-treated group versus 44% in the control group. Although treatment costs were somewhat increased, when they were coupled with the decreased mortality, intensive insulin therapy after AMI yielded a cost of EURO $24,100 per QALY gained (45).

In the area of revascularization strategies for patients with diabetes, the aforementioned ARTS trial compared multivessel percutaneous intervention with CABG. Total 1-year costs for patients with diabetes were $12,855 for stenting and $16,585 for CABG, more than 26% higher than the same costs in the nondiabetic cohort. Comorbid factors related to diabetes were a factor in the additional costs, and outcomes in patients with diabetes were generally worse than those in the nondiabetic cohort regardless of the revascularization method used. A cost advantage of $3,730 for stenting was found, despite greater need for repeat revascularization (11). Diabetes is associated with increased adverse events after both CABG and percutaneous coronary intervention. The comparative efficacy of each revascularization strategy was investigated in substudies (46,47), and the results are covered elsewhere in this text.

The Evaluation of Platelet IIb/IIIa Inhibitor for Stenting (EPISTENT) trial analyzed the cost-effectiveness of abciximab, a platelet glycoprotein IIb/IIIa inhibitor, in combination with stenting. When compared with stenting alone or with balloon angioplasty plus abciximab, a strategy of stenting plus abciximab was found to be cost-effective, with cost-effectiveness ratios of $5,291 and $6,213 per added YOL, respectively (48). Another study found that use of abciximab during routine medical care of high-risk patients (e.g., those with diabetes) reduced the incidence of ischemic events (death, MI, revascularization) by 40%, with a net 6-month cost of $2,400 and a cost-effectiveness ratio of $21,789 per event avoided (49).

Cerebrovascular Disease

Cerebrovascular disease is the third leading cause of death in the United States, and the total estimated costs of stroke are more than $45 billion annually. In patients with diabetes, ischemic stroke is estimated to cost $40,616 per event, whereas a transient ischemic attack costs $6,204 per event (Table 10-4). The average annual cost of stroke care in the presence of diabetes is estimated to be 3.5 times higher than stroke care in nondiabetics (44). Stroke involves a number of mechanisms, including atherosclerosis, vessel wall injury, and platelet aggregation. Diabetes affects all of these variables and therefore contributes to the risk for the major forms of ischemic stroke (50). Patients with diabetes are two to three times more likely to experience stroke, to have an adverse clinic outcome (7), and to require greater medical resources than patients without diabetes. Among diabetic patients who have had a stroke, 40% receive some level of inpatient care after discharge, and another 13% receive home health care (43).

Because stroke, like CAD, is associated with hypertension, atherosclerosis, and diabetes it-

self, comprehensive management of stroke in the patient with diabetes includes treatment of hypertension, dyslipidemia, and hyperglycemia, as well as antiplatelet therapy (51). As discussed in more detail later, the UKPDS showed a 44% reduction in relative risk for stroke in patients with diabetes whose blood pressure was well controlled (52). Furthermore, the Heart Outcomes Prevention Evaluation (HOPE) study provided evidence that treatment with the ACE inhibitor ramipril reduces the risk of stroke in high-risk patients by mechanisms other than lowering blood pressure. In fact, ramipril therapy achieved a 33% reduction in stroke among patients with diabetes. Based on the HOPE study, the American Heart Association guidelines for the primary prevention of stroke recommend ramipril to prevent stroke in patients with diabetes (53).

In regard to dyslipidemia, several 3-hydroxy-3-methylglutaryl coenzyme A (HMG-CoA) reductase inhibitor trials have shown consistent reduction in stroke risk with the use of these agents. From a surgical standpoint, for patients who have developed significant carotid artery stenosis, carotid endarterectomy may be indicated as a preventive measure. In these patients, the presence of diabetes is a predictor for a prolonged length of stay after surgery and therefore is likely to result in higher costs (54).

Peripheral Vascular Disease

Diabetes is the most common cause of lower-extremity amputation in the United States; more than 56,000 diabetes-related amputations are performed annually, and the risk of a leg amputation is 15 to 40 times greater among people with diabetes. The incidence of foot ulcers is reported to be 2% to 7% per year (55,56), relatively low compared with other complications. However, foot ulcer is a major cause of hospitalization, and it is the most frequent diabetic complication in developing countries. The cost of treatment can be high: in 1995, disease-attributable Medicare spending for patients with lower-extremity ulcers was $1.5 billion, and Ramsey et al. (55) found that, for 2 years after diagnosis, the attributable cost of diabetic foot ulcer care was $27,987. In both cases, the majority of spending was for inpatient stays. Lower-extremity amputation is estimated to cost $26,894 for the first amputation and $27,132 for the second (Table 10-4).

In addition to the high costs of disease-attributable care, morbidity, mortality, and excess care costs are substantial in patients with foot ulcers. For example, ulcers often progress to infections of the surrounding tissue, osteomyelitis, and amputation, and survival can be significantly reduced. The management of the diabetic foot is a complex problem: healing is limited by multiple factors, including cardiovascular disease, degree of metabolic control, and compliance. Inpatient care and topical treatment have been found to be the largest drivers of excess costs. Treatment of diabetic foot ulcers can involve primary healing, vascular reconstruction, or amputation. Due to the high costs associated with treatment and the varying efficacy among treatment options, some controversy exists as to the optimal choice of therapy. Amputation has been considered costly not only as a result of its direct costs, but also due to its consequences, both in follow-up care and in quality of life, and many authors advocate limb salvage if it is possible (57).

Microvascular Complications of Diabetes

Nephropathy

The prevalence of renal involvement in persons with diabetes is high; 25% to 50% of patients with type 1 diabetes develop microalbuminuria (58,59), and many of these patients go on to develop albuminuria and ESRD. In fact, diabetes is the leading cause of ESRD, and 28,000 people initiate treatment for ESRD annually. The relationship between hypertension, diabetes, and albuminuria has been well established. A significant percentage of diabetic patients are also hypertensive, and the proportion increases to as much as 90% in those with microalbuminuria or macroalbuminuria (60). Furthermore, the coexistence of albuminuria and hypertension markedly increases the mortality risk in persons with diabetes, by 11- to 18-fold in patients with type 1 diabetes and 5- to 8-fold in those with type 2 diabetes (61). Even without hypertension or proteinuria, mortality ratios are significantly increased

in patients with diabetes. Similarly, the incidence of comorbid conditions is increased in diabetic patients with nephropathy. For example, diabetic patients with nephropathy are at heightened risk for development of certain complications, with a 2- to 4-fold increase in the risk of stroke and a 5- to 10-fold increase in the risk for AMI (62). Management of ESRD is estimated to cost $53,659 annually per patient (Table 10-4), up to 4.3 times the cost of treating ESRD in a non-diabetic person, resulting in an excess of $15.6 billion spent in 1997 (39).

Due to the high cost of managing ESRD, prevention of ESRD or delay of its onset can result in significant cost savings. As previously discussed, good metabolic control is key to preventing the development of nephropathy. In addition, reductions in blood pressure have been shown to preserve renal function (63). Studies show that, independent of blood pressure reduction, ACE inhibitors slow the rate of progression of diabetic nephropathy to ESRD (64,65). As a consequence, ACE inhibitors reduce the cost of complications and have been found to be a cost-effective treatment for diabetic nephropathy. Rodby et al. (66) found that treatment with captopril for patients with diabetes and nephropathy resulted in absolute direct cost savings of $32,550 per patient with type 1 diabetes and $9,900 per patient with type 2 diabetes. Savings of indirect costs were even more pronounced, at $84,390 and $45,730 per patient with type 1 and type 2 diabetes, respectively. The aggregate direct cost savings were estimated to be $189 million per year in 1999 and $475 million per year in 2004, or a present value of $2.4 billion over 10 years (66). One analysis even suggested that a strategy of treating all cases of type 2 diabetes with ACE inhibitors should be considered, estimating a cost-effectiveness ratio of $7,500 per QALY gained when compared with screening for microalbuminuria (67). Angiotensin receptor blockers (ARBs) have also been shown to slow the progression of nephropathy, although their cost-effectiveness in patients with diabetes has not yet been established.

When patients do reach ESRD, dialysis or kidney transplantation may be considered in terms of both patient survival and cost savings. As with cardiovascular procedures, these treatment strategies are more costly in patients with diabetes. Cost-effectiveness ratios for patients with type 1 diabetes have been estimated to be as high as $317,746 per QALY for dialysis, $156,042 per QALY for kidney transplantation, and $123,923 per QALY for simultaneous pancreas-kidney transplantation (68). It is obvious from the high cost of these procedures that early therapy targeted toward prevention and management is desirable.

Retinopathy

Diabetes is the leading cause of blindness in the United States, and diabetic retinopathy will eventually develop in up to 80% of persons with diabetes. Each year, between 12,000 to 24,000 people in the country lose their sight due to diabetes (7). Treatment costs for macular edema and proliferative diabetic retinopathy are estimated to be $1,100 and $1,044, respectively, and the cost of blindness is even higher (Table 10-4). As with the other complications of diabetes, the risk for retinopathy and blindness can be related to the levels of glycemic and blood pressure control. As numerous studies have shown, once retinopathy is present, photocoagulation can significantly reduce the risk of developing visual loss due to diabetic retinopathy and macular edema (69). However, screening is vital to prevent visual loss, because diabetic retinopathy is often asymptomatic early in the course of the disease.

Previous cost-effectiveness analyses demonstrated that annual screening and treatment for diabetic retinopathy and macular edema are cost-effective interventions (70). Furthermore, such preventive treatment may even be cost-saving, with an estimated savings to the federal budget of $248 million to $472 million (depending on the level of care), or $975 per person enrolled in a screening program (71). As a result of these studies, provision of annual eye screening is now being used as a measure of quality of care. Unfortunately, compliance with this recommendation has been disappointing, with surveys suggesting annual screening rates of about 50% (72).

Management of Comorbidities of Diabetes

Hypertension

Total U. S. health care costs for the treatment of hypertension have been estimated at $15 billion per year (39). Up to 60% of persons with diabetes are hypertensive, and the coexistence of hypertension is an unfavorable prognostic factor; the mortality rate for hypertensive diabetics is three times that of normotensive diabetic patients. Patients with both diabetes and hypertension were found to incur much higher costs than patients with either disease alone ($13,446 per patient per year versus $8,493 for diabetes alone and $8,424 for hypertension alone) (73). Hospitalization costs contributed the greatest amount to total costs; disease specific costs were less than one quarter of total costs.

For many years, the blood pressure treatment goal for hypertensive patients has been 140/90 mm Hg or better. However, several authorities have espoused that patients with diabetes or renal impairment should have a lower target blood pressure than other individuals (74,75). The Sixth Report of the Joint National Committee on Prevention, Detection, Evaluation, and Treatment of High Blood Pressure (JNC VI) recommended a treatment goal of less than 130/85 mm Hg for such persons, and the American Diabetes Association recommended an even lower treatment goal of 130/80 mm Hg (76). Although achievement of this lower goal often requires the use of a multidrug regimen, the lowered JNC VI target was found to be cost-effective (Fig. 10-3) due to both an increase in life expectancy of 0.48 years and a decrease in total lifetime medical costs of $1,450 when blood pressure is reduced from 140/90 to 130/85 mm Hg (77). Moreover, the cost reduction was apparent across multiple diabetic complications (Fig. 10-4). Because life expectancy is increased and costs are decreased, the cost-effectiveness ratio for 60-year-olds (the average age of patients with type 2 diabetes in the United States) is negative, indicating overall cost savings. The ratios for other age groups, although they do not indicate cost savings, are also well within the range of cost-effectiveness.

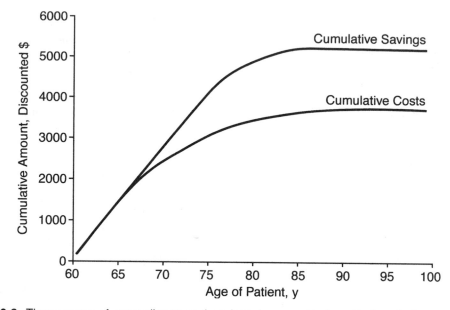

FIG. 10-3. Time course of expenditures and savings from avoided medical costs for a cohort of 60-year-old high-risk diabetic patients after treatment and achievement of a blood pressure goal of 130/85 mm Hg or lower. (From Elliott WJ, Weir DR, Black HR. Cost-effectiveness of the lower treatment goal [of JNC VI] for diabetic hypertensive patients. *Arch Intern Med* 2000;160:1277–1283, with permission from The American Medical Association.)

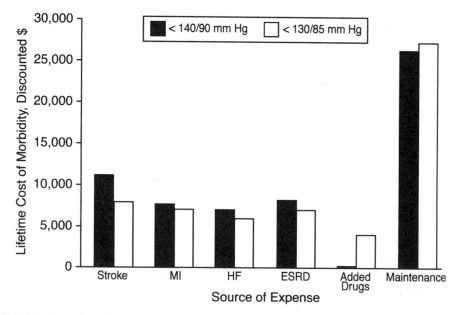

FIG. 10-4. Lifetime allocation of resources to a cohort of 60-year-old diabetic hypertensive patients (under baseline conditions) for each type of medical care outcome under two blood pressure goals: less than 140/90 mm Hg (as previously recommended) and less than 130/85 mm Hg (as recommended by the Sixth Report of the Joint National Committee on Prevention, Detection, Evaluation, and Treatment of High Blood Pressure [JNC VI]). (From Elliott WJ, Weir DR, Black HR. Cost-effectiveness of the lower treatment goal [of JNC VI] for diabetic hypertensive patients. *Arch Intern Med* 2000;160:1277–1283, with permission from The American Medical Association.)

Although the blood pressure goal analyzed in the UKPDS (150/85 mm Hg) was higher than the JNC recommendation, the UKPDS also found that a lower blood pressure target was cost-effective, and in fact resulted in cost savings, over the 8.4 years of therapy. Savings again resulted because the additional costs of the more intensive treatment strategy (using either captopril or atenolol) were overshadowed by the 34% reduction in risk of macrovascular complications (MI, stroke, PVD) and the 37% reduction in risk of microvascular disease progression (nephropathy and retinopathy) (52). Tight control increased the total costs of treatment by £740 while reducing the cost of complications by £949, a net savings of £209 per patient over the duration of the study (78). When based on resources used in standard practice rather than trial protocols, the net increase in cost for tight control was £237.

In a related study, UKPDS researchers analyzed specific antihypertensive classes, comparing the net cost of blood pressure control with captopril versus atenolol in patients with type 2 diabetes. Both drugs were found to be cost-effective, but there were cost differences between the two drug regimens. The mean cost of antihypertensive drugs over the trial period was £1,421 in the captopril group and £998 in the atenolol group, a difference of £423 in favor of atenolol. In contrast, the mean cost of antidiabetic drugs was £1,155 in the captopril group and £1,457 in the atenolol group, a difference of £302 in favor of captopril. This result was expected, because atenolol was previously shown to increase blood glucose and insulin, thus necessitating more drug therapy to control blood glucose. These figures yielded a modest mean difference in the total cost of therapy of £35 in favor of atenolol (79).

Surprisingly, costs of complications (e.g., hospitalizations, follow-up outpatient visits) were also different between the two groups, yielding a mean difference of £1,127 per patient in favor of atenolol. The lower costs for atenolol were due to both fewer hospitalizations and shorter lengths of stay. Therefore, treatment with atenolol resulted in both lower therapy costs and lower complication costs. Although ACE inhibition would seem preferable due to atenolol's effect on blood glucose, from an economic perspective atenolol remains a desirable antihypertensive agent. However, information on cost-effectiveness must be coupled with the numerous other beneficial effects of ACE inhibitors when individualizing antihypertensive therapy for diabetic patients.

Building on the UKPDS findings, the CDC also found intensified hypertension control, using either ACE inhibitors or β-blockers, to be cost-effective when compared with moderate control through diet and other drugs (28). Intensive control reduced the risk of stroke by 44% and also reduced the cumulative incidence of nephropathy and retinopathy. Although the more intensive intervention cost $3,708, the cost of complications was reduced by $4,836, leading to a net cost savings of $776, an increase of 0.3962 QALY and an incremental cost-effectiveness ratio of −$1,959 per QALY, indicating that intensive hypertension control with either ACE inhibitors or β-blockers is actually cost-saving (Table 10-2).

Although numerous other antihypertensive agents (e.g., ARBs, diuretics, calcium channel blockers) have been shown to be effective in decreasing cardiovascular events and in some cases possibly slowing the progression of retinopathy and nephropathy, the cost-effectiveness of these treatments in the diabetic population has not been fully established.

Dyslipidemia

Dyslipidemia is also quite common in individuals with diabetes, and its presence substantially increases the risk of cardiovascular disease. Trials such as the Multiple Risk Factor Intervention Trial (MRFIT) and the Framingham Study indicate that, for the same serum lipid levels, diabetics have a higher risk of CAD than do nondiabetics. The risk of MI in diabetic patients without CAD is comparable to the risk of MI in nondiabetics with CAD; Haffner et al. (80) found that the 7-year incidence of MI in nondiabetic subjects with prior MI was similar to that for diabetic subjects without prior MI (18.8% versus 20.2%, respectively) (80). However, despite the similarity in incidence, the fatality rates for MI are significantly higher in diabetic subjects.

As mentioned earlier, MI and cerebral vascular disease are more than twice as frequent among patients with diabetes as among those without the disease, and management of acute episodes in the diabetic population is particularly costly. Patients with diabetes are 15 times more likely to be admitted for PVD, and 6 to 10 times more likely to be admitted for CAD and cerebral vascular disease (81). Together, CAD and stroke account for approximately 80% of deaths in patients with diabetes; along with hypertension, they account for 33.3% of the total costs of diabetes. Furthermore, the occurrence of adverse events after revascularization is higher for patients with diabetes (82). Optimization of lipid management has an important impact on the vascular outcome of persons with diabetes.

Recent guidelines have recognized the value of aggressive management of blood lipids: the American Diabetes Association recommends an LDL cholesterol goal of less than 100 mg/dL for diabetic patients (83). In patients with diabetes, statins are recommended as first-line drug therapy for the treatment of dyslipidemia, and several studies suggest that patients with diabetes and CAD benefit from statin therapy through a reduction in the risk of coronary and other atherosclerotic events. The cost-effectiveness of simvastatin treatment in patients with diabetes and CAD has been demonstrated, and analysis indicates that it may be cost-effective to intervene with statin therapy in any patient who is at increased risk for CAD, including patients with diabetes (84).

In the Scandinavian Simvastatin Survival Study (85), simvastatin treatment reduced the incidence of cardiovascular events in patients with diabetes, hypercholesterolemia, and CAD. Simvastatin treatment during the 5.4 years of the trial cost $5,877 per patient; in patients with diabetes, the treatment reduced CAD-related hospitalizations by 40%, average length of stay by 2.4 days, and CAD-related hospital days by 55%. The end result of simvastatin therapy was a reduction in net hospital costs of $7,678, yielding a net cost savings of $1,801 per patient for the duration of the trial (85).

Using a model based on the results of the Scandinavian study and the Cholesterol and Recruitment Events (CARE) trial, Grover et al. (86) found that simvastatin treatment in patients with diabetes and CAD reduced the number of deaths from CAD, resulting in increased life expectancy ranging from 0.73 to 5.30 YOL saved, depending on patient demographics. The benefit of therapy was substantial for both men and women across a wide range of baseline LDL cholesterol values, and the cost-effectiveness ratios of simvastatin treatment ranged from $4,000 to $8,000 per YOL saved, much lower than the ratios for similar nondiabetic patients.

In addition, Grover's group found that simvastatin therapy as primary prevention in patients with diabetes but without symptomatic CAD was cost-effective (86). Among men, the cost-effectiveness of simvastatin therapy for primary prevention ranged from $4,000 to $10,000 per YOL saved (Fig. 10-5). Although the ratios were higher in women, they were still well within the accepted range of cost-effectiveness. Even among patients with diabetes who were without CAD and had near-normal lipid levels, the cost-effectiveness of simvastatin for primary prevention was evident, with ratios of $7,000 to $15,000 per YOL saved for men and $24,000 to $40,000 per YOL saved for women. In a separate study, Grover et al. (87) further found that the cost-effectiveness of primary prevention with simvastatin in diabetes patients without CAD, at ratios ranging from $5,063 to $14,156 per YOL saved, was similar to that for treatment of CAD patients without diabetes (87).

The CDC has also studied the cost-effectiveness of serum cholesterol reduction using pravastatin. A reduction in serum cholesterol reduced the risk of CAD by 31%, compared with no treatment. Pravastatin treatment resulted in an incremental total cost of $18,033 and an increase in QALY of 0.3475, yielding an incremental cost-effectiveness ratio of $51,889 per QALY (Table 10-2) (28).

ADMINISTRATIVE STRATEGIES TO REDUCE THE ECONOMIC BURDEN OF DIABETES

Effective management of diabetes includes not only the individual patient and health care professional but also consideration of the systems of care in which both patients and providers

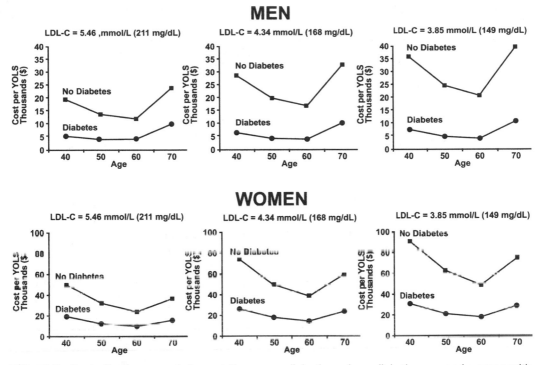

FIG. 10-5. Cost-effectiveness of simvastatin among diabetic and nondiabetic men and women with out cardiovascular disease, at various baseline low-density lipoprotein (LDL) cholesterol levels, after reductions of 35% in total cholesterol and 25% in LDL cholesterol and an 8% increase in high-density lipoprotein (HDL) cholesterol. (From Grover SA, Coupal L, Zowall H, et al. Cost-effectiveness of treating hyperlipidemia in the presence of diabetes: who should be treated? *Circulation* 2000;102:722–727, with permission.)

must operate. As noted by Glasgow et al. (88), the majority of care for patients with diabetes is problematic; this primarily stems from the acute illness model of care that still predominates in the United States. Given the importance of aligning incentives to improve care for patients with diabetes and to reduce diabetic complications, the alignment of provider reimbursement with quality outcomes should be considered as one economic tool to reduce the economic burden of diabetes in the country. This section discusses the role of payers in improving care and reducing the morbidity and mortality of diabetes.

Health care plans are increasingly challenged by employers to reduce costs and improve the quality of care for patients with diabetes. To assist in this regard, health plans have adopted multiple strategies, one of which involves measuring Health Plan Employer Data and Information Set (HEDIS) standards of care and rewarding physicians with high rates of compliance with them. Another involves the use of disease management vendors to improve the coordination of care in capitated health care plans. A brief description of each approach is provided here.

The National Committee for Quality Assurance developed HEDIS guidelines for the appropriate treatment of diabetes (Table 10-5). The standards include appropriate monitoring of HbA_{1C} to measure effective blood sugar control, laboratory monitoring for lipid concentrations and kidney function, and appropriate scheduling of retinal eye examinations. One performance goal, glycemic control, illustrates how administrative policies are currently being designed and implemented to align incentives with quality outcomes in diabetes (see later discussion).

TABLE 10-5. *Quality goals and HEDIS performance measure for treatment of diabetes*

Quality goal	HEDIS performance measure
Improved compliance with clinical guidelines Improved compliance with laboratory monitoring guidelines Improved compliance with chronic disease medication management guidelines	Increase compliance with HEDIS measures for diabetes: Hemoglobin A_{1C} Laboratory monitoring for low-density lipoproteins Retinal eye examinations Measurements for nephropathy

HEDIS, Health Plan Employer Data and Information Set.
Adapted from Diabetes quality improvement project initial measure set. Available at http://www.ncqa.org/DPRP/dqip2.htm.

Again, it has long been known that the HbA_{1C} level is a good marker for blood sugar control. The importance of blood sugar control in the appropriate management of patient costs cannot be overstated. The economic implications of poor blood sugar control also should not be underestimated.

As already discussed, results of the DCCT indicate that intensive glycemic control is beneficial in improving blood glucose control in patients with diabetes. In that trial, intensive glycemic control, compared with conventional therapy, delayed the onset and slowed the progression of diabetic complications in patients with type 1 diabetes mellitus, reducing the occurrence of retinopathy by 47%, microalbuminuria by 39%, clinical nephropathy by 54%, and neuropathy by 60% (29). The economic implications of these findings were also estimated: over the 3 years of the study, patients with diabetes and preexisting complications had fewer hospitalizations with intensive therapy than with conventional therapy. Menzin et al. (10) also showed through a retrospective database analysis that poor glycemic control, as measured by HbA_{1C} levels, was associated with greater health care costs over a 3-year period, particularly for patients with coexisting hypertension or heart disease or both. Because the DCCT did not continue long enough and was not designed to demonstrate reductions in the costly end-stage complications of diabetes (e.g. blindness, ESRD, lower-extremity amputations), a Monte Carlo simulation was performed to estimate the long-term economic implications of the two treatment strategies. The results of this simulation revealed a cost-effectiveness ratio of $28,661 per YOL gained (30).

Health plans may measure physicians' performance against the HEDIS criteria, and increasingly health plans are rewarding physicians whose clinical practice patterns reflect compliance with HEDIS standards. In areas where health maintenance organization (HMO) penetration is high, the use of both financial and nonfinancial incentives is increasing. Financial incentives may include, but are not limited to, increases in per-member monthly payments to physicians and quality bonuses distributed as a lump sum at the end of a physician's contracting cycle. Nonfinancial incentives include performance profiling and the publication of performance results. The ultimate goal is to increase the use of evidence-based recommendations to improve the quality of care and reduce health care costs through the prevention of diabetic complications.

Another tool used by health plans to reduce the cost of diabetes-related complications is the use of disease management programs. Disease management vendors identify patients who are at risk for diabetic complications through administrative database and decision rules. The cost-effectiveness of appropriate screening and patient risk stratification is important to the success of these programs. Risk stratification allows the disease management vendor to focus on those patients who are most at risk for adverse events. Once patients are identified, they are asked to enroll in the disease management program. The vendor then works with the physician to increase the patients' compliance with best care practices.

The effectiveness of these intensive case management programs is well documented. In one study, patients had more eye examinations, a reduced incidence of legal blindness, an increased number of foot examinations, and better blood pressure control (89). Another study reported that the disease management program resulted in improved glycemic control, increased monitoring and management of diabetic complications, and greater patient and provider satisfaction (90).

Barriers to the successful implementation of disease management programs for diabetes do exist; they include inadequate access to care and financial barriers to care. More than 25% of providers and administrators in one diabetes disease management program agreed that significant barriers include lack of affordability of home blood glucose and other laboratory monitoring equipment, lack of access to providers, lack of routine eye and foot examinations by the provider, lack of time for diabetes education, and language and cultural barriers (91).

CONCLUSION AND POLICY CONSIDERATION

The economic burden of diabetes is substantial and continues to increase. As a result of the disease and its complications, people with diabetes have more frequent and more intensive encounters with the health care system, even though significant cost reductions could be achieved through prevention or more effective management of the disease and its complications (3). Current incentives reward extensive resource utilization for the treatment of complications associated with diabetes and fail to recognize the value of preventive measures such as diabetes education and appropriate glycemic control. Until cost-effective strategies for the management of diabetes are recognized and rewarded, the aggregate growth in health care expenditures attributed to this patient population is likely to continue.

REFERENCES

1. Boyle JP, Honeycutt AA, Narayan KM, et al. Projection of diabetes burden through 2050: impact of changing demography and disease prevalence in the U.S. *Diabetes Care* 2001;24:1936–1940.
2. Mokdad AH, Bowman BA, Ford ES, et al. The continuing epidemic of obesity and diabetes in the United States. *JAMA* 2001;286:1195–1200.
3. Rubin RJ, Altman WM, Mendelson DN. Health care expenditures for people with diabetes mellitus, 1992. *J Clin Endocrinol Metab* 1994;78:809A–809F.
4. Druss BG, Marcus SC, Olfson M, et al. Comparing the national economic burden of five chronic conditions. *Health Aff (Millwood)* 2001;20:233–241.
5. Pagano E, Brunetti M, Tediosi F, et al. Costs of diabetes: a methodological analysis of the literature. *Pharmacoeconomics* 1999;15:583–595.
6. Gagliardino JJ, Williams R, Clark CM Jr. Using hospitalization rates to track the economic costs and benefits of improved diabetes care in the Americas: a proposal for health policy makers. *Diabetes Care* 2000;23:1844–1846.
7. American Diabetes Association. *Facts and Figures: Direct and Indirect Costs of Diabetes.* Available at http://www.diabetes.org/main/info/facts/impact/default2.jsp. Accessed June 19, 2002.
8. Basile F. The increasing prevalence of diabetes and its economic burden. *Am J Managed Care* 2000;6[Suppl 21]:S1077–S1081.
9. Bjork S. The cost of diabetes and diabetes care. *Diabetes Res Clin Pract* 2001;54[Suppl 1]:S13–S18.
10. Menzin J, Langley-Hawthorne C, Friedman M, et al. Potential short-term economic benefits of improved glycemic control: a managed care perspective. *Diabetes Care* 2001;24:51–5.
11. Abizaid A, Costa MA, Centemero M, et al. Clinical and economic impact of diabetes mellitus on percutaneous and surgical treatment of multivessel coronary disease patients: insights from the Arterial Revascularization Therapy Study (ARTS) trial. *Circulation* 2001;104:533–538.
12. Evans JM, MacDonald TM, Leese GP, et al. Impact of type 1 and type 2 diabetes on patterns and costs of drug prescribing: a population-based study. *Diabetes Care* 2000;23:770–774.
13. Ng YC, Jacobs P, Johnson JA. Productivity losses associated with diabetes in the US. *Diabetes Care* 2001;24:257–261.
14. Ramsey S, Summers KH, Leong SA, et al. Productivity and medical costs of diabetes in a large employer population. *Diabetes Care* 2002;25:23–29.
15. Laditka SB, Mastanduno MP, Laditka JN. Health care use of individuals with diabetes in an employer-based insurance population. *Arch Intern Med* 2001;161:1301–1308.
16. Ray NF, Thamer M, Taylor T, et al. Hospitalization and expenditures for the treatment of general medical conditions among the U.S. diabetic population in 1991. *J Clin Endocrinol Metab* 1996;81:3671–3679.
17. Hodgson TA, Cohen AJ. Medical care expenditures for diabetes, its chronic complications, and its comorbidities. *Prev Med* 1999;29:173–186.
18. Assal JP. Cost-effectiveness of diabetes education. *Pharmacoeconomics* 1995;8[Suppl 1]:68–71.
19. Kaplan RM, Davis WK. Evaluating the costs and benefits of outpatient diabetes education and nutrition counseling. *Diabetes Care* 1986;9:81–86.
20. The Diabetes-Heart Disease Link: Surveying Attitudes, Knowledge and Risk. Available at: http://www.diabetes.org/main/uedocuments/executivesummary.pdf.
21. Brown JB, Nichols GA, Glauber HS, et al. Type 2 diabetes: incremental medical care costs during the first 8 years after diagnosis. *Diabetes Care* 1999;22:1116–1124.
22. Kraut A, Walld R, Tate R, et al. Impact of diabetes on employment and income in Manitoba, Canada. *Diabetes Care* 2001;24:64–68.

23. Strutton DR, Stang PE, Erbey JR, et al. Estimated coronary heart disease attributable to insulin resistance in populations with and without type 2 diabetes mellitus. *Am J Managed Care* 2001;7:765–773.

24. Skyler JS. The economic burden of diabetes and the benefits of improved glycemic control: the potential role of a continuous glucose monitoring system. *Diabetes Technol Ther* 2000;2[Suppl 1]:S7–S12.

25. United Kingdom Prospective Diabetes Study Group. Cost-effectiveness of an intensive blood glucose control policy in patients with type 2 diabetes: economic analysis alongside randomised controlled trial (UKPDS 41). *BMJ* 2000;320:1373–1378.

26. Wagner EH, Sandhu N, Newton KM, et al. Effect of improved glycemic control on health care costs and utilization. *JAMA* 2001;285:182–189.

27. Gilmer TP, O'Connor PJ, Manning WG, et al. The cost to health plans of poor glycemic control. *Diabetes Care* 1997;20:1847–1853.

28. The Centers for Disease Control Diabetes Cost-Effectiveness Group. Cost-effectiveness of intensive glycemic control, intensified hypertension control, and serum cholesterol level reduction for type 2 diabetes. *JAMA* 2002;287:2542–2551.

29. The Diabetes Control and Complications Trial Research Group. Resource utilization and costs of care in the Diabetes Control and Complications Trial. *Diabetes Care* 1995;18:1468–1478.

30. The Diabetes Control and Complications Trial Research Group. Lifetime benefits and costs of intensive therapy as practiced in the Diabetes Control and Complications Trial. *JAMA* 1996;276:1409–1415.

31. Eastman RC, Javitt JC, Herman WH, et al. Model of complications of NIDDM: II. Analysis of the health benefits and cost-effectiveness of treating NIDDM with the goal of normoglycemia. *Diabetes Care* 1997;20:735–744.

32. McCulloch, D. Managing diabetes for improved health and economic outcomes. *Am J Managed Care* 2000;6[Suppl 21]:S1089–S1095.

33. Costa, B, Arroyo J, Sabate A. The economics of pharmacotherapy for diabetes mellitus. *Pharmacoeconomics* 1997;11:139–158.

34. Brown JB, Nichols GA, Glauber HS, et al. Health care costs associated with escalation of drug treatment in type 2 diabetes mellitus. *Am J Health-Syst Pharm* 2001;58:151–157.

35. Ramsdell JW, Grossman JA, Stephens JM, et al. A short-term cost-of-treatment model for type 2 diabetes: comparison of glipizide gastrointestinal therapeutic system, metformin, and acarbose. *Am J Manag Care* 1999;5:1007–1024.

36. Morris AD. The reality of type 2 diabetes treatment today. *Int J Clin Pract Suppl* 2001;121:32–35.

37. Nichols GA, Brown JB. The impact of cardiovascular disease on medical care costs in subjects with and without type 2 diabetes. *Diabetes Care* 2002;25:482–486.

38. Wingard DL, Barrett-Connor E. Heart disease and diabetes. In: Harris MI, ed. *Diabetes in America,* 2nd ed. Washington, DC: U. S. Government Printing Office, 1995:429–448.

39. American Diabetes Association. Economic consequences of diabetes mellitus in the U.S. in 1997. *Diabetes Care* 1998;21:296–309.

40. Weintraub WS, Mauldin PD, Becker E, et al. A comparison of the costs of and quality of life after coronary angioplasty or coronary surgery for multivessel coronary artery disease: results from the Emory Angioplasty Versus Surgery Trial (EAST). *Circulation* 1995;92:2831–2840.

41. Hlatky MA, Rogers WJ, Johnstone I, et al. Medical care costs and quality of life after randomization to coronary angioplasty or coronary bypass surgery. Bypass Angioplasty Revascularization Investigation (BARI) Investigators. *N Engl J Med* 1997;336:92–99.

42. Caro JJ, Ward AJ, O'Brien JA. Lifetime costs of complications resulting from type 2 diabetes in the U.S. *Diabetes Care* 2002;25:476–481.

43. O'Brien JA, Shomphe LA, Kavanagh PL, et al. Direct medical costs of complications resulting from type 2 diabetes in the U.S. *Diabetes Care* 1998;21:1122–1128.

44. Ramsey SD, Newton K, Blough D, et al. Patient-level estimates of the cost of complications in diabetes in a managed-care population. *Pharmacoeconomics* 1999;16:285–295.

45. Almbrand B, Johannesson M, Sjostrand B, et al. Cost-effectiveness of intense insulin treatment after acute myocardial infarction in patients with diabetes mellitus: results from the DIGAMI study. *Eur Heart J* 2000;21:733–739.

46. Influence of diabetes on 5-year mortality and morbidity in a randomized trial comparing CABG and PTCA in patients with multivessel disease: the Bypass Angioplasty Revascularization Investigation (BARI). *Circulation* 1997;96:1761–1769.

47. King SB, Kosinski AS, Guyton RA, et al. Eight year mortality in the Emory Angioplasty vs. Surgery Trial (EAST). *N Engl J Med* 1994;331:1044–1050.

48. Topol EJ, Mark DB, Lincoff AM, et al. Outcomes at 1 year and economic implications of platelet glycoprotein IIb/IIIa blockade in patients undergoing coronary stenting: results from a multicentre randomized trial. EPISTENT Investigators. Evaluation of Platelet IIb/IIIa Inhibitor for Stenting. *Lancet* 1999;354:2019–2024.

49. Reed SO, Mullins CD, Magder LS. Cost effectiveness of abciximab during routine medical practice. *Pharmacoeconomics* 2000;18:265–274.

50. Brass LM. The impact of cerebrovascular disease *Diabetes Obes Metab* 2000;2[Suppl 2]:S6–S10.

51. Sacco RL. Reducing the risk of stroke in diabetes: what have we learned that is new? *Diabetes Obes Metab* 2002;4[Suppl 1]:S27–S34.

52. United Kingdom Prospective Diabetes Study Group. Tight blood pressure control and risk of macrovascular and microvascular complications in type 2 diabetes: UKPDS 38. *BMJ* 1998;317:703–713.

53. Goldstein LB, Adams R, Becker K, et al. Primary prevention of ischemic stroke: a statement for healthcare professionals from the Stroke Council of the American Heart Association. *Stroke* 2001;32:280–299.

54. Roddy SP, Estes JM, Kwoun MO, et al. Factors predicting prolonged length of stay after carotid endarterectomy. *J Vasc Surg* 2000;32:550–554.

55. Ramsey SD, Newton K, Blough D, et al. Incidence, outcomes, and cost of foot ulcers in patients with diabetes. *Diabetes Care* 1999;22:382–387.

56. Harrington C, Zagari MJ, Corea J, et al. A cost analysis of diabetic lower-extremity ulcers. *Diabetes Care* 2000;23:1333–1338.

57. Ragnarson-Tennvall G, Apelqvist J. Cost-effective

management of diabetic foot ulcers: a review. *Pharmacoeconomics* 1997;12:42–53.

58. Andersen AR, Christiansen JS, Andersen JK, et al. Diabetic nephropathy in type 1 (insulin-dependent) diabetes: an epidemiological study. *Diabetologia* 1983;25:496–501.

59. Krolewski AS, Warram JH, Christlieb AR, et al. The changing natural history of nephropathy in type I diabetes. *Am J Med* 1985;78:785–794.

60. Tarnow L, Rossing P, Gall MA, et al. Prevalence of arterial hypertension in diabetic patients before and after the JNC-V. *Diabetes Care* 1994;17:1247–1251.

61. Wang SL, Head J, Stevens L, et al. Excess mortality and its relation to hypertension and proteinuria in diabetic patients: the World Health Organization multinational study of vascular disease in diabetes. *Diabetes Care* 1996;19:305–312.

62. Borch-Johnsen K. The costs of nephropathy in type II diabetes. *Pharmacoeconomics* 1995;8[Suppl 1]:40–45.

63. Parving HH, Andersen AR, Smidt UM, et al. Early aggressive antihypertensive treatment reduces rate of decline in kidney function in diabetic nephropathy. *Lancet* 1983;1:1175–1179.

64. Lewis EJ, Hunsicker LG, Bain RP, et al. The effect of angiotensin-converting-enzyme inhibition on diabetic nephropathy. The Collaborative Study Group. *N Engl J Med* 1993;329:1456–1462.

65. Ravid M, Lang R, Rachmani R, et al. Long-term renoprotective effect of angiotensin-converting enzyme inhibition in non-insulin-dependent diabetes mellitus: a 7-year follow-up study. *Arch Intern Med* 1996;156:286–289.

66. Rodby RA, Firth LM, Lewis EJ. An economic analysis of captopril in the treatment of diabetic nephropathy. The Collaborative Study Group. *Diabetes Care* 1996;19:1051–1061.

67. Golan L, Birkmeyer JD, Welch HG. The cost-effectiveness of treating all patients with type 2 diabetes with angiotensin-converting enzyme inhibitors. *Ann Intern Med* 1999;131:660–667.

68. Douzdjian V, Ferrara D, Silvestri G. Treatment strategies for insulin-dependent diabetics with ESRD: a cost-effectiveness decision analysis model. *Am J Kidney Dis* 1998;31:794–802.

69. The Diabetic Retinopathy Study Research Group. Photocoagulation treatment of proliferative diabetic retinopathy: clinical application of Diabetic Retinopathy Study (DRS) findings. DRS report number 8. *Ophthalmology* 1981;88:583–600.

70. Javitt JC, Aiello LP. Cost-effectiveness of detecting and treating diabetic retinopathy. *Ann Intern Med* 1996;124:164–169.

71. Javitt JC, Aiello LP, Chang Y, et al. Preventive eye care in people with diabetes is cost-saving to the federal government: implications for health-care reform. *Diabetes Care* 1994;17:909–917.

72. Brechner RJ, Cowie CC, Howie LJ, et al. Ophthalmic examination among adults with diagnosed diabetes mellitus. *JAMA* 1993;270:1714–1718.

73. Barrie W. Cost-effective therapy for hypertension. *West J Med* 1996;164:303–309.

74. National High Blood Pressure Education Program Working Group. Report on hypertension in diabetes. *Hypertension* 1994;23:145–158; discussion 159–160.

75. American Diabetes Association. Standards of medical care for patients with diabetes mellitus. *Diabetes Care* 2002;25[Suppl 1]:S33–S49.

76. The sixth report of the Joint National Committee on Prevention, Detection, Evaluation, and Treatment of High Blood Pressure. *Arch Intern Med* 1997;157:2413–2446.

77. Elliott WJ, Weir DR, Black HR. Cost-effectiveness of the lower treatment goal (of JNC VI) for diabetic hypertensive patients. Joint National Committee on Prevention, Detection, Evaluation, and Treatment of High Blood Pressure. *Arch Intern Med* 2000;160:1277–1283.

78. United Kingdom Prospective Diabetes Study Group. Cost effectiveness analysis of improved blood pressure control in hypertensive patients with type 2 diabetes: UKPDS 40. *BMJ* 1998;317:720–726.

79. Gray A, Clarke P, Raikou M, et al. An economic evaluation of atenolol vs. captopril in patients with type 2 diabetes (UKPDS 54). *Diabet Med* 2001;18:438–444.

80. Haffner SM, Lehto S, Ronnemaa T, et al. Mortality from coronary heart disease in subjects with type 2 diabetes and in nondiabetic subjects with and without prior myocardial infarction. *N Engl J Med* 1998;339:229–234.

81. Jacobs J, Sena M, Fox N. The cost of hospitalization for the late complications of diabetes in the United States. *Diabet Med* 1991;8 Spec No:S23–S29.

82. Weintraub WS, Stein B, Kosinski A, et al. Outcome of coronary bypass surgery versus coronary angioplasty in diabetic patients with multivessel coronary artery disease. *J Am Coll Cardiol* 1998;31:10–19.

83. American Diabetes Association. Management of dyslipidemia in adults with diabetes. *Diabetes Care* 2002;25[Suppl 1]:S74–S77.

84. Hay JW, Yu WM, Ashraf T. Pharmacoeconomics of lipid-lowering agents for primary and secondary prevention of coronary artery disease. *Pharmacoeconomics* 1999;15:47–74.

85. Herman WH, Alexander CM, Cook JR, et al. Effect of simvastatin treatment on cardiovascular resource utilization in impaired fasting glucose and diabetes: findings from the Scandinavian Simvastatin Survival Study. *Diabetes Care* 1999;22:1771–1778.

86. Grover SA, Coupal L, Zowall H, et al. Cost-effectiveness of treating hyperlipidemia in the presence of diabetes: who should be treated? *Circulation* 2000;102:722–727.

87. Grover SA, Coupal L, Zowall H, et al. How cost-effective is the treatment of dyslipidemia in patients with diabetes but without cardiovascular disease? *Diabetes Care* 2001;24:45–50.

88. Glasgow RE, Wagner EH, Kaplan RM, et al. If diabetes is a public health problem, why not treat it as one? A population-based approach to chronic illness. *Ann Behav Med* 1999;21:159–170.

89. Baker SB, Vallbona C, Pavlik V, et al. A diabetes control program in a public health care setting. *Public Health Rep* 1993;108:595–605.

90. Clark CM Jr, Snyder JW, Meek RL, et al. A systematic approach to risk stratification and intervention within a managed care environment improves diabetes outcomes and patient satisfaction. *Diabetes Care* 2001;24:1079–1086.

91. Chin MH, Cook S, Jin L, et al. Barriers to providing diabetes care in community health centers. *Diabetes Care* 2001;24:268–274.

Diabetes and Cardiovascular Disease
edited by Steven P. Marso and David M. Stern
Lippincott Williams & Wilkins, Philadelphia © 2004

11

Obesity

Mark W. Conard and Walker S. Carlos Poston

Department of Clinical Health Psychology, University of Missouri–Kansas City, Department of Clinical Health Outcomes Research, Mid America Heart Institute; Associate Professor, Department of Health Psychology, University of Missouri–Kansas City, Director, Behavioral Cardiology Research, Department of Cardiovascular Research, Saint Luke's Hospital, Kansas City, Missouri

SCOPE OF THE PROBLEM

Obesity is a significant health problem in the United States and other industrialized nations (1). It is a complex, multifaceted chronic disease that involves metabolic, physiologic, biochemical, genetic, behavioral, social, and cultural factors and results from an imbalance between energy expenditure and caloric intake (2). Traditionally, obesity has been defined as an excess of body fat: 25% body fat in men and 33% in women (3). Obesity is associated with greater risk for a number of health problems, including non-insulin-dependent (type 2) diabetes mellitus, hypertension, dyslipidemia, and cardiovascular disease (CVD) (1), and it has been found to be a modifiable and preventable risk factor for these and other medical conditions that can be treated by making lifestyle modifications.

In the year 2000, 64.5% of the adult population in the United States was overweight (i.e., had a body mass index [BMI] of 25 or higher), and 30.5% were obese (BMI, 30 or higher) (4). Secular trend data suggest that obesity prevalence has been increasing steadily over the last 30 years (1). According to the Centers for Disease Control and Prevention (5), 38.8 million adults in the United States were obese in 1999, including an estimated 19.6 million men and 19.2 million women. The highest prevalence rates were among minority groups, with 36.5% of African-American women and 33.3% of Mexican-American women meeting the criteria for obesity. In contrast, the lowest prevalence rates were found in Caucasian and African-American men (20.0% and 20.6%, respectively) (2). Whereas there is an epidemic of obesity in the United States, obesity is increasing worldwide at an alarming rate (6).

At the international level, it appears that the degree of obesity is linked to the levels of urbanization, economic development, and nutrition. Although women appear to have higher rates of obesity than men, being overweight is more common in men than in women (6). The prevalence of obesity appears to be linked to levels of urbanization and development in particular regions. In Africa, little information has been collected on obesity trends, but there has been an increase in the rates of obesity in the developing countries. For instance, in Mauritius the proportion of obese men increased from 3.4% to 5.3% and that of obese women from 10.4% to 15.2% over a 5-year period (6). In comparison, Brazil has undergone a transition from nutritional deficiencies to excess, as indicated by an increase in obesity across all groups of men (3.1% to 5.9%) and women (8.2% to 13.3%) over a 15-year period (6).

Obesity among children has also become an important public health concern, not only because there has been an alarming increase in the prevalence of pediatric obesity, with estimates ranging from 20% to 30% (7,8), but also because obese children are more likely to become obese adults (9) with a heightened risk of CVD (10). For example, the Bogalusa Heart Study found that there was a 50% increase over two decades in the rate of obesity among 6- to 11-year-olds, with the mean weight increasing 0.2 kg per year and mean skinfold thickness increasing by 0.15 mm per year (11). In addition, Schonfeld Warden et al. (12) reported that 80% of obese children become obese adults. Currently, there are approximately 22 million overweight children younger than 5 years of age worldwide. In the United States, approximately 22% of preschool children are overweight, and 10% are obese (13). Similar to the epidemiologic trends for adult-onset (type 2) diabetes mellitus, there is a disproportionate increase in childhood obesity among black and Hispanic children. In these two subgroups, there has been an approximate 20% increase in the prevalence of increased weight (14). Obese adolescents also appear to have an increased propensity for concomitant cardiovascular risk factors, including a heightened cardiovascular risk as adults (15). Obesity among young persons correlates with abnormalities in both systolic and diastolic blood pressure, elevated triglycerides, low levels of high-density lipoproteins (HDL), increased total cholesterol, diminished oxygen consumption, and a strong family history of precocious coronary heart disease (15). Importantly, there is a strong correlation between childhood obesity and the development of insulin resistance, impaired glucose tolerance (16), and type 2 diabetes mellitus (17). This trend has been noted worldwide. For instance, the incidence of type 2 diabetes among Japanese youth increased from 0.2 to 7.3 per 100,000 children per year between 1976 and 1995. This increase is probably attributable to a changing dietary pattern and increasing obesity among Japanese children (18).

In the United States, the costs of obesity were estimated to be $99.2 billion in 1995, with approximately $51.6 billion representing direct medical costs associated with the treatment of obesity-related diseases (1). These direct costs represented about 5.7% of the annual national health expenditure within the United States (19). The indirect costs, which represent the value of lost output (caused by morbidity and mortality), the effects of other medical conditions, and the personal and societal impacts of obesity, were

$47.6 billion (19). CVD and type 2 diabetes accounted for 48% and 17.5% of the indirect costs, respectively (20). The direct medical costs associated with diabetes in 1997 totaled $44.1 billion, with $11.8 billion due to excess prevalence of related chronic complications and $24.6 billion due to excess prevalence of general medical conditions (21).

In a study of the relationship between BMI and future health care costs, individuals with a BMI of 20 to 24.9 averaged costs of $7,673 for outpatient services, $5,460 for inpatient care, $2,450 for pharmacy services, and a total of $15,583 for all medical care over the 8-year investigation period (22). In contrast, for those with a BMI of 30 or higher, the average costs were substantially higher: $8,826 for outpatient services, $7,885 for inpatient care, and $5,000 for pharmacy services, leading to total medical costs of $21,711.

Other researchers reported that average annual total costs were 25% higher among individuals with a BMI of 30 to 34.9 (mild obesity) and 44% higher among those with a BMI of 35 or greater (moderate to severe obesity), compared with normal-weight individuals (23). Similar results were obtained by Pronk et al. (24), who found that the expected mean annualized costs were approximately 12% higher for individuals with a BMI of 30 to 34 and 19% higher for those with a BMI of 35 to 39, compared with normal-weight individuals.

ASSESSING OBESITY AND ITS PREVALENCE

Obese and overweight classifications are assessed routinely by determining an individual's waist circumference or BMI. These are quick methods of ascertaining the level of obesity and subsequent health risk. The BMI is calculated by dividing the individual's weight in kilograms by the square of the height in meters (1). BMI also can be calculated by dividing the weight in pounds by the square of the height in inches and multiplying the product by 704.5. Table 11-1 provides a BMI chart that is commonly used to assess obesity. BMI has been divided into classes to define underweight (BMI less than 18.5), normal

TABLE 11-1. *Body mass index (BMI) chart*

BMI	19	20	21	22	23	24	25	26	27	28	29	30	31	32	33	34	35
Height (in)								Weight (lb)									
58	91	96	100	105	110	115	119	124	129	134	138	143	148	153	158	162	167
59	94	99	104	109	114	119	124	128	133	138	143	148	153	158	163	168	173
60	97	102	107	112	118	123	128	133	138	143	148	153	158	163	168	174	179
61	100	106	111	116	122	127	132	137	143	148	153	158	164	169	174	180	185
62	104	109	115	120	126	131	136	142	147	153	158	164	169	175	180	186	191
63	107	113	118	124	130	135	141	146	152	158	163	169	175	180	186	191	197
64	110	116	122	128	134	140	145	151	157	163	169	174	180	186	192	197	204
65	114	120	126	132	138	144	150	156	162	168	174	180	186	192	198	204	210
66	118	124	130	136	142	148	155	161	167	173	179	186	192	198	204	210	216
67	121	127	134	140	146	153	159	166	172	178	185	191	198	204	211	217	223
68	125	131	138	144	151	158	164	171	177	184	190	197	203	210	216	223	230
69	128	135	142	149	155	162	169	176	182	189	196	203	209	216	223	230	236
70	132	139	146	153	160	167	174	181	188	195	202	209	216	222	229	236	243
71	136	143	150	157	165	172	179	186	193	200	208	215	222	229	236	243	250
72	140	147	154	162	169	177	184	191	199	206	213	221	228	235	242	250	258
73	144	151	159	166	174	182	189	197	204	212	219	227	235	242	250	257	265
74	148	155	163	171	179	186	194	202	210	218	225	233	241	249	256	264	272
75	152	160	168	176	184	192	200	208	216	224	232	240	248	256	264	272	279

National Institutes of Health. Clinical Guidelines on the Identification, Evaluation, and Treatment of Overweight and Obesity in Adults—The Evidence Report. *Obes Res* 1998;6 [Suppl 2]:51S–210S.

weight range (18.5 to 24.9), and overweight (25 to 29.9) individuals (Table 11-2).

Waist circumference is readily obtained, positively correlates with abdominal fat content (1), and provides a clinically acceptable measurement for determining central adiposity. For most adults with BMIs of 25 to 34.9, sex-specific cutoff points for abdominal girth have been determined to identify the increased relative risk for the development of obesity-related risk factors. A waist circumference greater than 102 cm (40 inch) in men or 88 cm (35 inch) in women appears to portend a heightened risk for the development of CVD risk factors (1).

Obesity, defined as a BMI greater than 30, is further divided into three classifications based on risk severity. Class I or mild obesity is defined as a BMI of 30.0 to 34.9. Class II or moder-

ate obesity is defined as a BMI of 35.0 to 39.9. Class III or severe obesity is defined as a BMI of 40 or higher (1). The advantages of using the BMI include its ease of use, its accuracy in measuring both weight and height, and its use of similar criteria independent of gender (2). However, the BMI has limitations, and clinical judgment should be used with certain individuals to avoid overestimating body fat in very muscular individuals or underestimating body fat in individuals who have lost muscle mass (1,25). For example, weight lifters have BMIs in the obese range due to their greater muscle mass, but they have lower body fat percentages. In addition, BMI categories have traditionally been restricted to individuals who are past puberty, and they are not accurate for children. However, researchers have examined the use of BMI in children using different cutoff points. For example, Sinha et al. (16) classified children whose BMIs were higher than the 95th percentile for age and sex as obese. Sinaiko et al. (26) used a broader range of BMI, 14 to 42. Both studies found BMI to be associated with insulin resistance, suggesting this value may, at least in part, correlate with obesity-related risk factors. Further research needs to be conducted to verify appropriate use of BMI and cutoff points in children.

TABLE 11-2. *Classification of obesity using body mass index (BMI)*

Category	BMI
Underweight	<18.5
Normal weight	18.5–24.9
Overweight	25–29.9
Mild obesity	30–34.9
Moderate obesity	35–39.9
Severe obesity	>40

OBESITY-ASSOCIATED COMORBIDITIES

Obesity contributes to an increased risk of multiple comorbid medical conditions (Table 11-3) (1,27–29). An individual with a BMI of 30 or higher is substantially more likely to have some comorbid condition than is an individual with a BMI between 19.0 and 24.9 (23). For example, obese patients are 1.7 times more likely to have heart disease, 2 times more likely to have hypertension, and 3 times more likely to have type 2 diabetes, compared with normal-weight individuals (23).

Type 2 Diabetes Mellitus

Type 2 diabetes mellitus is an emerging global health concern. Of the estimated 16 million persons with diabetes in the United States, a number that is projected to double within the next one to two decades, approximately 90% to 95% have type 2 diabetes. In addition, there are approximately 7 million undiagnosed cases of type 2 diabetes in the United States (30). Importantly, type 2 diabetes mellitus is frequently associated with insulin resistance, hypertension, dyslipidemia, advanced age, and obesity. The underpinnings of the increasing prevalence are not fully understood, but they probably are linked to the current obesity epidemic and the high levels of sedentary lifestyle in the United States. The prevalence of obesity is projected to increase sharply as the population ages (31–34). This increase in type 2 diabetes is substantially more common among overweight individuals older than 40 years of age, and the same trend is emerging in many developed and developing nations (34,35). According to the National Institutes of Health (NIH), among individuals diagnosed with type 2 diabetes, 67% have a BMI of 27 or greater, and 46% have a BMI of 30 or greater (36). Field et al. (37) found that a BMI of 35.0 or higher was associated with a 17-fold increased relative risk for development of diabetes in women (95% confidence interval [CI], 14.2 to 20.5) and a 23.4-fold increase in men (CI, 19.4 to 33.2), compared with individuals in the normal range of BMI. Those who were overweight were three times more likely to develop diabetes than those in the normal range of BMI.

Overweight and obesity contribute importantly to type 2 diabetes through increasing excess body fat and insulin resistance and possibly through accelerating the decline in insulin secretion that is required for development of clinical diabetes (38). At the insulin receptor site, the receptors are downregulated, resulting in a decrease in the number of these receptors across the membrane surface. This reduction causes a decrease in the binding of circulating insulin to receptors and impairs intercellular communication concerning insulin (39). At the postreceptor site, there is a reduction in the entrance of glucose into the cell and its use by insulin-sensitive cells, resulting in increased circulating glucose. This increase in blood glucose causes the pancreas to produce greater amounts of insulin as long as the person is overweight, eventually exhausting the pancreas and causing diabetes (40). After onset of type 2 diabetes, weight reduction still reduces insulin resistance and mitigates the metabolic risk factors associated with diabetes. Nonetheless, because of loss of beta-cell function, hyperglycemia may persist despite weight loss. In spite of these limitations, weight management in patients with type 2 diabetes must remain one component of risk factor management (38).

Type 2 diabetes mellitus affects many organ systems, often leading to blindness, renal failure, neuropathy, chronic skin changes, cerebrovascular disease, and CVD (36). In 2002, diabetes accounted for 43% of new cases of end-stage renal disease. CVD is more common in persons with type 2 diabetes than in nondiabetic individuals (41,42), with the relative risks for incident

TABLE 11-3. *Obesity-related comorbidities*

Type 2 diabetes
Hypertension
Dyslipidemia
Cardiovascular disease
Cerebrovascular disease
Gallbladder disorders
Certain cancers
Osteoarthritis
Insulin resistance
Sleep disorders
Respiratory disorders

coronary heart disease ranging from 1.7 to 3.1, depending on the epidemiologic data (30). Type 2 diabetes-related mortality is estimated to account for 17.2% of all deaths in the United States among persons 25 years of age or older (30). The risk of stroke is two to four times higher in people with diabetes (36). Diabetes also is the leading cause of new cases of blindness among adults 20 to 74 years old. Additionally, the complications of neuropathy due to diabetes can lead to amputations of legs, feet, and hands. Diabetes disrupts individuals' abilities to function and carry on activities of daily living.

Hypertension

The connection between obesity and hypertension has long been documented, yet the exact association is unknown (43). Much of the research has found that obesity and hypertension are linked through fluid retention and its effects on the body, resulting in hypertension. Several studies have quantified the impact of obesity on the risk for hypertension. Past research found that obese patients are two times more likely to be diagnosed with hypertension than are normal-weight individuals (23). More recently, the Framingham Heart Study found that both overweight and obesity were highly related to the risk of hypertension in both men and women (RR = 1.5 to 1.7 for overweight, 2.2 to 2.6 for obesity) (44). Other research has found that women who are overweight but not obese are at a higher risk for the development of hypertension than are women of normal weight (RR = 1.7; CI, 1.6 to 1.7) (37).

Understanding that obesity and hypertension are closely linked, researchers have examined the effect of weight reduction on hypertension (45). In phase II of the Trials of Hypertension Prevention (TOHP II), researchers attempted to understand the impact of weight loss on blood pressure by examining the changes seen in the most adherent subjects (45). Those subjects who lost the most weight (more than 4.4 kg) had a reduction of 5 mm Hg in systolic pressure and 7 mm Hg in diastolic pressure. For every 2 lb of body weight lost, there was a reduction of 1 mm Hg in systolic pressure and 1.4 mm Hg in diastolic

pressure. These findings demonstrate the health benefits of reducing weight in subjects with hypertension.

Cardiovascular Disease

Obesity increases the risks of developing CVD; however, there is some argument as to whether obesity is integral to CVD-related morbidity and mortality (28). There is little disagreement regarding the impact of obesity on other independent risk factors for CVD (i.e., hypertension, dyslipidemia, and diabetes) (28). The connection between obesity and CVD exists, as demonstrated in numerous studies such as the Framingham Heart Study. Wilson et al. (44) found that the age-adjusted relative risk for CVD was increased in overweight individuals (for men, RR = 1.21; CI, 1.05 to 1.40; for women, RR = 1.20; CI, 1.03 to 1.41) and in those who were obese (for men, RR = 1.46; CI, 1.20 to 1.77; for women, RR = 1.64; CI, 1.37 to 1.98). Additionally, Kenchaiah et al. (29) examined the impact of obesity on the development of heart failure. They found that the risk of heart failure was doubled for obese individuals (for men, RR = 1.90; CI, 1.30 to 2.79; for women, RR = 2.12; CI, 1.51 to 2.97).

Obesity increases the risk of CVD-related mortality by up to twofold as well (1,46). A study of patients with CAD found that a BMI greater than 35 was associated with a sevenfold increase in mortality risk (OR = 7.4, $p < .001$) (27). The leading cause of death for patients with type 2 diabetes (approximately 50%) is CVD. The risk of CVD-related mortality is approximately two to four times higher for individuals with type 2 diabetes than for nondiabetic persons (30,36). In fact, the presence of diabetes among women essentially abolishes the protection against CVD conferred by being female. Additionally, Field et al. (37) found that overweight women were significantly more likely to develop heart disease than were women in the normal range of BMI (RR = 1.4; CI, 1.2 to 1.5).

Dyslipidemia

Obesity tends to result in two lipid abnormalities: an increase in triglycerides and a decrease in HDL cholesterol (28). The increase in triglyceride levels is a consequence of both increased production from the liver and decreased clearance at the periphery. The increased productivity of the liver causes increased levels of very-low-density lipoproteins, which transport triglycerides (28). Additionally, there is a decrease in lipoprotein lipase, which hydrolyzes triglycerides. Both of these processes result in an increase in triglycerides. The low HDL cholesterol concentration acts in combination with mildly elevated or normal-range low-density lipoprotein (LDL) cholesterol to significantly increase the risks of CVD (28). The prevalence of abnormal cholesterol levels (240 mg/dL or higher) in the original Framingham Heart Study sample was approximately 30% to 45%, and those individuals with increased cholesterol levels (275 mg/dL or higher) had an increased risk of adverse outcomes regardless of whether they were healthy or had coronary artery disease (CAD) at baseline (47). Additionally, Field et al. (37) found that women who were overweight but not obese were significantly more likely than those with normal

weights to have high cholesterol levels (RR = 1.1; CI, 1.1 to 1.2).

Dyslipidemia is an additional and well-known risk factor for CVD (48), especially for individuals with type 2 diabetes (49). For instance, subjects with elevated cholesterol levels were found to have an increased risk of adverse outcomes whether they were healthy or diagnosed with CVD at baseline, including a risk ratio of 3.8 for reinfarction and 2.6 for CVD mortality (47). During 12 years of follow-up of the Framingham Heart Study cohort, 11% of the men and 4.7% of the women developed coronary heart disease (48).

Mortality

Increasing body mass is associated with greater mortality risk (1,37,50–53). For example, Calle et al. (50) found that Caucasian men and women in the highest BMI category had increased risks of death (RR = 2.58 for men, 2.00 for women). In addition, a high BMI was most predictive of CVD mortality, especially in men (RR = 2.90;

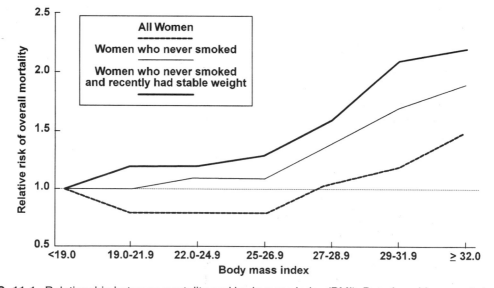

FIG. 11-1. Relationship between mortality and body mass index (BMI). Data from Manson et al. and the Nurses Health Study (52) suggest that when mortality risk is adjusted for disease-related health status and smoking, the leanest women (BMI <20) have the lowest mortality risk and that the mortality risk increases with increasing BMI. (Adapted with permission from World Health Organization [1998]. Obesity: preventing and managing the global epidemic. *Consultation on obesity report.*)

CI, 2.37 to 3.56). Further, in a study of Norwegian men, researchers found a J-shaped relationship between BMI and all-cause mortality, with individuals in the highest BMI categories having increased risk for death. For a BMI of 27 to 29.9, the relative risk was 1.31 (CI, 1.16 to 1.48), and for a BMI of 30 or higher, it was 1.64 (CI, 1.37 to 1.95) (51). Among women, a similar J-shaped association was discovered, with the relative risk of all-cause mortality increasing as categories of BMI increased: 1.2 for a BMI of 22.0 to 24.9, 1.3 for BMI 25.0 to 26.9, 1.6 for BMI 27.0 to 28.9, 2.1 for BMI 29.0 to 31.9, and 2.2 for BMI 32.0 or higher (p for trend, $<.001$) (52). Figure 11-1 provides a graphical representation of this relationship; the J shaped curve indicates that the mortality risk increases as the BMI increases. Although there appears to be ample evidence regarding the impact of obesity on the risk of mortality, there is considerable debate as to how strong the association is and whether the relationship is linear, J-shaped, or U-shaped (37,53). This controversy stems from whether studies examining this association were adequately controlled for various factors that may account for this relationship, including physical activity, smoking, and comorbid illnesses (53). Yet, studies that are controlled for potential confounding factors do find a positive relationship between increasing levels of obesity (i.e., high BMI) and mortality.

RISK FACTORS ASSOCIATED WITH OBESITY

Caloric Intake

One environmental risk factor contributing to obesity is a diet that is high in calories and fat. Americans eat approximately 150 more calories per day than they did 10 years ago (29). This increase in fat and calories, mainly from carbohydrates, affects the development of insulin resistance and CVD. Most notably, an increased amount of saturated fats consumed increases the incidence of insulin resistance, blood pressure, and cholesterol levels (54,55). In contrast, diets that increase monounsaturated fats improve the insulin resistance syndrome (55). Addition-

ally, there are consistent research findings linking insulin resistance to the development of CVD, indicating that the two have many similar risk factors and resulting disorders (54). These findings support the recommendation that lowering one's intake of saturated fats will lead to numerous health benefits.

Diet has long been discussed as a possible cause of diabetes, with caloric intake, carbohydrates, and fats considered to be leading dietary macronutrients affecting diabetes (34). However, a recent review of diet and type 2 diabetes (34) found that previous studies provided inconsistent results, and several did not demonstrate significant relationships between dietary carbohydrate or fiber intake and type 2 diabetes. Diets high in saturated fats have been associated consistently with an occurrence of type 2 diabetes (34).

The Health Professionals Follow-up Study examined the impact of diet on the development of type 2 diabetes (56). This study examined two types of dietary patterns: the prudent dietary pattern, which consisted of a higher consumption of vegetables, fruits, fish, poultry, and whole grains, and the Western dietary pattern, which consisted of a higher consumption of red meat, processed meat, French fries, high-fat dairy products, refined grains, sweets, and desserts. Van Dam et al. (56) found that the Western dietary pattern was associated with a substantially higher risk for type 2 diabetes (RR = 1.59; CI, 1.31 to 1.93; $p < .001$ for trend) and the prudent dietary pattern was associated with a moderately reduced risk for type 2 diabetes (RR = 0.84; CI, 0.7 to 1.0). In examining these multivariate relationships, the researchers controlled for numerous lifestyle factors, including physical activity, cigarette smoking, alcohol consumption, hypertension, and family history of type 2 diabetes.

There has been growing interest in the effect of adding or increasing omega-3 fatty acids to the diet. Rewers and Hamman (57) noted that diets high in omega-3 fatty acids appear to protect against the development of type 2 diabetes by lowering serum lipids, lipoproteins, platelet aggregation, blood pressure, and insulin resistance. Additionally, omega-3 fatty acids have been found to aid in the protection against CVD, its many comorbidities, and CVD mortality in similar ways (58,59). For instance, researchers have found that the effects of omega-3 fatty acids lead to improvements in lipids and lipoprotein metabolism and reductions in triglyceride levels, blood pressure, CAD progression, and heart rate. Omega-3 fatty acids are mainly derived from fish and fish oils but also can be found in some vegetable oils (58,59). In their review of the effects of omega-3 fatty acids in animals and humans, Mori and Beilin (59) noted that triglyceride levels are reduced by approximately 25% to 30%. Another impact of omega-3 fatty acids is on the progression of coronary heart disease (60). Research has shown slowed progression of the disease and, in some cases, more regression after 2 years. Other researchers found that omega-3 fatty acids combined with a weight loss program significantly decreased triglycerides by 38% ($p < .001$) and increased HDL$_2$ cholesterol by 24% ($p = .04$) (61). These results support the recommendations that omega-3 fatty acids should be incorporated into the diet of both healthy individuals and those who are at risk for CAD or who have established CAD (58,59).

Physical Inactivity

Americans have become increasingly sedentary in both work and leisure (1), such that 70% of adults are underactive and 50% do not exercise on a regular basis (62). As a result, 1 in 10 persons dies prematurely from chronic diseases associated with physical inactivity (63). This results in an annualized 250,000 premature deaths secondary to CAD, type 2 diabetes mellitus, and colon cancer. Physical activity results in measurable improvements in endothelium-dependent vasodilation, both in coronary arteries and in resistance vessels (64); improved glucose handling via improved insulin sensitivity, most likely mediated through the glucose transporter GLUT4 (65); and improved lipoprotein metabolism, with a reduction in circulating postprandial triglyceride levels (66). Physical inactivity is a readily modifiable risk factor, and when activity is increased, health is improved. For example, in the Nurses Health Study involving more than 72,000

women, brisk walking resulted in a 30% reduction in the incidence of coronary heart disease (67), stroke (68), and type 2 diabetes mellitus (69). Other studies have found that increased levels of physical activity are associated with a lower incidence of type 2 diabetes (57). This protective effect results from the prevention of insulin resistance, but some studies suggest that the effect differs depending on the level of insulin that was present when physical activity was initiated (57). The overall results from these studies suggest that increased physical activity decreases the risk of type 2 diabetes.

GENETICS OF OBESITY

A great deal of attention has been focused on the genetics of obesity. Like many chronic disorders, obesity is the final common pathway of the interplay of many genes and the environment. Genetic influences have been found to contribute to differences in resting metabolic rate (70), body fat distribution (71), and weight gain in response to overfeeding (72). The eighth (2001) update of the human obesity gene map indicates that obesity is a complex, polygenic disease (73). According to this update, 174 studies have reported a positive association to obesity phenotype, with variation in specific genes among 58 candidate genes located on all chromosomes except for Y. An increasing number of these studies are being done, and the resulting observations will, no doubt, increase the biochemical understanding of obesity. However, it should be noted that there have been no major shifts in the obesity gene pool to account for the epidemic of obesity during the last decade. Environmental factors, which interact with obesity-promoting genes, are therefore important to understanding the current increasing prevalence of obesity. Environmental factors are also readily modifiable and can have an immediate impact on the health of individual patients and society overall (74).

RISK FACTORS IN SPECIAL POPULATIONS

As previously noted, the prevalences of obesity and type 2 diabetes are higher among members of ethnic minority groups (2,30,75). This of special concern particularly in developing countries, where both diseases are on the increase. The epidemiologic underpinnings are unknown, but recent studies suggest that lower levels of income, education, and social class are associated with increased prevalence of type 2 diabetes (57) and obesity (76). In addition, urban residents have higher rates of type 2 diabetes, compared with residents of rural areas (57,77). For example, a study examining the prevalence of type 2 diabetes in Japan found that the age-adjusted prevalence in men was two times higher in an urban area than in a rural area (78). Singh et al. (79) discovered that the prevalences of type 2 diabetes and CAD were higher in urban areas of north India than in rural areas (type 2 diabetes, 6.0% versus 2.8%; CAD, 9.0% versus 3.2%).

Connected to socioeconomic status is a belief that acculturation to a Western lifestyle affects the incidence of type 2 diabetes, but studies examining this link have yielded inconsistent results (57). Other theories about this association contend that acculturation occurs more easily among individuals who appear less different from the dominant culture (e.g., lighter skinned African-Americans and Hispanics in the United States). Studies have shown that those who are the most acculturated and lighter skinned also have lowered risk of type 2 diabetes, compared with the least acculturated and darker-skinned individuals (57). The difficulty in separating out the confounding between acculturation and genetics is great and requires more clarification in future studies. Studies examining migrant groups also have found consistently high prevalence rates of type 2 diabetes, obesity, and other comorbid conditions with Westernization. These conditions are usually accompanied by increases in obesity, decreases in physical activity, and increases in fat and caloric intake (57,74,80).

TREATMENT STRATEGIES FOR OBESITY

An essential component in the management of obesity and type 2 diabetes is the modification of lifestyle. The focus is on creating realistic expectations for success and awareness of one's behaviors, increasing physical activity, and normalizing caloric consumption. In addition to lifestyle modifications, obesity pharmacotherapy and surgery are available.

Psychosocial Treatments

Seven basic lifestyle modification approaches are used to decrease caloric consumption and to increase physical activity: setting realistic goals, self-monitoring, stimulus control, cognitive restructuring, stress management, relapse prevention training, and social support (2).

Setting Realistic Goals

On average, a patient will lose 8% to 10% of his or her baseline weight in an intervention program, but most obese patients desire additional weight loss. Therefore, an important early treatment strategy is to assist patients in setting realistic weight loss goals. For example, a physician might encourage a patient to adopt small behavioral changes in eating and physical activity and to concentrate on the health benefits associated with these changes (2). This type of approach provides the patient with dual benefits: feelings of success for meeting short-term goals and movement toward the long-term goal of weight loss that can be maintained (2). These goals tend to be individualized to each patient's needs. Some examples of possible goals include not having second helpings at a meal, eating smaller portions, eating low-fat snacks during the day, exercising at least 15 minutes during the week, and taking a walk during work breaks. The goals can begin as small steps and progress to larger ones (e.g., increasing amounts of exercise) as the patient gains reinforcement from achieving the smaller goals.

Self-monitoring

A key lifestyle modification strategy is self-monitoring (2). Self-monitoring involves the systematic observation and recording of specific target behaviors, related feelings, and environmental cues (81). This technique is particularly useful for patients who are attempting weight loss, because it raises their awareness of their eating behaviors and physical activity levels, as well as what factors may be affecting these behaviors. Self-monitoring tools include (a) food diaries to record total caloric intake, total fat grams consumed, food groups used, and situations in which overeating is common; (b) physical activity logs to record the frequency, duration, and intensity of exercise and electronic devices that count the number of steps taken; and (c) weight scales or body composition measures to record changes in weight, body fat, or lean body mass (82).

Accuracy in self-reporting of behavior is desirable but does not usually occur, and absolute accuracy is not necessary (2). For example, patients tend to underestimate caloric consumption by about one third and to overestimate physical activity by about one half. Self-monitoring is beneficial even with some inaccuracy because it provides an increased awareness of eating and physical activity behaviors, possibly leading to an actionable change in eating and exercise habits (83,84). Self-monitoring strategies have been found to be consistently effective in improving treatment outcomes, and patients report that they are one of the most helpful tools in obesity management (81,85,86).

Stimulus Control

Stimulus control involves the identification and modification of environmental cues that contribute to overeating and inactivity (81). Once the environmental cues have been identified, patients can devise strategies to control them, which can be useful in maintaining long-term weight loss (87). Various techniques to help control common environmental cues include eating only at the kitchen table without watching television, keeping no snack foods in the house, and placing exercise clothes out the night before as a reminder to jog in the morning.

Cognitive Restructuring

Cognitive restructuring refers to encouraging patients to examine their inner thoughts, feelings, and beliefs about themselves and their weight and challenging them to modify those beliefs that

are inaccurate or counterproductive (87). This method is particularly useful with obese patients, because many of them have poor self-esteem and distorted body image. In addition, some obese patients are unrealistic about how much weight they can lose and about the benefits of weight loss (82). The goal of cognitive restructuring is to identify these self-defeating cognitions and to assist the patient in replacing them with more productive and affirming ones (2).

Stress Management

Stress management training is useful in the management of weight loss, because stress has been found to be a strong predictor of overeating and relapse (86,88). There are a number of techniques to manage stress and reduce associated sympathetic nervous system arousal. These techniques include diaphragmatic breathing, stress inoculation training, progressive muscle relaxation, and meditation (82). By reducing the stress response, an individual derives numerous benefits (e.g., more positive well-being, reduced autonomic tone), which may lead to less frequent stress-related eating and reduction in weight and cardiovascular risk factors.

Relapse Prevention

Relapse prevention training attempts to normalize lapses (i.e., breaks from an activity or dietary change program) as an acceptable part of weight-loss management (83,87). Relapse prevention teaches patients to accept lapses as inevitable and prepares them to manage lapses by minimizing the damage and getting back on the road to weight loss as quickly as possible. This technique lessens the chance that a full relapse will occur.

Social Support

Research has demonstrated that patients with high levels of positive social support tend to have greater success in achieving and maintaining weight losses than do those lacking in support (86). High levels of social support also improve adherence to obesity management programs (83,89). Improving social support can involve inclusion of family members and friends in the weight loss intervention, participation in community-based programs, involvement in outside social activities (e.g., university or community education courses, health clubs, church-related activities), or referrals to groups of individuals with similar goals (2,82). Social support helps patients become more self-accepting, develop new norms for interpersonal relationships, and manage stressful work- or family-related situations (86,87).

Increasing Physical Activity

The U. S. population has become increasingly sedentary in recent years. Physical activity is associated with improvements in a number of comorbid obesity-related medical conditions, including reduced risk for CVD and type 2 diabetes, reduced blood pressure, improved lipoprotein metabolism, and improved insulin sensitivity, and it is an important predictor of weight loss maintenance (1,62). The type, frequency, intensity, and duration of activity should be considered when adding physical activity to a weight loss program (2). The activities selected should be matched to the individual's physical and psychological limitations to ensure consistency and enhance adherence.

The American College of Sports Medicine (ACSM) has recommended specific guidelines for exercise-induced weight loss (90). These guidelines recommend that total energy intake be reduced by 500 to 1,000 kcal/day and that overweight and obese individuals increase their physical activity to a minimum of 150 minutes of moderate exercise per week. For long-term weight loss, the ACSM recommends increasing physical activity (e.g., 200 to 300 minutes per week or at least 2,000 kcal/week of leisure-time physical activity) (90). However, these goals may not be realistic for obese patients just beginning a weight loss program or for those limited by possible complications due to other illnesses (e.g., CVD). Obese patients should begin a program slowly, building to moderate levels of activity (e.g., brisk walking) for 30 to 40 minutes, three to five times per week (an expenditure of 150 to

225 kcal per session) (1). The focus of physical activity should be weight loss, with maximum physical exertion not required. Moderate-intensity lifestyle activity can be as effective as higher-intensity exertion in burning calories (2,91,92). Talking with patients about the benefits of moderate-intensity exercise and encouraging small increases in physical activity may lead to modest efforts that contribute to overall treatment adherence.

It is essential that all persons begin a physical activity regimen in consultation with their physician and health care team. Unfortunately, the term "exercise" often has many negative connotations for patients, resulting in a reluctance to begin the process of physical activity. Sedentary persons can derive significant health-related benefits from merely increasing their physical activity in daily living. The concept of "functional physical activity" diminishes the barriers to begin a lifestyle focused on healthy behavior rather than the activity of exercise. Examples include taking the stairs rather than the elevator, choosing the farthest parking spot rather than the closest, walking or bicycling short distances rather than driving, and beginning hobbies that increase physical activity (93).

Two subgroups that deserve special attention with respect to increasing physical activity are children and the elderly. Children have become increasingly sedentary. For example, it is estimated that approximately two thirds of Canadian children are below the level of physical activity thought to be requisite for optimal growth and development (94). Physical inactivity appears to be more common in female children and adolescents. This has resulted in a gradual decline in muscular strength, flexibility, and endurance. It follows that there has been a near-doubling of childhood obesity in recent decades (95). There remains a strong correlation between childhood obesity and hours spent watching television. The prevalence of obesity was lowest among children who watched less than 1 hour of television daily and was greatest among those who watched 4 or more hours daily (96).

Physical inactivity increases among the elderly and directly contributes to muscle wasting, bone loss, insulin resistance, diminished cardiac output, orthostatic intolerance, and diminished immune function. Although implementation of a regular physical activity program in elderly persons is challenging, a recent intervention program was found to increase weekly caloric expenditure among persons age 65 to 90 years of age by 46% (97). Therefore, it is neither too late nor too early to initiate healthy behavior such as a routine physical fitness program.

Sporadic counseling during routine scheduled office visits is not an effective method of increasing long-lasting physical activity (98). There are numerous barriers to implementing an effective clinical program resulting in an increase in physical activity. The three major barriers cited by physicians are inadequate time for counseling, lack of necessary skills and tools to provide counseling, and lack of reimbursement from health care insurance and managed care plans (99). Although brief recommendations are ineffectual, health care professionals can successfully implement an exercise-counseling regimen that results in improved activity. A comprehensive strategy, including office visits, telephone interviews, and newsletters totaling 22 contacts from the health care provider's office over 2 years, resulted in a marked improvement in regular physical activity (100). This increase in activity led to a 5% increase in maximal aerobic capacity, which would translate into a reduction of approximately 9% in all-cause mortality (101).

Modifying Diet

The U. S. Department of Agriculture (USDA) guidelines recommend that individuals reduce their calorie intake by 500 to 1,000 kcal/day from the current level, which will lead to a weight loss of 0.45 to 0.9 kg (1 to 2 lb) per week (1). According to these guidelines, women may follow a diet of 1,000 to 1,200 kcal/day, and men 1,200 to 1,600 kcal/day (1). A reduction of 500 calories per day will result in a loss of 1 lb/week (2). Determining an appropriate caloric intake, along with self-monitoring, enables patients to attain better control over their diet. However, knowing the amount of calories in a given meal is not easy. When in doubt, patients should focus on portion sizes, especially in regard to foods known to be high in fat content (2).

In addition to reducing calories, patients should be encouraged to lower the amount of fat and "empty calories" that they ingest. Previous research has found that lowering total dietary fat (especially saturated fat) and modifying caloric intake reduces CVD risk in obese diabetics (102). The Food Guide Pyramid (103) and the Exchange Lists for Meal Planning (104) can be helpful in determining which foods to eat and the number of servings that promote healthy eating. By following a balanced, reduced-calorie diet, with choices made according to USDA recommendations, patients are more likely to achieve and maintain their desired weight loss.

A specialized very-low-calorie diet (VLCD) is commonly used with severely obese individuals and consists of eating less than 800 kcal/day. Normally, VLCDs involve consuming a prepared liquid formula or only lean meat, fish, or fowl (105). These diets, although stringent, have been demonstrated to be safe if conducted under medical supervision. VLCDs have been found to be effective for short-term weight loss and rapid improvement in obesity-related medical conditions (106), with weight losses in the range of 9 kg (22.5 lb) in 12 weeks (105). VLCDs have been in existence since the 1920's but did not come into widespread use until the 1990's, when the formulations were improved with a better balance of nutrients and a higher quality of foods. VLCDs should generally be used for only those patients with a BMI greater than 30. VLCDs coupled with behavior modification strategies appear to be the most efficacious approach, resulting in magnified weight loss and a reduction in weight regain, compared with the use of a VLCD as the sole weight loss strategy. Pekkarinen and Mustajoki (107) found that results were significantly better when VLCDs were combined with behavior therapy than when VLCDs were used alone. In their study, patients using a combination of a VLCD plus a 16-week behavior modification program achieved significantly greater mean weight changes than did patients using only a VLCD (−22.9 kg versus −8.9 kg, respectively; $p < .001$). These results were still evident at the 5-year follow-up (−16.9 kg versus −4.9 kg, respectively; $p = .03$) (107). When combined with exercise, VLCDs have been shown to promote long-term maintenance of weight loss.

However, the long-term effects of VLCDs are discouraging, and many individuals regain their lost weight within 5 years (106).

Outcomes Associated with Lifestyle Modification

Incorporating lifestyle modification strategies into obesity management programs produces average weight losses of about 10 kg (22 lb) over 6 months (82). Intervention programs typically last 20 to 24 weeks and include multiple treatment strategies. Patients tend to maintain about two thirds of their initial weight loss 9 to 10 months after the termination of their treatment. Although a weight loss of 5% to 10% of initial weight can confer health benefits, it is not known how long these health benefits last or how quickly the gradual weight gain after treatment termination mitigates these benefits (1). Attrition rates are usually low (less than 18%). There is greater weight loss when multiple lifestyle modification strategies are used (1).

The Diabetes Prevention Project, a lifestyle intervention trial, compared a comprehensive lifestyle modification program with (initially) two other antidiabetic agents, metformin and troglitazone, in reducing the incidence of type 2 diabetes (108). The troglitazone arm was discontinued with the withdrawal of this agent from the market subsequent to severe and unexpected hepatotoxicity. The lifestyle modification program consisted of a 16-lesson curriculum covering diet, exercise, and behavior modification designed to teach the participants to eat a healthy, low-fat, low-calorie diet and to engage in moderate physical activity. The metformin group took an initial dose of 850 mg orally once daily; at 1 month, the dose was increased to 850 mg twice daily unless gastrointestinal side effects warranted a slower titration period (108).

Both groups showed reduced incidence of type 2 diabetes, but the results for the lifestyle modification group were much more pronounced than those for the metformin group. At follow-up, the incidence of type 2 diabetes was 4.8 cases per 100 person-years with lifestyle modification, compared with 7.8 cases per 100 person-years with metformin. The investigators reported that the lifestyle modification intervention reduced the incidence of type 2 diabetes by 58%, compared with 31% in the metformin group. Additionally, the average weight loss was 5.6 kg in the former group and 2.1 kg in the latter ($p < .001$), and half of the lifestyle modification group obtained a weight loss of 7% or more by the end of the program. Likewise, 74% of the lifestyle modification group had met the goal of at least 150 minutes of physical activity per week by the end of the program. When treatments were compared across various subgroups (sex, gender, age, ethnicity, BMI, and plasma glucose concentration), the lifestyle modification program was highly effective in all subgroups. However, lifestyle intervention was more advantageous than metformin in older individuals and in those with lower BMIs (108).

Pharmacotherapy

Although lifestyle modifications appear to be helpful for most obese patients, they do not ensure long-term weight-loss maintenance (82). Current NIH clinical guidelines view pharmacotherapy as an adjunct to lifestyle modification programs (1). Pharmacotherapy is appropriate for patients with a BMI of 30 or greater and for those with a BMI of 27 or greater in the presence of other comorbidities (hypertension, dyslipidemia, or type 2 diabetes) (1).

The effectiveness of drug therapy and behavior modification suggests an opportunity for enhanced weight reduction in subjects undergoing behavior modification therapy. In one study, behavior therapy alone or in combination with drug therapy resulted in greater weight loss than in a wait-list control group (10.9, 15.3, and 1.3 kg, respectively) (109). Obesity drugs, in conjunction with dietary programs, typically result in modest weight losses (2 to 10 kg) compared with placebo groups (1). A recent, comprehensive metaanalysis of randomized clinical trials of obesity medications found similar results: the incremental benefit of adding obesity medications to a lifestyle modification program was modest but clinically significant (110). No drug or class of drugs demonstrated clear superiority, and the effect of drug treatment was maximal within the first 6 months after initiation, with

TABLE 11-4. *List of obesity drugs*

Agent	DEA schedule	Action
Diethylpropion (Tenuate)	IV	Noradrenergic
Mazindol (Sanorex)	IV	Noradrenergic
Orlistat[a] (Xenical)	None	Lipase inhibitor
Phendimetrazine (Plegine)	III	Noradrenergic
Phentermine (Fastin)	IV	Noradrenergic
Phentermine resin (Ionamin)	IV	Noradrenergic
Phenylpropanolamine (Dexatrim)	Over-the-counter	Noradrenergic
Sibutramine[a] (Meridia)	IV	SNRI

DEA, Drug Enforcement Agency; SNRI, serotonergic noradrenergic reuptake inhibitor.
[a]Orlistat and sibutramine are the only drugs labeled by the U.S. Food and Drug Administration for long-term treatment of obesity.

weight loss being generally maintained for the duration of the treatment (82,110). The various medications for weight loss fall into two broad categories: appetite suppressants, which decrease intake through reducing appetite or increasing satiety, and drugs that decrease nutrient absorption (111). Table 11-4 lists examples of available obesity medications.

Noradrenergic Agents

Noradrenergic agents affect weight by suppressing a patient's appetite. Noradrenergic agents include phentermine resin (Ionamin), mazindol (Sanorex), phenylpropanolamine (Dexatrim), phendimetrazine (Plegine), and diethylpropion (Tenuate). When combined with dietary programs, these medications produce modest short-term weight losses compared with placebo. The U. S. Food and Drug Administration (FDA) has not approved any of these drugs for the long-term treatment of obesity (82). Side effects include increased heart rate and blood pressure, insomnia, constipation, and dry mouth (111).

Serotonin and Noradrenaline Reuptake Inhibition

Sibutramine (Meridia) is a serotonin and noradrenaline reuptake inhibitor. It is approved by the FDA for the long-term treatment of obesity. Sibutramine was developed initially as an antidepressant (112). However, weight loss was seen in depressed patients who were not actively attempting to lose weight (82). Clinical studies have shown that sibutramine produces losses of 4.7 to 7.6 kg (10.3 to 16.7 lb) in patients receiving

the drug, compared with placebo. Weight loss is dose dependent and reaches a plateau at 6 months (113,114). In more than 20 trials, weight loss was significantly greater among sibutramine-treated patients (who lost about 6% to 10% of body weight over 6 to 12 months) than among patients given the placebo (82).

Side effects of sibutramine include a mean increase in blood pressure of 1 to 3 mm Hg and a mean increase in heart rate of about 4 beats/minute, with a few patients experiencing a significant increase in blood pressure (113). These potentially clinically significant increases have been documented with an incidence of 2% relative to placebo in patients with uncomplicated obesity (2). Care should be taken when prescribing sibutramine for patients with a history of hypertension, and it should not be given to those with poorly controlled blood pressure. There have been no reported cases of ischemic coronary problems, arrhythmias, cerebrovascular difficulties, neurotoxicity, primary pulmonary hypertension, or valvular heart disease in patients taking sibutramine compared with placebo (2,113). Drug interactions occur with monoamine oxidase inhibitors (MAOIs), selective serotonin reuptake inhibitors (SSRIs), erythromycin, and ketoconazole (2).

Lipase Inhibition

Orlistat (Xenical) is a lipase inhibitor that works by reducing the body's absorption of dietary fat. It is a nonsystemic drug that blocks about 30% of dietary fat intake (115). Orlistat has been approved by the FDA for long-term use. One clinical study reported weight loss of about 5 kg

(11 lb) after 12 weeks of treatment with orlistat (360 mg/day), compared with a 2- to 3-kg loss (4.4 to 6.6 lb) in the placebo group (116). Weight loss appeared to be dose dependent, with lower doses producing smaller losses. Orlistat use has been associated with a reduction in circulating LDL and insulin levels (117). A number of 2-year randomized, double-blind, prospective studies have found that patients lose significantly more weight with orlistat than with placebo and improve their health profiles (2).

The contraindications for the use of orlistat include chronic malabsorption syndrome and cholestasis (2). Side effects include changes in bowel habits, such as oily or loose stools, the need to have a bowel movement quickly, bloating, and oily spotting. These side effects tend to occur when individuals consume more than 30% of calories from fat and can be minimized once patients lower the fat content of their diet to less than 30%. Orlistat reduces the absorption of fat-soluble vitamins A, D, E, and K as well as β-carotene. Patients taking orlistat should take a multivitamin supplement containing fat-soluble vitamins (2).

Because of the difficulty in maintaining weight loss over time, studies have been conducted on the role of pharmacologic treatments for weight loss maintenance. For example, orlistat-treated patients had significantly lower weight regains than did individuals randomly assigned to placebo treatment (118,119). Sibutramine is helpful in maintaining weight loss after a VLCD; 75% of patients taking sibutramine maintained 100% of their initial weight loss for 1 year, compared with only 42% of those taking placebo (120). James et al. (121) found that 43% of sibutramine-treated patients maintained a greater amount of their initial weight loss, compared with 16% of the placebo group. However, Yanovski and Yanovski (111) noted that none of the FDA-approved weight-loss medications has been studied for effectiveness and safety for weight maintenance over periods longer than 2 years.

Surgery

Past surgical treatments for obesity have included wiring the patient's jaw to lower caloric intake

and jejunoileal bypass to induce malabsorption. Both of these treatments were abandoned, jaw wiring due to lack of long-term efficacy and intestinal bypass surgery due to unacceptable side effects (122). Currently, gastric partitioning is used to decrease the intake of food by increasing satiety through reducing the size of the patient's stomach. The current NIH guidelines for surgical interventions indicate that this option is acceptable only for carefully selected patients with severe obesity (defined as a BMI of 40 or higher, or a BMI of 35 or higher with other comorbidities when less invasive techniques have failed to work) (1).

Because severely obese patients traditionally have not been helped by the more conservative interventions such as lifestyle modification (2), the surgical option is seen as a reasonable approach for those patients who are at increased risk for premature death and whose potential benefits from the procedure outweigh the risks involved (123). The effectiveness of surgical interventions has been well documented, with weight losses of 100 lb or more 12 months after surgery (2). Additionally, the prospective Swedish Obese Subjects (SOS) Intervention Study (124) is investigating the benefits of surgery for severely obese individuals. Preliminary results indicate that surgically treated patients had a significant decrease ($p < .001$) in the incidence of diabetes (0.2% versus 6.3%), hypertension (5.4% versus 13.6%), hyperinsulinemia (0.6% versus 6.3%), and hypertriglyceridemia (0.8% versus 1.7%) over 2 years (125). Furthermore, a greater number of the surgically treated patients discontinued the use of cardiovascular medications (RR = 0.69 at 2 years; RR = 0.77 at 6 years) and diabetes medications (RR = 0.56 at 2 years; RR = 0.71 at 6 years), compared with controls (126).

REVIEW OF OBESITY PREVENTION

Prevention includes the primary prevention of obesity itself, secondary prevention or avoidance of weight regain after weight loss, and prevention of further weight increases in obese patients who are unable to lose weight (127). It is likely that an individual who has developed type 2 diabetes is already obese or overweight, so these patients need to work on secondary preventative measures. The latter can decrease the impact of the effects of obesity on type 2 diabetes, making the disease more manageable. This is especially true in light of the fact that the two diseases have similar risk factors and have such devastating effects if left untreated.

Most strategies for the prevention of obesity have focused on modifying the obese patient's behaviors, focusing predominantly on altering diet and increasing physical activity. To prevent further weight gains or regains, the individual, in consultation with the physician, implements the appropriate lifestyle modifications discussed earlier, including a lower intake of calories and fatty foods and an increased amount of physical activity. Lifestyle modification has been found to be effective in reducing obesity and obesity-related effects, especially when multiple lifestyle modification strategies are used (1).

CONCLUSION

Obesity is becoming more prevalent around the world, and its complications are affecting the lives of numerous individuals. Obesity is now considered an epidemic in developed and developing countries, especially in light of the increased incidence of childhood obesity. Obesity is a complex, multifaceted disease that has no easy cure. It leads to many other illnesses, particularly type 2 diabetes and CVD. However, obesity is a risk factor that can be modified or prevented. This can be done by modifying one's lifestyle through healthy eating and an increased level of physical activity. By taking these actions, individuals with type 2 diabetes can lessen the impact that obesity has on their disease, including the resultant consequences related to diabetes.

REFERENCES

1. National Institutes of Health. Clinical Guidelines on the Identification, Evaluation, and Treatment of Overweight and Obesity in Adults—The Evidence Report. *Obes Res* 1998;6[Suppl 2]:51S–210S.
2. Foreyt JP, Pendleton VR. Management of obesity. *Prim Care Rep* 2000;6:19–30.
3. Bray GA. *Contemporary diagnosis and management of obesity.* Newton, PA: Handbooks in Health Care Co., 1998.
4. Flegal, KM, Carroll, MD, Ogden, CL, et al. Prevalence and trends in obesity among US adults, 1999–2000. *JAMA* 2002;288:1723–1727.
5. Centers for Disease Control and Prevention. *Prevalence of overweight and obesity among adults: United States, 1999.* CDC, 2000. Available at: http://www.cdc.gov/nchs/products/pubs/pubd/hestats/obese/obse99.htm. Accessed June 16, 2003.
6. World Health Organization. *Obesity: preventing and managing the global epidemic.* Geneva: World Health Organization, 1998.
7. Gortmaker SL, Dietz WH Jr, Sobol AM, et al. Increasing pediatric obesity in the United States. *Am J Dis Child* 1987;141:535–540.
8. Troiano RP, Flegal FM. Overweight children and adolescents: description, epidemiology, and demographics. *Pediatrics* 1998;101[Suppl]:497–504.
9. Serdula MK, Ivery D, Coates RJ, et al. Do obese children become obese adults? A review of the literature. *Prev Med* 1993;22:167–177.
10. Hoffmans MD, Kromhout D, de Lezenne Coulander C. The impact of body mass index of 78,612 18-year-old Dutch men on 32-year mortality from all causes. *J Clin Epidemiol* 1988;41:749–756.
11. Freedman DS, Srinivasan SR, Valdez RA, et al. Secular increases in relative weight and adiposity among children over two decades: the Bogalusa Heart Study. *Pediatrics* 1997;99:420–426.
12. Schonfeld-Warden N, Warden CH. Pediatric obesity: an overview of etiology and treatment. *Pediatr Clin North Am* 1997;44:339–361.
13. Deckelbaum RJ, Williams CL. Childhood obesity: the health issue. *Obes Res* 2001;9[Suppl 4]:239S–243S.
14. Strauss RS, Pollack HA. Epidemic increase in childhood overweight, 1986–1998. *JAMA* 2001;286:2845–2848.
15. Becque MD, Katch VL, Rocchini AP, et al. Coronary risk incidence of obese adolescents: reduction by exercise plus diet intervention. *Pediatrics* 1988;81:605–612.
16. Sinha R, Fisch G, Teague B, et al. Prevalence of impaired glucose intolerance among children and adolescents with marked obesity. *N Engl J Med* 2002;346:802–810.
17. Pinhas-Hamiel O, Dolan LM, Daniels SR, et al. Increased incidence of non-insulin-dependent diabetes mellitus among adolescents. *J Pediatr* 1996;128:608–615.
18. Kitagawa T, Owada M, Urakami T, et al. Increased incidence of non-insulin dependent diabetes mellitus among Japanese schoolchildren correlates with an increased intake of animal protein and fat. *Clin Pediatr* 1998;37:111–115.
19. Wolf AM, Colditz GA. Current estimates of the economic costs of obesity in the United States. *Obes Res* 1998;6:97–106.
20. Colditz G. Economic costs of obesity and inactivity. *Med Sci Sports Med* 1999;31:S663–S667.
21. American Diabetes Association. Economic consequences of diabetes mellitus in the U.S. in 1997. *Diabetes Care* 1998;21:296–309.

22. Thompson D, Brown JB, Nichols GA, et al. Body mass index and future healthcare costs: a retrospective cohort study. *Obes Res* 2001;9:210–218.

23. Quesenberry CP, Caan B, Joscobson A. Obesity, health services use, and health care costs among members of a health maintenance organization. *Arch Intern Med* 1998;158:466–472.

24. Pronk NP, Tan AW, O'Connor P. Obesity, fitness, willingness to communicate and health care costs. *Med Sci Sports Exer* 1999;31:1535–1543.

25. Poston WS, Forety JP. Body mass index: uses and limitations. *Strength and Conditioning Journal* 2002;24:15–17.

26. Sinaiko AR, Jacobs DR Jr, Steinberger J, et al. Insulin resistance syndrome in childhood: associations of the euglycemic insulin clamp and fasting insulin with fatness and other risk factors. *J Pediatr* 2001;139:700–707.

27. Ellis SG, Elliott J, Horrigan M, et al. Low-normal or excessive body mass index: newly identified and powerful risk factors for death and other complications with percutaneous coronary intervention. *Am J Cardiol* 1996;78:641–646.

28. Pi-Sunyer FX. The medical risks of obesity. *Obes Surg* 2002;12:6S–11S.

29. Kenchaiah S, Evans JC, Levy D, et al. Obesity and the risk of heart failure. *N Engl J Med* 2002;347:305–313.

30. Harris MI. Summary. In: Harris MI, Cowie CC, Stern MP, et al., eds. *Diabetes in America,* 2nd ed. Bethesda, MD: National Institutes of Health, National Diabetes and Digestive and Kidney Diseases, 2000:1–13.

31. Crespo CJ, Keteyian SJ, Heath GW, et al. Leisure-time physical activity among US adults. *Arch Intern Med* 1996;156:93–98.

32. Flegal KM, Carroll MD, Kuczmarski RJ, et al. Overweight and obesity in the United States: prevalence and trends, 1960–1994. *Int J Obes Rel Metab Disord* 1998;22:39–47.

33. Prevalence of leisure time and occupational physical activity among employed adults—United States, 1990. *MMWR Morb Mortal Wkly Rep* 2000;49:420–424.

34. Seidell JC. Obesity, insulin resistance and diabetes: a worldwide epidemic. *Br J Nutr* 2000;83:S5–S8.

35. Nathan DM, Meigs J, Singer DE. The epidemiology of CVD in type 2 diabetes mellitus: how sweet it is. . . or is it? *Lancet* 1997;350[Suppl 1]:4–9.

36. National Institute of Diabetes and Digestive and Kidney Diseases. *National Diabetes Statistics fact sheet: general information and national estimates on diabetes in the United States, 2000.* Bethesda, MD: U. S. Department of Health and Human Services, National Institutes of Health, 2002.

37. Field AE, Coakley EH, Must A, et al. Impact of overweight on the risk of developing common chronic diseases during a 10-year period. *Arch Intern Med* 2001;161:1581–1586.

38. Grundy SM, Garber A, Goldberg R, et al. Diabetes and CVD writing group VI: lifestyle and medical management of risk factors. *Circulation* 2002;105:e153–e158.

39. Kolterman OG, Insel J, Saekow M, et al. Mechanisms of insulin resistance in human obesity: evidence for receptor and postreceptor defects. *J Clin Invest* 1980;65:1272–1284.

40. Polonsky KS, Given BD, Hirsch L, et al. Quantitative study of insulin secretion and clearance in normal and obese subjects. *J Clin Invest* 1988;81:435–441.

41. Laakso M. Hyperglycemia and CVD in type 2 diabetes. *Diabetes* 1999;18:937–942.

42. Stamler J, Vaccaro, O, Neaton, JD, et al. Diabetes, other risk factors, and 12-yr cardiovascular mortality for men screened in the Multiple Risk Factor Intervention Trial. *Diabetes Care* 1993;16:434–444.

43. Rocchini AP. Obesity hypertension. *Am J Hypertens* 2001;15:50S–52S.

44. Wilson PW, D'Agostino RB, Sullivan L, et al. Overweight and obesity as determinants of cardiovascular risk. *Arch Intern Med* 2002;162:1867–1872.

45. Stevens VJ, Obarazanek E, Cook NR, et al. Long-term weight loss and changes in blood pressure results of the Trials of Hypertension Prevention, phase II. *Ann Intern Med* 2001;134:1–11.

46. Singh PN, Linstead KD. Body mass and 26-year risk of mortality from specific disease among women who never smoked. *Epidemiology* 1998;9:246–254.

47. Kannel WB. Range of serum cholesterol values in the population developing coronary artery disease. *Am J Cardiol* 1995;76:69C–77C.

48. Lloyd-Jones DM, O'Donnell CJ, D'Agostino RB, et al. Applicability of cholesterol-lowering primary prevention trials to a general population. *Arch Intern Med* 2001;161:949–954.

49. Ryden L. Managing cardiovascular risk in patients with diabetes. *Heart* 2000;84:123–125.

50. Calle EE, Thun MJ, Petrelli JM, et al. Body-mass index and mortality in a prospective cohort of US adults. *N Engl J Med* 1999;341:1097–1105.

51. Meyer HE, Søgaard AJ, Tverdal A, et al. Body mass index and mortality: the influence of physical activity and smoking. *Med Sci Sports Exer* 2002;34:1065–1070.

52. Manson JE, Willett WC, Stampfer MJ, et al. Body weight and mortality among women. *JAMA* 1995;333:677–685.

53. Solomon CG, Manson JE. Obesity and mortality: a review of the epidemiologic data. *Am J Clin Nutr* 1997;66[4 Suppl]:1044S–1050S.

54. Liu S, Manson JE. Dietary carbohydrates, physical inactivity, obesity, and the "metabolic syndrome" as predictors of coronary heart disease. *Curr Opin Lipidol* 2001;12:395–404.

55. Rivellese AA, De Natale C, Lilli S. Type of dietary fat and insulin resistance. *Ann N Y Acad Sci* 2002;967:329–335.

56. van Dam RM, Rimm EB, Willett WC, et al. Dietary patterns and risk for type 2 diabetes mellitus in US men. *Ann Intern Med* 2002;136:201–209.

57. Rewers M, Hamman RF. Risk factors for non-insulin-dependent diabetes. In: Harris MI, Cowie CC, Stern MP, et al., eds. *Diabetes in America,* 2nd ed. Bethesda, MD: National Institutes of Health, National Diabetes and Digestive and Kidney Diseases, 2000:179–196.

58. Holub BJ. Clinical nutrition: 4. Omega-3 fatty acids in cardiovascular care. *Can Med Assoc J* 2002;165:608–615.

59. Mori TA, Beilin LJ. Long-chain omega 3 fatty acids, blood lipids and cardiovascular risk reduction. *Curr Opin Lipidol* 2001;12:11–17.

60. von Schacky C, Angerer P, Kothny W, et al. The effect of dietary omega-3 fatty acids on coronary atherosclerosis:

a randomized, double-blind, placebo-controlled trial. *Ann Intern Med* 1999;130:554–562.

61. Mori TA, Bao DQ, Burke V, et al. Dietary fish as a major component of a weight-loss diet: effect on serum lipids, glucose, and insulin metabolism in overweight hypertensive subjects. *Am J Clin Nutr* 1999;70:817–825.

62. Centers for Disease Control and Prevention. *Physical activity and health: a report of the Surgeon General.* Atlanta, GA: U. S. Department of Health and Human Services, 1996. Available at: http:/www.cdc.gov/nccdphp/sgr/sgr.htm. Accessed June 16, 2003.

63. Hahn RA, Teutsch SM, Rothenberg RB, et al. Excess deaths from nine chronic diseases in the United States, 1986. *JAMA* 1990;264:2654–2659.

64. Hambrecht R, Wolf A, Gielen S, et al. Effects of exercise on coronary endothelial function in patients with coronary artery disease. *N Engl J Med* 2000;342:454–460.

65. Goodyear LJ, Kahn BB. Exercise, glucose transport, and insulin sensitivity. *Ann Rev Med* 1998;49:235–261.

66. Herd SL, Kiens B, Boobis LH, et al. Moderate exercise, postprandial lipemia, and skeletal muscle lipoprotein lipase activity. *Metabolism* 2001;50:756–762.

67. Manson JE, Hu FB, Rich-Edwards JW, et al. A prospective study of walking as compared with vigorous exercise in the prevention of coronary heart disease in women. *N Engl J Med* 1999;341:650–658.

68. Hu FB, Stampfer MJ, Colditz GA, et al. Physical activity and risk of stroke in women. *JAMA* 2000;283:2961–2967.

69. Hu FB, Sigal RJ, Rich-Edwards JW, et al. Walking compared with vigorous physical activity and risk of type 2 diabetes in women: a prospective study. *JAMA* 1999;282:1433–1439.

70. Rice T, Tremblay A, Deriaz O, et al. A major gene for resting metabolic rate unassociated with body composition: results from the Quebec Family Study. *Obes Res* 1996;4:441–449.

71. Bouchard C, Perusse L, Rice T, et al. The genetics of human obesity. In: Bray GA, Bouchard C, James WPT, eds. *Handbook of obesity.* New York: Marcel Dekker, 1998:157–190.

72. Bouchard C, Tremblay A, Despres JP, et al. The response to long-term overfeeding in identical twins. *N Engl J Med* 1990;322:1477–1482.

73. Rankinen T, Perusse L, Weisnagel SJ, et al. The human obesity gene map: the 2001 update. *Obes Res* 2002;10:196–243.

74. Poston WS 2nd, Foreyt JP. Obesity is an environmental issue. *Atherosclerosis* 1999;146:201–209.

·75. Libman I, Arslanian SA. Type II diabetes mellitus: no longer just adults. *Pediatr Ann* 1999;28:589–593.

76. Connolly VM, Kesson CM. Socioeconomic status and clustering of CVD risk factors in diabetic patients. *Diabetes Care* 1996;19:419–422.

77. Sobngwi E, Mauvis-Jarvis F, Vexiau P, et al. Diabetes in Africans. Part I: epidemiology and clinical specificities. *Diabetes Metab* 2001;27:628–634.

78. Sekikawa A, Eguchi H, Tominaga M, et al. Prevalence of type 2 diabetes mellitus and impaired glucose tolerance in a rural area of Japan. The Funagata diabetes study. *J Diabetes Complications* 2000;14:78–83.

79. Singh RB, Bajaj S, Niaz MA, et al. Prevalence of type 2 diabetes mellitus and risk of hypertension and coronary artery disease in rural and urban population with low rates of obesity. *Int J Cardiol* 1998;66:65–72.

80. Poston WS 2nd, Haddock K, Olvera NE, et al. Evaluation of a culturally appropriate intervention to increase physical activity. *Am J Health Behav* 2001;25:396–406.

81. Baker RC, Kirschenbaum DS. Self-monitoring may be necessary for successful weight control. *Behav Ther* 1993;24:377–394.

82. Poston WS 2nd, Foreyt JP. Successful management of the obese patient. *J Am Fam Physician* 2000;61:3615–3622.

83. Foreyt JP, Goodrick GK. Factors common in successful therapy for the obese patient. *Med Sci Sports Exercise* 1991;23:292–297.

84. Foreyt JP, Poston WSC. Building better compliance: factors and methods common to achieving a healthy lifestyle. In: Gotto AM, et al., eds. *Drugs affecting lipid metabolism: risk factors and future direction.* Dordrecht, The Netherlands: Kluwer Academic Publishers, 1996:489–496.

85. Boutelle KN, Kirschenbaum DS. Further support for consistent self-monitoring as a vital component of successful weight control. *Obes Res* 1998;6:219–224.

86. Kayman S, Bruvold W, Stern JS. Maintenance and relapse after weight loss in women: behavioral aspects. *Am J Clin Nutr* 1990;52:800–807.

87. Foreyt JP, Goodrick GK. Evidence for success of behavior modification in weight loss and control. *Ann Intern Med* 1993;119:698–701.

88. Pendleton VR, Willems E, Swank P, et al. Negative stress and the outcome of treatment for binge eating. *Eating Disord* 2001;9:351–360.

89. Klem ML, Wing RR, Simkin-Silverman L, et al. The psychological consequences of weight gain prevention in healthy, premenopausal women. *Int J Eating Disord* 1997;21:167–174.

90. American College of Sports Medicine. Appropriate intervention strategies for weight loss and prevention of weight regain for adults *Med Sci Sports Exer* 2001;33:2145–2156.

91. Andersen RE, Wadden TA, Bartlett SJ, et al. Effects of lifestyle activity vs. structured aerobic exercise in obese women: a randomized trial. *JAMA* 1999;281:335–340.

92. Dunn AL, Marcus BH, Kampert JB, et al. Comparison of lifestyle and structured interventions to increase physical activity and cardiorespiratory fitness: a randomized trial. *JAMA* 1999;281:327–334.

93. Chakravarthy MV, Joyner MJ, Booth FW. An obligation for primary care physicians to prescribe physical activity to sedentary patients to reduce the risk of chronic health conditions. *Mayo Clinic Proc* 2002;77:165–173.

94. Canadian Fitness and Lifestyle Research Institute. Available at: http://www.heart-health.ns.ca/hpc/downloads/children_and_inactivity.doc. Accessed June 16, 2003.

95. Mokdad AH, Bowman BA, Ford ES, et al. The continuing epidemics of obesity and diabetes in the United States. *JAMA* 2001;286:1195–1200.

96. Crespo CJ, Smit E, Troiano RP, et al. Televsision watching, energy intake, and obesity in US children: results in from the third National Health and Nutrition

Examination Survey, 1988–1994. *Arch Pediatr Adolesc Med* 2001;155:360–365.

97. Stewart AL, Verboncoeur CJ, McLellan BY, et al. Physical activity outcomes of CHAMPS II: a physical activity promotion program for older adults. *J Gerontol A Biol Sci Med Sci* 2001;56:M465–M470.

98. Lawlor DA, Hanratty B. The effect of physical activity advice given in routine primary care consultations: a systematic review. *J Public Health Med* 2001;23:219–226.

99. Petrella RJ, Wight D. An office-based instrument for exercise counseling and prescriptions in primary care: the Step Exercise Prescription (STEP). *Arch Family Med* 2000;9:339–344.

100. Writing Group for the Activity Counseling Trial Research Group. Effects of physical activity counseling in primary care. *JAMA* 2001;286:677–687.

101. Blair SN, Kohl HW, Barlow CE, et al. Changes in physical fitness and all-cause mortality: a prospective study of healthy and unhealthy men. *JAMA* 1995;273:1093–1098.

102. Foreyt JP, Poston WS 2nd. The challenge of diet, exercise and lifestyle modification in the management of the obese diabetic patient. *Int J Obes* 1999;23:S5–S11.

103. U. S. Department of Agriculture. *The food guide pyramid.* Home and Garden Bulletin no. 252. Washington, DC: U. S. Government Printing Office, 1992.

104. American Dietetic Association and American Diabetes Association. *Exchange lists for weight management.* Chicago: American Dietetic Association, 1989.

105. Van Gaal LF. Dietary treatment for obesity. In: Bray GA, Bouchard C, James WPT, eds. *Handbook of obesity.* New York: Marcel Dekker, 1998:875–891.

106. National Task Force on the Prevention and Treatment of Obesity. Very low-calorie diets. *JAMA* 1993;270:967–974.

107. Pekkarinen T, Mustajoki P. Comparison of behavior therapy with and without very-low-energy diet in the treatment of morbid obesity. *Arch Intern Med* 1997;157:1581–1585.

108. Diabetes Prevention Program Research Group. Reduction in the incidence of type 2 diabetes with lifestyle intervention or metformin. *N Engl J Med* 2002;348:393–403.

109. Craighead LW, Stunkard AJ, O'Brien RM. Behavior therapy and pharmacotherapy for obesity. *Arch Gen Psychiatry* 1981;38:763–768.

110. Haddock CK, Poston WS 2nd, Dill PL, et al. Pharmacotherapy for obesity: a quantitative analysis of four decades of published randomized clinical trials. *Int J Obes* 2002;26:262–273.

111. Yanovski SZ, Yanovski JA. Drug therapy: obesity. *N Engl J Med* 2002;346:591–602.

112. Luque CA, Rey JA. Sibutramine: a serotonin-norepinephrine reuptake-inhibitor for the treatment of obesity. *Ann Pharmacother* 1999;31:968–978.

113. Lean ME. Sibutramine: a review of clinical efficacy. *Int J Obes Rel Metab Disord* 1997;21[Suppl 1]:S30–S36.

114. Seagle HM, Bessesen DH, Hill JO. Effects of sibutramine on resting metabolic rate and weight loss in overweight women. *Obes Res* 1998;6:115–121.

115. Hvizdos KM, Markham A. Orlistat: a review of its use in the management of obesity. *Drugs* 1999;58:743–760.

116. Drent ML, Larsson I, William-Olsson T, et al. Orlistat (RO 18-0647), a lipase inhibitor, in the treatment of human obesity: a multiple dose study. *Int J Obes Rel Metab Disord* 1995;19:221–226.

117. Davidson MH, Hauptman J, DiGirolamo M, et al. Weight control and risk factor reduction in obese subjects treated for 2 years with orlistat: a randomized controlled trial. *JAMA* 1999;281:235–242.

118. Hill JO, Hauptman J, Anderson JW, et al. Orlistat, a lipase inhibitor, for weight maintenance after conventional dieting: a 1-year study. *Am J Clin Nutr* 1999;69:1108–1116.

119. Sjöstrom L, Rissanen A, Andersen T, et al. Randomised placebo-controlled trial of orlistat for weight loss and prevention of weight regain in obese patients. *Lancet* 1998;352:167–173.

120. Apfelbaum M, Vague P, Ziegler O, et al. Long-term maintenance of weight loss after a very-low calorie diet: a randomized blinded trial of the efficacy and tolerability of sibutramine. *Am J Med* 1999;106:179–184.

121. James WP, Astrup A, Finer N, et al. Effect of sibutramine on weight maintenance after weight loss: a randomised trial. *Lancet* 2000;356:2119–2125.

122. Gray DS. Obesity. In: Wiess BD, ed. *Twenty common problems in primary care.* New York: McGraw-Hill, 1999:27–50.

123. National Institutes of Health Consensus Development Conference Statement. Gastrointestinal surgery for severe obesity. *Am J Clin Nutr* 1992;55:615S–619S.

124. Sjöström L, Larsson B, Backman L, et al. Swedish obese subjects (SOS): recruitment for an intervention study and a selected description of the obese state. *Int J Obes Rel Metab Disord* 1992;16:465–479.

125. Sjöström CD, Lissner L, Wedel H, et al. Reduction in incidence of diabetes, hypertension and lipid disturbances after intentional weight loss induced by bariatric surgery: the SOS Intervention Study. *Obes Res* 1999;7:477–484.

126. Ågren G, Narbo K, Näslund I, et al. Long-term effects of weight loss on pharmaceutical costs in obese subjects: a report from the SOS Intervention Study. *Int J Obes* 2002;226:184–192.

127. Jeffery RW. Prevention of obesity. In: Bray GA, Bouchard C, James WPT, eds. *Handbook of obesity.* New York: Marcel Dekker, 1998:819–830.

Diabetes and Cardiovascular Disease
edited by Steven P. Marso and David M. Stern
Lippincott Williams & Wilkins, Philadelphia © 2004

12

Diabetes Treatment

William L. Isley

Medical Director, Lipid and Diabetes Research Center, Saint Luke's Hospital, Associate Professor, Department of Medicine, University of Missouri–Kansas, Kansas City, Missouri

Diabetes mellitus is a group of metabolic disorders that are characterized by hyperglycemia and associated with chronic microvascular (eye and kidney), neuropathic (metabolic and microvascular), and macrovascular complications. Almost 11 million Americans have diagnosed diabetes mellitus, and an additional 5.5 million remain undiagnosed (1). Diabetes prevalence is increasing worldwide. In the United States, increased prevalence of non-insulin-dependent (type 2) diabetes mellitus is associated with greater societal obesity, aging, and an increasing proportion of highly susceptible minority group members in the population. The economic burden of diabetes mellitus was approximately $98 billion in 1997 (2). More than half of medical expenditures related to diabetes mellitus result from hospitalizations for cardiovascular disease (3). Although diabetes is the leading cause of blindness in adults age 20 to 74 years and the leading contributor to the development of end-stage renal disease, a cardiovascular event is responsible for 75% of deaths in individuals with type 2 diabetes mellitus (4). Because more than 90% of diabetes cases are type 2, the majority of information within this chapter is geared toward this form of glucose intolerance.

The treatment of diabetes is aimed at three goals: elimination of symptoms of hyperglycemia, prevention of microvascular complications, and prevention of macrovascular complications, all without producing excess hypoglycemia or other untoward effects. Modern diabetes management attempts to allow the patient to manage the disease, rather than have diabetes manage the patient. Although much progress has been made in the past 20 years in the treatment of hyperglycemia and the prevention and treatment of attendant microvascular complications, one of the disappointments of modern medicine has been the finding that glycemic control has only a modest effect on cardiovascular risk (5). There are several possible reasons for this result: (a) glycemia may have been reduced sufficiently in clinical trials to affect microvascular complications but not enough to substantively change macrovascular risk; (b) treatment of the insulin resistance syndrome *per se* (or perhaps of other pathophysiologic abnormalities) rather than glycemic therapy alone is necessary to reduce cardiovascular risk; and (c) hyperglycemia exacerbates the effects of typical risk factors (including dyslipidemia, hypertension, and a procoagulant state) and aggressive treatment of these risk factors is necessary to reduce cardiovascular risk. The first possibility is being addressed by the Action to Control Cardiovascular Risk in Diabetes Study (ACCORD) (1), in which investigators are attempting to achieve a mean hemoglobin A_{1C} (HbA_{1C}) level of 6%, approximately 1% lower than that in other glycemic intervention trials. The second possibility is being addressed by the Bypass Angioplasty Revascularization Intervention Type 2 Diabetes Study (BARI 2D) (6), wherein insulin sensitizers are used exclusively as initial therapy in one group of patients, and insulin augmentation therapies (sulfonylureas and insulin) are used in the other group. Findings in the obese metformin subgroup from the United Kingdom Prospective Diabetes Study (UKPDS) (7), would lend some credence to the insulin sensitizer strategy (see later discussion). Supportive evidence for the last possibility is already available from numerous lipid and hypertension trials in which diabetic subjects have been enrolled. In such trials, diabetic subjects often were found to have a greater beneficial effect from lipid therapy or blood pressure control than their nondiabetic counterparts (8,9). Treatment of other cardiovascular risk factors is discussed in other chapters of this book and cannot be overemphasized. For too long, therapy for diabetes has been overly focused on glycemia. Global risk management is vital to reduce both microvascular and macrovascular risks.

CLASSIFICATION AND PATHOGENESIS

The American Diabetes Association (ADA) adopted new nomenclature for diabetes mellitus in 1997 (10). Insulin-dependent (type 1, or juvenile-onset) diabetes mellitus is characterized by absolute deficiency of insulin. This is usually due to immune-mediated destruction of pancreatic beta cells. Because these patients often present with marked symptoms (polyuria, polydipsia, polyphagia, weight loss, and "metabolic bankruptcy"), it was presumed until recently that patients developed this disease in a matter of days. However, it is now known that there is a long preclinical period associated with the appearance of immune markers and beta-cell destruction. Occasionally a patient with type 1 diabetes mellitus comes to medical attention with hyperglycemia before the development of ketoacidosis. Frank diabetes does not occur until about 90% of beta cells are destroyed. These patients often have a transient remission (the so-called honeymoon phase) when they still produce some insulin and glycemia is relatively easy to control. Ultimately, multiple insulin injections will be necessary to achieve adequate glycemic control. Typical type 1 diabetes mellitus is more common in non-Hispanic whites than in other population groups. Type 1 diabetes is one of the few disorders that predisposes young

people to coronary heart disease, eliminating the usual hormonal protection associated with the premenopausal state in women (11). The diagnosis of type 1 diabetes is usually made when the patient presents with typical symptoms and a random plasma glucose concentration measurement is greater than 200 mg/dL. Type 1 diabetes appears to occur in genetically susceptible individuals after some environmental trigger (e.g., viral infection) that initiates the autoimmune destructive process. Insulin sensitivity is normal in patients with type 1 diabetes mellitus.

Type 2 diabetes (also called adult-onset or maturity-onset diabetes) is a heterogeneous disorder characterized by the presence of both insulin resistance and *relative* insulin deficiency, though some patients may predominantly have insulin deficiency (12). Insulin resistance is manifested by a decrease in skeletal muscle uptake of glucose, particularly in the postprandial state; dysregulation of hepatic glucose production; and an increase in fat breakdown (lipolysis) that results in elevated plasma free fatty acid levels. This last abnormality is associated with the characteristic dyslipidemia of type 2 diabetes mellitus: a high level of triglycerides and a low concentration of high-density lipoprotein cholesterol (HDL-C). It is possible that increased plasma free fatty acids may lead to hyperglycemia by stimulating hepatic glucose production and producing muscle insulin resistance as a primary defect (13). This theory is presently being intensely investigated.

Beta cell dysfunction in type 2 diabetes is progressive and contributes to worsening blood glucose control with time (14). The concept that insulin resistance is the primary defect, with hyperinsulinemia a secondary result, may be too simplistic. Work in Pima Indians revealed subtle defects in timing of insulin release long before deterioration of glucose tolerance occurred (15). The "proximal defect" in type 2 diabetes is unknown, although both insulin resistance and insulin deficiency appear to be heritable to some extent, whereas insulin resistance is clearly promoted by the usual (more than 80%) coexistence of obesity in these patients. Insulin resistance alone does not cause diabetes, because multiple disorders (obesity, polycystic ovary disease, hypertension) are associated with insulin resistance but not necessarily glucose intolerance.

Type 2 diabetes mellitus occurs when a diabetogenic lifestyle (excessive calories, inadequate caloric expenditure, and obesity) is superimposed on a susceptible genotype. The weight gain necessary for the development of significant insulin resistance appears to vary among racial and ethnic groups. For example, overweight patients from the Indian subcontinent are, at most, mildly overweight by Western standards, but they may be very insulin resistant. Also, the high prevalence of type 2 diabetes mellitus in Native American populations is usually associated with marked obesity. Whereas type 2 diabetes mellitus has classically been viewed as a disease of older individuals, with increasing societal obesity it is now often seen in teenagers and even prepubertal children, particularly in susceptible minority populations. Therefore, age at onset may not be helpful in discerning the pathophysiology involved in an individual patient's glucose intolerance.

Because the natural history of type 2 diabetes mellitus is the ultimate development of insulin deficiency (albeit not complete), the classification of a patient as "insulin dependent," based on the use of insulin injections alone, is to be avoided. Classification can usually be made on the basis of the clinical history (Table 12-1), but occasionally serologic tests for specific antibodies (anti-glutamic acid decarboxylase [anti-GAD], islet cell and insulin antibodies), or assessment of endogenous insulin production by measurement of C peptide after ingestion of a standard liquid meal or glucagon injection, is needed to accurately determine the patient's type of diabetes mellitus.

In type 2 diabetes mellitus, increased cardiovascular risk appears to begin before the development of frank hyperglycemia, possibly due to the effects of insulin resistance. It now appears that hyperinsulinemia is a secondary phenomenon and is not causative of increased atherosclerotic risk. Stern et al. (16) developed the "ticking clock" hypothesis of complications, asserting that the clock starts ticking for microvascular (eye and kidney) risk at the onset of hyperglycemia, whereas for macrovascular risk it starts ticking at some antecedent point, presumably with the onset of insulin resistance (16). Because many patients with type 2 diabetes are asymptomatic for a prolonged period, precise identification of the onset of hyperglycemia is usually impossible.

Insulin resistance is associated with multiple metabolic abnormalities (small, dense low-density lipoprotein [LDL] particles, low HDL-C levels, elevated remnant lipoproteins), prothrombotic markers (elevated type-1 plasminogen activator inhibitor [PAI-1]), and increased inflammatory markers. Most patients with type 2 diabetes have many or all of the components of the so-called insulin resistance syndrome (also known as the metabolic syndrome, the dysmetabolic syndrome, or syndrome X). (17).

Although some patients present with typical symptoms (as in type 1 diabetes mellitus,

TABLE 12-1. *Differentiating type 1 from type 2 diabetes mellitus*

	Type 1 diabetes mellitus	Type 2 diabetes mellitus
Race/ethnicity	Less common in minorities	More common in minorities
Age	<30 yr	Any age in minorities; usually >30 yr in non-Hispanic whites
Body habitus	Lean	Obese or history of obesity
Family history	Usually negative for type 1 diabetes mellitus	Often positive for type 2 diabetes mellitus
Onset	Often fulminant	Often asymptomatic
Ketoacidosis in the absence of intercurrent illness	Yes	No
Response to oral drugs	Brief or no response to secretagogues	Most respond for years
Need for insulin	Usually immediate	Years after diagnosis

TABLE 12-2. *Diagnosis of diabetes mellitus[a]*

Symptoms of diabetes plus a random plasma glucose
  ≥200 mg/dL
or
Fasting plasma glucose ≥126 mg/dL
or
2-hr plasma glucose ≥200 mg/dL during an OGTT
Other categories of glucose intolerance
  IFG (fasting plasma glucose >110 mg/dL,
    <126 mg/dL)
  IGT (2-hr plasma glucose on OGTT >140 mg/dL,
    <200 mg/dL)

IFG, impaired fasting glucose; IGT, impaired glucose
tolerance; OGTT, oral glucose (75 g) tolerance test.
[a]Abnormal tests repeated for confirmation.

but usually less severe), type 2 diabetes mellitus is often discovered on "routine" blood work or in the evaluation of neuropathy or dyslipidemia. Acanthosis nigricans is common in dark skinned populations with type 2 diabetes mellitus. The diagnostic criteria for diabetes mellitus are summarized in Table 12-2. The fasting plasma glucose criterion is the one most often used in the United States. In nonpregnant individuals, oral glucose tolerance tests are rarely necessary as a diagnostic tool for diabetes, although vigorous advocates for this diagnostic procedure still abound in Europe (18). Glucose values determined on serum from standard chemistry profiles may be up to 15% lower than plasma values, so gray top tubes (containing sodium fluoride) should be used if the diagnosis of diabetes is being considered. Capillary whole-blood glucose values are not recommended to diagnose diabetes mellitus. Hemoglobin A_{1C} (HbA_{1C}) measurements are not sensitive enough to detect diabetes but are the gold standard for long-term glycemic monitoring.

An extensive discussion of the less common types of diabetes is beyond the scope of this chapter. However, clinicians should be aware of what is presently called type 1 diabetes mellitus idiopathic (10). Patients with this disorder are usually young African-Americans with intermittent insulin deficiency. Such patients often are obese, often have acanthosis nigricans, frequently have a positive family history for type 2 diabetes, and lack the autoimmune markers of typical type 1 diabetes mellitus. With the exception of bouts

of insulin deficiency, manifested by diabetic ketoacidosis or hyperglycemic hyperosmolar nonketotic syndromes, the best treatment for such patients may be to consider them to have a form of type 2 diabetes. Clinicians should also be aware of postpancreatitic diabetes, which behaves more like type 1 diabetes, although insulin requirements are often less and pancreatic function may recover over time. Finally, steroid-induced diabetes, manifested by insulin resistance, is seen commonly in adults treated with systemic glucocorticoids.

Impaired glucose tolerance (IGT) and impaired fasting glucose (IFG) are terms used to describe patients whose plasma glucose levels are higher than normal but not diagnostic of diabetes mellitus (see Table 12-2). These disorders are associated with increased risk for the future development of diabetes mellitus. At the time of this writing, the utility of these diagnostic categories is being hotly debated, with IGT favored by Europeans (18) and IFG used in the United States, primarily because its determination does not require the use of the oral glucose tolerance test. Values measured after oral glucose challenge are better predictors of cardiovascular risk and therefore are favored by those who are interested in cardiovascular epidemiology (19).

TREATMENT

Rationale for Glycemic Therapy

The role of glucose control in diabetic complications was a matter of intense debate until relatively recently. The "glucose hypothesis" was finally accepted with the publication of the Diabetes Control and Complications Trial (DCCT) in 1993. The relevant clinical trials related to the role of glycemia in complications are summarized in Table 12-3.

Diabetes Control and Complications Trial

The DCCT (20) enrolled 1,441 patients with type 1 diabetes mellitus; about half had no evidence of microvascular disease (primary prevention), and the other half had evidence of early

TABLE 12-3. *Major clinical end-point trials in diabetes mellitus*

Trial (ref. no.)	Type of diabetes	Therapy	Mean length of study (yr)	Difference in HbA$_{1C}$
DCCT (20)	1	Intensive insulin vs. conventional insulin	6.5	7.2% vs. 9.1%
UKPDS (21)	2	Sulfonylureas, insulin, or metformin vs. minimalistic therapy	10	7.0% vs. 7.9%
Kumamoto (26)	2[a]	Intensive insulin vs. conventional insulin	6	7.1% vs. 9.4%
DIGAMI[b] (27)	2	Intensive insulin vs. conventional insulin	3.4	6.7% vs. 7.8%

[a]Patients not obese by American standards.
[b]Patients with acute myocardial infarction.

microvascular disease (secondary prevention). The patients were randomly assigned to receive either conventional therapy or intensive therapy. Conventional therapy at that time comprised one or two shots of insulin daily and infrequent self-monitoring of blood glucose (SMBG), with no attempt to change therapy based on SMBG readings. Intensive therapy consisted of three or more injections of insulin daily or insulin pump, with frequent SMBG and alteration of insulin therapy based on SMBG results, plus frequent contact with a health professional. After 6.5 years of mean follow-up with a difference in HbA$_{1C}$ between the two groups of about 2% (approximately 9% versus about 7%), retinopathy was decreased by 76% in the primary prevention cohort, and among those with retinopathy in the secondary prevention group, progression was reduced by 54%. Neuropathy was decreased by 60% in both groups combined. Microalbuminuria was decreased by 39%, and macroproteinuria was reduced by 54% with intensive therapy. Hypoglycemia was more common and weight gain was greater with intensive therapy. A non-statistically significant reduction in coronary events was seen in the intensively treated group compared with the conventional group, although the event rate in the study population was low.

United Kingdom Prospective Diabetes Study

The UKPDS (21) was a landmark study for the care of patients with type 2 diabetes mellitus, confirming the importance of glycemic control

for reducing the risk of microvascular complications. More than 5,000 patients with newly diagnosed type 2 diabetes entered the study. Patients were monitored for an average of 10 years. The major portion of the study assessed conventional therapy (i.e., no drug therapy unless the patient was symptomatic or had a fasting plasma glucose level higher than 270 mg/dL) versus intensive therapy (which started with either sulfonylureas or insulin and aimed at keeping the fasting plasma glucose concentration at lower than 108 mg/dL). In a subset of obese patients, metformin was used as the primary therapeutic agent.

Significant findings included the following:

1. Even "early" in the course of disease, beta cell function is already significantly compromised (about 50% of normal), with further loss of function regardless of initial therapy.
2. Microvascular complications (predominantly the need for laser photocoagulation on retinal lesions) are reduced by 25% when the median HbA$_{1C}$ is 7% compared with 7.9%.
3. As was shown in the DCCT, there is a continuous relationship between glycemia and microvascular complications. There was a 35% reduction in risk for each 1% decrement in HbA$_{1C}$. There is no glycemic threshold for microvascular disease (22).
4. Glycemic control has minimal effect on macrovascular disease risk. Excess macrovascular risk appears to be related to conventional risk factors such as dyslipidemia and hypertension.

5. Sulfonylureas and insulin therapy do not increase macrovascular disease risk. The assurance of cardiovascular safety was important because of the specter of possible toxicity seen in the University Diabetes Group Project (UGDP) of the 1960's, in which the use of tolbutamide, a short-acting, low-potency, first-generation sulfonylurea, was associated with excess cardiovascular risk. (Additionally, the UGDP was carried out before the availability of SMBG and HbA$_{1C}$ measurements.)
6. Metformin reduces macrovascular risk in obese patients (23).
7. Vigorous blood pressure control reduces microvascular and macrovascular events (24). The relative effects of blood pressure lowering may be greater than those of glycemic control. There was no evidence for a threshold systolic blood pressure greater than 130 mm Hg for protection against complications (25).

Kumamoto Study

In the Kumamoto Study, 102 Japanese patients with type 2 diabetes mellitus (who were nonobese by American standards but overweight by Japanese norms) were monitored for 6 years of treatment with intensive insulin versus one or two shots of intermediate-acting insulin daily (26). Patients without complications and those with early microvascular complications were enrolled. A HbA$_{1C}$ difference of 2.3% (7.1% versus 9.4%) resulted in a 69% reduction in retinopathy progression and a 70% reduction in nephropathy progression.

Diabetes Mellitus, Insulin Glucose Infusion in Acute Myocardial Infarction (DIGAMI) Study

Among 620 Swedish patients with acute myocardial infarction in the Diabetes Mellitus, Insulin Glucose Infusion in Acute Myocardial Infarction (DIGAMI) Study, half received intravenous insulin and glucose followed by intensive insulin therapy, and the other half received conventional therapy (27). At 1 year, the mortality rate was reduced 30% in the intensive treatment group. Recent studies in other ill patients (discussed later) have suggested that intravenous insulin therapy, with very tight glycemic control, may have salutatory benefits on mediators of disease other than glycemia (28). Longer follow-up (mean, 3.5 years) showed similar risk reductions, with the effect being most marked in patients who had not previously received insulin.

General Approach to Treatment

Appropriate care requires goal setting for glycemia, blood pressure, and lipid levels; regular monitoring of complications; dietary and exercise modifications; medications; appropriate SMBG; and laboratory assessment of glycemia and other parameters (29). Patient education by qualified personnel is of utmost importance to ensure understanding, cooperation, and compliance with the therapeutic regimen.

Unless the risk outweighs the benefit (as in elderly patients, patients with advanced complications, and patients with other advanced disease), an HbA$_{1C}$ target of less than 7%, as recommended by the ADA, is appropriate. Some groups now advocate more stringent goals (HbA$_{1C}$ lower than 6.5%) (30). On balance, more stringent goals require more vigorous therapy (earlier use of oral combinations and earlier and greater use of insulin). Such strategies are associated with increased costs, probable increased weight gain, and more potential drug toxicity. Although it is unclear to me what the optimal glycemic treatment goal should be for most patients, it is probably wise to achieve the lowest HbA$_{1C}$ possible, if this goal is readily and easily achievable (i.e., oral monotherapy or dual oral combination therapy if no significant side effects). This scenario is usually present only early after diagnosis. Recommendations for various glycemic goals are given in Table 12-4.

Routine yearly monitoring for eye and kidney disease is recommended through dilated eye examinations and microalbuminuria screening. Regular foot examinations and simple neurologic assessments are vital to reduce amputations.

The advent of SMBG in the early 1980's revolutionized the treatment of diabetes mellitus, allowing patients to know their blood glucose

TABLE 12-4. *Therapeutic goals in patients with diabetes mellitus*

Parameter	Goal	Suggested action level
HbA$_{1C}$ (%)	<7%	>8%
Fasting capillary glucose (mg/dL)	80–120 mg/dL	<80, >140 mg/dL
Bedtime capillary glucose (mg/dL)	100–140 mg/dL	<100, >160 mg/dL
Low-density lipoprotein-cholesterol (mg/dL)	<100 mg/dL	
High-density lipoprotein-cholesterol (mg/dL)	>45 mg/dL (men)	
	>55 mg/dL (women)	
Triglycerides (mg/dL)	<150 mg/dL	
Blood pressure (mm Hg)	<130/<80 mm Hg	

Data from American Diabetes Association. Standards of medical care for patients with diabetes mellitus. *Diabetes Care* 2002;25:213–229.

concentration at any moment easily and relatively inexpensively. Frequent SMBG is necessary to achieve near-normal blood glucose concentrations without inducing hypoglycemia in patients with type 1 diabetes (31). The more intense the insulin regimen is, the more frequent the SMBG needs to be (four or more times daily in patients taking multiple insulin injections per day). The utility and optimal frequency of SMBG for patients with type 2 diabetes mellitus is unresolved (32). Frequency of monitoring in type 2 diabetes should be sufficient to facilitate reaching glucose goals, but patients must be empowered to change their therapeutic regimen (lifestyle and medications) in response to test results or no meaningful change is likely to be effected. Intensive SMBG in type 2 diabetes (only in patients taking insulin) is preferable; less frequent monitoring in patients taking insulin secretagogues (to detect and avoid hypoglycemia) and minimal monitoring in patients taking other agents (which generally do not cause hypoglycemia) are acceptable.

Therapeutic Lifestyle: Diet and Exercise

Medical nutrition therapy is recommended for all persons with diabetes mellitus (33). For individuals with type 1 diabetes, the focus is on balancing carbohydrate intake with insulin and exercise to achieve and maintain a healthy body weight. Young, active adults with type 1 diabetes are often underfed by the typical 1,800-calorie ADA diet and may require 2,500 to 3,500 calories per day. The role of an experienced nutritionist in dealing with these patients cannot be overemphasized. Although the point is still debated, a diet that is high in carbohydrates (with modest simple sugar intake in the context of a mixed meal), low in fats (especially low in saturated fat), and low in cholesterol is appropriate in most situations. Carbohydrate counting is a particularly useful strategy for estimating meal insulin requirements in patients with type 1 diabetes mellitus. Snacking to prevent hypoglycemia is rarely necessary with the availability of SMBG and modern insulin therapy.

Most patients with type 2 diabetes mellitus are obese and need caloric restriction. Rather than a set diabetic diet that a patient is unlikely to follow, the health care team should advocate a diet using foods that are within the financial reach and cultural milieu of the patient. Bedtime and between-meal snacks are not usually needed if pharmacologic management is appropriate. High-carbohydrate, low-fat diets are usually recommended except for patients with very high triglyceride levels. In these situations, isocaloric substitution of monounsaturates for carbohydrate may be beneficial for achieving glycemic and lipid goals.

In general, most patients with diabetes mellitus benefit from increased activity (34). Management of vigorous exercise sessions in patients with type 1 diabetes mellitus must be guided by frequent SMBG. In patients with type 2 diabetes, aerobic exercise can be expected to improve insulin resistance and may improve glycemia markedly in some patients. Older patients, patients with long-standing disease, patients with multiple risk factors, and patients with previous evidence of atherosclerotic disease should have a thorough cardiovascular evaluation, probably including a stress-perfusion imaging study, before beginning a significant exercise regime.

Efforts at weight loss have their greatest effect on glycemia early in the course of type 2 diabetes mellitus. In patients with long-standing type 2 diabetes, sudden weight loss is probably more indicative of insulinopenia and poor glycemic control than sudden compliance to diet and exercise.

Pharmacologic Therapy

Type 1 Diabetes Mellitus

The only effective drug treatment for type 1 diabetes mellitus is insulin (35). Although the newer insulin preparations and delivery methods are still imperfect, they offer closer replication of normal physiology than did those of just a few years ago. Insulin preparations are categorized according to their strength, onset, and duration of action. Modifications to the insulin molecule (insulin analogs) impart beneficial alterations in pharmacokinetic properties. In the United States, human insulins, obtained by the use of recombinant DNA technology, and insulin analogs similarly manufactured, are used almost exclusively.

Simplistically speaking, normal insulin secretion can be broken down into (a) a relatively constant background ("basal") level of insulin for fasting and postabsorptive periods and (b) prandial ("bolus") spikes of insulin after eating (Fig. 12-1) (36). Insulin sensitivity and nonprandial insulin secretion are not constant throughout the day, rendering the basal concept somewhat inaccurate, but in most clinical situations this approach provides a useful paradigm for understanding and applying insulin treatment for type 1 diabetes mellitus. The other basic principle to consider, when using exogenous insulin, is that the timing of insulin onset, peak, and duration of effect must match meal patterns and exercise schedules to achieve near-normal blood glucose values throughout the day.

The basal-bolus concept is an attempt to replicate normal insulin physiology with a combination of intermediate or long-acting insulin to give the basal component and short-acting insulin to give the bolus component. Various strategies have been used for the basal component, including once- or twice-daily neutral protamine Hagedorn (NPH), lente, or ultralente insulin and

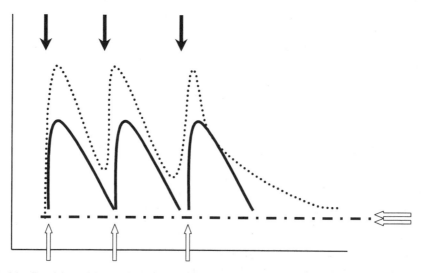

FIG. 12-1. Idealized basal-bolus insulin concept for insulin treatment of diabetes mellitus. Heavy arrows mark meals. The dotted line indicates normal insulin secretion. The dashed line and double light arrow represent "basal insulin therapy" (injection given once or twice daily). Solid lines and single light arrows represent "bolus insulin therapy" (injection given preprandially).

once-daily insulin glargine. Once-daily regimens are usually administered at bedtime to ensure adequate insulinization during sleep and control of the fasting glucose concentration in the morning. Because the duration of insulin action is 10 to 20 hours, most patients require two shots per day of any of these preparations except insulin glargine (which has a duration of action of approximately 24 hours). Furthermore, the peak of activity (except for insulin glargine) is generally 4 to 8 hours after injection (although ultralente has less of a peak in activity than does NPH or lente), so the patient must plan his or her life and meals by the timing of these peaks. For these reasons, many patients with type 1 diabetes mellitus use insulin glargine as a relatively "peakless," long-acting insulin for basal insulin therapy.

The bolus insulin component is given before meals with regular insulin, lispro insulin, or insulin aspart. The rapid onset of action (15 minutes), early peak (1 to 2 hours) and short time course of lispro insulin and insulin aspart more closely replicate the normal physiology. This approach allows the patient to vary the amount of insulin injected, depending on the preprandial SMBG level, the anticipated activity (e.g., upcoming exercise may reduce the insulin requirement), and anticipated carbohydrate intake. Many patients have a prescribed preprandial dose of insulin, which they vary by use of a sliding scale. This type of adjusted-scale insulin (known as variable-dose prandial insulin or insulin algorithm) is intended to optimize the insulin regimen. Carbohydrate counting is a very effective tool for determining the amount of insulin to be injected preprandially. Regular insulin has traditionally been used for bolus injections before meals, but it has a slow onset and a much longer duration of activity than the typical postmeal endogenous rise in insulin. Therefore, lispro and aspart, two insulin analogs with rapid onset of activity and much shorter duration, have been developed. These agents can be given immediately before eating, whereas with regular insulin a 20- to 30-minute lag time is necessary to match the effect on ingested carbohydrates.

Insulin pumps are a high-tech way of administering basal-bolus insulin therapy. For many patients with type 1 diabetes mellitus, this approach provides the most flexibility and control (37). To use these devices optimally, however, greater attention to detail and more frequent SMBG are usually necessary. Patients who assume that they can "plug it in and forget it" are doomed to failure in controlling their diabetes.

As a rough estimate of insulin requirements, patients may start on approximately 0.6 U/kg per day, with basal insulin being 45% of the total dose and prandial insulin given as 25% of the total dose before breakfast, 15% before lunch, and 15% before supper. Type 1 diabetics usually require 0.5 to 1.0 U/kg per day. The need for significantly higher amounts of insulin suggests the presence of insulin antibodies or insulin resistance.

Intensive (basal-bolus) therapy for all cases of type 1 diabetes in adults is recommended at the time of diagnosis, to reinforce the importance of glycemic control from the outset rather than change strategies, over time, due to lack of control. Occasionally a patient with an extended honeymoon period needs less intense therapy initially but should be converted to basal-bolus therapy at the onset of glycemic liability. Because prepubertal children are generally spared microvascular complications, less intense regimens are often used in the pediatric population. Regardless of the regimen chosen, gross adjustments in the total insulin dose can be made based on HbA_{1C} measurements and symptoms such as polyuria, polydipsia, and weight gain or loss. Finer insulin adjustments can be based on the results of frequent SMBG.

There is sufficient variability of insulin absorption from anatomic region to region that traditional injection rotation schemes can cause significant swings in blood glucose levels. The most consistent absorption of insulin is from the abdomen, which is the preferred site of insulin injection. Giving insulin into a limb and then exercising that limb is to be avoided. Erratic SMBG results may indicate insulin absorption problems (e.g., repeated insulin administration into an area of lipohypertrophy that markedly slows absorption) or poor injection techniques.

Hypoglycemia is the result of not matching carbohydrate intake with insulin action. This may occur if meals are skipped, carbohydrate intake is inadequate, or the timing of eating does not concur with the peaks of administered insulin. Basal-bolus regimens that administer prandial insulin only with meals and that base dosing on anticipated carbohydrate intake obviate many of these problems.

Overtreatment with insulin is a common problem. The answer to all high blood sugar levels is not necessarily more insulin, because the patient may be insulinopenic or may be "rebounding" from a previous low sugar level and treating it with excessive amounts of carbohydrate. Fastidious SMBG, particularly during the night (or selected use of continuous glucose monitoring) will help sort out this clinical dilemma. Far too many patients have elevated glucose readings and are treated with more insulin, resulting in more hypoglycemia and weight gain. Marked weight gain is a clue that patients are receiving too much insulin (overinsulinization).

Patients with type 1 diabetes mellitus are absolutely insulinopenic but have normal insulin sensitivity. Patients with type 2 diabetes have varying degrees of insulin resistance. Therefore, a change in insulin dose of only 1 U may have a dramatic effect on glucose concentrations in a patient with type 1 diabetes, whereas a change of 10 U may have little effect on glucose in some patients with type 2 diabetes mellitus. Large changes in insulin dosage in patients with type 1 diabetes are not usually indicated unless the patient's blood glucose control is very poor.

SMBG is essential for the management of insulin therapy. Morning fasting blood sugar concentrations are usually the result of the basal insulin component. Other premeal glucose concentrations may be related to both the basal component and the previous premeal insulin dose, as well as carbohydrate ingestion. Glycemic excursions with meals are related to the amount and type of carbohydrate intake and the bolus of prandial insulin administered.

After several years of type 1 diabetes, hypoglycemia unawareness may develop, either as the result of autonomic neuropathy or because of extremely frequent hypoglycemia. If the former is the case, a less stringent glycemic goal may be in order, because such patients may have no warning before the development of seizures or coma. In patients with hypoglycemia-induced hypoglycemia unawareness, vigorous monitoring and a reduction in insulin dose usually solve the problem. Oral glucose ingestion or injection of glucagon is used to treat hypoglycemia.

Type 2 Diabetes Mellitus

The last few years have seen an explosion in the treatment armamentarium for type 2 diabetes mellitus. Insulin secretagogues (sulfonylureas and other agents), biguanides, peroxisome proliferator agonist receptor-γ (PPAR-γ) agonists (thiazolidinediones or glitazones), α-glucosidase inhibitors, and insulin are now used in the treatment of this condition. The following paragraphs review individual classes of agents and then discuss a general therapeutic strategy.

Sulfonylureas. Sulfonylureas exert their hypoglycemic action by stimulating pancreatic secretion of insulin (38). These agents bind to the pancreatic beta-cell plasma membrane associated with the adenosine triphosphate (ATP)-dependent K^+ channel. On binding, sulfonylureas close these channels, causing depolarization of the membrane and opening of the voltage-dependent Ca^{2+} channels, resulting in an increase in insulin secretion.

Whereas all sulfonylureas are equally effective in lowering blood glucose when administered in equipotent doses, usually only second-generation agents are used in the United States, because of their decreased propensity for drug interactions. The most common side effect of sulfonylureas is hypoglycemia. Individuals who are at high risk for hypoglycemia (e.g., elderly individuals, those with renal insufficiency or advanced liver disease) should be given a low dose of a shorter-acting agent, or other short-acting secretagogue, or insulin to minimize this risk. Mild weight gain is common with sulfonylurea therapy, probably as a result of reduction in glycosuria.

Animal and limited human studies suggest that glyburide (by binding to the ATP-dependent K^+ channel in the heart) inhibits cardiac preischemic conditioning, possibly increasing myocardial damage during ischemic episodes. Glimepiride and meglitinides exhibit little binding to the cardiac K^+ channels. Although some authorities suggest that the latter agents should be the preferred insulin secretagogues (because of this interaction), many clinicians doubt the significance of these findings. The lack of increased cardiac events in patients treated with glyburide in the UKPDS is reassuring in this debate.

Starting doses of the commonly used sulfonylureas are as follows: glimepiride, 1 mg; glipizide, 5 mg; glipizide XL, 2.5 to 5 mg; and glyburide, 2.5 to 5 mg. Lower dosages are recommended for elderly patients and for those who have compromised renal or hepatic function. The dosage can be titrated every 1 to 2 weeks to achieve glycemic goals. Because half-maximal doses provide maximum glycemic efficacy in most patients, half-maximal doses (glimepiride, 4 mg; glipizide, 10 mg b.i.d.; glipizide XL, 10 mg; and glyburide, 10 mg) are often the maximum used, particularly for patients taking insulin sensitizers.

Meglitinides. The meglitinide class of oral agents lowers glucose by binding to the sulfonylurea receptor, but with a much shorter binding time (39,40). With repaglinide and nateglinide, insulin release is glucose dependent and diminishes at low blood glucose concentrations, reducing the potential for severe hypoglycemia. Meal-related insulin secretion is more physiologic with these agents, producing greater effects on postprandial glucose concentrations but less on fasting glycemia. These agents are particularly useful for patients who are at increased risk for hypoglycemia, such as elderly individuals and those with renal disease.

Biguanides. Metformin is the only biguanide available in the United States (41). Phenformin was removed from the market by the U. S. Food and Drug Administration (FDA) in 1977 due to its propensity to cause lactic acidosis. When metformin is administered according to the manufacturer's recommendations, the risk for lactic acidosis is extremely small. Metformin reduces hepatic glucose production and often induces mild anorexia, facilitating weight loss. Insulin must be present for metformin to work. Metformin produces modest favorable effects on the lipid profile. The positive affect of metformin on cardiovascular risk, as demonstrated for obese

patients in the UKPDS, has cemented its role as the mainstay of oral glycemic therapy in obese patients with type 2 diabetes mellitus.

With the expiration of the patent for metformin in the United States, an extended-release version (Glucophage XR) and a combination tablet with glyburide (Glucovance) have become available. Glycemic efficacy with the extended-release formulation may not be equivalent to that achieved with the immediate-release product. Furthermore, for unclear reasons, the positive effects seen on serum triglycerides with immediate-release metformin have not been reported with the extended-release product. Because the positive cardiovascular effects in the UKPDS were seen with the immediate-release product and these effects may be related to the gastrointestinal side effects and resultant anorexia, immediate-release metformin should be the standard, unless patients are truly intolerant of the drug. Most patients deemed intolerant to the immediate-release form are taking the drug before meals or without initial slow titration. With proper patient education, tolerability can be achieved in many of these patients. The major advantage of the combination product is patient convenience.

The most common adverse effects with metformin are nausea, vomiting, and diarrhea. Anorexia or a metallic taste is also frequently reported. These side effects are dose dependent and can be minimized by titrating the dose slowly and by taking the medication with food or, if need be, at the end of the meal.

Metformin can be initiated with immediate-release tablets, at 500 mg twice daily with meals or 850 mg once a day, and increased by 500 mg weekly or 850 mg every 2 weeks to a total of 2,000 mg/day. The maximum recommended dose is 2,550 mg/day, but the maximum glycemic efficacy seems to be at 2,000 mg/day in most patients. Metformin should not be given to patients with renal insufficiency (serum creatinine greater than 1.3 mg/dL for women or 1.4 mg/dL for men), significant liver dysfunction, or *decompensated* congestive heart failure. Treated heart failure that is hemodynamically stable is not considered to be a contraindication by most practitioners. The drug should be used with caution, if at all, in persons older than 75 years of age.

Metformin should be omitted for 48 hours after radiocontrast administration until normal renal function is confirmed.

Metformin XR can be initiated with 500 mg with the evening meal and increased by 500 mg weekly to a maximum dosage of 2,000 mg/day. If suboptimal glycemic control is achieved with 2,000 mg administered once daily, 1,000 mg given twice daily with meals can be considered.

Peroxisome Proliferator-activated Receptor-γ Agonists. Rosiglitazone and pioglitazone are the two available thiazolidinediones (glitazones). Glitazones are the first group of agents targeted to activate PPARγ (42). Many nonglitazone PPARγ agonists and agents that activate both PPARα and PPARγ are currently under development. PPARγ agonists reduce insulin resistance in the periphery (i.e., they sensitize fat and muscle to the actions of insulin). Whether the effects on muscle are primary or are secondary to reductions of free fatty acids is unknown. Effects of PPARγ agonists on cardiovascular risk factors are listed in Table 12-5 (43). Insulin must be present for these agents to work. Although concentrations of triglycerides and HDL-C often improve with these agents, LDL-cholesterol may actually increase, at least in the short term. Early data possibly suggest beta-cell preservation in patients using glitazones early in the course of disease (44). Whether this finding will be confirmed in long-term studies of large numbers of patients remains to be seen.

The onset of action of these drugs is slow, with 2 to 3 months required to demonstrate full effect.

TABLE 12-5. *Effects of PPARγ agents on cardiovascular risk factors*

Decreased triglycerides
Increased high-density lipoprotein-cholesterol
Decreased plasminogen activator inhibitor-1 and
  fibrinogen
Decreased visceral fat
Decreased blood pressure
Decreased microalbuminuria
Decreased intima-medial thickness
Improved vascular function

Data from Parulkar AA, Pendergrass ML, Granda-Ayala R, et al. Nonhypoglycemic effects of thiazolidinediones. *Ann Intern Med* 2001;134:61–71.

Monotherapy is often ineffective unless the drugs are given very early in the course of disease, when sufficient beta-cell function and hyperinsulinemia are present. The dosage for rosiglitazone is 4 mg to 8 mg daily, either as a single dose, or with half the dose given twice daily. There are some data suggesting slightly greater efficacy with twice-daily therapy; however, given the mechanism of action of these drugs, it is difficult to believe that twice-daily dosing is necessary. The dosage for pioglitazone is 15 to 45 mg once daily. Both drugs should be given with food in the morning.

Edema and weight gain can be very problematic in patients taking glitazones, particularly if they are taken in conjunction with insulin or insulin secretagogues. Hemodilution, with a resulting decrease in hemoglobin and hematocrit, is common. Weight gains of more than 10 kg are not unusual, and some patients have massive weight gain (more than 30 to 40 kg). It is hard to imagine that these effects are merely the result of changes in energy balance (i.e., less glycosuria with improved glycemic control). Fat mobilization from the visceral compartment to the periphery and differentiation of preadipocytes into adipocytes may be a cause of weight gain, unexplained by simple changes in energy balance. The patients with the best glycemic response often have the most weight gain. Fluid retention may induce or worsen congestive heart failure in patients with left ventricular compromise. A recent report associated glitazone twice as often as other antidiabetic agents with the development of congestive heart failure (45). Glitazones have not been tested in patients with New York Heart Association class III or IV heart failure. Therefore, initiation of glitazone therapy in a patient with an ejection fraction lower than 35%, regardless of the patient's symptoms, seems unwarranted. Although animal and *in vitro* studies suggest antiatherogenic activities of these drugs, it will be years before the results of clinical trials are available to prove that such a promise is actually fulfilled.

The newer glitazones (rosiglitazone and pioglitazone) do not appear to have the severe liver toxicity that led to the withdrawal from the market of the first drug in this class, troglitazone. However, very rare case reports of less fulminant liver disease have surfaced (46). Liver function test monitoring is still recommended if these agents are used. On initiation of therapy with pioglitazone or rosiglitazone, baseline liver function tests (minimally, aspartate transaminase [AST] and alanine transaminase [ALT] measurements) should be obtained. This testing should be repeated every other month for the first 12 months and periodically thereafter. Neither drug should be instituted if the baseline AST or ALT exceeds 2.5 times the upper limit of normal, and either should be discontinued if the AST or ALT exceeds 3 times the upper limit of normal or if signs or symptoms of liver injury become evident.

Practically speaking, edema and weight gain are the usual reasons for stopping therapy with glitazones. These side effects are particularly problematic in patients who are receiving concomitant insulin secretagogues or insulin therapy. The cause of the edema is unknown, and it may sometimes be refractory to diuretics. Anecdotal reports suggest that maximal inhibition of the renin-angiotensin system before initiation of therapy may prevent the development of edema. Weight gain of more than 10 to 15 kg should prompt discontinuation of the glitazone agents, which usually results in some loss of weight.

α-Glucosidase Inhibitors. α-Glucosidase inhibitors (acarbose and miglitol) prevent the breakdown of sucrose and complex carbohydrates in the small intestine, prolonging the absorption of carbohydrates (47). The net effect from this action is to reduce postprandial blood glucose rise with no effect on fasting glucose concentrations. These agents have a modest effect on HbA_{1C}.

Flatulence is a very common side effect and greatly limits the use of these agents. α-Glucosidase inhibitors should be titrated very slowly to reduce gastrointestinal intolerance. Usually therapy is started with one-half to one pill of the smallest dose with the biggest meal and titrated slowly, over time, to a full tablet (25 to 100 mg) with every meal. If a patient develops hypoglycemia while taking an α-glucosidase inhibitor, oral glucose (or parenteral glucose or glucagon) must be given, because the drug

will inhibit the breakdown of more complex sugar molecules in the gut. Liver function abnormalities have been seen with high doses of acarbose.

Practical Drug Therapy (Including Insulin Therapy). Patients experiencing symptoms may initially require treatment with insulin or insulin secretagogues to eliminate symptoms, because these agents produce the most rapid reduction in blood glucose concentrations (35,38,48). Such therapy also reduces "glucose toxicity," a reversible form of insulin resistance and inadequate insulin secretion. Otherwise, patients with an HbA_{1C} lower than 7% are usually treated with therapeutic lifestyle measures. Those with an HbA_{1C} of 7% to 8% are initially treated with single oral agents. Depending on motivation and adherence to therapeutic lifestyle changes, most patients with an HbA_{1C} higher than 9% require therapy with two or more agents to reach glycemic goals. Of the oral agents, insulin secretagogues produce the most rapid effect on glycemia, followed by metformin.

The best initial oral therapy for patients with type 2 diabetes mellitus is widely debated. With the exception of α-glucosidase inhibitors, which are less efficacious, all other therapies are about equally efficacious as initial oral monotherapy. Differences reported in the literature often relate to the population studied, such as greater HbA_{1C} reductions with monotherapy in drug-naïve and more markedly hyperglycemic patients. If one subscribes to the theory that insulin resistance is the proximal pathophysiologic defect and specific treatment thereof may reduce cardiovascular risk, then the use of insulin sensitizers will be emphasized, particularly early in the course of disease. However, if the practitioner believes that both insulin resistance and beta-cell dysfunction are part and parcel of the disease process, a two-pronged approach, using an insulin sensitizer and an insulin secretagogue, would be rational therapy.

Furthermore, arguments based on presumed pathophysiology often ignore well-done clinical end-point trials. Based on the UKPDS, progressive beta-cell dysfunction appears to be inherent to the disease process in type 2 diabetes mellitus and not a result of the use of insulin secretagogues. The same study confirmed the safety of this class of agents as well as insulin therapy for this disease. Furthermore, the only positive results for oral therapies in cardiovascular prevention are from the UKPDS substudy of metformin in obese patients. Because glitazones are associated with weight gain rather than weight loss, it is uncertain whether the results obtained with metformin in the UKPDS can be extrapolated to similar patients treated with thiazolidinediones. The disconcerting results (increased cardiac events) of "early addition" of metformin to existing maximal-dose sulfonylurea therapy (compared with sulfonylureas alone) in UKPDS have been called into question based on other analyses. (Perhaps there were fewer than the expected number of events in the sulfonylurea-alone group, rather than more events in the combination group [21].) Seeming confirmatory findings in some epidemiologic analyses most likely suggest that *maximal-dose* sulfonylurea therapy should not be used in combination with metformin. Hypoglycemia occurs not infrequently when insulin sensitizers are added to sulfonylureas. Given that the maximum efficacy of sulfonylureas in most patients is at half the maximum dose, it is reasonable to routinely reduce the dose of sulfonylureas to no more than half the maximum recommended dose whenever metformin or a glitazone is started.

Lastly, the startling mortality reductions seen with insulin as primary therapy in DIGAMI should make insulin an attractive therapeutic option. Furthermore, insulin therapy generally produces the maximal reduction in HbA_{1C}. As stated previously, there is no clinical evidence (despite some theoretical concerns to the contrary) that insulin, either endogenous or given exogenously, is

atherogenic. Some endocrinologists have opined that the major problem with insulin resistance is the resistance of physicians and patients to use insulin. Insulin therapy is generally underutilized in the management of type 2 diabetes mellitus. Addition of an insulin sensitizer to insulin will further facilitate glycemic control in many patients.

Based on the results of the UKPDS and the safety record, I usually start obese patients (i.e., those weighing more than 120% of their ideal body weight) on metformin initially and titrate to at least 2,000 mg/day (48). Patients who are at near-normal weights may be treated with insulin secretagogues. Failure of initial therapy should result in drug addition rather than substitution. Therapeutic substitution should be reserved for drug side effects. A proposed therapeutic scheme is listed in Table 12-6. Thiazolidinediones may be substituted if the patient is intolerant of, or has a contraindication to, metformin.

Some authorities believe strongly that insulin resistance should be addressed aggressively with insulin sensitizers early in the course of disease, because the ravages of insulin resistance on the cardiovascular system are presumably already taking their toll. If such a strategy is adopted, initial treatment with metformin and a glitazone is not unreasonable. However, no clinical outcome studies using this strategy have been completed. Care must be exercised in extrapolating to glitazones the positive cardiovascular effects demonstrated with metformin treatment in the UKPDS, because the two drug groups have different mechanisms of actions and different side effects. Particularly, the significant weight gain and fluid retention often seen with glitazones should give one pause in their use. Because of the frequency of troublesome side effects with

TABLE 12-6. *Overview of initial treatment of type 2 diabetes mellitus*

Clinical picture	Initial treatment	Add	Add
Normal weight	Secretagogue	Metformin	Insulin
Obese	Metformin	Secretagogue	Glitazone
Severely insulin resistant	Metformin	Glitazone	Secretagogue
Elderly	Short-acting secretagogue or insulin	—	—

Data from Oki JC, Isley WL. Diabetes mellitus. In: Dipiro JT, Talbert RL, Yee GC, et al., eds. *Pharmacotherapy: a pathophysiologic approach*, 5th ed. New York: McGraw-Hill, 2002:1335–1358.

glitazones and the lack of clinical trial end-point data, reserving early therapy with these agents for patients with marked evidence of the insulin resistance syndrome (triglycerides greater than 300 mg/dL, HDL-C below 30 mg/dL) seems prudent.

α-Glucosidase inhibitors can be used as monotherapy in patients at high risk for hypoglycemia, in patients manifesting primarily postprandial hyperglycemia, and in combination with virtually any other drug. However, compliance with these agents is poor in most patients.

After two oral drugs have failed to achieve the desired results, addition of a third class of oral agents can be considered (49). In fact, the FDA has recently approved oral triple therapy with a glitazone, metformin, and a sulfonylurea. An alternative would be to add bedtime insulin (NPH or insulin glargine) to oral agents.

Virtually all patients with type 2 diabetes ultimately become insulinopenic and require insulin therapy. Patients are often "transitioned" to insulin with the use of a bedtime injection of intermediate or long acting insulin, retaining oral agents primarily for control during the day (30,31). The insulin dose is started at approximately 0.2 U/kg and increased as needed to achieve fasting glucose targets. The insulin primarily reduces hepatic glucose production overnight, thus decreasing the morning fasting glucose concentration. Compared with multiple insulin injections, this strategy leads to less hyperinsulinemia during the day and is associated with less weight gain. A long-acting insulin preparation (e.g., insulin glargine) will also have some effect throughout the day. An alternative strategy, which is particularly useful in more obese patients and in patients consuming a very large evening meal, is to use a premixed insulin combination (NPH and regular or lispro or aspart insulin) before the evening meal (52). The reduction of the "baseline" glucose with such strategies allows for more optimal use of the various oral agents for daytime glycemic control. Because most patients are insulin resistant, at least one insulin sensitizer is commonly used with insulin therapy. The initial use of metformin as an insulin sensitizer in this situation,

with glitazones reserved for patients who are unable to take metformin, is a reasonable approach. Combination sensitizer therapy may prove useful in patients with evidence of marked insulin resistance.

Patients with type 2 diabetes mellitus are usually well buffered against hypoglycemia. However, patients receiving bedtime insulin injections should be monitored for hypoglycemia by asking about nocturnal sweating, palpitations, and nightmares and by prescribing SMBG. Failure of glycemic control in such patients, particularly when one of the oral agents is an insulin secretagogue, usually implies that there is insufficient pancreatic beta-cell function and that a more complete "insulin substitution" regimen should be begun.

When bedtime insulin plus daytime oral medications fail, a conventional insulin regimen of multiple doses with or without an insulin sensitizer can be tried. Concerns and problems with insulin administration, as addressed in the section on type 1 diabetes, generally are germane to the therapy of type 2 diabetes. However, patients with type 2 diabetes mellitus rarely have hypoglycemia unawareness, and they are better buffered against hypoglycemia. Also, the variability of insulin resistance means that insulin doses may range from 0.5 to 2.5 U/kg or more. Because most of these patients have some degree of residual insulin secretion, twice-daily injections of NPH and regular insulin can frequently be used to achieve adequate glycemic control. Weight gain is mild with insulin monotherapy and may be blunted by the concomitant use of metformin (53). Glitazones added to insulin usually result in rather significant weight gain despite the ability to use a lower dose of insulin (54). More vigorous insulin regimens will be needed (typically, a four-shot daily basal-bolus regimen) as patients become even more insulinopenic.

The availability of short-acting insulin secretagogues, very short-acting insulin, and α-glucosidase inhibitors, all of which target postprandial glycemia, has reminded practitioners that glycemic control is a function of fasting and preprandial glycemia and postprandial glycemic excursions (55). It remains to be seen whether targeting of after-meal glucose excursions has a greater effect on macrovascular complication risk than more conventional strategies do. Targeting of postprandial glucose values may be critical, given that epidemiologic studies show that glucose measurements obtained after glucose challenge are better predictors of macrovascular disease risk than are fasting glucose levels (56). However, new recommendations, suggesting that postprandial glucose targets be equivalent to essentially normal glucose values, do not take into account the fact that the therapeutic tools are not available to achieve these goals in most patients.

As stated previously, vigorous treatment of all cardiovascular risk factors is vital. Glucocentricity is unacceptable diabetes management in the 21st century. Data management of multiple parameters (SMBG data, HbA$_{1C}$, lipids, blood pressure, microalbuminuria) is mandatory. Computerized medical records are helpful for this purpose.

SPECIAL SITUATIONS

Prevention of Diabetes Mellitus

Efforts to prevent type 1 diabetes mellitus with immunosuppressive drugs (57) or insulin therapy (58) have been unsuccessful. Modest lifestyle changes (exercise and diet-induced weight loss) have proved quite successful in the prevention of type 2 diabetes mellitus in high-risk individuals. The recently published Diabetes Primary Prevention trial results (59) showed a 58% reduction in the development of type 2 diabetes. In the same study, low-dose metformin reduced the development of diabetes by 31%. Troglitazone has been shown to reduce subsequent development of type 2 diabetes mellitus in women with a history of gestational diabetes (60). Acarbose was recently shown to reduce diabetes by 25% in high-risk patients (61). Other pharmacologic prevention trials are in progress.

Acute Myocardial Infarction

Results of the DIGAMI study, previously discussed, suggest that tight glycemic control, with intravenous insulin infusion and multiple daily insulin injections reduce mortality in patients with acute myocardial infarction. A recently published study of critically ill surgical patients (most of whom were not even diabetic) showed reductions of approximately 40% in mortality when glucose was very tightly regulated (lower than 108 mg/dL), further suggesting that ill patients may be best cared for by rigorous glucose control (62). It has been hypothesized that the effects of such therapy are related to effects of insulin *per se,* rather than being necessarily a reflection of blood glucose levels.

Perioperative Management

Surgical patients may experience worsening of glycemia due to increased release of counter-regulatory (anti-insulin) hormones (63). Patients taking oral agents may need transient therapy with insulin to control blood glucose. In patients who require insulin, scheduled doses of insulin or continuous insulin infusions are preferred. The typical sliding-scale insulin approach is without scientific support (64) and is actually admitting defeat, because the glucose level soars due to no therapy, then plummets with zealous short-acting insulin therapy. The reason that more patients are not harmed from this strategy is that most patients have type 2 diabetes and are relatively resistant to ketosis and well buffered against hypoglycemia. Many patients with type 1 diabetes in the past were allowed to develop diabetic ketoacidosis because their insulin was omitted, or were made profoundly hypoglycemic by large doses of regular insulin. For patients who can eat soon after surgery, the time-honored approach of giving half of the usual morning NPH insulin dose with 5% dextrose in water intravenously is acceptable, with resumption of scheduled insulin, perhaps at reduced doses, within the first day. For patients requiring more prolonged periods without oral nutrition and for those undergoing major surgery, continuous insulin infusion is preferred. Vigorous glycemic control in the postoperative state appears to reduce morality (64), as described previously. Metformin should be discontinued temporarily after any major surgery, until it is clear that the patient is hemodynamically stable and normal renal function is documented.

THE FUTURE OF DIABETIC TREATMENT

Novel innovations in the treatment of diabetes mellitus are currently being developed and investigated. This section discusses new means of insulin delivery and new doses of drugs for the treatment of both type 1 and type 2 diabetes mellitus.

The "holy grail" of insulin delivery is a noninjectable system. Closest to market is pulmonary inhaled insulin (65,66), although recent concerns about lung toxicity have arisen and it remains to be seen whether this obstacle can be overcome. Other oral means of insulin delivery are in development, including absorption through the buccal mucosa and through the gastrointestinal tract (67). These latter approaches are clearly years away from use by practicing physicians and their patients.

Beta-cell and whole-pancreas transplantation have been used in highly selected patients with type 1 diabetes mellitus who were already receiving or would be receiving immunosuppressive medications after kidney transplantation (68). It is my view that such approaches will continue to be limited by the availability of organs, incompatibility issues, and problems of immunosuppression.

The major emphasis of drug development in type 2 diabetes mellitus has been to improve and expand the role of insulin sensitizers, particularly PPARγ agonists. Glitazone and nonglitazone dual and triple agonists (for PPARα and PPARδ as well as PPARγ) are in development and may prove very useful for lipid treatment (lowering triglycerides and increasing HDL-C) as well as glycemic improvement (69). Because such agents also have pleiotropic effects (e.g., reduced inflammation, reduced blood pressure), they have a potential to modulate diabetes cardiovascular complications. However, the drugs in development so far continue to be plagued by the complications of weight gain and edema. Whether agents can be developed that do not have these shortcomings remains to be seen. Perhaps

drugs that are differential agonists and antagonists (akin to selective receptor modulators such as raloxifene for the estrogen receptor) will ultimately solve this dilemma.

Lastly, a novel approach with possible benefits for both major kinds of diabetes are the glucagon-like peptide 1 (GLP-1) analogs and agents that inhibit the breakdown of this endogenous hormone (dipeptidyl peptidase IV inhibitors) (70). Such agents may restore beta-cell function and improve glycemia by multiple mechanisms. These drugs are currently being investigated in phase I and II clinical trials.

REFERENCES

1. Boyle JP, Honeycutt AA, Narayan KM, et al. Projection of diabetes burden through 2050: impact of changing demography and disease prevalence in the U.S. *Diabetes Care* 2001;24:1936–1940.
2. American Diabetes Association. Economic consequences of diabetes mellitus in the U.S. in 1997. *Diabetes Care* 1998;21:296–309.
3. Nichols GA, Brown JB. The impact of cardiovascular disease on medical care costs in subjects with and without type 2 diabetes. *Diabetes Care* 2002;25:482–486.
4. Grundy SM, Benjamin IJ, Burke GL, et al. Diabetes and cardiovascular disease: a statement for healthcare professionals from the American Heart Association. *Circulation* 1999;100.1134–1146.
5. Haffner SM. Management of dyslipidemia in adults with diabetes. *Diabetes Care* 1998;21:160–178.
6. Bardsley JK, Passaro M. ABCs of diabetes research. *Clin Diabetes* 2002;20:5–8.
7. United Kingdom Prospective Diabetes Study Group. Effect of intensive blood-glucose control with metformin on complications in overweight patients with type 2 diabetes (UKPDS 34). *Lancet* 1998;352:854 865.
8. Haffner SM, Alexander CM, Cook TJ, et al. Reduced coronary events in simvastatin-treated patients with coronary heart disease and diabetes or impaired fasting glucose levels: subgroup analyses in the Scandinavian Simvastatin Survival Study. *Arch Intern Med* 1999;159:2661–2667.
9. Hansson L, Zanchetti A, Carruthers SG, et al. Effects of intensive blood-pressure lowering and low-dose aspirin in patients with hypertension: principal results of the Hypertension Optimal Treatment (HOT) randomised trial. HOT Study Group. *Lancet* 1998;351:1755–1762.
10. Report of the Expert Committee on the Diagnosis and Classification of Diabetes Mellitus. *Diabetes Care* 2002;25:5–20.
11. Leaf DA. Women and coronary artery disease: gender confers no immunity. *Postgrad Med* 1990;87:55–60.
12. DeFronzo RA, Bonadonna RC, Ferrannini E. Pathogenesis of NIDDM: a balanced overview. *Diabetes Care* 1992;15:318–368.
13. Boden G. Pathogenesis of type 2 diabetes. *Clin Endocrinol Metab North Am* 2002;30:801–815.

14. Turner RC, Cull CA, Frighi V. Glycemic control with diet, sulfonylurea, metformin, or insulin in patients with type 2 diabetes mellitus: progressive requirement for multiple therapies (UKPDS 49). UK Prospective Diabetes Study (UKPDS) Group. *JAMA* 1999;281:2005–2012.

15. Weyer C, Pratley RE, Tataranni PA. Role of insulin resistance and insulin secretory dysfunction in the pathogenesis of type 2 diabetes mellitus: lessons from cross-sectional, prospective, and longitudinal studies in Pima Indians. *Curr Opin Endocrinol Metab* 2002;9:130–138.

16. Haffner SM, Stern MP, Hazuda HP, et al. Cardiovascular risk factors in confirmed prediabetic individuals: does the clock for coronary heart disease start ticking before the onset of clinical diabetes? *JAMA* 1990;263:2893–2898.

17. Reaven GM. Role of insulin resistance in human disease (syndrome X): an expanded definition. *Annu Rev Med* 1993;44:121–131.

18. Borch-Johnsen K. The new classification of diabetes mellitus and IGT: a critical approach. *Exp Clin Endocrinol Diabetes* 2001;109[Suppl 2]:S86–S93.

19. Thompson WG. Early recognition and treatment of glucose abnormalities to prevent type 2 diabetes mellitus and coronary heart disease. *Mayo Clin Proc* 2001;76:1137–1143.

20. Diabetes Control and Complications Trial Research Group. The effect of intensive treatment of diabetes on the development and progression of long-term complications in insulin-dependent diabetes mellitus. *N Engl J Med* 1993;329:977–986.

21. United Kingdom Prospective Diabetes Study Group. Intensive blood-glucose control with sulphonylureas or insulin compared with conventional treatment and risk of complications in patients with type 2 diabetes (UKPDS 33). *Lancet* 1998;352:837–853.

22. Stratton IM, Adler AI, Neil HA. Association of glycaemia with macrovascular and microvascular complications of type 2 diabetes (UKPDS 35): prospective observational study. *BMJ* 2000;321:405–412.

23. United Kingdom Prospective Diabetes Study Group. Effect of intensive blood-glucose control with metformin on complications in overweight patients with type 2 diabetes (UKPDS 34). *Lancet* 1998;352:854–865.

24. Adler AI, Stratton IM, Neil HA. Association of systolic blood pressure with macrovascular and microvascular complications of type 2 diabetes (UKPDS 36): prospective observational study. *BMJ* 2000;321:412–419.

25. United Kingdom Prospective Diabetes Study Group. Efficacy of atenolol and captopril in reducing risk of macrovascular and microvascular complications in type 2 diabetes: UKPDS 39. *BMJ* 1998;317:713–720.

26. Ohkubo Y, Kishikawa H, Araki E, et al. Intensive insulin therapy prevents the progression of diabetic microvascular complications in Japanese patients with non-insulin-dependent diabetes mellitus: a randomized prospective 6-year study. *Diabetes Res Clin Pract* 1995;28:103–117.

27. Malmberg K, Diabetes Mellitus, Insulin Glucose Infusion in Acute Myocardial Infarction (DIGAMI) Study Group. Prospective randomized study of intensive insulin treatment on long-term survival after acute myocar-dial infarction in patients with diabetes mellitus. *BMJ* 1997;314:1512–1515.

28. Hirsch IB, Coviello A. Intensive insulin therapy in critically ill patients [Letter]. *N Engl J Med* 2002;346:1586–1588.

29. American Diabetes Association. Standards of medical care for patients with diabetes mellitus. *Diabetes Care* 2002;25:213–229.

30. American Association of Clinical Endocrinologists. Medical Guidelines for the Management of Diabetes Mellitus: the AACE system of intensive diabetes self-management—2000 update. *Endocr Pract* 2000;6:43–84.

31. Self-monitoring of blood glucose. American Diabetes Association. *Diabetes Care* 1994;17:81–86.

32. Norris SL, Engelgau MM, Narayan KM. Effectiveness of self-management training in type 2 diabetes: a systematic review of randomized controlled trials. *Diabetes Care* 2001;24:561–587.

33. Evidence-based nutrition principles and recommendations for the treatment and prevention of diabetes and related complications. *Diabetes Care* 2002;25:50–60.

34. American Diabetes Association. Diabetes mellitus and exercise. *Diabetes Care* 2002;25:64–68.

35. Oki JC, Isley WL. Diabetes mellitus. In: Dipiro JT, Talbert RL, Yee GC, et al, eds. *Pharmacotherapy: a pathophysiologic approach,* 5th ed. New York: McGraw-Hill, 2002:1335–1358.

36. Strowig S, Raskin P. Intensive management of insulin-dependent diabetes mellitus. In: Porte D Jr, Sherwin RS. *Ellenberg and Rifkin's diabetes mellitus,* 5th ed. Stamford, CT: Appleton & Lange, 1997:709–733.

37. Reynolds LR. Reemergence of insulin pump therapy in the 1990s. *South Med J* 2000;93:1157–1161.

38. Lebovitz HE. Oral therapies for diabetic hyperglycemia. *Clin Endocrinol Metab* 2001;30:909–933.

39. Culy CR, Jarvis B. Repaglinide: a review of its therapeutic use in type 2 diabetes mellitus. *Drugs* 2001;61:1625–1660.

40. Levien TL, Baker DE, Campbell RK, et al. Nateglinide therapy for type 2 diabetes mellitus. *Ann Pharmacother* 2001;35:1426–1434.

41. Inzucchi SE. Oral antihyperglycemic therapy for type 2 diabetes: scientific review. *JAMA* 2002;287:360–372.

42. Lebovitz HE, Banerji MA. Insulin resistance and its treatment by thiazolidinediones. *Recent Prog Horm Res* 2001;56:265–294.

43. Parulkar AA, Pendergrass ML, Granda-Ayala R, et al. Nonhypoglycemic effects of thiazolidinediones. *Ann Intern Med* 2001;134:61–71.

44. Lebovitz HE, Dole JF, Patwardhan R, et al. Rosiglitazone monotherapy is effective in patients with type 2 diabetes. *J Clin Endocrinol Metab* 2001;86:280–288.

45. Delea TE, Hagiwara M, Edelsberg JS, et al. *Thiazolidinediones are associated with increased risk of heart failure in patients with type 2 diabetes.* Presented at the American Diabetes Association 62nd Annual Scientific Session, San Francisco, 2002.

46. Isley WL, Oki JC. Hepatotoxicity of thiazolidinediones. *Diabetes Obes Metab* 2001;3:389–392.

47. Mooradian AD, Thurman JE. Drug therapy of postprandial hyperglycemia. *Drugs* 1999;57:19–29.

48. DeFronzo RA. Pharmacologic therapy for type 2 diabetes mellitus. *Ann Intern Med* 1999;131:281–303

49. Yale JF, Valiquett TR, Ghazzi MN, et al. The effect of a thiazolidinedione drug, troglitazone, on glycemia in patients with type 2 diabetes mellitus poorly controlled with sulfonylurea and metformin: a multicenter, randomized, double-blind, placebo-controlled trial. *Ann Intern Med* 2001;134:737–745.

50. Shank ML, Del Prato S, DeFronzo RA. Bedtime insulin/daytime glipizide: effective therapy for sulfonylurea failures in NIDDM. *Diabetes* 1995;44:165–172.

51. Yki-Jarvinen H, Ryysy L, Nikkila K. Comparison of bedtime insulin regimens in patients with type 2 diabetes mellitus: a randomized, controlled trial. *Ann Intern Med* 1999;130:389–396.

52. Riddle MC, Schneider J. Beginning insulin treatment of obese patients with evening 70/30 insulin plus glimepiride versus insulin alone. Glimepiride Combination Group. *Diabetes Care* 1998;21:1052–1057.

53. Aviles-Santa L, Sinding J, Raskin P. Effects of metformin in patients with poorly controlled, insulin-treated type 2 diabetes mellitus: a randomized, double-blind, placebo-controlled trial. *Ann Intern Med* 1999;131:182–188.

54. Raskin P, Rendell M, Riddle MC, et al. A randomized trial of rosiglitazone therapy in patients with inadequately controlled insulin-treated type 2 diabetes. *Diabetes Care* 2001;24:1226–1232.

55. Bastyr EJ 3rd, Stuart CA, Brodows RG. Therapy focused on lowering postprandial glucose, not fasting glucose, may be superior for lowering HbA1c. IOEZ Study Group. *Diabetes Care* 2000;23:1236–1241.

56. Glucose tolerance and mortality: comparison of WHO and American Diabetes Association diagnostic criteria. The DECODE study group. European Diabetes Epidemiology Group Diabetes Epidemiology: Collaborative analysis of diagnostic criteria in Europe. *Lancet* 1999;354:617–621.

57. Schernthaner G. Progress in the immunointervention of type-1 diabetes mellitus. *Horm Metab Res* 1995;27:547–554.

58. Diabetes Prevention Trial–Type 1 Diabetes Study Group. Effects of insulin in relatives of patients with type 1 diabetes mellitus. *N Engl J Med* 2002;346:1685–1691.

59. Knowler WC, Barrett-Connor E, Fowler SE, et al. Diabetes Prevention Program Research Group. Reduction in the incidence of type 2 diabetes with lifestyle intervention or metformin. *N Engl J Med* 2002;346:393–403.

60. Buchanan T, Xiang A, Peters R, et al. *Prevention of type 2 diabetes by treatment of insulin resistance: comparison of early vs. late intervention in the TRIPOD study.* Presented at the American Diabetes Association 62nd Annual Scientific Session, San Francisco, 2002.

61. Chiasson JL, Josse RG, Gomis R, et al. , for the STOP-NIDDM Trial Research Group. Acarbose for prevention of type 2 diabetes mellitus: the STOP-NIDDM randomised trial. *Lancet* 2002;359:2072–2077.

62. Van den Berghe G, Wouters P, Weekers F, et al. Intensive insulin therapy in critically ill patients. *N Engl J Med* 2001;345:1359–1367.

63. Jacober SJ, Sowers JR. An update on perioperative management of diabetes. *Arch Intern Med* 1999;159:2405–2411.

64. Lorber DL. Sliding scale insulin. *Diabetes Care* 2001;24:2011–2012.

65. Skyler JS, Cefalu WT, Kourides IA, et al. Efficacy of inhaled human insulin in type 1 diabetes mellitus: a randomised proof-of-concept study. *Lancet* 2001;357:331–335.

66. Cefalu WT, Skyler JS, Kourides IA, et al. Inhaled human insulin treatment in patients with type 2 diabetes mellitus. *Ann Intern Med* 2001;134:203–207.

67. Cefalu WT. Novel routes of insulin delivery for patients with type 1 or type 2 diabetes. *Ann Med* 2001;33:579–586.

68. White SA, Kimber R, Veitch PS, et al. Surgical treatment of diabetes mellitus by islet cell and pancreas transplantation. *Postgrad Med J* 2001;77:383–387.

69. Brand CL, Sturis J, Gotfredsen CF, et al. Dual PPARα/γ activation provides enhanced improvement of insulin sensitivity and glycemic control in ZDF rats. *Am J Physiol Endocrinol Metab* 2003;284:E841–E854.

70. Drucker DJ. Therapeutic potential of dipeptidyl peptidase IV inhibitors for the treatment of type 2 diabetes. *Expert Opin Investig Drugs* 2003;12:87–100.

Diabetes and Cardiovascular Disease
edited by Steven P. Marso and David M. Stern
Lippincott Williams & Wilkins, Philadelphia © 2004

13

Endothelial Dysfunction

Joshua A. Beckman

*Instructor of Medicine, Department of Medicine, Harvard Medical School, Associate
Attending Physician, Department of Medicine, Brigham and Women's Hospital, Boston,
Massachusetts*

The characterization of diabetes mellitus derives from observed abnormalities in carbohydrate metabolism that stem from a relative or complete absence of insulin. In contrast to this operational definition, the dysmetabolism inherent in diabetes arises from abnormalities in adipose storage, lipid metabolism, protein biochemistry, and signal transduction in addition to carbohydrate metabolism. Indeed, of this wide range of abnormalities, each has important effects on vascular function to an extent far greater than any other of the demonstrated risk factors. Among the well-established cardiovascular risk factors, only non-insulin-dependent (type 2) diabetes mellitus carries the same risk for myocardial infarction as prior myocardial infarction itself (1). The affects of diabetes mellitus on the vasculature may be thought of as a cascade of assaults, each providing specific insult, with the aggregate yielding an environment permissive for the development of atherosclerosis.

Recognition of the importance of diabetes in cardiovascular disease has been increasing recently (2). The confluence of increasing ponderosity and increasing age of the population is serving to dramatically increase the rate of type 2 diabetes mellitus, which accounts for more than 90% of all cases of diabetes in the United States (3,4). Although the importance of diabetes in microvascular disease has been well known for years, the frequency of clinical events, rate of hospitalization, and mortality rate are dramatically higher for macrovascular disease (5).

THE ENDOTHELIUM

Numerous plausible biologic mechanisms have been put forward to explain the early development of atherosclerosis and the exceptionally poor outcome of patients with diabetes mellitus and cardiovascular disease. Patients with type 2 diabetes have early development of abnormal endothelial function, platelet hyperactivity, aggressive atherosclerosis, a propensity for adverse arterial remodeling, enhanced cellular and matrix proliferation after arterial injury, and impaired fibrinolysis with a tendency for thrombosis and inflammation (2). As a result, the diabetic state leads to profound arteriopathy. Perhaps the earliest demonstrable manifestation is that of endothelial dysfunction.

Until the seminal experiments of Furchgott and Zawadzki in 1980 (6), the endothelium was commonly thought to be a relatively inert barrier lining the inner walls of blood vessels. Although the function of the endothelial cell layer continues to be actively investigated, it has become clear that the endothelium plays a crucial role in vascular homeostasis, modulating blood flow, delivery of nutrients and removal of waste, thrombosis and coagulation, inflammation, leukocyte trafficking, and vascular smooth muscle cell proliferation and migration. Loss of normal endothelial cellular function, thought to be an early marker for the development of atherosclerosis, is associated with diabetes mellitus and provides a key link between the dysmetabolism of diabetes mellitus and the development of both microvascular and macro-vascular disease states resulting in end-organ damage, including nephropathy, retinopathy, neuropathy, myocardial infarction, stroke, and death.

ENDOTHELIAL REGULATION

Endothelial regulation occurs through the production of important autocrine and paracrine substances that regulate the structure and function of vascular cells (Fig. 13-1). Among other factors, the control of the vascular microenvironment relies on a balance between vasodilators and vasoconstrictors, between coagulants and anticoagulants, and among modulators of platelet activity (Table 13-1). Nitric oxide (NO), probably the best-characterized endothelium-derived factor, is constitutively produced by endothe-lial nitric oxide synthase (eNOS) and is a potent vasodilator (7). NO production may be influenced by a wide variety of chemical and biomechanical stimuli, allowing the fine modulation of its release (7). The two best-characterized endothelium-derived vasoconstrictors, endothelin (ET) and angiotensin II, antagonize the effects of NO and allow the endothelium to regulate vascular homeostasis (8).

Constitutive release of NO by healthy endothelium importantly regulates vascular tone in both muscular conduit vessels and resistance arterioles (9), with some contribution from a secondary vasodilator, prostacyclin (10), and the vasoconstrictors angiotensin II (11) and ET (12). In healthy subjects, endothelial release of NO causes vasodilation in both peripheral and coronary arteries. In the setting of risk factors for atherosclerosis, including diabetes mellitus

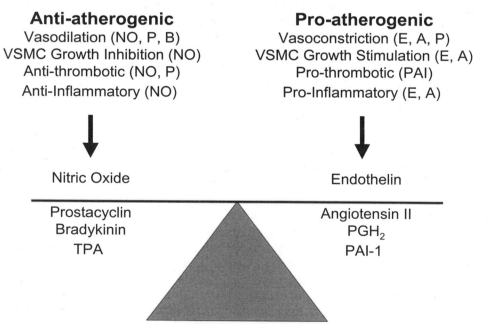

FIG. 13-1. The endothelium elaborates many mediators that regulate vascular function. Depending on the clinical scenario, the elaborated factors may slow or enhance vascular dysfunction. Important factors are listed and grouped according to their atherogenic tendency. A, angiotensin II; B, bradykinin; E, endothelin; NO, nitric oxide; P, prostacyclin; PAI-1, plasminogen activator inhibitor-1; PGH_2, prostaglandin H_2; TPA, tissue plasminogen activator.

TABLE 13-1. *Activity of endothelium-derived mediators*

Mediator	Vasodilation	Inflammation	Thrombosis	Proliferation of vascular smooth muscle cells
Nitric oxide	↑	↓	↓	↓
Prostacyclin	↑	—	↓	↓
Endothelium-derived hyperpolarizing factors	↑	—	—	—
Endothelin	↓	↑	↑	↑
Angiotensin II	↓	↑	↑	↑
Superoxide anion	↓	↑	—	↑
Bradykinin	↑	↓	—	—
Prostaglandin H_2	↓	—	—	—

↑, increases; ↓, decreases.

specifically, and in atherosclerosis *per se,* the vasodilation in peripheral arteries is attenuated and there is paradoxical constriction in coronary arteries (13,14).

Measurement of the bioavailability of NO in humans is accomplished through NO's vasodilatory role. eNOS may be stimulated by infusing agonists such as acetylcholine, methacholine, serotonin, or substance P to measure receptor-mediated release of NO in limb resistance vessels and coronary arteries or by increasing shear stress using sphygmomanometric cuffs to create a reactive hyperemic stimulus in limb conduit vessels (15,16). Determining the vasodilatory response to the stimulus allows comparison between healthy subjects and patient groups. Patients with atherosclerosis and its risk factors, including diabetes mellitus in particular, have a diminished vasodilatory capacity (17,18). This diminished vasodilatory capacity is commonly described as endothelial dysfunction and can be demonstrated in subjects with both insulin-dependent (type 1) and type 2 diabetes mellitus (18,19).

Although endothelial dysfunction in humans is typically measured as diminished vasodilation, the diminished bioavailability of NO and the production of proatherogenic peptides such as ET promote multiple atherogenic processes in addition to vasoconstriction. Endothelium-derived mediators, particularly NO, regulate vessel inflammation and thrombosis through pleiotropic interactions with leukocytes and platelets. The attraction of leukocytes into the subintima represents an important component of athero-genesis. Endothelial cells produce chemokines and cytokines to attract and increase the interaction between leukocyte adhesion molecules, thereby increasing white blood cell rolling, vessel wall adhesion, and subendothelial diapedesis (20). NO antagonizes these processes through its antagonism of intracellular proinflammatory transcription factors. The endothelium also regulates hemostasis through the production of coagulation factors and modulation of platelet activity (21). Elaboration of NO inhibits platelet binding and activation (22,23).

How does endothelial dysfunction participate in the development of atherosclerosis? Impaired endothelial function precedes clinically detectable atherosclerosis and creates an environment permissive for atherogenesis. Decreased endothelium-derived NO increases the process of inflammation, including the production of chemokines, cytokines, and leukocyte adhesion molecules; enhances vascular smooth muscle proliferation and migration; causes platelet activation; may participate in intravascular neovascularization; and enhances adverse lipid modification (24). Moreover, once atherosclerotic lesions have developed, endothelial dysfunction may exacerbate lesion progression and the development of clinical events. Impaired endothelium may abnormally reduce vascular perfusion, produce factors that decrease plaque stability, and increase the risk of plaque rupture. Endothelial dysfunction *per se* can predict the presence of significant coronary artery disease (25) and can provide prognostic information concerning the likelihood of events in patients with coronary artery disease, both over time (26) and after noncardiac surgery (27). Thus, abnormal endothelial function in diabetes augments atherosclerosis development, progression, and clinical event frequency and severity (2).

CLINICAL ASSESSMENT OF ENDOTHELIAL FUNCTION

The vascular architecture essentially consists of three layers: intima, media, and adventitia. The majority of work in intact humans has focused on characterizing the inner lining of the intima, the endothelium. Although no gold standard exists for the clinical quantification of endothelial function, several modalities are used to quantify vascular reactivity. Initially, endothelium-dependent relaxation was invasively assessed with the use of acetylcholine in the human coronary circulation (14). Endothelial function is determined invasively through quantitative coronary angiography or a Doppler flow wire. In the former method, epicardial lumen diameter is measured after administration of an endothelium-dependent vasodilator such as acetylcholine or serotonin. A Doppler flow wire assesses the microvascular endothelial function by measuring coronary flow reserve. The major limitation with these modalities is that they require invasive cannulation of coronary arteries. Therefore, minimally invasive strategies have been developed to assess endothelial function. One such technique employs high-resolution ultrasonography to measure flow-mediated dilation. This method was first applied clinically in the early 1990's (28); it depends on hyperemic-mediated dilation of the brachial artery and has been shown to have an acceptable reliability with respect to measurement of flow-mediated dilation (17,28–32). In this model, the artery of interest, usually the brachial or superficial femoral artery, is occluded with the use of a cuff inflation protocol for 4 to 5 minutes. The diameter of the target artery is measured on a two-dimensional ultrasound image at rest and after hyperemia. This model is the most common method for the noninvasive detection of endothelial dysfunction and has been demonstrated in many disease states, including hypertension (31) and type 2 diabetes (33), and among persons at risk for coronary artery disease (34).

Another noninvasive tool to assess endothelial function is venous-occlusion plethysmography. In this model, forearm blood flow (FBF) is measured in response to endothelium-dependent vasodilators, such as methacholine, and endothelium-independent vasodilators, such as verapamil (35). This technique has been used to evaluate FBF in patients with diabetes mellitus. Although basal FBF appears to be similar among persons with and without diabetes, the vasodilator response is attenuated in diabetic subjects compared with controls (19,36).

Other tools to evaluate endothelium clinically include measurement of intimal medial thickness, determination of pulse wave velocity, and the use of positron emission tomography (37).

MECHANISMS OF ENDOTHELIAL DYSFUNCTION IN DIABETES

The biologic drivers of impaired endothelial function among subjects with type 2 diabetes are varied but are undoubtedly linked to NO regulation; they include diminished NO production, increased inactivation by reactive oxygen species (ROS), and impaired signal transduction. Dysregulation and elevation of blood glucose was the earliest recognized pathologic process in diabetes mellitus and remains an important therapeutic target. The endothelium is a very sensitive sensor for elevations in blood glucose. Abnormalities in endothelial function in healthy human beings *in vivo* develop rapidly (as early as 6 hours) in response to hyperglycemia (38,39). The rapidity of these functional changes positions the endothelium as an early barometer for the pathophysiology associated with hyperglycemia and diabetes. Why does the endothelium uniquely express these changes so rapidly among the cellular components of the vasculature? The answer may lie, in part, in the persistent expression of glucose transporter 1 (GLUT1) in endothelial cells despite ambient hyperglycemia (40). Indeed, vascular endothelial cells maintain an intracellular glucose concentration mirroring that found in the extracellular environment, whereas vascular smooth muscle cells decrease glucose transport to maintain a normal intracellular glucose concentration (41).

Hyperglycemia

Of the many recognized abnormalities caused by hyperglycemia, the shift in production of ROS from NO to superoxide anion represents a central process with diverse pathogenic effects. In fact, endothelial cells probably are the primary source of vascular oxidative stress in diabetes mellitus (42). Recent data have indicated that the earliest source of superoxide anion from hyperglycemia begins within the endothelial cell. Hyperglycemia causes the electron transport chain in the mitochondria to generate superoxide anion instead of donating electrons for the production of adenosine triphosphate (ATP) (43). This process initiates and supports an ever-increasing dedication of cellular machinery to the production of ROS in general and superoxide anion in particular. Mitochondrial production of superoxide anion causes the activation of protein kinase C (PKC), which in turn activates cytosolic production of superoxide anion by reduced nicotinamide adenine dinucleotide phosphate (NADPH) oxidase (44). Increases in cytosolic production of superoxide anion attenuate the normal physiologic function of eNOS by increasing the production of peroxynitrite anion to oxidize the eNOS cofactor tetrahydrobiopterin and cause preferential production of superoxide anion instead of NO by eNOS (45). Increased hexosamine pathway activity, resulting from increased mitochondrial superoxide anion production, further diminishes eNOS production of NO by inhibiting the phosphorylation of an eNOS activation site by the protein kinase akt (46). In addition to enhanced intracellular and extracellular enzymatic production of superoxide anion, xanthine oxidase liberation (most likely from the liver) augments oxidative stress in the extracellular space (47–49).

Hyperglycemia also increases other sources of oxidative stress, including intracellular production of advanced glycation end products (AGEs) and activation of the endothelial receptor for AGE (RAGE). Increased intracellular concentrations of glucose foster the development of AGEs and typically occur within about 1 week after the initiation of hyperglycemia (50). Although a component of AGEs is formed extracellularly, the predominant location for their generation is probably intracellular. They can develop as a result of auto-oxidation of glucose, decomposition of the Amadori product, or fragmentation of the glyceraldehyde-3-phosphate to methylglyoxal (51). A subsequent reaction with the amino groups of intracellular and extracellular proteins forms the AGEs (50). Functional abnormalities arise in response to intracellular protein modification and activation of RAGE (52). AGEs can produce ROS and also can increase intracellular enzymatic production of ROS via activation of RAGE (53,54).

Increases in glucose concentration also increase the concentration of diacylglycerol (55). Diacylglycerol causes the preferential endothelial activation of PKC-β and -δ (56,57). Controlling glycemia or increasing the catabolism of diacylglycerol, or both, eliminates activation of PKC, suggesting the importance of this pathway of activation *in vivo* (58,59). In fact, in healthy humans, inhibition of PKC-β prevented endothelial dysfunction in response to hyperglycemia (60). The importance of this pathway can be found in PKC's effects of augmenting insulin resistance and increasing oxidative stress (44,61). Thus, hyperglycemia may participate importantly in the regulation of insulin resistance (62).

Increased Free Fatty Acid Concentration

Insulin resistance and the commensurate liberation of free fatty acids also augment the oxidative stress burden and diminish the bioavailability of NO (63). Arising from increased release from adipose tissue and decreased skeletal muscle uptake (64), increased plasma free fatty acids augment oxidative stress by increasing the production of small, dense, oxidized low-density lipoprotein (LDL) (65,66) and by directly affecting the endothelium (61). In the endothelium, free fatty acids cause membrane translocation and activation of PKC, antagonize the phosphatidylinositol-3-kinase (PI3) pathway (an eNOS stimulator), augment the production of ET-1 (most likely through the augmentation of mitogen-activated protein [MAP] kinase activation), and increase the production of ROS (61,63,67–69).

Insulin Resistance

Most individuals with type 2 diabetes exhibit insulin resistance (70), which is characterized by impaired glucose disposal mediated at the peripheral tissue level, initial hyperinsulinemia, and typical clinical characteristics including central adiposity, dyslipidemia, and hypertension. Insulin resistance often precedes the onset of overt hyperglycemia by years to decades, and it plays a deterministic role in the development of macrovascular disease. Although peripheral resistance to insulin continues, in time beta-cell failure ensues, resulting in further hyperglycemia and a decrease in circulating insulin levels. Insulin resistance occurs in many tissues, including the endothelium. Supporting the concept of a systemic process, the extent of insulin resistance correlates with both glucose disposal and endothelium-dependent vasodilation (71). In healthy subjects, insulin acts as an endothelium-dependent vasodilator, increasing the production of NO in both the basal and the stimulated state (72–74). In contradistinction, persons with diabetes have markedly abnormal endothelial function. Specifically, in subjects with either insulin resistance or overt type 2 diabetes, insulin-mediated endothelium-dependent vasodilation is impaired (72,75). Endothelial dysfunction also is manifested in the early stages of diabetes (18,76,77); it precedes the onset of microalbuminuria (78); and it is evident among persons with impaired glucose tolerance and among first-degree relatives of persons with type 2 diabetes mellitus (79). Furthermore, in patients with type 2 diabetes, impaired glucose tolerance and first-degree relatives of persons with type 2 diabetes have increased circulating markers of endothelial dysfunction, including soluble vascular cell adhesion molecule (sVCAM), soluble intercellular cell adhesion molecule (sICAM), ET-1, and von Willebrand factor. These data support the notion that macrovascular risk occurs well before the development of overt diabetes mellitus. Although there is clearly a clustering of

cardiovascular risk factors before the development of diabetes, it remains likely that insulin resistance syndrome and/or the prediabetic state contributes to substantial vascular risk beyond traditional risk factors. This pathobiologic link of insulin resistance and type 2 diabetes with endothelial function suggests that pharmacologic improvements in insulin resistance may result in improved endothelium-dependent vasodilation. This proof of concept has been demonstrated with the insulin-sensitizing agents troglitazone and metformin (80,81).

Endothelial cell insulin receptor activation stimulates two major intracellular signaling pathways, the PI3 kinase and MAP kinase pathways (82). Stimulation of the PI3 kinase pathway increases the activity of eNOS and commensurate NO production, leading to insulin-mediated increases in endothelium-dependent vasodilation (83). Increased concentrations of free fatty acids, however, impair this pathway (67) and decrease both glucose disposal and eNOS activity (83). In the setting of insulin resistance, preferential activation of the MAP kinase pathway by insulin decreases NO production and results in increased production of ET, augmented inflammation, and an increased tendency to coagulation (84–86). Thus, insulin resistance, created by disturbances in carbohydrate and lipid metabolism, changes endothelial signaling pathways to promote atherogenesis.

ENDOTHELIAL DYSFUNCTION IN DIABETES

The metabolic disturbances described earlier change endothelial cell activity and have consequences that affect the capacity of blood vessels to resist the development of atherosclerosis. Each important function, including modulation of vascular tone, regulation of vessel inflammation, and inhibition of thrombosis, is impaired in diabetes, creating a permissive environment for atherogenesis.

Vasomotor Function

Increases in the production of alternative ROS, especially superoxide anion, decrease

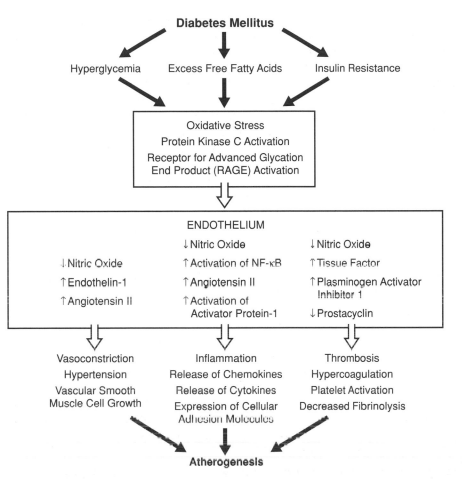

FIG. 13-2. Endothelial dysfunction and atherogenesis. The dysmetabolism in diabetes mellitus converts endothelial cell activity from an inhibitor of atherosclerosis to a participant in the process. Activation of these systems promotes vasoconstriction, inflammation, and thrombosis. (From Beckman JA, Creager MA, Libby P. Diabetes and atherosclerosis: epidemiology, pathophysiology, and management. *JAMA* 2002;287:2572, with permission.)

the bioavailability of endothelium-derived NO (Fig. 13-2). Superoxide anion and NO react in a diffusion-limited reaction to form peroxynitrite (87). Although peroxynitrite modestly causes vasodilation (88), endothelium-dependent vasodilation is impaired in resistance and conduit vessels among patients with type 1 and type 2 diabetes mellitus without evident vascular disease (18,19,89,90). Therefore, both receptor and shear stress-stimulated production of NO are impaired. Additionally, increases in oxidative stress inhibit the production of secondary vasodilators (e.g., prostacyclin) to diminish the tendency to vasorelaxation (91).

Vascular tone is further perturbed by the increase in vasoconstrictor peptides, including ET-1 and angiotensin II. As a result of insulin resistance, increased oxidative stress, as mediated by oxidized LDL (92), activation of PKC (56), ligand-receptor interaction between AGEs and RAGE (93), and preferential stimulation of MAP kinase over PI3 kinase combine to increase ET production (68,69). ET acts via the ET-A receptor to mediate contraction of vascular smooth muscle. In addition to its affects on vascular tone, ET stimulates the renin-angiotensin system, induces vascular smooth muscle hypertrophy, and augments sodium and volume retention (94).

Clinical and experimental data support the prominence of angiotensin II in the development and progression of atherosclerosis. Antagonism of renin-angiotensin activation has well-documented vascular benefits in diabetes (95). Moreover, the entire renin-angiotensin system is recapitulated within each endothelial cell (96). Increased angiotensin II activity has been demonstrated in diabetes mellitus and may result, in part, from hyperglycemia-mediated diminished endothelium-derived NO (97) or from activation of a lectin-like receptor by oxidized LDL (98). Angiotensin II counteracts many of the beneficial effects of NO by decreasing endothelium-dependent vasodilation, augmenting coagulation and platelet activation, increasing inflammation, and promoting the growth and migration of smooth muscle cells (99). Many of these effects may occur as a result of an angiotensin II-mediated increase in oxidative stress (100). Some investigators have shown that inhibition of the renin-angiotensin system and blockade of angiotensin II receptors improves endothelial function in resistance and conduit vessels in type 1 and type 2 diabetes, although others have reported no improvement (101–106). The relative importance of angiotensin II and other vasoconstrictors, including prostanoids and norepinephrine, on endothelial function *per se* and on atherosclerosis in general remains under active investigation (107–109).

Inflammation

Over the last decade, it has become recognized that inflammation characterizes the process of atherogenesis (110,111), and inflammation has recently been linked with the development of diabetes and insulin resistance (112,113). The process of atherosclerosis is initiated via migration of T lymphocytes into the vascular intima (111). These cells secrete cytokines and chemokines, recruiting monocytes and vascular smooth muscle cells, which, on reaching the subendothelium, scavenge oxidized LDL, become foam cells, and, in their accumulation, become fatty streaks (110). Each of these early atherogenic processes is facilitated by endothelial dysfunction. Augmented oxidative stress, RAGE activation,

PKC activation, decreased NO, and increased ET activate the transcription factors nuclear factor κB (NFκB) and activator protein-1 (AP-1) (114–116). These factors increase gene expression and transcription of proinflammatory cytokines and chemokines, increase the production of leukocyte adhesion molecules on the endothelial cell surface, and increase inflammatory mediator content within atherosclerotic lesions—processes that foster atherogenesis (117–119). Modulation of the cytokine axis, whether with pharmacologic agents (120) or by reducing visceral adiposity (121), results in improvement in endothelial function and a reduction in circulating cytokines and soluble markers of endothelial cellular activation.

Diabetes exacerbates the progression and development of clinical events as well. The mature atherosclerotic plaque is characterized by a lipid pool protected from the circulation by a fibrous cap. In diabetes, endothelial cells increase their production of matrix metalloproteinases and of cytokines that decrease the synthesis of collagen by vascular smooth muscle cells (122,123). As collagen production is diminished and extant fibrous cap collagen is metabolized, the risk of plaque rupture increases.

Thrombosis

On plaque rupture, the clinical severity of the event depends on the extent of thrombus formation and vessel occlusion. Diabetic endothelial cells augment the production of tissue factor, a power coagulant found in atherosclerotic lesions (124). Moreover, the dysfunctional endothelium adversely affects coagulation within the lumen as well. Diabetic endothelium has decreased expression of thrombomodulin, an important component of the protein C anticoagulation system; increased production of plasminogen activator inhibitor-1 (PAI-1), which decreases fibrinolytic capacity; and, because of diminished NO and prostacyclin, a decreased capacity to antagonize platelet activation and aggregation (125–127). Each of these insults may potentiate the severity of thrombus formation after plaque rupture and make the development of arterial occlusion and clinical events more likely.

CONCLUSION

The endothelial cell, which links the vasculature to the rest of the body, is first to be affected by the changes seen in diabetes and quickly begins to change its function in response. The multipronged assault from the varying components of dysmetabolism cause alterations in the elaboration of endothelium-derived mediators and increases in oxygen-derived free radical production. The repercussions of these effects include attenuated vasomotor function, increased inflammation, thrombosis and coagulation, and impaired function of other vascular cellular constituents, including leukocytes, platelets, and vascular smooth muscle cells, creating an environment permissive for the development and progression of atherosclerosis (2). Overall, diabetes adversely changes the role of the endothelial cell from atherogenesis antagonist to avid participant in the process.

REFERENCES

1. Haffner SM, et al. Mortality from coronary heart disease in subjects with type 2 diabetes and in nondiabetic subjects with and without prior myocardial infarction. *N Engl J Med* 1998;338:229–234.
2. Beckman JA, Creager MA, Libby P. Diabetes and atherosclerosis: epidemiology, pathophysiology, and management. *JAMA* 2002;287:2570–2581.
3. Mokdad AH, et al. The spread of the obesity epidemic in the United States, 1991–1998. *JAMA* 1999;282:1519–1522.
4. Mokdad AH, et al. The continuing increase of diabetes in the US. *Diabetes Care* 2001;24:412.
5. United Kingdom Prospective Diabetes Study Group. Intensive blood-glucose control with sulphonylureas or insulin compared with conventional treatment and risk of complications in patients with type 2 diabetes (UKPDS 33). *Lancet* 1998;352:837–853.
6. Furchgott RF, Zawadzki JV. The obligatory role of endothelial cells in the relaxation of arterial smooth muscle by acetylcholine. *Nature* 1980;288:373–376.
7. Moncada S, Higgs A. The L-arginine-nitric oxide pathway. *N Engl J Med* 1993;329:2002–2012.
8. Luft FC. Proinflammatory effects of angiotensin II and endothelin: targets for progression of cardiovascular and renal diseases. *Curr Opin Nephrol Hypertens* 2002;11:59–66.
9. Rees DD, Palmer RM, Moncada S. Role of endothelium-derived nitric oxide in the regulation of blood pressure. *Proc Natl Acad Sci U S A* 1989;86:3375–3378.
10. Duffy SJ, et al. Contribution of vasodilator prostanoids and nitric oxide to resting flow, metabolic vasodilation, and flow-mediated dilation in human coronary circulation. *Circulation* 1999;100:1951–1957.
11. Webb DJ, et al. Regulation of regional vascular tone: the role of angiotensin conversion in human forearm resistance vessels. *J Hypertens Suppl* 1988;6:S57–S59.
12. Haynes WG, et al. Systemic endothelin receptor blockade decreases peripheral vascular resistance and blood pressure in humans. *Circulation* 1996;93:1860–1870.
13. Lieberman EH, et al. Flow-induced vasodilation of the human brachial artery is impaired in patients 40 years of age with coronary artery disease. *Am J Cardiol* 1996;78:1210–1214.
14. Ludmer PL, et al. Paradoxical vasoconstriction induced by acetylcholine in atherosclerotic coronary arteries. *N Engl J Med* 1986;315:1046–1051.
15. Corretti MC, et al. Guidelines for the ultrasound assessment of endothelial-dependent flow-mediated vasodilation of the brachial artery: a report of the International Brachial Artery Reactivity Task Force. *J Am Coll Cardiol* 2002;39:257–265.
16. Playford DA, Watts GF. Special article: non-invasive measurement of endothelial function. *Clin Exp Pharmacol Physiol* 1998;25:640–643.
17. Anderson TJ, et al. Close relation of endothelial function in the human coronary and peripheral circulations. *J Am Coll Cardiol* 1995;26:1235–1241.
18. Williams SB, et al. Impaired nitric oxide-mediated vasodilation in patients with non-insulin-dependent diabetes mellitus. *J Am Coll Cardiol* 1996;27:567–574.
19. Johnstone MT, et al. Impaired endothelium-dependent vasodilation in patients with insulin-dependent diabetes mellitus. *Circulation* 1993;88:2510–2516.
20. Rosenfeld ME. Cellular mechanisms in the development of atherosclerosis. *Diabetes Res Clin Pract* 1996;30[Suppl]:1–11.
21. Gross PL, Aird WC. The endothelium and thrombosis. *Semin Thromb Hemost* 2000;26:463–478.
22. Radomski MW, Palmer RM, Moncada S. The role of nitric oxide and cGMP in platelet adhesion to vascular endothelium. *Biochem Biophys Res Commun* 1987;148:1482–1489.
23. Diodati JG, et al. Effect of atherosclerosis on endothelium-dependent inhibition of platelet activation in humans. *Circulation* 1998;98:17–24.
24. Vallance P, Chan N. Endothelial function and nitric oxide: clinical relevance. *Heart* 2001;85:342–350.
25. Kuvin JT, et al. Peripheral vascular endothelial function testing as a noninvasive indicator of coronary artery disease. *J Am Coll Cardiol* 2001;38:1843–1849.
26. Heitzer T, et al. Endothelial dysfunction, oxidative stress, and risk of cardiovascular events in patients with coronary artery disease. *Circulation* 2001;104:2673–2678.
27. Gokce N, et al. Risk stratification for postoperative cardiovascular events via noninvasive assessment of endothelial function: a prospective study. *Circulation* 2002;105:1567–1572.
28. Celermajer DS, et al. Non-invasive detection of endothelial dysfunction in children and adults at risk of atherosclerosis. *Lancet* 1992;340:1111–1115.
29. Corretti MC, Plotnick GD, Vogel RA. Technical aspects of evaluating brachial artery vasodilatation using high-frequency ultrasound. *Am J Physiol* 1995;268:H1397–H1404.

30. Celermajer DS, et al. Cigarette smoking is associated with dose-related and potentially reversible impairment of endothelium-dependent dilation in healthy young adults. *Circulation* 1993;88:2149–2155.

31. Li J, et al. Non-invasive detection of endothelial dysfunction in patients with essential hypertension. *Int J Cardiol* 1997;61:165–169.

32. Enderle MD, et al. Comparison of peripheral endothelial dysfunction and intimal media thickness in patients with suspected coronary artery disease. *Heart* 1998;80:349–354.

33. Veves A, et al. Aerobic exercise capacity remains normal despite impaired endothelial function in the micro- and macrocirculation of physically active IDDM patients. *Diabetes* 1997;46:1846–1852.

34. Clarkson P, et al. Endothelium-dependent dilatation is impaired in young healthy subjects with a family history of premature coronary disease. *Circulation* 1997;96:3378–3383.

35. Hokanson DE, Sumner DS, Strandness DE Jr. An electrically calibrated plethysmograph for direct measurement of limb blood flow. *IEEE Trans Biomed Eng* 1975;22:25–29.

36. Smits P, et al. Endothelium-dependent vascular relaxation in patients with type I diabetes. *Diabetes* 1993;42:148–153.

37. Beanlands RS, et al. Noninvasive quantification of regional myocardial flow reserve in patients with coronary atherosclerosis using nitrogen-13 ammonia positron emission tomography: determination of extent of altered vascular reactivity. *J Am Coll Cardiol* 1995;26:1465–1475.

38. Williams SB, et al. Acute hyperglycemia attenuates endothelium-dependent vasodilation in humans in vivo. *Circulation* 1998;97:1695–1701.

39. Beckman JA, et al. Ascorbate restores endothelium-dependent vasodilation impaired by acute hyperglycemia in humans. *Circulation* 2001;103:1618–1623.

40. Mandarino LJ, Finlayson J, Hassell JR. High glucose downregulates glucose transport activity in retinal capillary pericytes but not endothelial cells. *Invest Ophthalmol Vis Sci* 1994;35:964–972.

41. Kaiser N, et al. Differential regulation of glucose transport and transporters by glucose in vascular endothelial and smooth muscle cells. *Diabetes* 1993;42:80–89.

42. Guzik TJ, et al. Mechanisms of increased vascular superoxide production in human diabetes mellitus: role of NAD(P)H oxidase and endothelial nitric oxide synthase. *Circulation* 2002;105:1656–1662.

43. Nishikawa T, et al. Normalizing mitochondrial superoxide production blocks three pathways of hyperglycaemic damage. *Nature* 2000;404:787–790.

44. Hink U, et al. Mechanisms underlying endothelial dysfunction in diabetes mellitus. *Circ Res* 2001;88:E14–E22.

45. Milstien S, Katusic Z. Oxidation of tetrahydrobiopterin by peroxynitrite: implications for vascular endothelial function. *Biochem Biophys Res Commun* 1999;263:681–684.

46. Du XL, et al. Hyperglycemia inhibits endothelial nitric oxide synthase activity by posttranslational modification at the Akt site. *J Clin Invest* 2001;108:1341–1348.

47. Butler R, et al. Allopurinol normalizes endothelial dysfunction in type 2 diabetics with mild hypertension. *Hypertension* 2000;35:746–751.

48. Cai H, Harrison DG. Endothelial dysfunction in cardiovascular diseases: the role of oxidant stress. *Circ Res* 2000;87:840–844.

49. Desco MC, et al. Xanthine oxidase is involved in free radical production in type 1 diabetes: protection by allopurinol. *Diabetes* 2002;51:1118–1124.

50. Brownlee M. Biochemistry and molecular cell biology of diabetic complications. *Nature* 2001;414:813–820.

51. Thornalley PJ. The glyoxalase system: new developments towards functional characterization of a metabolic pathway fundamental to biological life. *Biochem J* 1990;269:1–11.

52. Schmidt AM, et al. Activation of receptor for advanced glycation end products: a mechanism for chronic vascular dysfunction in diabetic vasculopathy and atherosclerosis. *Circ Res* 1999;84:489–497.

53. Wautier MP, et al. Activation of NADPH oxidase by AGE links oxidant stress to altered gene expression via RAGE. *Am J Physiol Endocrinol Metab* 2001;280:E685–E694.

54. Schmidt AM, et al. Cellular receptors for advanced glycation end products: implications for induction of oxidant stress and cellular dysfunction in the pathogenesis of vascular lesions. *Arterioscler Thromb* 1994;14:1521–1528.

55. Xia P, et al. Characterization of the mechanism for the chronic activation of diacylglycerol-protein kinase C pathway in diabetes and hypergalactosemia. *Diabetes* 1994;43:1122–1129.

56. Park JY, et al. Induction of endothelin-1 expression by glucose: an effect of protein kinase C activation. *Diabetes* 2000;49:1239–1248.

57. Inoguchi T, et al. Preferential elevation of protein kinase C isoform beta II and diacylglycerol levels in the aorta and heart of diabetic rats: differential reversibility to glycemic control by islet cell transplantation. *Proc Natl Acad Sci U S A* 1992;89:11059–11063.

58. Kunisaki M, et al. Vitamin E normalizes diacylglycerol-protein kinase C activation induced by hyperglycemia in rat vascular tissues. *Diabetes* 1996;45[Suppl 3]:S117–S119.

59. Inoguchi T, et al. Insulin's effect on protein kinase C and diacylglycerol induced by diabetes and glucose in vascular tissues. *Am J Physiol* 1994;267:E369–E379.

60. Beckman JA, et al. Inhibition of protein kinase C beta prevents impaired endothelium-dependent vasodilation caused by hyperglycemia in humans. *Circ Res* 2002;90:107–111.

61. Inoguchi T, et al. High glucose level and free fatty acid stimulate reactive oxygen species production through protein kinase C–dependent activation of NAD(P)H oxidase in cultured vascular cells. *Diabetes* 2000;49:1939–1945.

62. Vuorinen-Markkola H, Koivisto VA, Yki-Jarvinen H. Mechanisms of hyperglycemia-induced insulin resistance in whole body and skeletal muscle of type I diabetic patients. *Diabetes* 1992;41:571–580.

63. Pleiner J, et al. FFA-induced endothelial dysfunction can be corrected by vitamin C. *J Clin Endocrinol Metab* 2002;87:2913–2917.

64. Blaak EE, et al. Plasma FFA utilization and fatty acid-binding protein content are diminished in type 2

diabetic muscle. *Am J Physiol Endocrinol Metab* 2000;279:E146–E154.

65. Sniderman AD, Scantlebury T, Cianflone K. Hypertriglyceridemic hyperApo B: the unappreciated atherogenic dyslipoproteinemia in type 2 diabetes mellitus. *Ann Intern Med* 2001;135:447–459.

66. Hart CM, Tolson JK, Block ER. Supplemental fatty acids alter lipid peroxidation and oxidant injury in endothelial cells. *Am J Physiol* 1991;260:L481–L488.

67. Dresner A, et al. Effects of free fatty acids on glucose transport and IRS-1-associated phosphatidylinositol 3-kinase activity. *J Clin Invest* 1999;103:253–259.

68. Irving RJ, et al. Activation of the endothelin system in insulin resistance. *QJM* 2001;94:321–326.

69. Mather K, Anderson TJ, Verma S. Insulin action in the vasculature: physiology and pathophysiology. *J Vasc Res* 2001;38:415–422.

70. Haffner SM, et al. Insulin-resistant prediabetic subjects have more atherogenic risk factors than insulin-sensitive prediabetic subjects: implications for preventing coronary heart disease during the prediabetic state. *Circulation* 2000;101:975–980.

71. Mather K, et al. Evidence for physiological coupling of insulin-mediated glucose metabolism and limb blood flow. *Am J Physiol Endocrinol Metab* 2000;279:E1264–E1270.

72. Laakso M, et al. Decreased effect of insulin to stimulate skeletal muscle blood flow in obese man: a novel mechanism for insulin resistance. *J Clin Invest* 1990;85:1844–1852.

73. Scherrer U, et al. Nitric oxide release accounts for insulin's vascular effects in humans. *J Clin Invest* 1994;94:2511–2515.

74. Steinberg HO, et al. Insulin-mediated skeletal muscle vasodilation is nitric oxide dependent: a novel action of insulin to increase nitric oxide release. *J Clin Invest* 1994;94:1172–1179.

75. Laakso M, et al. Impaired insulin-mediated skeletal muscle blood flow in patients with NIDDM. *Diabetes* 1992;41:1076–1083.

76. McVeigh GE, et al. Impaired endothelium-dependent and independent vasodilation in patients with type 2 (non-insulin-dependent) diabetes mellitus. *Diabetologia* 1992;35:771–776.

77. Morris SJ, Shore AC, Tooke JE. Responses of the skin microcirculation to acetylcholine and sodium nitroprusside in patients with NIDDM. *Diabetologia* 1995;38:1337–1344.

78. Lim SC, et al. Soluble intercellular adhesion molecule, vascular cell adhesion molecule, and impaired microvascular reactivity are early markers of vasculopathy in type 2 diabetic individuals without microalbuminuria. *Diabetes Care* 1999;22:1865–1870.

79. Saito Y, et al. Increased plasma endothelin level in patients with essential hypertension. *N Engl J Med* 1990;322:205.

80. Watanabe Y, et al. Troglitazone improves endothelial dysfunction in patients with insulin resistance. *J Atheroscler Thromb* 2000;7:159–163.

81. Mather KJ, Verma S, Anderson TJ. Improved endothelial function with metformin in type 2 diabetes mellitus. *J Am Coll Cardiol* 2001;37:1344–1350.

82. Hsueh WA, Law RE. Insulin signaling in the arterial wall. *Am J Cardiol* 1999;84:21J–24J.

83. Zeng G, Quon MJ. Insulin-stimulated production of nitric oxide is inhibited by wortmannin: direct measurement in vascular endothelial cells. *J Clin Invest* 1996;98:894–898.

84. Montagnani M, et al. Inhibition of phosphatidylinositol 3-kinase enhances mitogenic actions of insulin in endothelial cells. *J Biol Chem* 2002;277:1794–1799.

85. Oliver FJ, et al. Stimulation of endothelin-1 gene expression by insulin in endothelial cells. *J Biol Chem* 1991;266:23251–23256.

86. Ferri C, et al. Insulin stimulates endothelin-1 secretion from human endothelial cells and modulates its circulating levels in vivo. *J Clin Endocrinol Metab* 1995;80:829–835.

87. Beckman JS, Koppenol WH. Nitric oxide, superoxide, and peroxynitrite: the good, the bad, and ugly. *Am J Physiol* 1996;272:C1424–C1437.

88. Graves JE, Lewis SJ, Kooy NW. Peroxynitrite-mediated vasorelaxation: evidence against the formation of circulating S-nitrosothiols. *Am J Physiol* 1998;274:H1001–H1008.

89. Tan KC, et al. Advanced glycation end products and endothelial dysfunction in type 2 diabetes. *Diabetes Care* 2002;25:1055–1059.

90. Dogra G, et al. Endothelium-dependent and independent vasodilation studies at normoglycaemia in type I diabetes mellitus with and without microalbuminuria. *Diabetologia* 2001;44:593–601.

91. Zou M, Yesilkaya A, Ullrich V. Peroxynitrite inactivates prostacyclin synthase by heme-thiolate-catalyzed tyrosine nitration. *Drug Metab Rev* 1999;31:343–349.

92. Achmad TH, et al. Oxidized low density lipoprotein acts on endothelial cells in culture to enhance endothelin secretion and monocyte migration. *Methods Find Exp Clin Pharmacol* 1997;19:153–159.

93. Quehenberger P, et al. Endothelin 1 transcription is controlled by nuclear factor-kappaB in AGE-stimulated cultured endothelial cells. *Diabetes* 2000;49:1561–1570.

94. Hopfner RL, Gopalakrishnan V. Endothelin: emerging role in diabetic vascular complications. *Diabetologia* 1999;42:1383–1394.

95. Heart Outcomes Prevention Evaluation Study Investigators. Effects of ramipril on cardiovascular and microvascular outcomes in people with diabetes mellitus: results of the HOPE study and Micro-HOPE substudy. *Lancet* 2000;355:253–259.

96. Dzau VJ, et al. The relevance of tissue angiotensin-converting enzyme: manifestations in mechanistic and endpoint data. *Am J Cardiol* 2001;88[Suppl]:1L–20L.

97. Arima S, et al. High glucose augments angiotensin II action by inhibiting NO synthesis in in vitro microperfused rabbit afferent arterioles. *Kidney Int* 1995;48:683–689.

98. Mehta JL, Li D. Identification, regulation and function of a novel lectin-like oxidized low-density lipoprotein receptor. *J Am Coll Cardiol* 2002;39:1429–1435.

99. Weiss D, Sorescu D, Taylor WR. Angiotensin II and atherosclerosis. *Am J Cardiol* 2001;87:25C–32C.

100. Rajagopalan S, et al. Angiotensin II-mediated hypertension in the rat increases vascular superoxide production via membrane NADH/NADPH oxidase activation: contribution to alterations of vasomotor tone. *J Clin Invest* 1996;97:1916–1923.

101. O'Driscoll G, et al. Improvement in endothelial function by angiotensin converting enzyme inhibition in insulin-dependent diabetes mellitus. *J Clin Invest* 1997;100:678–684.

102. O'Driscoll G, et al. Improvement in endothelial function by angiotensin-converting enzyme inhibition in non-insulin-dependent diabetes mellitus. *J Am Coll Cardiol* 1999;33:1506–1511.

103. Cheetham C, et al. Losartan, an angiotensin type 1 receptor antagonist, improves endothelial function in non-insulin-dependent diabetes. *J Am Coll Cardiol* 2000;36:1461–1466.

104. Cheetham C, et al. Losartan, an angiotensin type I receptor antagonist, improves conduit vessel endothelial function in type II diabetes. *Clin Sci (Lond)* 2001;100:13–17.

105. Mullen MJ, et al. Effect of enalapril on endothelial function in young insulin-dependent diabetic patients: a randomized, double-blind study. *J Am Coll Cardiol* 1998;31:1330–1335.

106. Schalkwijk CG, et al. ACE-inhibition modulates some endothelial functions in healthy subjects and in normotensive type 1 diabetic patients. *Eur J Clin Invest* 2000;30:853–860.

107. Tesfamariam B, et al. Elevated glucose promotes generation of endothelium-derived vasoconstrictor prostanoids in rabbit aorta. *J Clin Invest* 1990;85:929–932.

108. Hogikyan RV, et al. Heightened norepinephrine-mediated vasoconstriction in type 2 diabetes. *Metabolism* 1999;48:1536–1541.

109. Christlieb AR, et al. Vascular reactivity to angiotensin II and to norepinephrine in diabetic subjects. *Diabetes* 1976;25:268–274.

110. Ross R. Atherosclerosis is an inflammatory disease. *Am Heart J* 1999;138:S419–S420.

111. Libby P. Changing concepts of atherogenesis. *J Intern Med* 2000;247:349–358.

112. Pradhan AD, et al. C-reactive protein, interleukin 6, and risk of developing type 2 diabetes mellitus. *JAMA* 2001;286:327–334.

113. Festa A, et al. Chronic subclinical inflammation as part of the insulin resistance syndrome: the Insulin Resistance Atherosclerosis Study (IRAS). *Circulation* 2000;102:42–47.

114. Zeiher AM, et al. Nitric oxide modulates the expression of monocyte chemoattractant protein 1 in cultured human endothelial cells. *Circ Res* 1995;76:980–986.

115. Nomura S, et al. Significance of chemokines and activated platelets in patients with diabetes. *Clin Exp Immunol* 2000;121:437–443.

116. Dichtl W, et al. Very low-density lipoprotein activates nuclear factor-kappaB in endothelial cells. *Circ Res* 1999;84:1085–1094.

117. Mohamed AK, et al. The role of oxidative stress and NF-kappaB activation in late diabetic complications. *Biofactors* 1999;10:157–167.

118. Collins T, Cybulsky MI. NF-kappaB: pivotal mediator or innocent bystander in atherogenesis? *J Clin Invest* 2001;107:255–264.

119. Li C, Xu Q. Mechanical stress-initiated signal transductions in vascular smooth muscle cells. *Cell Signal* 2000;12:435–445.

120. Fichtlscherer S, et al. Elevated C-reactive protein levels and impaired endothelial vasoreactivity in patients with coronary artery disease. *Circulation* 2000;102:1000–1006.

121. Ziccardi P, et al. Reduction of inflammatory cytokine concentrations and improvement of endothelial functions in obese women after weight loss over one year. *Circulation* 2002;105:804–809.

122. Hussain MJ, et al. Elevated serum levels of macrophage-derived cytokines precede and accompany the onset of IDDM. *Diabetologia* 1996;39:60–69.

123. Uemura S, et al. Diabetes mellitus enhances vascular matrix metalloproteinase activity: role of oxidative stress. *Circ Res* 2001;88:1291–1298.

124. Kario K, et al. Activation of tissue factor-induced coagulation and endothelial cell dysfunction in non-insulin-dependent diabetic patients with microalbuminuria. *Arterioscler Thromb Vasc Biol* 1995;15:1114–1120.

125. Ren S, et al. Impact of diabetes-associated lipoproteins on generation of fibrinolytic regulators from vascular endothelial cells. *J Clin Endocrinol Metab* 2002;87:286–291.

126. Hafer-Macko CE, et al. Thrombomodulin deficiency in human diabetic nerve microvasculature. *Diabetes* 2002;51:1957–1963.

127. Vinik AI, et al. Platelet dysfunction in type 2 diabetes. *Diabetes Care* 2001;24:1476–1485.

Diabetes and Cardiovascular Disease
edited by Steven P. Marso and David M. Stern
Lippincott Williams & Wilkins, Philadelphia © 2004

14

Platelet Dysfunction

Robert Kelly and Steven R. Steinhubl

Cardiology Fellow, Division of Cardiology, University of North Carolina, University of North Carolina Hospital; Associate Professor, Division of Cardiology, University of North Carolina, Associate Professor, University of North Carolina Hospital, Chapel Hill, North Carolina

ROLE OF PLATELETS IN ATHEROTHROMBOTIC DISEASE

Platelets are small, anucleated, discoid cells that circulate in the blood and participate in hemostasis. Their main function is to plug holes in damaged blood vessel walls. They do this by undergoing a change in shape, adhering to subendothelial surfaces, secreting the contents of intracellular organelles, and aggregating to form a thrombus in response to stimuli generated in the endothelium of damaged blood vessels. These aggregatory stimuli include thrombin, collagen, and epinephrine (which are exogenous to the platelet) and agents such as adenosine diphosphate (ADP), which is secreted from platelet storage granules, and thromboxane A_2 (TXA_2), which is synthesized by the platelets during activation (Fig. 14-1) (1).

During aggregation, platelets secrete coagulation and growth factors that are needed for wound healing. Platelet activation results in changes in the level of expression of surface glycoproteins (GPs), both integrins and nonintegrins, that act as receptors for platelet agonists and for adhesive proteins involved in platelet aggregation. After platelet activation, P-selectin (GMP-140) is one of multiple proteins that translocates to the plasma membrane. The GPIIb/IIIa complex on the plasma membrane undergoes a conformational change that exposes a fibrinogen-binding site (Fig. 14-2) (2).

Antiaggregatory factors, namely prostacyclin (prostaglandin I_2, or PGI_2) and endothelium-derived relaxing factor (nitric oxide, or NO), are released by intact vascular endothelium and antagonize the effect of proaggregants so that thrombi do not form in healthy sections of blood vessels.

In atherosclerosis, platelet activity is increased, with local factors favoring thrombus formation. The localized activation of platelets also enhances the inflammatory response. On granule release, platelets provide the microenvironment with growth factors, such as platelet-derived growth factor (PGDF), and proinflammatory molecules, such as CD40 ligand, which contributes to the migration and proliferation of smooth muscle cells and macrophages. CD40 ligand on platelets binds with endothelium, leading to the secretion of chemokines (e.g., monocyte chemoattractant protein-1) and expression of adhesion molecules (Fig. 14-3) (3).

This binding generates the signals that recruit inflammatory cells (e.g., matrix metalloproteinases, tissue factor) to the site of vascular injury and promote the extravasation of leukocytes to the inner layer of the vessel wall. Platelets that accumulate at the site of arterial injury can directly recruit monocytes to the vessel wall through the binding of monocyte surface P-selectin glycoprotein ligand-1 (PSGL-1) to platelet surface P-selectin and monocyte surface Mac-1 (CD11b/CD18) to platelet surface GPIb/IX/V complex (3).

Diabetes, with its associated hyperglycemia and hyperinsulinemia, can lead to abnormalities in potentially all of the mechanisms regulating

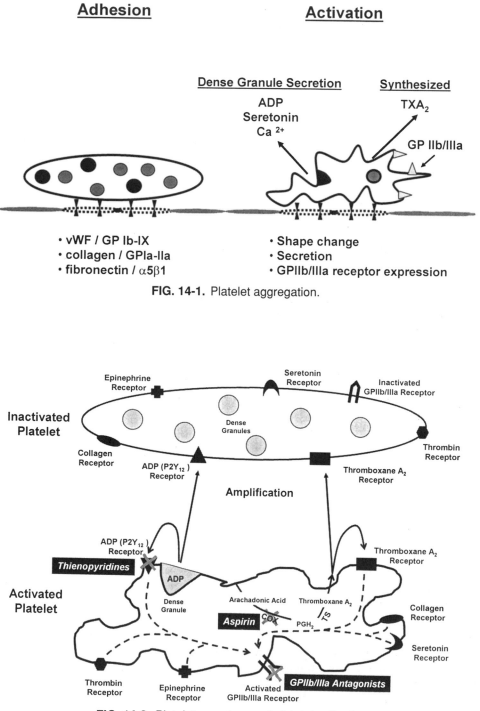

FIG. 14-1. Platelet aggregation.

FIG. 14-2. Platelet receptors and platelet activation.

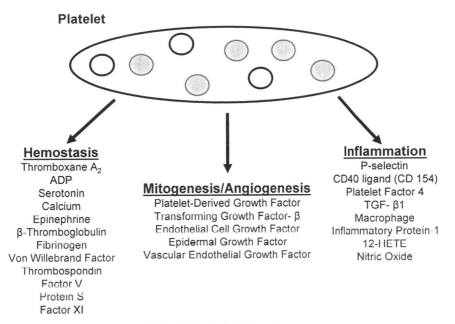

FIG. 14-3. Platelet functions.

platelet function—platelet-agonist interaction, platelet-vessel wall interaction, platelet-platelet interaction, platelet secretion and platelet-coagulant protein interaction—many of which have been identified in the peripheral blood of patients with coronary artery disease (CAD).

PLATELETS IN DIABETES MELLITUS

Diabetes mellitus (DM) is associated with accelerated atherosclerosis and with an increased incidence of cardiovascular events (4–6). This increased risk of events is partly due to an increased prevalence of hypertension and hyperlipidemia among diabetic patients, but it may also be due to a variety of abnormalities in diabetic platelets (Fig. 14-4).

Anatomic Features	Physiologic Features
↑Platelet size	↑Platelet aggregation
Large platelet shape	↑*In vivo* activation
↑Glycoprotein receptor density	↑Membrane thromboxane
Membrane fluidity	↑Glycoprotein receptor binding
	Platelet contents
	Nonenzymatic glycation

FIG. 14-4. Anatomy and physiologic features of platelets in diabetes.

Anatomic Differences in Platelets

Platelet Size

Diabetic platelets are larger than those of nondiabetic patients (7). This may occur as the result of stem cell dysfunction of the megakaryocytic series and progenitor cells in diabetes patients, but also it may occur in response to chronic activation (8). Platelets in diabetic patients have increased potency to adhere and aggregate, and the increased platelet size is also associated with an increased risk of stroke in DM (9). Similarly, mean platelet volume (MPV) is increased in diabetic patients, which is likely to be a marker of increased activation, but this appears to be unrelated to the level of hemoglobin A_{1C} (HbA$_{1C}$), the patient's age, or the fasting blood glucose concentration (10). Increased platelet volume is associated with retinopathy and activated coagulation in these patients (11).

Glycoprotein Density

Between 20% and 26% more GPs per platelet are observed in patients with type 1 or type 2 diabetes, which may be due to larger platelet size

(12). The abnormal expression of GPs in DM is reflected by increases in platelet volume, with a significant shift of the volume distribution to larger platelets (12). The cause is unknown, but there is some evidence that insulin has a direct effect on the proliferation and differentiation of cultured megakaryocytes, which may partly explain the altered megakaryocytothrombopoiesis that is seen in diabetes (13).

Platelet Membrane

The platelet membrane of patients with DM shows reduced lipid fluidity, so receptors are more exposed to the external environment and may contribute to the hypersensitivity of these platelets (14).

Physiologic Differences in Platelets

Platelet Aggregation

Platelets isolated from patients with DM show increased adhesiveness (15,16), exhibit more spontaneous aggregation (17), and are hyperaggregable in response to agonists *in vitro* (i.e., ADP, epinephrine, thrombin, low-density lipoproteins [LDL], glucose, and collagen) (18,19). It is unclear at present whether the platelet abnormalities are intrinsic to the platelet or are a consequence of circulating factors that affect platelet function, as has been demonstrated for insulin immune-complexes (20).

In Vivo *Platelet Activation*

In vivo platelet activation occurs with elevated levels of protein kinase C-α, Rho A, and phosphatidylinositol-3-kinase (PI3 kinase) in diabetic patients who have microangiopathy despite good glycemia control (21). This suggests that platelet second-messenger molecules activate platelet hyperfunction independent of metabolic control. Further evidence for increased *in vivo* platelet activation comes from flow cytometry studies, which show enhanced expression of CD62 (P-selectin), thrombospondin (α-granule activity) and GP53 activity to platelets

isolated from newly diagnosed diabetics, especially those with vascular complications, compared with controls (22).

Production of Arachidonic Acid and Thromboxane

Higher concentrations of arachidonate are found in the phospholipid membranes of DM platelets compared with normal controls (23). Increased conversion of arachidonic acid through the platelet cyclooxygenase pathway produces aggregating eicosanoids such as TXA_2 and prostaglandin H_2. The hyperaggregability of platelets appears to be independent of ADP and arachidonic acid pathways, and it is not diminished after 7 days of insulin therapy, which normalizes glucose but not the lipid profile (24,25). It has been suggested that a "feedback" circle is set up, in which vascular disease may lead to platelet damage, and altered platelet function may contribute to vascular disease (25).

Increased release of vasoconstrictors (e.g., TXA_2) from activated platelets is regulated in part by metabolic control (26). Elevated TXA_2 production may be due to lower antioxidant levels of glutathione (GSH) and GSH peroxidase in DM (27). Elevated TXA_2 enhances platelet turnover and increases fibrinogen binding (11). Some reports have shown that normalization of blood glucose can switch off this platelet hypersensitivity (28,29). In animal models of diabetes, enhanced platelet aggregation and TXA_2 synthesis were detected within days after rats were made diabetic with streptozotocin, before vascular disease was evident (30). Vascular disease is promoted by platelet activation and release of mitogens that stimulate vascular smooth muscle cell proliferation, further suggesting that platelets may play a role in the etiology of atherosclerosis.

Glycoprotein Receptor Binding

Platelet hypersensitivity to ADP, as shown in the diabetic animal model, increases fibrinogen binding, which may reflect an increase in the number of fibrinogen-binding receptors or in their affinity for fibrinogen. The enhanced early binding of fibrinogen to its receptor on the platelet surface results from the diabetic state itself rather than from the administration of insulin or the mechanisms through which diabetes occurs. This so-called platelet/clotting factor role (initiating intrinsic pathway, activating factor X, prothrombin production) is increased in diabetic patients with retinopathy, compared with normal controls (31). Some authors have also suggested that platelets of patients with DM produce a greater number of free radicals than do platelets of nondiabetic patients (32,33), and others have pointed to the question of a platelet aggregation enhancing factor. There is evidence that platelets of diabetic patients have greater growth-promoting activity on smooth muscle cells in culture, a function that relates to metabolic control (34,35).

Platelet Content

As a consequence of increased platelet activation in diabetes, there is an increase in production of von Willebrand factor and factor VIII antigen, leading to enhanced platelet aggregation (36). Platelets from plasma of DM patients release more α-granule contents (platelet factor 4, β-thromboglobulin), and lower levels of PDGF and serotonin are found in diabetic patients compared with controls, suggesting increased release of α and amine storage granules (37,38).

ETIOLOGY OF PLATELET ABNORMALITIES IN DIABETES

Nonenzymatic Glycation of Platelet Membranes

Glycation of platelet membrane proteins is significantly increased in DM. Membrane GPs IIb and IIIa participate in nonenzymatic glycation, and this activity may relate to the number of lysine residues in these proteins that are available for glycation (39). The increased glycation of GPIIb/IIIa may lead to increased platelet aggregation, which is related to altered platelet membrane fluidity (40).

Platelet Vasodilatation

In addition to increased platelet activation in diabetes, there is evidence that platelets have an impaired ability to mediate vasodilatation (vasomotor tone). This may be due to high glucose concentrations, and it is both time and concentration dependent. Similar platelet-vessel alterations have been found in patients with hypercholesterolemia (41). There appear to be two negative feedback loops: one that counteracts vasoconstriction associated with intraarterial platelet aggregation and another that moderates platelet aggregation and thrombus formation (42).

MECHANISM OF PLATELET ABNORMALITIES IN DIABETES MELLITUS

Figure 14-5 depicts the etiology of platelet abnormalities in diabetes.

Primary Receptor Abnormalities

Platelet plug formation is normally prevented by PGI_2 and NO, which combine to prevent platelet adherence to normal endothelium and platelet aggregation (43). In diabetics, there is decreased production of PGI_2 (44) and decreased synthesis and release of NO (45). PGI_2 levels can be normalized by glycemia control (46). Hyperglycemia inhibits NO production by blocking nitric oxide synthase (NOS) activation and increasing superoxide (peroxynitrite) production in endothelial cells (47). In vascular disease patients with diabetes, there is less platelet response and sensitivity to NO and PGI_2 (48,49). Reduced sensitivity of coronary vascular smooth muscle

- Primary receptor abnormality
- Endothelial dysfunction
- Increased sensitivity to agonist
- Advanced glycation end products (AGE) and their receptors (RAGE)
- Oxidative stress
- Inflammation
- Insulin resistance

FIG. 14-5. Etiology of platelet abnormalities in diabetes.

to NO has been suggested in ischemic heart disease (50).

A variety of reasons may be put forth to explain the decrease in platelet sensitivity to PGI_2 and NO. One possible explanation is decreased PGI_2 receptor activity. This has been described in CAD but not in DM (49,51,52). Some studies have suggested changes in G proteins in diabetes (52). The presence of decreased G_1 in platelet membranes from type 2 diabetics correlates with reduced stimulation of adenylate cyclase in response to activation of the PGI_2 receptor by PGE_1 (53). Kahn (54) reported that there is overexpression of ras-related G protein in skeletal muscle in type 2 DM, and Nolan et al. (54) found a 10-fold increase in the translocation of rap1B to the cytoskeleton in activated platelets from patients with type 2 DM in the absence of a concomitant increase in the expression of rap1B. It is possible that defective posttranslational processing of proteins in DM leads to inappropriate activity or subcellular localization of the proteins.

Endothelial Dysfunction

Endothelial dysfunction may influence platelet aggregation in DM by enhancing von Willebrand factor activity. This activity reflects endothelial damage and may be reduced by insulin *in vitro*. Abnormal endothelial function combines with platelet dysfunction to accelerate atherosclerosis. There is evidence in vascular endothelium that nonesterified fatty acids impair the insulin effect on glucose uptake long before hyperglycemia appears (55). This increases insulin resistance. Microscopically, there is evidence of abnormal microvasculature before metabolic abnormalities appear.

Clinical studies in diabetics with acute coronary syndromes confirm the link between platelet activation and endothelial dysfunction, with increased P-selectin (platelet activation) in DM patients up to 6 weeks after myocardial infarction (MI) (56). This finding is backed up by laboratory data, which show that glucose and insulin modulate the capacity of endothelial cells to express P-selectin and to bind to monocytes, suggesting that hyperglycemia may be implicated in vascular disease in DM (57).

Increased Platelet Sensitivity to Agonists

Inositol phospholipid turnover and calcium release occur early in the platelet response, before the arachidonic acid response, and are influenced by free magnesium concentrations. These parameters may predict platelet thrombosis (58). Free magnesium correlates with blood glucose, cholesterol, apolipoprotein B, hypertension, insulin resistance, and left ventricular hypertrophy. Increasing the intracellular calcium and reducing the magnesium are associated with more platelet aggregation in type 2 DM. G-protein binding that links agonists with platelets is calcium dependent. Phosphoinositide turnover increases in type 2 DM but is reduced in type 1 DM, for reasons that are unclear. It causes platelet aggregation in both settings.

Platelets in type 1 diabetics with poor glycemic control have increased calcium levels compared with controls. Thrombin-induced calcium is elevated only during tight glycemic control. Basal and collagen-stimulated calcium levels are increased in type 2 DM compared with controls. There is a suggestion that a compensatory response to other pathways is responsible for the differences between type 1 and type 2 DM. Changes in type 1 DM platelet calcium were not affected by acute alterations in *in vitro* glucose concentrations, indicating that glucose does not affect platelet aggregation directly (27,59).

Products and Receptors of Advanced Glycosylation

Advanced glycation end products (AGE) are terminal adducts of a nonenzymatic reaction between glucose and amino groups of protein that accumulate at an accelerated rate in tissues of DM patients. The extent of glycosylation of platelet membrane proteins in DM relates to reduced membrane fluidity, and this may contribute to platelet hyperfunction. In addition, enhanced glycosylation of subendothelial proteins quenches endothelial NO and reduces platelet inhibition (45). Platelet membrane fluidity is also altered by the plasma lipoprotein profile (60). There is an increase in LDL platelet aggregation in type 1 DM (61).

AGEs are formed in the presence of hyperglycemia. They form at the lysine side-chain end of proteins. Receptors for AGE (RAGE) have recently been described (62). Engagement of RAGE can activate inflammation of endothelial cells, smooth muscle cells, and macrophages, causing atherosclerosis. In addition, RAGE binds cytokines of the S100/calgranulin family, linking glycosylation with inflammation. Blocking of RAGE reduces the formation of atheroma in mice.

AGEs stimulate endothelial cells. This stimulation is mediated by RAGE and its signal transducers, both of which are increased in DM. A positive feedback loop occurs when RAGE is occupied by AGE; RAGE expression is increased, giving rise to chronic inflammation. Interestingly, RAGE activation is also seen in normoglycemic atherosclerosis, especially with the formation of carboxymethyl-lysine (CML) products (63,64). This suggests that AGEs may occur in atherosclerosis independently of blood sugar levels. AGE glycation is related to oxidant stress. Higher AGE concentrations occur during high redox oxidized states (e.g., renal failure, ischemia). High redox oxidized states are driven by myeloperoxidases found in neutrophils, which in active atherosclerotic lesions may generate continuous inflammation.

It is thought that AGEs increase platelet aggregation by 40% to 50% through an oxidative stress mechanism (AGE-generated superoxide radicals). Superoxide anions are already known to increase platelet aggregation (65,66). However, although receptors (RAGE) are found on endothelial cells and monocytes, they have not been found on platelets.

In diabetes, the prooxidant, lipid-rich environment contributes to elevated AGE-RAGE. In the absence of RAGE, AGE is inert. In diabetes, RAGE generates a redox oxidized state, reduces antioxidant levels of glutathione, activates nuclear factor κB (NFκB, a signal transducer central to inflammatory responses), and activates vascular cell adhesion molecule (VCAM) in chronic stages. DM modulates an intracellular redox state and the expression of redox-sensitive inflammatory genes within the vessel wall. The gene encoding RAGE is located on chromosome 6 at the NFκB site and is part of the human leukocyte antigen (HLA) class II/III subtype.

AGE formation correlates with elevated HbA$_{1C}$ and a higher incidence of nephropathy, retinopathy, and neuropathy in DM. It is unknown whether reduction of AGE would improve these conditions. In terms of CAD, tight metabolic control does not correlate with significant reductions in acute events (67,68), but modification of risk factors with other treatments, such as 3-hydroxy-3-methylglutaryl coenzyme A (HMG-CoA) reductase inhibitors (69), angiotensin-converting enzyme (ACE) inhibitors (70), aspirin, and clopidogrel (71) can reduce the incidence of MI in DM. RAGE appears to have a role in DM beyond blood sugar control that involves platelet-leukocyte, platelet-endothelium interactions and inflammation, but further research is needed to clarify its importance in the process and complications of DM.

Oxidative Stress and Platelet Activation

Hyperglycemia contributes to oxidative stress, as manifested by lipid peroxidation in vascular walls (lipid hydroperoxides, thiobarbiturate). Oxidation results in increased production of AGE.

Isoprostanes

F$_2$-Isoprostanes are nonenzymatic products of arachidonic acid that form *in situ* on esterified phospholipids and are subsequently released, in free form, by the action of phospholipases. They are a useful marker of oxidative stress. In diabetes, F$_2$-isoprostanes are elevated. This is related to glycemic control and lipid peroxidation (72). 8-iso-PGF$_{2\alpha}$ induces vasoconstriction and modulates platelet adhesion (73,74). Isoprostane inhibits the antiaggregatory effects of NO and causes dose-dependent, irreversible platelet aggregation in the presence of collagen, ADP, arachidonic acid and PGH$_2$/TXA$_2$ analogs. Gopaul et al. (75) showed that there is three times as much 8-epi-PGF$_{2\alpha}$ in type 2 diabetics as in normal controls (75). Isoprostanes are elevated in type 1 and type 2 DM. Metabolic control can reduce isoprostane production, suggesting that glycemic control regulates oxidative stress.

The role of lipid peroxidation in DM is unknown. However, lipid peroxidation is not affected by aspirin, and studies in platelets suggest that increasing lipid peroxidation causes enhanced platelet aggregation (75).

Auto-oxidation and Enediol Ions

Glucose may undergo auto-oxidation, forming enediol radical ions (76). These ions enhance lipid oxidation and increase platelet activation. In addition, the dicarbyl groups can form AGE, which depends on metal ion availability (e.g., copper). AGEs enhance human platelet aggregation *ex vivo*. AGE formation on proteins and lipids contributes to lipid peroxidation and platelet activation.

Matrix Metalloproteinases

DM enhances the activity of vascular matrix metalloproteinases (MMPs) in endothelial cells (77). This effect is dependent on glucose levels and oxidative stress. MMPs are zinc- and calcium-dependent endopeptidases that promote cell migration and tissue remodeling in monocytes and vascular smooth muscle cells. They are synthesized in atheromatous plaques, especially at the shoulder regions of blood vessels, and are found in increased amounts in acute coronary syndromes or unstable angina and during plaque rupture, as well as in DM (78). MMPs are also found in platelets. MMP9 predicts albuminuria in DM (a marker of outcome in DM after percutaneous transluminal coronary angioplasty) (79). MMP9 is required for angiogenesis to promote continuous growth of atherosclerotic lesions. MMP gene expression is increased by cytokines and growth factors.

Inflammation and Platelets

DM is characterized by an increase in cytokines and acute phase reactants (e.g., fibrinogen, oroso-mucoid, haptoglobulin, α_1-antitrypsin. Removal of the sialic acid component of acute phase glycoprotein causes insulin resistance (80). However, the source of inflammation in DM is unclear.

Hyperglycemia activates inflammatory cytokines (81). DM may represent an activated immune system with ongoing cytokine-mediated acute phase responses. Furthermore, C-reactive protein (CRP) and interleukin-6 (IL-6) have been associated with an increased risk of developing type 2 DM (82). Increased levels of IL-6 and tumor necrosis factor-α (TNF-α) have been reported in patients with type 2 DM and insulin resistance. Hyperglycemia appears to increase IL-6, IL-18, and TNF by an oxidative stress mechanism. The peak glucose levels, rather than continuous hyperglycemia, predict the inflammatory response. IL-6 correlates with HbA$_{1C}$ levels and the presence of diabetic nephropathy and predicts the risk of future cardiac events in type 2 DM. IL-18 has been found in human atheromata. It appears to regulate IL-6, intracellular adhesion molecule-1 (ICAM-1), and MMPs 1, 9, and 13 in the process of atherosclerosis. Increased IL-18 messenger RNA expression has been found in symptomatic rather than asymptomatic plaques, suggesting a role for IL-18 in plaque stability.

The link between platelet activation and inflammation may lie in the presence of these inflammatory markers in platelets. Platelets express CD154 (CD40 ligand) when activated, illustrating a potential interaction between proinflammatory and prothrombotic pathways (83). Moreover, it was recently shown that leukocyte binding and migration across a carpet of platelets adherent to diseased or injured intima are dependent on the leukocyte integrin Mac-1 and on platelet GPIbα (84). CD40 ligand binds leucocytes and stimulates tissue factor expression. It induces inflammatory signals in cells of vascular walls. Glycoprotein IIb/IIIa engagement on platelets upregulates expression of CD40 and CD62 (P-selectin) (85). In patients at risk for DM, there is evidence supporting the presence of inflammation before the onset of metabolic abnormalities (7,12); this finding might support an inflammatory hypothesis as to the cause of increased platelet activation in DM.

Insulin Resistance and Platelet Activity

Insulin resistance increases platelet aggregation, platelet adhesion, von Willebrand factor, factor VIII, tissue plasminogen activator (tPA), and fibrinogen. The European Concerted Action on Thrombosis Study confirmed the link between atherosclerosis, insulin resistance, and thrombotic factors (86). Central to fatal events is plaque rupture and adherence of platelets. Platelets retain a functional insulin receptor that is capable of binding insulin and of autophosphorylation (87). Insulin is thought to reduce platelet responses to agonists such as ADP, collagen, and thrombin. It downregulates the number of α_2-adrenergic receptors on platelets (88). In diabetics, there is reduced insulin sensitivity, with decreased platelet insulin receptor number and affinity (89). In nondiabetic patients with acute coronary syndromes, there is reduced insulin and PGI$_2$ binding to platelets. The impaired response to PGI$_2$ improves with insulin administration (90,91). In this instance, insulin increases the number of PGI$_2$ binding sites on platelets, which increases the cyclic adenosine monophosphate (cAMP) response to PGI$_2$. This is seen in patients with ischemic heart disease (92).

These studies emphasize the importance of insulin in maintaining normal platelet sensitivity to PGI$_2$ and may suggest a way in which platelets are more active in DM. Insulin in patients with insulin resistance impairs the inhibition of platelet aggregation in response to proaggregatory agents in obese subjects rather than lean subjects (59). Resistance of diabetic platelets to the inhibitory action of insulin is borne out by the relative resistance of people with DM to measures taken to reduce CAD (93).

CLINICAL IMPORTANCE

Antiplatelet Therapies in Diabetes Mellitus

Current antiplatelet therapy consists of aspirin, thienopyridines (clopidogrel and ticlopidine), and glycoprotein IIb/IIIa receptor antagonists (Table 14-1). All patients with type 2 diabetes should be taking aspirin. Clopidogrel, with or without aspirin, should be considered in high-risk groups. The recently published American College of Cardiology/American Heart Association (AHA/ACC) guidelines advise that all DM patients undergoing percutaneous coronary

TABLE 14-1. *Therapies affecting platelet function in diabetes*

Medication	Platelet aggregation/ adhesion	Proven cardiac mortality benefit in all patients	Independent cardiovascular mortality benefit in diabetes mellitus	Authors/study (ref. no.)
Aspirin	↓	Yes	Unknown	
Clopidogrel	↓	Yes	Probably	Bhatt et al. (98)
Ticlopidine	↓	No	Unknown	
GIIb/IIIa complex	↓	Yes	Yes	Bhatt et al. (108)
Glucose control	↔	Yes	Yes	DIGAMI (119)
Metformin	↓	No	Unknown	
Sulfonylureas	↓	May increase mortality	No	
PPAR	↓?	Ongoing study	Unknown	
Statins	↓	Yes	Yes	CARE (144)
ACE inhibitors	↓	Yes	Yes	HOPE (136), MICROHOPE
Angiotensin II blockers	↓	No	Unknown	
Antioxidants	↔	Equivocal	Unknown	

↓, reduces/inhibits; ↔, no effect/equivocal effect; ACE, angiotensin-converting enzyme; PPAR, peroxisome proliferator activated receptor.

intervention (PCI) should receive GPIIb/IIIa antagonists (94).

Aspirin

Aspirin reduces vascular events in all CAD patients by 25% to 34% (93). In this context, 75 to 100 mg/day is recommended to suppress TXA_2 and to reduce bleeding side effects. The importance of aspirin in DM is emphasized by the fact that the risk of future cardiac events is as high in DM patients as it is in non-DM patients who have previously had an MI (5). The Hypertension Optimal Treatment (HOT) study showed that aspirin is more beneficial to diabetics than to nondiabetics (95). The American Diabetic Association recommends that DM patients older than 30 years of age who have evidence of large-vessel disease receive 80 to 325 mg of aspirin daily. The benefit of aspirin in DM is also emphasized by the 27% reduction in MI among patients in the Early Treatment Diabetic Retinopathy Study (ETDRS) (96). Kodama et al. (97) also showed that aspirin reduces carotid intima thickness progression in DM. Therefore, the evidence supports aspirin use in all DM patients older than 30 years of age at a dose between 80 and 325 mg/day.

Thienopyridines

Clopidogrel and ticlopidine block ADP-induced platelet aggregation and activation. The benefit of clopidogrel compared with aspirin was established in the Clopidogrel versus Aspirin in Patients at Risk of Ischaemic Events (CAPRIE) study (71). Clopidogrel reduced the risk of stroke, MI, or vascular death by 8.7% in high-risk patients.

In DM patients, the benefit of clopidogrel was even greater, with a 13.1% reduction in adverse cardiac events (98). The combination of clopidogrel and aspirin provides synergistic antiplatelet protection. The clinical benefit of this combination was proved in the Clopidogrel in Unstable Angina to Prevent Recurrent Events study (CURE) and Clopidogrel for the Reduction of Events During Observation (CREDO) trials (99,100). The 20% to 30% relative risk reduction in the combined end point of death/MI and stroke achieved in these trials with combination therapy, compared with aspirin alone, was similar in diabetic and nondiabetic patients. Further evaluation is pending with the Clopidogrel for High Atherothrombotic Risk and Ischaemic Stabilization, Management and Avoidance (CHARISMA) trial, which will directly evaluate clopidogrel treatment in high-risk patients, a high percentage of whom have DM, with anticipated follow-up of 3 to 4 years (101).

Glycoprotein Receptor Antagonists

GPIIb/IIIa receptor antagonists include abciximab, tirofiban, and eptifibatide. Abciximab and eptifibatide are approved and recommended for DM patients undergoing PCI. These agents appear to be beneficial only when given in the short term and intravenously. Oral equivalent agents have had disappointing results in patients undergoing PCI. This may be due, in part, to their partial agonist effect, which leads to increased platelet activation (102).

The evidence base for GPIIb/IIIa antagonists comes from the ESPRIT (eptifibatide) (103), EPISTENT/EPILOG (abciximab) (104,105), and TARGET (abciximab versus tirofiban) (106) trials. In patients undergoing PCI, GPIIb/IIIa agents reduced multiple adverse cardiovascular events (MACE) by 20% to 43%. The outcome in these studies was linked to inhibition of platelet aggregation (107–109). DM patients benefit especially from this treatment, which is not surprising, because the GPIIb/IIIa receptor contributes directly to platelet hyperreactivity in DM. It is noteworthy that platelet activity is markedly increased at the time of PCI in diabetic patients, compared with nondiabetic patients (110). In the EPILOG study, DM patients had a greater reduction in MACE and better outcome with higher doses of heparin than did non-DM patients (105).

At adequate doses, each of the GPIIb/IIIa antagonists has also been found to inhibit soluble CD40 ligand, which may provide the basis for an antiinflammatory role for these drugs as well as an antithrombotic one (111). Furthermore, suboptimal doses of GPIIb/IIIa agents could potentially be proinflammatory (111).

Role of Other Therapies

Glucose-Insulin-Potassium Therapy

Glucose control in the short term reduces TXA_2 but does not change platelet aggregation (112). Insulin therapy for patients with acute MI reduced death and nonfatal MI by 28% in both diabetic and nondiabetic patients (113,114). Glycemic control (keeping HbA_{1C} lower than 7%) reduces MACE after PCI in DM patients (115). Interestingly, the Diabetes Control and Complications Trial (DCCT) showed that glycemic control did not significantly reduce vascular mortality despite clear evidence of reduced platelet thromboxane production with metabolic improvement (116,117). Therefore, it is questionable whether strict glucose control can improve platelet hypercoagulability (118,119). On the other hand, insulin inhibits platelet aggregation (120). The clinical relevance of these findings is still under debate.

Oral Hypoglycemic Agents

Metformin reduces platelet superoxide anion production in DM (121). Sulfonylurea drugs suppress platelet aggregation, platelet production of phospholipase C, plasminogen activator, and diacylglycerol production, which affects protein kinase C and phosphatidylinositol-3-kinase (PI3 kinase) (122). Controversy surrounds the use of sulfonylurea drugs, because the University Groups Diabetes Program (UGDP) study showed increased mortality in patients taking this treatment. In a recent analysis of the Bypass Angioplasty Revascularization Investigation (BARI), patients with DM who were taking sulfonylureas had better outcomes after coronary artery bypass grafting than after PCI (123). This result may have been biased by the fact that these patients received left internal mammary artery grafts. There is also an issue concerning K^+ATP channels and myocardial preconditioning and the fact that sulfonylureas may protect against this. The link between K^+ATPase channels and platelet aggregation is unknown at present.

Peroxisome Proliferator-activated Receptor Drugs (Thiazolinediones)

Troglitazone improves insulin resistance. Its structure is similar to vitamin E, and it inhibits platelet aggregation by suppressing thrombin-induced activation of phosphoinositide signaling in platelets (via protein kinase C and PI3 kinase). Pioglitazone lacks the vitamin E structure and does not inhibit platelet aggregation. Troglitazone and pioglitazone both inhibit protein kinase, but only troglitazone inhibits platelet aggregation (124).

Rosiglitazone is associated with reduced progression to chronic nephropathy and is protective against endothelial dysfunction in animal models. Rosiglitazone reduces CRP (125), MMP, TNF (126), and urine albumin and is associated with better outcome in DM. Troglitazone slows carotid intima thickening in DM patients. The role of rosiglitazone in preventing adverse ischemic events and their role in patients undergoing PCI will be addressed in an upcoming PCI trial. An interesting point is that rosiglitazone has recently been shown to increase cholesterol levels in the presence of statin treatment in patients with DM. The thiazolinediones have a modest effect in the overall lipoprotein profile. Overall, there is a small but measurable increase in LDL. However, there seems to be a shift in concentration from a predominant small, oxidized, atherogenic LDL pool to a more buoyant, light LDL particle pool. (Troglitazone has recently been withdrawn from use due to unacceptable hepatic effects.)

Statins

Statins significantly reduce morbidity and mortality in DM patients with CAD (127). In addition to reducing cholesterol, they have pleiotropic effects: they stabilize plaque, regenerate endothelium, reduce new vessel occlusions, reduce platelet aggregation and thrombus formation, and reduce CRP (128–132). Simvastatin has antiinflammatory effects (133) and can act as an immune modulator (134). Pravastatin induces inhibition of platelet aggregation and expression of thromboxanes (TXB_2) and α-granule membrane protein (GMP-140). This occurs within 8 weeks after initiation of treatment for hypercholesterolemia (135). Ongoing studies (Collaborative Atorvastatin Diabetes Study and Atorvastatin Study in Preventing Endpoints in NIDDM in high-risk patients and diabetics) are looking at ischemic outcomes with statin therapy (136).

Angiotensin-converting Enzyme Inhibitors and Angiotensin II Receptor Antagonists

ACE inhibitors improve outcomes in high-risk patients including diabetics. The Heart Outcomes Prevention Evaluation (HOPE) and MICRO-HOPE studies showed 25% reduction in mortality (70) and 34% reduction in onset of new cases of DM, in addition to a reduction in the progression of atherosclerosis (137,138). ACE inhibitors inhibit platelet aggregation by 16%, compared with 23% inhibition achieved with aspirin and clopidogrel (139).

Angiotensin II receptor antagonists interact with TXA_2 and PGH_2 receptors on platelets. Valsartan and losartan reduce platelet aggregation, but candesartan does not (140). This effect is optimal at higher doses. Angiotensin II antagonists reduce progression of nephropathy in DM patients. Valsartan reduces intima media thickening in rabbits (141).

Antioxidants

Vitamin E scavenges free radicals and can downregulate thromboxane generation. It decreases TXA_2 metabolite production by 50%. Vitamins E and C were shown to improve outcomes in angina patients in the Cambridge Heart Antioxidant Study (CHAOS) (142). In the Harvard Intravascular Ultrasound trial, vitamins E and C reduced the progression of coronary atherosclerosis at 1 year (143). In the Gruppo Italiano per lo Studio della Sopravvivenza nell'Infarto Miocardico (GISSI) prevention trial, vitamin E had no effect on cardiovascular events (144). Similarly, in the HOPE study, the addition of vitamin E to ACE inhibitor therapy had no benefit in reducing MIs or cardiovascular accidents in high-risk patients, including diabetic patients

(70,138). Antioxidants also include allopurinol and acetylcysteine, which have been shown to normalize isoprostanes, a marker of oxidative stress in DM platelets. Ongoing studies (SuVi-MAX, MAX, and WHS) are currently trying to clarify these issues surrounding antioxidant therapies in CAD (136).

CONCLUSION

DM, a well established independent risk factor for future cardiovascular events, is characterized by elevated glucose substrate, increased platelet aggregation, and increased adhesion between platelets and with leukocytes, monocytes, endothelium, and macrophages. Diabetic platelets are larger, have more GP receptors, bind differently to agonists, and are more active than platelets in other CAD populations. Altered glycemia does contribute to platelet hyperresponsiveness but it is not the sole cause of it; in fact, platelets themselves may cause the vascular complications of diabetes, and with inflammation and oxidative stress, platelets may even contribute to the DM itself. The etiology linking atherosclerosis and abnormal DM platelet activity is a complex combination of primary platelet receptor abnormalities, agonist binding, endothelial dysfunction, inflammation, oxidative stress, megakaryocyte activity, AGEs and their receptors, and insulin resistance. Antiplatelet therapies significantly improve clinical outcomes in DM patients. Adjuvant therapies such as ACE inhibitors and statins have important pleiotropic benefits, and blood sugar management is essential, although its direct effect on platelet activity does not appear to be as significant as that of antiplatelet drugs. Finally, genetic medicine may help to identify the cause and treatment of some of the platelet abnormalities seen in DM patients.

REFERENCES

1. Fitzgerald DJ. Vascular biology of thrombosis: the role of platelet-vessel wall adhesion. *Neurology* 2001;57 [Suppl 2]:S1–S4.
2. Coller BS, Peerschke EI, Scudder LE, et al. A murine monoclonal antibody that completely blocks the binding of fibrinogen to platelets produces a thrombasthenic-like state in normal platelets and binds

to glycoproteins IIb and/or IIIa. *J Clin Invest* 1983; 72:325–338.

3. Sarma J, Laan CA, Alam S, et al. Increased platelet binding to circulating monocytes in acute coronary syndromes. *Circulation* 2002;105:2166–2171.

4. Donnan PT, Boyle DI, Broomhall J, et al. Prognosis following first acute myocardial infarction in type II diabetes: a comparative population study. *Diabet Med* 2002;19:448–455.

5. Haffner SM, Lehto MD, Ronnemaa T, et al. Mortality from coronary heart disease in subjects with type 2 diabetes and in nondiabetic subjects with and without prior myocardial infarction. *N Engl J Med* 1998;339:229–234.

6. Abizaid A, Costa M, Centemero M, et al. Clinical and economic impact of diabetes mellitus on percutaneous and surgical treatment of multivessel coronary disease patients. *Circulation* 2001;104:533–538.

7. Tschoepe D, Langer E, Schauseil S, et al. Increased platelet volume: sign of impaired thrombopoiesis in diabetes mellitus. *Klin Wochenschr* 1989;67:253–259.

8. Brown AS, Hong Y, deBelder A, et al. Megakaryocyte ploidy and platelet changes in human diabetes and atherosclerosis. *Arterioscler Thromb Vasc Biol* 1997;17:802–807.

9. D'Erasmo E, Albierti G, Celi FS. Platelet count, mean platelet volume and their relation to prognosis in cerebral infarction. *J Int Med* 1990;227:11–14.

10. Sharpe PC, Trinick T. Mean platelet volume in diabetes mellitus. *QJM* 1993;86:739–742.

11. Koneti Rao A, Goldberg RE, Walsh P. Evidence for relationship between platelet coagulant hyperactivity and platelet volume. *J Lab Clin Med* 1984;103:82–91.

12. Tschoepe D, Roesen P, Kaufmann L, et al. Evidence for abnormal platelet glycoprotein expression in diabetes mellitus. *Eur J Clin Invest* 1990;20:166–170.

13. Watanabe Y. Effect of insulin on murine megakaryocytopoiesis in a liquid culture system. *Cell Struct Funct* 1987;12:311–316.

14. Winocour PD, Watala C, Perry DW, et al. Decreased platelet membrane fluidity due to glycation or acetylation of membrane proteins. *Thromb Haemost* 1992;68:577–582.

15. Shaw S, Pegrum GD, Wolff SS, et al. Platelet adhesiveness in diabetes mellitus. *J Clin Pathol* 1967;20:845–847.

16. Mayne EE, Bridges JM, Weaver JA. Platelet adhesiveness, plasma fibrinogen and factor VIII levels in diabetes mellitus. *Diabetologia* 1970;6:436–440.

17. Menys VS, Bhatnagar D, Mackness MI, et al. Spontaneous platelet aggregation in whole blood is increased in non-insulin dependent diabetes mellitus and in female but not male patients with primary dyslipidaemia. *Atherosclerosis* 1995;112:115–122.

18. Butkus A, Skrinska VA, Schumacker P, et al. Thromboxane production and platelet aggregation in diabetic patients with clinical complications. *Thromb Res* 1980;19:211–223.

19. Catalano DG, Averna M, Notarbartolo A, et al. Thromboxane biosynthesis and platelet function in type II diabetes mellitus. *N Engl J Med* 1990;322:1769–1774.

20. Park JY, Kim SA, Kim SJ, et al. Circulating immune complexes in diabetic patients. *Yonsei Med J* 1985;26:35–38.

21. Kajita K, Ischizuka T, Miura A, et al. Increased platelet aggregation in diabetic patients with microangiopathy despite good glycaemic control. *Platelets* 2001;12:343–351.

22. Tschoepe D, Driesch E, Schwippert B, et al. Activated platelets in subjects at increased risk of IDDM. Deutsche Nikotinamid Interventionsstudie (DENIS) Study Group. *Diabetologia* 1997;40:573–577.

23. Morita I, Takahashi R, Ito H, et al. Increased arachidonic acid content in platelet phospholipids from diabetic patients. *Prostaglandins Leukot Med* 1983;11:33–41.

24. Van Zile J, Kilpatrick M, Laimins M, et al. Platelet aggregation and release of ATP after incubation with soluble immune complexes purified from the serum of diabetic patients. *Diabetes* 1981;30:575–579.

25. Colwell JA. Antiplatelet drugs and the prevention of macrovascular disease in diabetes mellitus. *Metabolism* 1992;41:7–10.

26. Davi G, Catalano I, Averna M, et al. Thromboxane biosynthesis and platelet function in type II diabetes mellitus. *N Engl J Med* 1990;322:1769–1774.

27. Mazzanti L, Mutus B. Diabetes induced alterations in platelet metabolism. *Clin Biochem* 1997;7:509–515.

28. McDonald JW, Duprue J, Rodger NW, et al. Comparison of platelet thromboxane synthesis in diabetic patients on conventional insulin therapy and continuous insulin infusions. *Thromb Res* 1982;28:705–712.

29. Brownlee M, Cerami A. The biochemistry of the complications of diabetes mellitus. *Annu Rev Biochem* 1981;50:385–432.

30. Gerrard JM, Stuart MJ, Rao MJ, et al. Alterations in the balance of prostaglandin and thromboxane synthesis in diabetic rats. *J Lab Clin Med* 1980;95:950–958.

31. Winocour PD, Perry DW, Hatton MW, et al. The hypersensitivity to thrombin of platelets from diabetic rats is not due to increased thrombin binding. *Thromb Res* 1991;61:469–475.

32. Kitagawa S, Fujisawa H, Kametani F, et al. Generation of active oxygen species in platelets. *Free Radic Res Commun* 1992;15:319–324.

33. Iuliano L, Pedersen JZ, Pratico D, et al. Role of hydroxyl radicals in the activation of human platelets. *Eur J Biochem* 1994;221:695–704.

34. Sugimoto H, Franks DJ, Lecavalier L, et al. Therapeutic modulation of growth promoting activity in platelets from diabetic patients. *Diabetes* 1987;36:667–672.

35. Koschinsky T, Bunting CE, Rutter R, et al. Vascular growth factors and the development of macrovascular disease in diabetes mellitus. *Diabetes Metab* 1987;13:318–325.

36. Colwell JA, Winocour PD, Lopes-Virella M, et al. New concepts about the pathogenesis of atherosclerosis in diabetes mellitus. *Am J Med* 1983;75:67–80.

37. Guillausseau PJ, Dupuy E, Bryckaert MC, et al. Platelet derived growth factor in type I diabetes mellitus. *Eur J Clin Invest* 1989;19:172–175.

38. Barradas MA, Gill DS, Fonseca VA, et al. Intraplatelet serotonin in patients with diabetes mellitus and peripheral vascular disease. *Eur J Clin Invest* 1988;18:399–404.

39. Cohen I, Burk D, Fullerton RJ, et al. Nonenzymatic glycation of human blood platelet proteins. *Thromb Res* 1989;55:341–349.

40. Sampietro T, Lenzi S, Cecchetti P, et al. Nonenzymatic glycation of human platelet membrane proteins in vitro and in vivo. *Clin Chem* 1986;32:1328–1331.

41. Kaul S, Waack BJ, Padgett RC, et al. Altered vascular responses to platelets from hypercholesterolaemic humans. *Circ Res* 1993;72:737–743.

42. Oskarsson HJ, Hofmeyer TG. Platelets from patients with diabetes mellitus have impaired ability to mediate vasodilation. *J Am Coll Cardiol* 1996;27:1464–1470.

43. Gryglewski RJ, Botting RM, Vane JR. Mediators produced by the endothelial cell. *Hypertension* 1988;12:530–548.

44. Harrison HE, Reece AH, Johnson M. Effect of insulin treatment on prostacyclin in experimental diabetes. *Diabetologia* 1980;18:65–68.

45. Bucala R, Tracey KJ, Cerami A. Advanced glycosylation products quench nitric oxide and mediate defective endothelium-dependent vasodilation in experimental diabetes. *J Clin Invest* 1991;87:432–438.

46. Lazarowski ER, Winegar DA, Nolan RD, et al. Effect of protein kinase A on inositide metabolism and rap 1 G-protein in human erythroleukaemia cells. *J Biol Chem* 1990;265:13118–13123.

47. DeVriese AS, Verbeuren TJ, VandeVoorde J, et al. Endothelial dysfunction in diabetes. *Br J Pharmacol* 2000;130:963–974.

48. Akai T, Naka K, Okuda K, et al. Decreased sensitivity of platelets to prostacyclin in patients with diabetes mellitus. *Horm Metab Res* 1983;15:523–526.

49. Nolan RD, Platt KH, Loose PG. The resistance to nitric oxide inhibition of platelet aggregation is due to decreased phosphorylation of rap 1B in platelets of NIDDM compared with control subjects. *Diabetes* 1994;43[Suppl 1]:101a.

50. Forstermann U, Mugge A, Alheid U, et al. Selective attenuation of endothelium mediated vasodilation in atherosclerotic human coronary arteries. *Circ Res* 1988;62:185–190.

51. Chin JH, Azhar S, Hoffman BB. Inactivation of endothelial-derived relaxing factor by oxidised lipoproteins. *J Clin Invest* 1992;89:10–18.

52. Bastyr EJ III, Lu J, Stowe R, et al. Low molecular weight GTP-binding proteins are altered in platelet hyperaggregation in IDDM. *Oncogene* 1993;8:515–518.

53. Livingstone C, McLellan AR, McGregor M, et al. Altered G-protein expression and adenylate cyclase activity in platelets of NIDDM male subjects. *Biochim Biophys Acta* 1991;1096:127–133.

54. Nolan RD, Burch M, Salter LM, et al. Abnormalities in the distribution of rap 1B platelets of NIDDM. *Diabetes* 1993;42:72a.

55. Steinberg HO, Baron AD. Vascular function, insulin resistance and fatty acids. *Diabetologia* 2002;45;623–634.

56. Mulvihill N, Foley JB, Murphy RT, et al. Enhanced endothelial activation in diabetic patients with unstable angina and non-Q-wave myocardial infarction. *Diabet Med* 2001;18:979–983.

57. Puente-Navazo MD, Chettab K, Duhault J, et al. Glucose and insulin modulate the capacity of endothelial cells to express P-selectin and bind a monocytic cell line. *Thromb Haemost* 2001;86:680–685.

58. Shechter M, Merz CN, Paul-Labrador MJ, et al. Blood glucose and platelet-dependent thrombosis in patients with coronary artery disease. *J Am Coll Cardiol* 2000;35:300–307.

59. Vinik A, Erbas T, Nolan R, et al. Platelet dysfunction in type 2 diabetes. *Diabetes Care* 2001;24:1476–1485.

60. Winocour PD, Bryszewska M, Watala C, et al. Reduced membrane fluidity in platelets from diabetic patients. *Diabetes* 1990;39:241–244.

61. Watanabe G, Saito Y, Madaule P, et al. Protein kinase N (PKN) and PKN related protein rhophilin as targets of small GTPase rho. *Science* 1996;271:645–647.

62. Stern DM, Yan SD, Yan SF, et al. Receptor for advanced glycation end products (RAGE) and the complications of diabetes. *Ageing Res Rev* 2002;1:1–15.

63. Palinski W, Koschinsky T, Butler SW, et al. Immunological evidence for the presence of advanced glycosylation end products in atherosclerotic lesions of euglycaemic rabbits. *Arterioscler Thromb Vasc Biol* 1995;15:571–582.

64. Sakata N, Imanaga Y, Meng J, et al. Immunohistochemical localization of different epitopes of advanced glycation end products in human atherosclerotic lesions. *Atherosclerosis* 1998;141:61–75.

65. Del Principe D, Menichelli A, De Matteis W, et al. Hydrogen peroxide has a role in the aggregation of human platelets. *FEBS Lett* 1985;185:142–146.

66. Harlan JM, Callahan KS. Role of hydrogen peroxide in the neutrophil-mediated release of prostacyclin from cultured endothelial cells. *J Clin Invest* 1984;74:442–448.

67. Stratton IM, Adler AI, Neil HA, et al. Association of glycaemia with macrovascular and microvascular complications of type 2 diabetes (UKPDS 35). *BMJ* 2000;321:405–412.

68. Goldner MG, Knatterud GL, Prout TE. Effects of hypoglycaemic agents on vascular complications in patients with adult onset diabetes. *JAMA* 1971;218:1400–1410.

69. Scandinavian Simvastatin Survival Study Group. Randomised trial of cholesterol lowering in 4444 with coronary heart disease. *Lancet* 1994;344:1383–1389.

70. Gerstein HC. Reduction of cardiovascular events and microvascular complications in diabetes with ACE inhibitor treatment: HOPE and MICROHOPE. *Diabetes Metab Res Rev* 2002;18[Suppl 3]:S82–S85.

71. Jarvis B, Simpson K. Clopidogrel: a review of its use in the prevention of atherothrombosis. *Drugs* 2000;60:347–377.

72. Davi G, Ciabattoni G, Consoli A, et al. In vivo formation of 8-iso-prostaglandin F2alpha and platelet activation in diabetes mellitus. *Circulation* 1999;99:224–229.

73. Takahashi K, Nammour TM, Fukunaga M, et al. A series of prostaglandin F2-like compounds are produced in vivo in humans by a non-cyclooxygenase free radical catalysed mechanism. *Proc Natl Acad Sci U S A* 1990;87:9383–9387.

74. Morrow JD, Minton TA, Roberts LJ, et al. The F2 isoprostane 8-epi-PGF2 alpha, a potent agonist of the vascular thromboxane/endoperoxide receptor, is a

platelet thromboxane/endoperoxide receptor antagonist. *Prostaglandins* 1992;44:155–163.

75. Gopaul NK, Anggard EE, Mallet AI, et al. Plasma 8-iso-PGF 2 alpha levels are elevated in individuals with non-insulin dependent diabetes mellitus. *FEBS Lett* 1995;368:225–229.

76. Keaney JF, Loscalzo J. Diabetes, oxidative stress and platelet activation. *Circulation* 1999;99:189–191.

77. Uemura S, Matsushita H, Li W, et al. Diabetes mellitus enhances vascular matrix metalloproteinase activity: role of oxidative stress. *Circ Res* 2001;88:1291–1298.

78. Dobos V, Anstadt MP, Hutchinson J, et al. Evidence for matrix metalloproteinase induction/activation system in arterial vasculature and decreased synthesis and activity in diabetes. *Diabetes* 2002;51:3063–3068.

79. Ebihara I, Nakamura T, Shimada N, et al. Increased plasma MMP-9 concentrations precede the development of microalbuminuria in non-insulin dependent diabetes mellitus. *Am J Kidney Dis* 1998;32:544–550.

80. Schmidt MI, Dunoon R, Sharrett AR, et al. Markers of inflammation and prediction of diabetes mellitus in adults (ARIC Study). *Lancet* 1999;353:1649–1652.

81. Esposito K, Nappo F, Marfella R, et al. Inflammatory cytokine concentrations are acutely increased by hyperglycaemia in humans. *Circulation* 2002;106:2067–2072.

82. Pradhan AD, Manson JE, Rifai N, et al. C-reactive protein, interleukin 6, and risk of developing diabetes mellitus. *JAMA* 2001;286:327–334.

83. Libby P, Simon DI. Inflammation and thrombosis: the clot thickens. *Circulation* 2001;103:1718–1720.

84. Simon DI, Chen Z, Xu H, et al. Platelet glycoprotein 1b alpha is a counter receptor for the leukocyte integrin Mac-1 (CD11B/CD18). *J Exp Med* 2000;192:193–204.

85. May AE, Kalsch T, Massberg S, et al. Engagement of glycoprotein IIb/IIIa on platelets upregulates CD40L and triggers CD4OL dependent matrix degradation by endothelial cells. *Circulation* 2002;106:2111–2117.

86. Juhan-Vague I, Thompson SG, Jespersen J. Involvement of the haemostatic system in the insulin resistance syndrome. The ECAT angina pectoris study group. *Arterioscler Thromb* 1993;13:1865–1873.

87. Falcon C, Pfliegler G, Deckmyn H, et al. The platelet insulin receptor. *Biochem Biophys Res Commun* 1988;157:1190–1196.

88. Abrahm DR, Hollingsworth PJ, Smith CB, et al. Decreased alpha 2 adrenergic receptors on platelet membranes from diabetic patients with autonomic neuropathy and orthostatic hypotension. *J Clin Endoc Metab* 1986;63:906–912.

89. Udvardy M, Pfliegler G, Rak K. Platelet insulin receptor determination in NIDDM. *Experientia* 1985;41:422–423.

90. Khan NN, Mueller HS, Sinha AK, et al. Restoration by insulin of impaired prostaglandin E1/12 receptor activity of platelets in acute ischaemic heart disease. *Circ Res* 1991;68:245–254.

91. Kahn NN, Najeeb MA, Ishaq M, et al. Normalisation of impaired response of platelets to PGE 1/12 and synthesis of PGI2 by insulin in unstable angina pectoris and in acute myocardial infarction. *Am J Cardiol* 1992;70:582–586.

92. Kahn NN, Bauman WA, Sinha AK. Transient decrease of binding of insulin to platelets in acute ischaemic heart disease. *Am J Med Sci* 1994;307:21–26.

93. The Platelet Aspirin Trialist Group. Collaborative review of randomised trials of antiplatelet therapy. *BMJ* 1994;308:81–106.

94. Smith SC Jr, Dove JT, Jacobs AK, et al. ACC/AHA Guidelines for Percutaneous Coronary Intervention. *J Am Coll Cardiol* 2001;37:2215–2239.

95. Grossman E, Goldbourt U. Hypertension Optimal Treatment (HOT) trial. *Lancet* 1998;352:572; author reply, 574–575.

96. Early Treatment Diabetic Retinopathy Study Research Group. Effects of aspirin treatment on diabetic retinopathy. ETDRS report number 8. *Ophthalmology* 1991;98[5 Suppl]:757–765.

97. Kodama M, Yamasaki Y, Sakamoto K, et al. Antiplatelet drugs attenuate progression of carotid intima-media thickness in subjects with type 2 diabetes. *Thromb Res* 2000;97:239–245.

98. Bhatt DL, Marso SP, Hirsch AT, et al. Amplified benefit of clopidogrel versus aspirin in patients with diabetes mellitus. *Am J Cardiol* 2002;90:625–628.

99. Budaj A, Yusuf S, Mehta SR, et al. Benefit of clopidogrel in patients with acute coronary syndromes without ST-segment elevation in various risk groups. *Circulation* 2002;106:1622–1626.

100. Steinhubl SR, Berger PB, Mann JT 3rd, et al. Early and sustained dual oral antiplatelet therapy following percutaneous coronary intervention: a randomized controlled trial. *JAMA* 2002;288:2411–2420.

101. CHARISMA trial: Clopidogrel for High Atherothrombotic Risk and Ischaemic Stabilization, Management and Avoidance. Personal communication from study investigators (Bhatt DP, Topol E, et al.), 2003.

102. Cox D, Smith R, Quinn M, et al. Evidence of platelet activation during treatment with a GPIIb/IIIa antagonist in patients presenting with acute coronary syndromes. *J Am Coll Cardiol* 2000;36:1514–1519.

103. O'Shea JC, Buller CE, Cantor WJ, et al. Long-term efficacy of platelet glycoprotein IIb/IIIa integrin blockade with eptifibatide in coronary stent intervention. *JAMA* 2002;287:618–621.

104. Randomised placebo-controlled and balloon-angioplasty-controlled trial to assess safety of coronary stenting with use of platelet glycoprotein-IIb/IIIa blockade. The Evaluation of Platelet IIb/IIIa Inhibitor for Stenting (EPISTENT) investigators. *Lancet* 1998;352:87–92.

105. Roe MT, Moliterno DJ. Abciximab prevents ischemic complications during angioplasty. The Evaluation in PTCA to Improve Long-Term Outcome with Abciximab GP IIb/IIIa Blockade (EPILOG) trial. *Cleve Clin J Med* 1998;65:267–272.

106. Roffi M, Moliterno DJ, Meier B, et al. Impact of different platelet glycoprotein IIb/IIIa receptor inhibitors among diabetic patients undergoing percutaneous coronary intervention: do Tirofiban and ReoPro Give Similar Efficacy Outcomes Trial (TARGET) 1-year follow-up. *Circulation* 2002;105:2730–2736.

107. Marso SP, Lincoff AM, Ellis SG, et al. Optimizing the percutaneous interventional outcomes for patients with diabetes mellitus: results of the EPISTENT (Evaluation of Platelet IIb/IIIa Inhibitor for Stenting Trial) diabetic substudy. *Circulation* 1999;100:2477–2784.

108. Bhatt DL, Marso SP, Lincoff AM, et al. Abciximab reduces mortality in diabetic patients following percutaneous coronary intervention. *J Am Coll Cardiol* 2000;35:922–928.

109. Kleiman NS, Lincoff AM, Kereiakes DJ, et al. Diabetes mellitus, glycoprotein IIb/IIIa blockade, and heparin: evidence for a complex interaction in a multicenter trial. EPILOG Investigators. *Circulation* 1998;97:1912–1920.

110. Kabbani SS, Watkins MW, Ashikaga T, et al. Platelet reactivity characterized prospectively: a determinant of outcome 90 days after percutaneous coronary intervention. *Circulation* 2001;104:181–186.

111. Nannizzi-Alaimo L, Alves VL, Phillips DR. Inhibitory effects of glycoprotein IIb/IIIa antagonists and aspirin on the release of soluble CD40 ligand during platelet stimulation. *Circulation* 2003;107:1123–1128.

112. Mayfield RK, Halushka PV, Wohltmann HJ, et al. Platelet function during continuous insulin infusion treatment in insulin-dependent diabetic patients. *Diabetes* 1985;34:1127–1133.

113. Malmberg K, Norhammar A, Ryden L. Insulin treatment post myocardial infarction: the DIGAMI study. *Adv Exp Med Biol* 2001;498:279–284.

114. Davies MJ, Lawrence IG. DIGAMI (Diabetes Mellitus, Insulin Glucose Infusion in Acute Myocardial Infarction): theory and practice. *Diabetes Obes Metab* 2002;4:289–295.

115. Otsuka Y, Miyazaki S, Okumura H, et al. Abnormal glucose tolerance, not small vessel diameter, is a determinant of long-term prognosis in patients treated with balloon coronary angioplasty. *Eur Heart J* 2000;21:1790–1796.

116. Aoki I, Shimoyama K, Aoki N, et al. Platelet-dependent thrombin generation in patients with diabetes mellitus: effects of glycemic control on coagulability in diabetes. *J Am Coll Cardiol* 1996;27:560–566.

117. Chrisholm DJ. The Diabetes Control and Complications Trial (DCCT): a milestone in diabetes management. *Med J Aust* 1993;159:721–723.

118. Emanuele N, Azad N, Abraira C, et al. Effect of intensive glycemic control on fibrinogen, lipids, and lipoproteins: Veterans Affairs Cooperative Study in Type II Diabetes Mellitus. *Arch Intern Med* 1998;158:2485–2490.

119. Roshan B, Tofler GH, Weinrauch LA, et al. Improved glycemic control and platelet function abnormalities in diabetic patients with microvascular disease. *Metabolism* 2000;49:88–91.

120. Trovati M, Massucco P, Mattiello L, et al. Insulin increases guanosine-3′,5′-cyclic monophosphate in human platelets: a mechanism involved in the insulin antiaggregating effect. *Diabetes* 1994;43:1015–1019.

121. Gargiulo P, Caccese D, Pignatelli P, et al. Metformin decreases platelet superoxide anion production in diabetic patients. *Diabetes Metab Res Rev* 2002;18:156–159.

122. Ishizuka T, Taniguchi O, Yamamoto M, et al. Thrombin-induced platelet aggregation, phosphoinositide metabolism and protein phosphorylation in NIDDM patients treated by diet, sulphonylurea or insulin. *Diabetologia* 1994;37:632–638.

123. O'Keefe JH, Blackstone EH, Sergeant P, et al. The optimal mode of coronary revascularization for diabetic patients: a risk-adjusted long-term study comparing coronary angioplasty and coronary bypass surgery. *Eur Heart J* 1998;19:1696–1703.

124. Ishizuka T, Itaya S, Wada H, et al. Differential effect of the antidiabetic thiazolidinediones troglitazone and pioglitazone on human platelet aggregation mechanism. *Diabetes* 1998;47:1494–1500.

125. Haffner SM, Greenberg AS, Weston WM, et al. Effect of rosiglitazone treatment on nontraditional markers of cardiovascular disease in patients with type 2 diabetes mellitus. *Circulation* 2002;106:679–684.

126. Meier CA, Chicheportiche R, Juge-Aubry CE, et al. Regulation of the interleukin-1 receptor antagonist in THP-1 cells by ligands of the peroxisome proliferator-activated receptor gamma. *Cytokine* 2002;18:320–328.

127. Steiner G. Lipid intervention trials in diabetes. *Diabetes Care* 2000;23[Suppl 2]:B49–B53.

128. van de Ree MA, Huisman MV, Princen HM, et al. Strong decrease of high sensitivity C-reactive protein with high-dose atorvastatin in patients with type 2 diabetes mellitus. *Atherosclerosis* 2003;166:129–135.

129. Treasure CB, Klein JL, Weintraub WS, et al. Beneficial effects of cholesterol-lowering therapy on the coronary endothelium in patients with coronary artery disease. *N Engl J Med* 1995;332:481–487.

130. Katznelson S, Ramirez A, Perez R, et al. Pravastatin and cyclosporine inhibit platelet-derived growth factor-stimulated vascular smooth muscle cell mitogenesis: an investigation of mechanisms. *Transplant Proc* 1998;30:998–999.

131. Negre-Aminou P, van Vliet AK, van Erck M, et al. Inhibition of proliferation of human smooth muscle cells by various HMG-CoA reductase inhibitors: comparison with other human cell types. *Biochim Biophys Acta* 1997;1345:259–268.

132. Rosenson RS, Lowe GD. Effects of lipids and lipoproteins on thrombosis and rheology. *Atherosclerosis* 1998;140:271–280.

133. Sparrow CP, Burton CA, Hernandez M, et al. Simvastatin has anti-inflammatory and antiatherosclerotic activities independent of plasma cholesterol lowering. *Arterioscler Thromb Vasc Biol* 2001;21:115–121.

134. Kwak B, Mulhaupt F, Myit S, et al. Statins as a newly recognized type of immunomodulator. *Nat Med* 2000;6:1399–1402.

135. Ma LP, Nie DN, Hsu SX, et al. Inhibition of platelet aggregation and expression of alpha granule membrane protein 140 and thromboxane B2 with pravastatin therapy for hypercholesterolemia. *J Assoc Acad Minor Phys* 2002;13:23–26.

136. Haffner S. Clinical trials and guidelines for lipid management in the diabetic patient; www.lipidsonline.org.

137. Yusuf S, Sleight P, Pogue J, et al. Effects of an angiotensin-converting-enzyme inhibitor, ramipril, on cardiovascular events in high-risk patients. The Heart Outcomes Prevention Evaluation Study Investigators. *N Engl J Med* 2000;342:145–153.

138. Lonn E, Yusuf S, Dzavik V, et al. Effects of ramipril and vitamin E on atherosclerosis: the Study to Evaluate Carotid Ultrasound Changes in Patients Treated with Ramipril and Vitamin E (SECURE). *Circulation* 2001;103:919–925.

139. Bauriedel G, Skowasch D, Schneider M, et al. Antiplatelet effects of angiotensin-converting enzyme inhibitors compared with aspirin and clopidogrel:

a pilot study with whole-blood aggregometry. *Am Heart J* 2003;145:343–348.

140. Nunez A, Gomez J, Zalba LR, et al. Losartan inhibits in vitro platelet activation: comparison with candesartan and valsartan. *J Renin Angiotensin Aldosterone Syst* 2000;1:175–179.

141. de las Heras N, Aragoncillo P, Maeso R, et al. AT(1) receptor antagonism reduces endothelial dysfunction and intimal thickening in atherosclerotic rabbits. *Hypertension* 1999;34:969–975.

142. Stephens NG, Parsons A, Schofield PM, et al. Randomised controlled trial of vitamin E in patients with coronary disease: Cambridge Heart Antioxidant Study (CHAOS). *Lancet* 1996;347:781–786.

143. Salonen JT. Clinical trials testing cardiovascular benefits of antioxidant supplementation. *Free Radic Res* 2002;36:1299–1306.

144. Marchioli R, Schweiger C, Tavazzi L, et al. Efficacy of n-3 polyunsaturated fatty acids after myocardial infarction: results of GISSI-Prevenzione trial. Gruppo Italiano per lo Studio della Sopravvivenza nell'Infarto Miocardico. *Lipids* 2001;36[Suppl]:S119–S126.

145. Kreisberg RA. Diabetic dyslipidemia. *Am J Cardiol* 1998;82:67U–73U; discussion, 85U–86U.

Diabetes and Cardiovascular Disease
edited by Steven P. Marso and David M. Stern
Lippincott Williams & Wilkins, Philadelphia © 2004

15

Diabetes, Impaired Fibrinolysis, and Thrombosis

Peter J. Grant and Lucinda K. M. Summers

Professor of Medicine, Academic Unit of Molecular Vascular Medicine, Leeds General Infirmary; Senior Lecturer, Academic Unit of Molecular Vascular Medicine, University of Leeds, Honorary Consultant, Diabetes Center, Leeds General Infirmary, Leeds, West Yorkshire, United Kingdom

DIABETES AND CORONARY ARTERY DISEASE

Diabetes is a common metabolic condition that is characterized by fasting hyperglycemia and the development of chronic vascular complications. It affects between 1% and 10% of most populations, although in some areas of the world up to 50% of the population has diabetes (1). It has been known for many years that the development of diabetes mellitus is associated with increased risks for cardiovascular, cerebrovascular, and peripheral vascular disease (2) (Tables 15-1 and 15-2). Men with diabetes have a twofold to threefold increase in the incidence of coronary artery disease (CAD), compared with nondiabetics, and women have a threefold to fivefold increase (2,3) (Table 15-2). The Multiple Risk Factor Intervention Trial (MRFIT) revealed that CAD was the major cause of death in men with diabetes and was responsible for approximately 40% of deaths over a 16-year period (4). Even with adjustment for risk factors such as age, race, income, cholesterol concentration, systolic blood pressure, and cigarette smoking, the risk of death from CAD was three times greater in diabetic men (5). For all participants, cholesterol concentration, systolic blood pressure, and cigarette smoking were predictors of CAD mortality, but for men with diabetes the absolute risk of death from CAD increased more steeply with each risk factor (5).

Diabetes is associated with greater progression of CAD (6) and a higher mortality rate from CAD (7–9). Interventions such as percutaneous transluminal coronary angioplasty (10–12) and coronary stenting (13) tend to be less successful, and a higher mortality rate is reported after coronary artery bypass grafting in diabetics (14), although not all studies are in agreement on this issue (12). Overall, approximately 70% of deaths in subjects with diabetes are due to cardiovascular disease, and a large proportion of the inpatient budget in the United Kingdom spent on diabetes relates to the management of cardiovascular disease.

Although insulin-dependent (type 1) and non-insulin-dependent (type 2) diabetes mellitus have differing etiologies, they share a similar burden of macrovascular complications. Results from the Diabetes Control and Complications Trial (DCCT) and United Kingdom Prospective Diabetes Study (UKPDS) indicate that hyperglycemia and glycosylation are important determinants of microvascular disorders; however, the evidence in relation to cardiovascular disease is less clear. MRFIT emphasized the importance of risk factor clustering in the pathogenesis of myocardial infarction (MI) and that enhanced vascular risk occurs in diabetic patients under such conditions. Type 2 subjects who are insulin resistant make up around 85% of type 2 diabetics, and such individuals tend to cluster atherothrombotic risk factors, as shown in Table 15-3. The

TABLE 15-1. *Incidence over a 7-year period of myocardial infarction in people with type 2 diabetes compared with the general population[a]*

Event	Type 2 diabetes (%)	General population (%)
First myocardial infarction	20.2	3.5
Subsequent myocardial infarction	45	18.8

[a]People with type 2 diabetes have approximately the same risk of myocardial infarction as people without diabetes who have already had a myocardial infarction.

Data from Haffner SM, Lehto S, Ronnemaa T, et al. Mortality from coronary heart disease in 1059 subjects with type 2 diabetes and in 1373 nondiabetic subjects with and without prior myocardial infarction. *N Engl J Med* 1998;339:229–234.

development of microalbuminuria in both type 1 and type 2 diabetes promotes similar risk clustering, which is further enhanced by the presence of hypertension, oxidized lipoproteins, and glycosylation. This knowledge should move clinicians away from a purely glucocentric view of the pathogenesis of macrovascular disease and toward an understanding of the complexity of vascular risk and the implications for its prevention and management. This chapter discusses the prothrombotic and impaired fibrinolytic changes reported in relation to diabetes.

MECHANISMS OF THROMBOSIS

The biochemical processes that regulate the formation and subsequent lysis of a clot are complex and depend on a wide variety of interrelated metabolic reactions (Fig. 15-1).

Coagulation

Thrombi formed in the coronary artery form a platelet-rich fibrin network with a minor contribution from other plasma proteins and white blood cells. When coronary artery wall plaques rupture, constituents of the vessel wall (e.g., collagen) are exposed to blood. This promotes adhesion of platelets and release of activated tissue factor from damaged cells (reviewed by Morrissey [15]), which initiates activation of the intrinsic and extrinsic coagulation pathways, leading to thrombin generation. The conversion of prothrombin is governed by the generation of activated factor X, which in turn is regulated by the action of the intrinsic pathway (factors XII, XI, IX, and VIII) and the extrinsic pathway (tissue factor and factor VII). Thrombin acts to convert fibrinogen to soluble fibrin and then to fibrinolysis-resistant cross-linked fibrin, the latter reaction being dependent on thrombin activation of factor XIII (reviewed by Lorand [16]). Factor XIII is a protransglutaminase that catalyses covalent cross-linking of the γ and α chains of fibrin(ogen) to a stable structure that is resistant to physical and chemical insults (17).

Inhibitors of Coagulation

With the exception of tissue factor, which is released from damaged cells in its active form, coagulation factors circulate in the inactive state and are activated in a coagulation cascade. A complex feedback system limits the generation

TABLE 15-2. *Mean annual age-adjusted incidence per 1,000 subjects of manifestations of atherosclerotic disease*

Event or condition	Men		Women	
	Diabetes	No diabetes	Diabetes	No diabetes
Coronary artery disease	24.8	14.9	17.8	6.9
Intermittent claudication	12.6	3.3	11.4	2.2
Cerebrovascular accident	4.7	1.9	6.2	1.7
Cardiovascular disease[a]	39.1	19.1	27.2	10.2
Death from cardiovascular disease	17.4	8.5	17.0	3.6

[a]Cardiovascular disease includes atherosclerotic disease and congestive heart failure. The subjects were men and women in the Framingham cohort between 45 and 74 years old.

Data from Kannel WB, McGee DL. Diabetes and cardiovascular disease: the Framingham study. *JAMA* 1979;241:2035–2038.

TABLE 15-3. *Features of insulin resistance*

Metabolic features	Thrombolytic/fibrinolytic features
Hyperglycemia	↑ Plasminogen activator inhibitor-1 (PAI-1)
Hyperinsulinemia	↑ Fibrinogen
Hypertension	↑ Factor VII
Hypertriglyceridemia	↑ von Willebrand factor
Hyperuricemia	
↓ High-density lipoprotein-cholesterol	
↑ Small, dense low-density lipoproteins	

of thrombin. Tissue factor pathway inhibitor (TFPI), as its name implies, inhibits the tissue factor pathway. Thrombin also suppresses the co-agulation cascade by binding to thrombomodulin on the endothelial cell surface. Protein C is activated by this complex; together with protein S, it inactivates factors Va and VIIIa. Binding to thrombomodulin causes thrombin to lose its pro-coagulant functions. Thrombin is also specifically inhibited by antithrombin III.

Fibrinolysis

The fibrinolytic cascade consists of activa-tors and inhibitors that regulate the conversion of plasminogen to plasmin. Plasminogen, tis-sue plasminogen activator (tPA), and urinary-type plasminogen activator (uPA) are the major plasma fibrinolytic components. Although tPA and uPA are both synthesized in the endothe-lium, tPA is the primary plasminogen activator

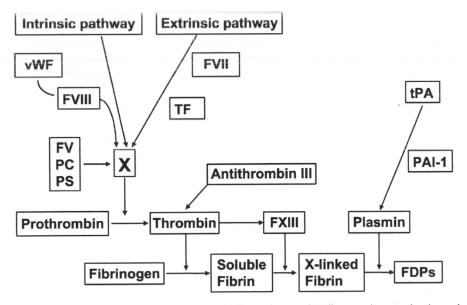

FIG. 15-1. Important components of the metabolic pathways leading to the production of cross-linked fibrin and its subsequent breakdown by the fibrinolytic system. The intrinsic and extrinsic pathways represent a simplified version of the coagulation cascade leading to the production of the prothrombinase complex, which initiates the conversion of prothrombin to thrombin. The production of cross-linked fibrin from fibrinogen is dependent on complex interactions between thrombin, fibrinogen, and thrombin-activated factor XIII. The cross-linked fibrin forms the basis of an established clot, and lysis and remodeling are principally regulated by fibrin and plasma from plasminogen.

in the vasculature. The enzyme responsible for the degradation of fibrin is plasmin, and the conversion of plasminogen to plasmin is crucial to the development of lytic activity, a reaction regulated by tPA and uPA. Both activators are quenched in the circulation by the binding of their fast-acting inhibitor, plasminogen activator inhibitor-1 (PAI-1), which exists in the circulation in excess. The main circulating inhibitors of fibrinolysis are PAI-1 and α_2-antiplasmin. PAI-1 is a rapid-acting inhibitor of both tPA and uPA (18), whereas α_2-antiplasmin is a specific inhibitor of plasmin and is covalently bound to polymerizing fibrin by activated factor XIII (19).

Activated PAI-1 is synthesized in platelets, vascular endothelial cells (20,21), liver, and adipose tissue (22). PAI-1 is released on the platelet surface when platelets are stimulated by thrombin, preventing premature lysis of the blood clot. Thrombin also stimulates endothelial cells to synthesize PAI-1 (23). Upon generation of free thrombin, there is a rapid local increase in the circulating PAI-1 concentration (21), which binds to tPA or uPA in a 1:1 ratio to form a stable complex (24) that is removed from the circulation by hepatic cells (25). Active PAI-1 has a half-life of 30 minutes (20), but it is stabilized by binding to vitronectin, a plasma protein (26).

Mechanisms of Fibrinolysis

Plasmin is formed when plasminogen on the surface of the fibrin clot is partially cleaved by tPA or uPA (27). Cross-linked fibrin binds plasminogen, plasmin, and tPA and allows these reactions to proceed unhindered by the effects of PAI-1. Polymerization of fibrin increases the activation of fibrin-bound plasminogen by tPA, and new binding sites for plasminogen on fibrin are revealed by the subsequent degradation of fibrin (28), resulting in increased fibrinolysis. Clinically, the importance of these processes lies in the fact that fibrinolysis is localized to the site of thrombus formation; systemic fibrino(geno)lysis does not occur under normal circumstances.

THE COAGULATION AND FIBRINOLYTIC PATHWAYS AND CARDIOVASCULAR RISK

Fibrinogen

Prospective studies have demonstrated a strong relationship between fibrinogen and the development of both cardiovascular and cerebrovascular disease (29). Fibrinogen was more strongly associated with cardiovascular disease than was cholesterol in the Northwick Park Heart Study (30). The Prospective Cardiovascular Munster (PROCAM) (31) and Gothenburg (32) studies showed that increased fibrinogen concentrations were associated with an increased risk of CAD. Plasma fibrinogen relates to vascular disorders in case-control studies (33,34), indicating that elevated fibrinogen increases risk of cardiovascular disease in diabetic subjects.

Factor VII

The Northwick Park Heart Study reported that increased factor VII was associated with fatal but not with nonfatal MI in a prospective study of middle-aged men (35). These findings were partially supported in the PROCAM study, although there was only a trend toward an association (31). However, there are conflicting data, and it remains unclear whether factor VII concentrations predict vascular risk (37). Other case-control studies have shown associations between factor VII and vascular disease, and the Progetto Lombardo Aterotrombosi (PLAT) study reported an association between factor VII and carotid intimal thickening (38).

Von Willebrand Factor

Von Willebrand factor (vWF) is elevated in the presence of microalbuminuria (39–42). There are indications that levels of vWF are lower before the development of microalbuminuria (41) and may predict its development (40). vWF was reported to predict deterioration of neuropathy in a mixed group of predominantly type 1 subjects (43) and was found to be elevated in type 1 subjects with retinopathy (44). These results must be viewed with a degree of caution, because there are complex clinical relationships between microvascular and macrovascular disease that may confuse the issue. However, vWF consistently appears as a risk marker for arterial disease, and increased levels in both type 1 and type 2 diabetics probably indicate endothelial cell and vascular damage.

Fibrinolysis

The Northwick Park Heart Study reported that global suppression of fibrinolysis was related to subsequent risk of MI (35). Hamsten et al. (45) found that levels of PAI-1 activity 3 months after a first MI in young men predicted recurrent MI. The Physicians Heart Study described tPA as being independently associated with stroke in a large study of American physicians (46). Clinical studies point toward PAI-1 as having an important role in heart disease in type 2 diabetes. Diabetic survivors of MI have higher levels of both tPA antigen and PAI 1 activity, compared with nondiabetic MI survivors and controls (47). A study using directional coronary atherectomy in type 2 diabetic subjects and controls reported higher concentrations of PAI-1 with lower levels of urokinase in atheroma from diabetic subjects (48). The authors speculated that these findings might relate to insulin resis-

tance and suggested that the new generation of insulin sensitizers might modify these changes.

DIABETES AND COAGULATION FACTORS

Multiple abnormalities of coagulation factors and inhibitors of the activated pathway have been described in relation to both type 1 and type 2 diabetes. The major changes observed are shown in Table 15-4.

Fibrinogen

Levels of fibrinogen are reported to be increased in type 1 diabetic subjects, compared with nondiabetic controls (49 52), although generally not to the same extent as in type 2 diabetes. In identical twins discordant for type 1 diabetes, the diabetic twin had increased systolic blood pressure and elevated fibrinogen levels, compared with the nondiabetic twin (50). Type 1 subjects without complications have elevated fibrinogen (51), and studies suggest that elevated fibrinogen is associated with the diabetic state rather than occurring secondary to the development of vascular complications. In a large study of type 2 diabetic patients, 50% had a plasma fibrinogen greater than 3.5 g/L (53), and many other studies have reported similar findings (54–59).

TABLE 15-4. *Effects of type 1 and type 2 diabetes on thrombotic and antithrombotic factors[a]*

Factor	Type 1 diabetes (ref. no.)	Type 2 diabetes (ref. no.)
Thrombotic		
Fibrinogen	? ↑ (50) or ↓ (220)	↑
Factor VII coagulant activity	? ↑ (87) or ↓ (50)	↑
von Willebrand factor	↑	↑
Antithrombotic		
Antithrombin III activity	↓	? ↓ (no data)
Protein C	→ (87,88) or ↓ (85)	→ (86) or ↑ (90,91)
Protein S	→ (88) or ↑ (92)	→ (93) or ↑ (93)
Thrombomodulin	↑	↑
Tissue factor pathway inhibitor (TFPI) activity	↑	Probably ↑

[a]In people with type 1 diabetes, fibrinogen, factor VII and protein S concentrations may be increased only in those with microalbuminuria. Antithrombin III activity has been shown to be decreased by hyperglycemia in people with type 1 diabetes and in people without diabetes and may therefore be decreased in type 2 diabetes. Similarly, tissue factor pathway inhibitor activity was increased with hyperglycemia together with hyperinsulinemia in people without diabetes, suggesting that activity may also be increased in people with type 2 diabetes.

Factor VII

Several studies have reported increased concentrations of factor VII in type 2 diabetes in the absence of complications (55,60–62) and in the presence of microalbuminuria (61). In type 1 diabetic subjects, factor VII is elevated in the presence of microalbuminuria (63), although it is not clear whether factor VII is increased in uncomplicated type 1 diabetes. Factor VII has been reported as being lower in female type 1 patients (64) and higher in male type 2 diabetic subjects (60,64). However, there have been inconsistent findings in this area, and another study in type 2 diabetic subjects reported that levels in women were 25% higher (65). Among first-degree relatives of type 2 subjects, higher levels of factor VII were found in the group as a whole, with a trend toward increased concentrations of factor VII in women (66). Because factor VII appears to be related to features of the insulin resistance syndrome and is increased in women with the polycystic ovary syndrome, it may be that menopausal status explains the differences between female type 1 and type 2 subjects.

Von Willebrand Factor

vWF is a circulating glycoprotein that has two main functions: it acts as a carrier protein for factor VIII and as a platelet/collagen ligand. In the latter role, vWF acts as an adhesion molecule to promote platelet adhesion by binding to the platelet glycoprotein GPIb/IX receptor and exposed subendothelial collagen. Elevated concentrations of vWF occur in both type 1 (67) and type 2 (62,68) diabetics.

METABOLIC DETERMINANTS OF COAGULATION FACTORS IN DIABETES

Fibrinogen

There is evidence that fibrinogen is weakly associated with features of the insulin resistance syndrome (66,69), and both glycosylated hemoglobin (53) and body mass index (59) have been related to increased fibrinogen concentra-

tions. The latter findings are described in nondiabetic subjects (70,71). Possibly the most important association with elevated fibrinogen is diabetic nephropathy. Diabetic subjects with albuminuria and otherwise normal renal function, as well as those with frank renal impairment, are at markedly increased risk for MI. Several studies have demonstrated consistent increases in plasma fibrinogen in type 1 and type 2 diabetic subjects with microalbuminuria (39,52,53,72,73). Similar findings have been reported in American Indians with diabetes and nephropathy (74). Although microalbuminuria appears to be associated with increased cardiovascular disease in the nondiabetic population (75), a study of hemostatic changes in hypertensive nondiabetic subjects with microalbuminuria showed weaker relationships with vWF and fibrinogen than would be expected in the diabetic population (76). These findings imply that microalbuminuria and the associated changes in fibrinogen are not directly related, but rather independently associated with another factor or factors, possibly protein glycosylation or ambient glucose concentration.

Factor VII

The major determinants of factor VII concentrations in diabetes appear to be gender, microalbuminuria, and some features of the insulin resistance syndrome. In nondiabetic populations there is evidence that levels of factor VII are related to cholesterol and, to a greater extent, triglyceride levels (77–79), observations that may help to explain some of the relationships between factor VII and vascular disease. In a study of type 2 diabetic patients characterized for features of insulin resistance, factor VII concentrations correlated strongly with total cholesterol, insulin, and triglycerides and to a lesser extent with age and body mass index (80). These findings, together with observations in first-degree relatives of type 2 diabetics (70), indicate that elevated factor VII clusters with insulin resistance in a manner similar to that described for PAI-1.

Von Willebrand Factor

As already stated, vWF is increased in the presence of microalbuminuria (39–42), and increasing vWF concentrations may predict the development of microalbuminuria (40). There is less evidence to support inclusion of vWF in the insulin resistance syndrome, because vWF levels appear to be unrelated to this condition (66).

DIABETES AND INHIBITORS OF THROMBOSIS

Antithrombin III

Antithrombin III is the most important inhibitor of thrombin activity, and levels are reduced by hyperglycemia in both type 1 diabetics (81) and nondiabetic subjects (82). When euglycemia was established by insulin infusion in subjects with type 1 diabetes, antithrombin III activity returned to normal (81). The decrease in activity with hyperglycemia is likely to be the result of glycation; *in vitro* studies have shown that increased glycation of antithrombin III impairs its thrombin-inhibiting activity (83), and *in vivo* studies have shown an inverse correlation between antithrombin III activity and HbA_{1c} and plasma glucose concentration (84).

Protein C

In type 1 diabetes, some studies have found decreased protein C concentrations (85), which are normalized by restoration of euglycemia (86). Others have found no difference in protein C concentrations between type 1 diabetics and healthy controls (87,88). Similarly, in a study comparing type 2 diabetic subjects and healthy controls, no difference in protein C activity was found (89), but type 2 diabetes was found to be associated with increased activation of protein C in other studies (90,91).

Protein S

In type 1 diabetes, protein S is increased with microalbuminuria (92) but not otherwise (88).

In subjects with type 2 diabetes compared with healthy controls, total protein S antigen was increased but free protein S concentrations were not (93).

Thrombomodulin

Increased thrombomodulin concentrations have been reported in type 1 diabetes (94). Studies have shown increased thrombomodulin in type 2 diabetes and with microalbuminuria (91,95). It has been suggested that this is a reflection of widespread vascular damage present in patients with nephropathy (95).

Tissue Factor Pathway Inhibitor Activity

TFPI is increased in type 1 diabetes (96,97). It is probable that TFPI is also increased in type 2 diabetes, because concentrations are increased by hyperglycemia combined with hyperinsulinemia in clamp studies in nondiabetic subjects (98).

DIABETES AND FIBRINOLYSIS

Fibrinolytic activity is decreased in type 1 and type 2 diabetes (99); given the prothrombotic changes present in many diabetic subjects, this results in an increased tendency for stable thrombus formation in the event of a ruptured coronary artery plaque. Increased tPA concentrations are associated with a risk of CAD, although the opposite might be expected because tPA is a fibrinolytic factor. However, this association is abolished once known risk factors are taken into account, so tPA is likely to be a risk marker rather than a cause of atherosclerotic disease (100,101). There is conflicting evidence with regard to concentrations of tPA in type 1 diabetes, with various studies showing that levels are normal (102), increased (103), and decreased (104). It appears that tPA concentrations are probably normal in type 2 diabetes (105), although one small study found that concentrations were increased (106).

Impaired fibrinolysis is mainly due to increased concentrations of PAI-1, which are found in both type 1 (87,88) and type 2 (99,105) diabetic subjects. PAI-1 concentrations are increased further in women with type 2 diabetes, which may contribute to their susceptibility to CAD (107).

Metabolic Determinants of PAI-1 Concentrations in Diabetic Subjects

Glucose stimulates PAI-1 expression in human vascular endothelial (108) and smooth muscle cells (109,110) *in vitro*, although not in cultured human hepatoma cells (111). Insulin and PAI-1 concentrations are correlated *in vivo* (112–114). This finding, together with the fact that insulin has been shown to stimulate the synthesis of PAI-1 from hepatocytes *in vitro* (115), led to the view that insulin directly stimulated PAI-1 production and that the hyperinsulinemia characteristic of type 2 diabetes was responsible for the increase in PAI-1 concentrations. However, this appears not to be the whole explanation, because control of hyperglycemia in type 2 diabetes with insulin therapy decreases PAI-1 concentrations (116,117). It has been suggested that increased PAI-1 concentrations are secondary to increased levels of proinsulin and split proinsulin (118), rather than insulin itself, because these insulin precursors induce time- and concentration-dependent increases in PAI-1 expression in cultured porcine aortic endothelial cells. *In vivo* studies in patients with type 2 diabetes support this argument. Improvement in glycemic control with insulin therapy results in decreased PAI-1 concentrations that correlate with decreased proinsulin concentrations (117,119), whereas improved control using sulfonylureas results in increased concentrations of PAI-1 and proinsulin (119).

On the basis of *in vitro* work showing that very low-density lipoprotein (VLDL)-triglyceride, insulin, and nonesterified fatty acids synergistically increase PAI-1 expression by human hepatoma cells (120), it has been proposed that PAI-1 concentrations increase in response to a combination of several features of insulin resistance, rather than hyperglycemia or hyperinsulinemia alone. Several studies in healthy volunteers showed that infusion of insulin with maintenance of eu-

glycemia does not cause an increase in PAI-1 (121,122). PAI-1 concentrations were also unaffected by combined hyperglycemia and hyperinsulinemia (121). In the same study, PAI-1 concentrations were unchanged by simultaneous insulin, glucose, and intralipid infusions (121). However, another study showed that hyperinsulinemia, hypertriglyceridemia, and hyperglycemia generated by dextrose and intralipid infusions resulted in increased PAI-1 concentrations, whereas saline infusion or euglycemic-hyperinsulinemic clamping did not (123). The findings of the latter study support the *in vitro* work, suggesting that PAI-1 concentrations are increased by a combination of several features of insulin resistance.

In view of the association of type 2 diabetes with obesity, the increased PAI-1 concentrations found in type 2 diabetes could be explained if adipose tissue were a major source of PAI-1. One indication that adipose tissue is a significant producer of PAI-1 is that weight loss induced by energy intake restriction in elderly, obese people decreased PAI-1 concentrations (124). PAI-1 messenger RNA (mRNA) expression in adipocytes is increased up to fivefold in obese mice, and insulin injection into lean mice increased PAI-1 in adipocytes (125). PAI-1 is expressed in human adipocytes *in vitro,* and this expression is stimulated by exogenous tumor necrosis factor-α (TNF-α) (126). These findings were confirmed *in vivo* by a study showing that adipose PAI-1 production correlates with plasma TNF-α and PAI-1 concentrations, suggesting that adipose tissue may be an important site of PAI-1 synthesis (127). Because TNF-α concentrations are chronically increased in insulin resistance, these findings may explain part of the link between insulin resistance and increased PAI-1. Other factors may also be involved; transforming growth factor-β, which is released from activated platelets, has been shown to stimulate PAI-1 production by mouse adipocytes *in vitro* (128), and PAI-1 mRNA expression and activity in human adipose tissue fragments is increased by incubation with interleukin-1β (129).

In addition to stimulating PAI-1 production in adipocytes, TNF-α has been shown to increase PAI-1 mRNA concentrations in cultured human microvascular endothelial cells, as have epidermal growth factor (130) and hepatocyte growth factor (131). The addition of transforming growth factor-β or TNF-α to cultured bovine aortic endothelial cells also increased PAI-1 mRNA (132). As a result of these *in vitro* studies, it was suggested that these factors have effects on PAI-1 gene transcription (132). As already mentioned, TNF-α concentrations are chronically increased in insulin resistance, and these findings therefore have potential clinical relevance.

GENETIC AND ENVIRONMENTAL INFLUENCES

Heritability Studies

A number of studies have attempted to estimate the relative contributions of environmental and genetic factors to the development of risk factors for CAD. The San Antonio Family Heart Study estimated the heritability of fasting glucose concentrations as 18% and that of fasting insulin concentrations as 35% (133). Recently, the heritabilities of many different hemostatic factors were estimated from a large twin study (Table 15-5). Quantitative genetic model fitting showed that between 41% and 75% of the variation in concentrations of fibrinogen, factor VII, vWF, factor XIII A-subunit, factor XIII B-subunit, and PAI-1 was the result of genetic factors (134). The heritability of factor XIII activity was higher, at 82% (134). The heritability estimate for fibrinogen from this twin study

largely agrees with the estimates from other family studies (135,136). vWF concentrations are determined to a large extent by ABO blood group. Those with blood group O have the lowest concentrations of vWF, and a small twin study found that up to 30% of the genetic variance can be attributed to the effect of blood group (137).

Genotype Association Studies

Fibrinogen

Although a family study in apparently healthy subjects showed that the influence of known polymorphisms on fibrinogen concentration was negligible (138), the Etude Cas-Temoins sur l'Infarctus du Myocarde (ECTIM) found that polymorphisms of the β-fibrinogen gene were associated with an increased plasma fibrinogen concentration and with the severity of CAD found during coronary angiography (139). However, there was no direct association with the incidence of myocardial infarction (139). Several other studies have also reported links between various polymorphisms and CAD, but two large studies showing an association between genotype and fibrinogen concentration failed to find a relationship between genotype and disease (140,141). A small study in people with type 2 diabetes showed that there was a higher prevalence of the G allele of the −455 G/A polymorphism in those with CAD (142). These disparate findings are partly explained by the fact that fibrinogen is an acute phase reactant and concentrations therefore vary widely in populations.

TABLE 15-5. *Estimates (and 95% confidence interval) of genetic and environmental variance for hemostatic factors*

Hemostatic factor	Additive genetic variance	Common environmental variance	Unique environmental variance
Fibrinogen	0.44 (0.32–0.54)		0.56 (0.46–0.68)
Factor VII	0.63 (0.50–0.72)		0.37 (0.28–0.50)
von Willebrand factor	0.75 (0.68–0.80)		0.25 (0.20–0.32)
Factor XIII A-subunit	0.64 (0.54–0.71)		0.36 (0.29–0.46)
Factor XIII B-subunit	0.41 (0.19–0.62)	0.26 (0.08–0.42)	0.33 (0.26–0.43)
Factor XIII activity	0.82 (0.76–0.86)		0.18 (0.14–0.24)
Tissue plasminogen activator	0.62 (0.53–0.69)		0.38 (0.31–0.47)
Plasminogen activator inhibitor-1	0.60 (0.51–0.68)		0.40 (0.32–0.49)

Data from a large twin study (de Lange M, Snieder H, Ariens RA. The genetics of hemostasis: a twin study. *Lancet* 2001;357:101–105).

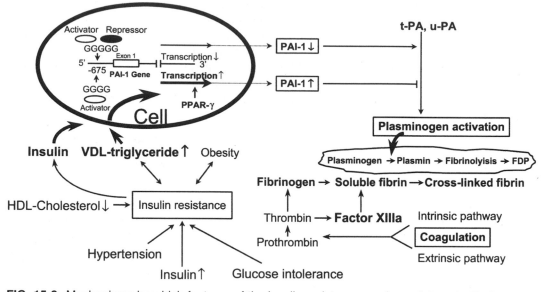

FIG. 15-2. Mechanisms by which features of the insulin resistance syndrome interact with the gene for plasminogen activator inhibitor-1 (PAI-1) to increase circulating levels of PAI-1. These simplified pathways provide insight into the processes by which prothrombotic proteins are recruited into the insulin resistance syndrome to create an atherothrombotic cluster.

Plasminogen Activator Inhibitor-1

Several polymorphisms of the human PAI-1 gene have been described, but there is conflicting evidence on the importance of these polymorphisms in determining PAI-1 concentrations. Homozygotes for the most common polymorphism, a single-base-pair change in the promoter region (4G/4G), have been described as having plasma PAI-1 concentrations that are increased by 25% compared with individuals who are homozygous for the 5G allele (143,144). However, other studies found that genetic polymorphisms had a negligible effect on PAI-1 concentrations (145,146) and that features of insulin resistance were the major determinant (147).

In a study of type 2 diabetes, subjects with the 4G/4G genotype had increased PAI-1 concentrations compared with those with the 5G/5G genotype at a given level of triglyceride, suggesting a genotype-specific interaction (148). Supportive evidence for this finding came with identification of a VLDL response element in the promoter region of the PAI-1 gene adjacent to the 4G/5G site (149). Also, HepG2 cells exposed to VLDL release more PAI-1 antigen and activity, an effect

that is augmented by the addition of insulin (150). These data suggest that insulin resistance, especially via the effects of triglycerides, increases the production and release of PAI-1, thereby increasing the risk of CAD in type 2 diabetes (Fig 15-2).

Von Willebrand Factor

vWF has been estimated to have a high heritability (134), but analysis of the 3′ region found polymorphisms that account for no more than 20% of the variability in concentration (151). A study in type 2 diabetics showed that vWF concentrations were not related to a restriction fragment length polymorphism in exon 12 of the vWF gene (152), whereas a study in people with type 1 diabetes and proliferative retinopathy found that the Thr789Ala polymorphism was associated with CAD (153).

Factor VII

Studies of the factor VII gene have demonstrated two sites in linkage disequilibrium that relate to circulating levels of factor VII, a promoter decanucleotide repeat and a single-base change at position R353Q in exon 8 (154). Several studies have demonstrated a relationship between circulating factor VII and dyslipidemia. In a study of patients with CAD, those homozygous for the insertion at the R353Q site had significantly higher levels of factor VII, although there was no relationship between possession of a particular genotype or FVII:C level (factor VII coagulant activity) and either extent of atheroma or a past history of AMI (155). Similar results were obtained in the ECTIM study (155).

Factor XIII

A common polymorphism in the factor XIII A-subunit, Val34Leu, was found to have little effect on factor XIII concentration (154) but did accelerate the activation of factor XIII by thrombin, thereby affecting the structure of the cross-linked fibrin clot (155). This polymorphism has attracted interest as a potential risk factor for thrombosis in both the venous and arterial systems. It is probable that this polymorphism, because of its effect on factor XIII activity, explains the high heritability of factor XIII activity (134). The B-subunit, on the other hand, serves mainly as a carrier of the A subunit in plasma and has a lower heritability. As well as a genetic effect, a common environmental influence for factor XIII B-subunit has been reported, explaining about 25% of the variance (134). This finding, in adult twins, may reflect shared fetal or early-life environmental effects (156) or the continuation of lifestyle habits acquired in childhood. In a study comparing type 2 diabetics, their first-degree relatives, and healthy controls, factor XIII activity increased in each group with the presence of the Val34Leu polymorphism but did not seem to be related to factor XIII A- or B-subunit concentrations across the groups (157).

Summary

In spite of the large number of studies looking for a genetic basis for CAD, few genetic risk factors have been identified, and there have been many inconsistent findings. Studies have often been too small to detect interactions between genetic polymorphisms and environmental changes. Also, frequently an apparent paradox has occurred: a firm relationship is found between the gene and the protein and between the protein and the disease, but no relationship between the gene and the disease. The link between the gene and the disease must therefore depend on the quantitative contribution of heritability to the phenotype. Because it is extremely unlikely that a single genetic polymorphism is the major determinant of CAD, future studies need to be designed to investigate the links between genetic polymorphisms and acquired environmental risk factors.

AN INTEGRATED VIEW OF VASCULAR RISK IN DIABETIC SUBJECTS

Any explanation of cardiovascular risk in relation to diabetes must take into account the underlying pathophysiology of the different presentations of this condition (Fig. 15-3). It is clear that type 1 diabetes is a condition characterized by beta-cell dysfunction and an absolute requirement for insulin, and that type 2 diabetes is generally characterized by the presence of insulin resistance and a variable degree of beta-cell dysfunction. In addition, a small proportion of type 2 subjects are relatively insulin sensitive at presentation. Despite the differences between type 1 and type 2 diabetes, both are associated with fasting hyperglycemia and a marked increase in cardiovascular risk.

For many years a case has been developed to argue that insulin-resistant type 2 diabetics cluster atheromatous risk factors, including hyperglycemia, relative hyperinsulinemia, hypertriglyceridemia, low HDL-cholesterol, and systolic hypertension. More recently, it has become apparent that complex gene/environment interactions recruit prothrombotic risk factors into this syndrome, including elevated PAI-1, factor VII, and fibrinogen, to create an atherothrombotic risk cluster that mirrors the changes in arterial disease. Evidence has accumulated to indicate that there is a considerable familial element to this syndrome, with young insulin-resistant subjects being prone to develop both early vascular disease and type 2 diabetes. Twin and family studies indicate there is genetic pleiotropy

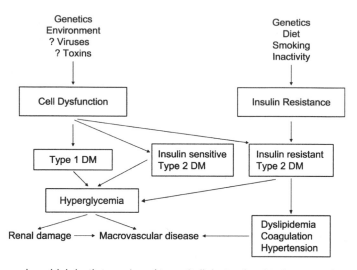

FIG. 15-3. Pathways by which both type 1 and type 2 diabetes lead to increased macrovascular risk.

between insulin resistance and some features of the atherothrombotic cluster. These findings support the common soil hypothesis, which states that type 2 diabetes and cardiovascular disease are the same condition with common genetic and environmental antecedents. With up to 25% of the population insulin resistant and increasing levels of obesity in the West, the public health challenges to prevent cardiovascular disorders become ever more pressing.

The atherothrombotic risk clustering associated with insulin resistance links well with the results of the MRFIT study but raises questions as to the pathogenesis of cardiovascular disease in the non-insulin-resistant type 1 population. The results of the San Antonio study in Mexican-Americans indicate clearly that the small number of non-insulin-resistant type 2 diabetic subjects do not cluster atherothrombotic risk and have the same risk profile (other than hyperglycemia) as a control population. Although not studied formally, the synthesis of studies in this area suggests that clustering of risk similarly does not occur in uncomplicated type 1 diabetes. Nevertheless, approximately 25% of juvenile-onset type 1 diabetic patients die from cardiovascular disease by 55 years of age. Several explanations may account for this finding. Although hyperglycemia is the predominant risk in early type 1 diabetes and clinical

studies indicate that glucose and glycation are more strongly related to microvascular disease, exposure to hyperglycemia is much longer in type 1 diabetes. This probably has an effect on vascular risk through glycation and other processes, increasing the effect of other acquired risk factors (e.g., hypercholesterolemia, hypertension, smoking) as they develop through life. In addition, the development of microalbuminuria and frank renal damage in both type 1 and type 2 diabetes is accompanied by an insulin-resistant state with similar risk clustering, which further enhances vascular mortality. Clinical observations indicate that lifestyle changes that ameliorate insulin resistance affect both vascular risk and onset of diabetes, and prospective studies have demonstrated that management of glycemia, blood pressure, and lipids are paramount in reducing vascular risk. These observations reflect much of our understanding of the complex interrelationships among lifestyle, insulin resistance, classic risk factors, and endothelial dysfunction that, in various combinations, seem to underpin vascular risk associated with both type 1 and type 2 diabetes. Although much remains to be discovered in relation to the pathogenesis of vascular disorders in diabetes, it remains clear that abnormalities in hemostatic processes are a common feature in both complicated type 1 and insulin-resistant type 2 diabetics and contribute to macrovascular risk.

TREATMENT STRATEGIES AND THROMBOTIC RISK

Over the last 10 years, the management of diabetes and prevention of vascular risk has developed an evidence base to assist us in our decision making. This has been in large part due to large-scale epidemiologic and interventional trials that have emphasized the tight relationship between diabetes and vascular risk. Therapeutic strategies are available to manage type 2 diabetes, prevent CAD, or both. The following section outlines the

effects of these treatments and treatment strategies on the hemostatic process. The main findings are shown in Table 15-6.

PRIMARY AND SECONDARY PREVENTION OF CORONARY ARTERY DISEASE

Lifestyle Change

Obesity is associated with increased concentrations of fibrinogen and PAI-1. Most patients with type 2 diabetes are overweight or obese. Dietary intervention resulting in weight loss has been shown to decrease PAI-1 concentrations in obese women, and these changes persisted

TABLE 15-6. *Drugs used in diabetic subjects for prevention or treatment of coronary artery disease and their effects on thrombosis and fibrinolysis*

Drug	Effect on thrombotic factors	Effect on fibrinolytic factors and inhibitors
Metformin	↓ Factor XIII concentration and activity Interferes with factor XIII activation and fibrin polymerization ↓ Factor VII ? fibrinogen	↓ PAI-1 concentration and activity ↓ tPA
Troglitazone (? other thiazolidinediones)	No data	↓ PAI-1 concentration and activity
Fibrates	↓ Fibrinogen ↓ Factor VIIc	↓ PAI-1 synthesis *in vitro,* not confirmed *in vivo*
HMG-CoA reductase inhibitors	May ↑ fibrinogen	↓ tPA ↓ PAI-1
Aspirin	Does not ↓ platelet hypersensitivity to thrombin *In vitro*	↓ PAI-1
Platelet glycoprotein inhibitors IIb/IIIa	No data	No data
ACE inhibitors	Data inconclusive[a]	↓ PAI-1 concentration and activity[b]
Angiotensin II antagonists	Data inconclusive[c]	May ↓ PAI-1 concentration and activity[d]
β-Blockers	Data inconclusive[e]	Data inconclusive[e]
Estrogen (in postmenopausal women)	Slight ↑ factor VII concentration	↓ PAI-1 concentration

ACE, angiotensin-converting enzyme; HMG-CoA, 3-hydroxy-3-methylglutaryl coenzyme A; PAI-1, plasminogen activator inhibitor-1; tPA, tissue plasminogen activator.

[a]Perindopril decreased fibrinogen concentrations in one study but not in another, and quinapril had no effect on fibrinogen, factor VII, or von Willebrand factor.

[b]PAI-1 concentration and activity decreased with ramipril, imidapril, and enalapril but not with trandolapril or quinapril.

[c]One study showed that losartan decreased fibrinogen concentrations; another, smaller and shorter study showed no effect.

[d]*In vitro* work suggests that PAI-1 synthesis is decreased, and several studies with losartan and irbesartan confirm this *in vivo*. However, in two studies losartan had no effect.

[e]Several studies show beneficial effects on fibrinogen and PAI-1, but other studies show no effect.

if the weight loss was maintained (158,159). Use of orlistat had no additional benefit on PAI-1 concentrations (159). Massive weight reduction in morbidly obese individuals after surgery resulted in decreased concentrations of not only PAI-1 but also fibrinogen and factor VII (160). Regular exercise should also be recommended to patients with diabetes. Post-MI patients who underwent 1 month of physical training had decreased concentrations of fibrinogen, vWF, and PAI-1 (161). PAI-1 concentrations were also decreased by regular exercise, although the association was no longer significant after adjustment for variables relating to insulin resistance, such as body mass index, waist-hip ratio, age, and triglyceride concentration (162). Patients should be advised to stop smoking, a major cause of CAD that is associated with increased fibrinogen concentrations (163).

Glycemic Control

Although intensive treatment of type 2 diabetes with sulfonylureas or insulin in the UKPDS did not significantly decrease the incidence of macrovascular disease, treatment of overweight patients with metformin decreased all-cause mortality and the incidence of stroke (164). One explanation for this finding may be the effects of metformin on the clotting system. *In vitro* work has suggested that metformin interferes with factor XIII activation and fibrin polymerization (165), and a 12-week course of metformin was shown to decrease factor XIII concentrations and activity (165). Another reason for expecting metformin to be beneficial in the prevention or treatment of macrovascular disease in type 2 diabetes is that it has been shown to decrease PAI-1 concentrations and activity (166). *In vitro* studies on human subcutaneous adipocytes (167), endothelial cells, and aortic smooth muscle cells (168) have shown that troglitazone decreases production of PAI-1. *In vivo* studies have shown that troglitazone markedly decreases PAI-1 concentrations and activity in women with polycystic ovary syndrome and impaired glucose tolerance (169). Troglitazone also decreased PAI-1 con-

centrations in several studies of patients with type 2 diabetes (170–172). Troglitazone is no longer licensed for use due to hepatotoxicity, but two other thiazolidinediones, rosiglitazone and pioglitazone, are now available. It is not yet clear whether these other thiazolidinediones have similar effects on PAI-1, but if this is a class effect, peroxisome proliferator-activated receptor-γ (PPARγ) may be involved in regulation of the PAI-1 gene.

Lipid-lowering

Fibrate treatment (fenofibrate, bezafibrate, or gemfibrozil) in patients with primary hypercholesterolemia has been shown to decrease fibrinogen concentrations independently of lipid-lowering effects, whereas treatment with 3-hydroxy-3-methylglutaryl coenzyme A (HMG-CoA) reductase inhibitor (simvastatin or pravastatin) had no effect (173). In people with type 2 diabetes, fenofibrate has also been demonstrated to decrease fibrinogen concentrations, but atorvastatin had no effect (174). Fibrates may also decrease factor VII coagulant activity (175). Experiments in rodents and *in vitro* work on monkey hepatocytes showed that fibrates decrease PAI-1 synthesis (176,177), although this finding was not confirmed *in vivo* in patients with primary hyperlipidemia treated with ciprofibrate or gemfibrozil (178). The Diabetes Atherosclerosis Intervention Study (DAIS) showed that fenofibrate treatment of people with type 2 diabetes decreased the angiographic progression of CAD (179), but as yet there are no data on the effect of fibrates on morbidity or mortality from CAD in diabetes. HMG-CoA reductase inhibitors may actually result in increased fibrinogen concentrations in the nondiabetic population (180), and certainly do not seem to reduce fibrinogen concentrations in people with type 2 diabetes (181). Factor VII concentrations in type 2 diabetics are also not affected by treatment with HMG-CoA reductase inhibitors (182). In an *in vitro* study, HMG-CoA reductase inhibitors decreased mRNA concentrations for PAI-1 in endothelial and smooth muscle cells and increased tPA mRNA concentrations in smooth muscle cells (183). All of the drugs studied, apart from pravastatin, decreased PAI-1 production from human vascular endothelial and smooth muscle cells, although not from HepG$_2$ cells (183). Also, apart from pravastatin, the HMG-CoA reductase inhibitors increased tPA production in human smooth muscle cells, although only simvastatin and lovastatin increased production in endothelial cells (183). Although pravastatin had little effect on PAI-1 production *in vitro*, there is some evidence that it decreased plasma PAI-1 concentrations *in vivo* (184–186). Again, in contrast to the *in vitro* work, *in vivo* studies in patients with hypercholesterolemia showed that HMG-CoA reductase inhibitors decreased concentrations of tPA (183).

In spite of the mixed results of HMG-CoA reductase inhibitors on thrombotic and fibrinolytic risk factors, post-hoc analysis of the Scandinavian Simvastatin Survival Study showed that cholesterol-lowering with simvastatin in the subgroup with diabetes decreased the risk of MI or other atherosclerotic events (187). Analysis of results from the West of Scotland Coronary Prevention Study (WOSCOPS) showed that pravastatin benefited those with diabetes (188). It was also suggested that the clinical benefit of treating people with diabetes may be greater than for the nondiabetic population, because diabetic subjects are at a much greater risk for CAD (187,188). In view of the evidence already discussed, it is likely that these effects are not mediated through effects on the coagulation system.

Aspirin and Platelet Glycoprotein IIb/IIIa Inhibitor

The use of aspirin in people with type 1 or 2 diabetes has been advocated by some as primary prevention against CAD. However, experiments in diabetic rats showed that aspirin does not reduce the hypersensitivity of platelets to thrombin (189), suggesting that aspirin therapy may not have the desired effect. However, two *in vivo* studies suggest that aspirin may decrease PAI-1 concentrations (190,191). Metaanalysis of several large trials showed that patients with diabetes who have acute coronary syndromes (unstable angina or non-ST-elevation MI) may benefit from the use of platelet glycoprotein IIb/IIIa inhibitors, particularly if they are undergoing percutaneous coronary interventions (192).

Angiotensin-converting Enzyme Inhibitors and Angiotensin II Antagonists

The Heart Outcomes Prevention Evaluation (HOPE) study showed that ramipril decreased the incidence of stroke, MI, and death from cardiovascular disease in the large group of diabetic patients with one other risk factor for CAD (193). The decrease in cardiovascular events was greater than could be attributed to the blood pressure lowering effects of ramipril alone, suggesting that ramipril has a vasculoprotective effect via another mechanism. One possible mechanism is that effects on the renin-angiotensin system may regulate the vascular thrombotic or fibrinolytic systems. An indication that the renin-angiotensin system may regulate the vascular fibrinolytic system is that both PAI-1 concentrations and activity were decreased in patients with acute anterior MI treated with ramipril (194). The angiotensin-converting enzyme (ACE) inhibitors imidapril and enalapril have also been shown to decrease PAI-1 concentrations in diabetic rats (195). However, treatment with trandolapril for 1 year did not decrease tPA or PAI-1 concentrations in patients with AMI (196), and quinapril given to normotensive type 1 diabetic patients for 5 weeks did not decrease PAI-1 concentrations (197). It may be, therefore, that the decrease in PAI-1 concentrations and activity seen with certain ACE inhibitors is not as a result of a class effect but rather an effect of those particular agents.

There are few data on the effects of ACE inhibitors on thrombotic factors, and the available data conflict. Perindopril decreased fibrinogen concentrations in one study of overweight hypertensive patients (198), although not in another group of hypertensives (199). Quinapril did not affect concentrations of fibrinogen, factor VII, or vWF in hypertensive subjects (200). Similarly, there are few data available on the effects of angiotensin II antagonists on the coagulation system. In one small study, a 6-week course of losartan did not reduce fibrinogen concentrations (198), but in another study, a 6-month course of irbesartan did decrease fibrinogen concentrations (201). Other investigations have shown that angiotensin II stimulates PAI-1 synthesis in cultured human vascular endothelial cells (202). It would therefore be expected that angiotensin II antagonists would decrease PAI-1 concentrations, and *in vitro* studies on human vascular endothelial (202), smooth muscle cells (203), and adipocytes (204) have demonstrated that angiotensin II antagonists prevent the angiotensin II-stimulated increase in PAI-1 protein and mRNA. As would be predicted from these data, *in vivo* studies of losartan in hypertensive subjects (205) and in patients with heart failure (206) demonstrated a reduction in PAI-1 concentrations and activity, as did a study using irbesartan in hypertensives (201). However, in other studies losartan did not decrease PAI-1 concentrations or activity (207,208).

β-Blockers

The UKPDS showed the importance of controlling blood pressure in patients with diabetes for the prevention of microvascular complications (209). ACE inhibitors and β-blockers seemed to be equally effective (209). It is probable that β-blockers also increase survival rates in people with diabetes and CAD (210,211). The effects of β-blockers on the thrombotic and fibrinolytic systems are uncertain, with some studies showing beneficial effects on fibrinogen and PAI-1 (201,212) and other studies showing no effect (213,214).

Estrogen Replacement in Postmenopausal Women

PAI-1 concentrations increase in women after the menopause (215), a possible explanation for the relative protection against CAD in premenopausal women. Estrogen replacement, alone or with progesterone, decreased PAI-1 by up to 50% in postmenopausal women (215–217), although it may also have slightly increased factor VII concentrations (217).

CONCLUSION

The development of either type 1 or type 2 diabetes is associated with a marked increase in vascular risk affecting both microvascular and macrovascular arterial trees. Considerable evidence has emerged to support the role of conventional risk factors in the pathogenesis of these conditions, although it is equally clear that they do not explain all the increased vascular risk associated with diabetes. The coagulation and fibrinolytic cascades have acquired a more important position in vascular risk because of three developments: (a) awareness that thrombosis is an important component of plaque rupture and atherothrombotic vascular occlusion; (b) evidence that hemostatic markers are increased in subjects at vascular risk and that these increases predict future vascular risk; and (c) the fact that some of the most potent primary and secondary prevention strategies involve interventions that modify thrombotic risk. Increasingly these developments are being applied to diabetes mellitus as we become aware of the central role of hemostatic changes in the development of vascular risk in this condition. Both type 1 and type 2 diabetes are associated with alterations in thrombotic risk that become more marked in the presence of renal damage. In type 2 diabetes, underlying insulin resistance seems to be a major determinant of thrombotic risk, with evidence linking increased concentrations of PAI-1, fibrinogen, and factor VII to this metabolic abnormality. The effects of oxidized lipoproteins, hyperglycemia and glycosylation, and abnormalities in endothelial cell function all contribute to the development of a prothrombotic, vasoconstrictive phenotype that contributes to increased vascular risk in diabetic subjects. The observation that therapeutic interventions in diabetes can ameliorate some of the thrombotic risk indicates that we should begin to tailor our management to include beneficial effects on thrombotic risk as one treatment objective. The increasing sophistication of this approach, coupled with the development of novel antithrombotic/profibrinolytic pharmacologic agents, will increase our ability to manage the life-threatening vascular complications associated with diabetes.

REFERENCES

1. World Health Organization. *Prevention of diabetes, 2002.* WHO Technical Report Series No.844. Geneva, World Health Organization.
2. Kannel WB, McGee DL. Diabetes and cardiovascular disease: the Framingham study. *JAMA* 1979;241:2035–2038.
3. Kannel WB, McGee DL. Diabetes and cardiovascular risk factors: the Framingham study. *Circulation* 1979;59:8–13.
4. Vaccaro O, Stamler J, Neaton JD. Sixteen-year coronary mortality in black and white men with diabetes screened for the Multiple Risk Factor Intervention Trial (MRFIT). *Int J Epidemiol* 1998;27:636–641.
5. Stamler J, Vaccaro O, Neaton JD, et al. Diabetes, other risk factors, and 12-yr cardiovascular mortality for men screened in the Multiple Risk Factor Intervention Trial 1. *Diabetes Care* 1993;16:434–444.
6. Alderman EL, Corley SD, Fisher LD, et al. Five-year angiographic follow-up of factors associated with progression of coronary artery disease in the Coronary Artery Surgery Study (CASS). CASS Participating Investigators and Staff. *J Am Coll Cardiol* 1993;22:1141–1154.
7. Gillum RF, Mussolino ME, Madans JH. Diabetes mellitus, coronary heart disease incidence, and death from all causes in African American and European American women: the NHANES I epidemiologic follow-up study. *J Clin Epidemiol* 2000;53:511–518.
8. Lotufo PA, Gaziano JM, Chae CU, et al. Diabetes and all-cause and coronary heart disease mortality among US male physicians. *Arch Intern Med* 2001;161:242–247.
9. Morrish NJ, Wang SL, Stevens LK, et al. Mortality and causes of death in the WHO Multinational Study of Vascular Disease in Diabetes. *Diabetologia* 2001;44[Suppl 2]:S14–S21.
10. Kurbaan AS, Bowker TJ, Ilsley CD, et al. Difference in the mortality of the CABRI diabetic and nondiabetic populations and its relation to coronary artery disease and the revascularization mode. *Am J Cardiol* 2001;87:947–950.
11. Niles NW, McGrath PD, Malenka D, et al. Survival of patients with diabetes and multivessel coronary artery disease after surgical or percutaneous coronary revascularization: results of a large regional prospective study. Northern New England Cardiovascular Disease Study Group. *J Am Coll Cardiol* 2001;37:1008–1015.
12. Anonymous. Influence of diabetes on 5-year mortality and morbidity in a randomized trial comparing CABG and PTCA in patients with multivessel disease: the Bypass Angioplasty Revascularization Investigation (BARI). *Circulation* 1997;96:1761–1769.
13. Abizaid A, Costa MA, Centemero M. Clinical and economic impact of diabetes mellitus on percutaneous and surgical treatment of multivessel coronary disease patients: insights from the Arterial Revascularization Therapy Study (ARTS) trial. *Circulation* 2001;104:533–538.
14. Herlitz J, Wognsen GB, Emanuelsson H, et al. Mortality and morbidity in diabetic and nondiabetic patients during a 2-year period after coronary artery bypass grafting. *Diabetes Care* 1996;19:698–703.
15. Morrissey JH. Tissue factor: an enzyme cofactor and a true receptor. *Thromb Haemost* 2001;86:66–74.
16. Lorand L. Factor XIII: structure, activation, and interactions with fibrinogen and fibrin. *Ann N Y Acad Sci* 2001;936:291–311.
17. Mosesson MW, Siebenlist KR, Meh DA. The structure and biological features of fibrinogen and fibrin. *Ann N Y Acad Sci* 2001;936:11–30.
18. Sprengers ED, Kluft C. Plasminogen activator inhibitors. *Blood* 1987;69:381–387.
19. Ichinose A, Tamaki T, Aoki N. Factor XIII-mediated cross-linking of NH2-terminal peptide of alpha 2-plasmin inhibitor to fibrin. *FEBS Lett* 1983;153:369–371.
20. Kooistra T, Sprengers ED, van Hinsbergh VW. Rapid inactivation of the plasminogen-activator inhibitor upon secretion from cultured human endothelial cells. *Biochem J* 1986;239:497–503.
21. Sprengers ED, Akkerman JW, Jansen BG. Blood platelet plasminogen activator inhibitor: two different pools of endothelial cell type plasminogen activator inhibitor in human blood. *Thromb Haemost* 1986;55:325–329.
22. Loskutoff DJ, Samad F. The adipocyte and hemostatic balance in obesity: studies of PAI-1. *Arterioscler Thromb Vasc Biol* 1998;18(1):1–6.
23. Gelehrter TD, Sznycer-Laszuk R. Thrombin induction of plasminogen activator-inhibitor in cultured human endothelial cells. *J Clin Invest* 1986;77:165–169.
24. Lindahl TL, Ohlsson PI, Wiman B. The mechanism of the reaction between human plasminogen-activator inhibitor 1 and tissue plasminogen activator. *Biochem J* 1990;265:109–113.
25. Owensby DA, Morton PA, Wun TC, et al. Binding of plasminogen activator inhibitor type-1 to extracellular matrix of Hep G2 cells. evidence that the binding protein is vitronectin. *J Biol Chem* 1991;266:4334–4340.
26. Declerck PJ, De Mol M, Alessi MC, et al. Purification and characterization of a plasminogen activator inhibitor 1 binding protein from human plasma. identification as a multimeric form of S protein (vitronectin). *J Biol Chem* 1988;263:15454–15461.
27. Hoylaerts M, Rijken DC, Lijnen HR, et al. Kinetics of the activation of plasminogen by human tissue plasminogen activator: role of fibrin. *J Biol Chem* 1982;257:2912–2919.
28. Higgins DL, Vehar GA. Interaction of one-chain and two-chain tissue plasminogen activator with intact and plasmin-degraded fibrin. *Biochemistry* 1987;26:7786–7791.
29. Ernst E, Resch KL. Fibrinogen as a cardiovascular risk factor: a meta-analysis and review of the literature. *Ann Intern Med* 1993;118:956–963.
30. Meade TW, Brozovic M, Chakrabarti RR, et al. Haemostatic function and ischaemic heart disease: principal results of the Northwick Park Heart Study. *Lancet* 1986;2:533–537.
31. Heinrich J, Balleisen L, Schulte H, et al. Fibrinogen and factor VII in the prediction of coronary risk: results from the PROCAM study in healthy men. *Arterioscler Thromb* 1994;14:54–59.
32. Wilhelmsen L, Svardsudd K, Korsan-Bengtsen K, et al. Fibrinogen as a risk factor for stroke and myocardial infarction. *N Engl J Med* 1984;311:501–505.

33. Kannel WB, D'Agostino RB, Belanger AJ. Update on fibrinogen as a cardiovascular risk factor. *Ann Epidemiol* 1992;2:457–466.

34. Violi F, Criqui M, Longoni A, et al. Relation between risk factors and cardiovascular complications in patients with peripheral vascular disease: results from the ADEP study. *Atherosclerosis* 1996;120:25–35.

35. Meade TW, North WR, Chakrabarti R, et al. Haemostatic function and cardiovascular death: early results of a prospective study. *Lancet* 1980;1:1050–1054.

36. [Removed]

37. Lane DA, Grant PJ. Role of hemostatic gene polymorphisms in venous and arterial thrombotic disease. *Blood* 2000;95:1517–1532.

38. Cortellaro M, Baldassarre D, Cofrancesco E, et al. Relation between hemostatic variables and increase of common carotid intima-media thickness in patients with peripheral arterial disease. *Stroke* 1996;27:450–454.

39. Knobl P, Schernthaner G, Schnack C, et al. Thrombogenic factors are related to urinary albumin excretion rate in type 1 (insulin-dependent) and type 2 (non-insulin-dependent) diabetic patients. *Diabetologia* 1993;36:1045–1050.

40. Myrup B, Mathiesen ER, Ronn B, et al. Endothelial function and serum lipids in the course of developing microalbuminuria in insulin-dependent diabetes mellitus. *Diabetes Res* 1994;26:33–39.

41. Stehouwer CD, Fischer HR, van Kuijk AW, et al. Endothelial dysfunction precedes development of microalbuminuria in IDDM. *Diabetes* 1995;44:561–564.

42. Yaqoob M, Patrick AW, McClelland P, et al. Relationship between markers of endothelial dysfunction, oxidant injury and tubular damage in patients with insulin-dependent diabetes mellitus. *Clin Sci* 1993;85:557–562.

43. Plater ME, Ford I, Dent MT, et al. Elevated von Willebrand factor antigen predicts deterioration in diabetic peripheral nerve function. *Diabetologia* 1996;39:336–343.

44. Morise T, Takeuchi Y, Kawano M, et al. Increased plasma levels of immunoreactive endothelin and von Willebrand factor in NIDDM patients. *Diabetes Care* 1995;18:87–89.

45. Hamsten A, de Faire U, Walldius G, et al. Plasminogen activator inhibitor in plasma: risk factor for recurrent myocardial infarction. *Lancet* 1987;2:3–9.

46. Ridker PM, Hennekens CH, Stampfer MJ, et al. Prospective study of endogenous tissue plasminogen activator and risk of stroke. *Lancet* 1994;343:940–943.

47. Gray RP, Panahloo A, Mohamed-Ali V, et al. Proinsulin-like molecules and plasminogen activator inhibitor type 1 (PAI-1) activity in diabetic and non-diabetic subjects with and without myocardial infarction. *Atherosclerosis* 1997;130:171–178.

48. Sobel BE, Woodcock-Mitchell J, Schneider DJ, et al. Increased plasminogen activator inhibitor type 1 in coronary artery atherectomy specimens from type 2 diabetic compared with nondiabetic patients: a potential factor predisposing to thrombosis and its persistence. *Circulation* 1998;97:2213–2221.

49. Carmassi F, Morale M, Puccetti R, et al. Coagulation and fibrinolytic system impairment in insulin dependent diabetes mellitus. *Thromb Res* 1992;67:643–654.

50. Dubrey SW, Reaveley DR, Seed M, et al. Risk factors for cardiovascular disease in IDDM: a study of identical twins. *Diabetes* 1994;43:831–835.

51. Kwaan HC. Changes in blood coagulation, platelet function, and plasminogen-plasmin system in diabetes. *Diabetes* 1992;41[Suppl 2]:32–35.

52. Lee P, Jenkins A, Bourke C, et al. Prothrombotic and antithrombotic factors are elevated in patients with type 1 diabetes complicated by microalbuminuria. *Diabet Med* 1993;10:122–128.

53. Colwell JA, Lyons TJ, Klein RL, et al. New concepts about the pathogenesis in type II diabetic patients. In: Levin M, ed. *The diabetic foot,* 5th ed. St Louis: Mosby, 1993:79–114.

54. Acang N, Jalil FD. Hypercoagulation in diabetes mellitus. *Southeast Asian J Trop Med Public Health* 1993;24[Suppl 1]:263–266.

55. Avellone G, Di Garbo V, Cordova R, et al. Blood coagulation and fibrinolysis in obese NIDDM patients. *Diabetes Res* 1994;25:85–92.

56. Ganda OP, Arkin CF. Hyperfibrinogenemia: an important risk factor for vascular complications in diabetes. *Diabetes Care* 1992;15:1245–1250.

57. Lee AJ, Lowe GD, Woodward M, et al. Fibrinogen in relation to personal history of prevalent hypertension, diabetes, stroke, intermittent claudication, coronary heart disease, and family history: the Scottish Heart Health Study. *Br Heart J* 1993;69:338–342.

58. Morishita E, Nakao S, Asakura H, et al. Hypercoagulability and high lipoprotein(a) levels in patients with aplastic anemia receiving cyclosporine. *Blood Coagul Fibrinolysis* 1996;7:609–614.

59. Vanninen E, Laitinen J, Uusitupa M. Physical activity and fibrinogen concentration in newly diagnosed NIDDM. *Diabetes Care* 1994;17:1031–1038.

60. Donders SH, Lustermans FA, van Wersch JW. Glycometabolic control, lipids, and coagulation parameters in patients with non-insulin-dependent diabetes mellitus. *Int J Clin Lab Res* 1993;23:155–159.

61. Kario K, Matsuo T, Kobayashi H. Activation of tissue factor-induced coagulation and endothelial cell dysfunction in non-insulin-dependent diabetic patients with microalbuminuria. *Arterioscler Thromb Vasc Biol* 1995;15:1114–1120.

62. Knobl P, Schernthaner G, Schnack C, et al. Haemostatic abnormalities persist despite glycaemic improvement by insulin therapy in lean type 2 diabetic patients. *Thromb Haemost* 1994;71:692–697.

63. Gruden G, Cavallo-Perin P, Bazzan M, et al. PAI-1 and factor VII activity are higher in IDDM patients with microalbuminuria. *Diabetes* 1994;43:426–429.

64. van Wersch JW. A chromogenic assay for coagulation factor VII: analytical performance characteristics and application in several diseases. *Int J Clin Lab Res* 1993;23:221–224.

65. Mansfield MW, Heywood DM, Grant PJ. Sex differences in coagulation and fibrinolysis in white subjects with non-insulin-dependent diabetes mellitus. *Arterioscler Thromb Vasc Biol* 1996;16:160–164.

66. Mansfield MW, Heywood DM, Grant PJ. Circulating levels of factor VII, fibrinogen, and von Willebrand factor and features of insulin resistance in first-degree relatives of patients with NIDDM. *Circulation* 1996;94:2171–2176.

67. el Khawand C, Jamart J, Donckier J, et al. Hemostasis

variables in type I diabetic patients without demonstrable vascular complications. *Diabetes Care* 1993;16: 1137–1145.

68. Heywood DM, Mansfield MW, Grant PJ. Levels of von Willebrand factor, insulin resistance syndrome, and a common vWF gene polymorphism in non-insulin-dependent (type 2) diabetes mellitus. *Diabet Med* 1996;13:720–725.

69. Burchfiel CM, Curb JD, Sharp DS, et al. Distribution and correlates of insulin in elderly men: the Honolulu Heart Program. *Arterioscler Thromb Vasc Biol* 1995;15:2213–2221.

70. Meade TW, Chakrabarti R, Haines AP, et al. Characteristics affecting fibrinolytic activity and plasma fibrinogen concentrations. *Br Med J* 1979;1:153–156.

71. Montgomery HE, Clarkson P, Nwose OM, et al. The acute rise in plasma fibrinogen concentration with exercise is influenced by the G-453-A polymorphism of the beta-fibrinogen gene. *Arterioscler Thromb Vasc Biol* 1996;16:386–391.

72. Jones SL, Close CF, Mattock MB, et al. Plasma lipid and coagulation factor concentrations in insulin dependent diabetics with microalbuminuria. *BMJ* 1989;298:487–490.

73. Schleiffer T, Hellstern P, Freitag M, et al. Plasminogen activator inhibitor 1 activity and lipoprotein(a) in nephropathic patients with non-insulin-dependent diabetes mellitus versus patients with nondiabetic nephropathy. *Haemostasis* 1994;24:49–54.

74. Robbins DC, Knowler WC, Lee ET, et al. Regional differences in albuminuria among American Indians: an epidemic of renal disease. *Kidney Int* 1996;49:557–563.

75. Yudkin JS, Forrest RD, Jackson CA. Microalbuminuria as predictor of vascular disease in non-diabetic subjects. Islington Diabetes Survey. *Lancet* 1988;2:530–533.

76. Agewall S, Fagerberg B, Attvall S, et al. Microalbuminuria, insulin sensitivity and haemostatic factors in non-diabetic treated hypertensive men. Risk Factor Intervention Study Group. *J Intern Med* 1995;237:195–203.

77. Miller GJ, Walter SJ, Stirling Y, et al. Assay of factor VII activity by two techniques: evidence for increased conversion of VII to alpha VIIa in hyperlipidaemia, with possible implications for ischaemic heart disease. *Br J Haematol* 1985;59:249–258.

78. Miller GJ, Martin JC, Mitropoulos KA, et al. Plasma factor VII is activated by postprandial triglyceridaemia, irrespective of dietary fat composition. *Atherosclerosis* 1991;86:163–171.

79. Simpson HC, Mann JI, Meade TW, et al. Hypertriglyceridaemia and hypercoagulability. *Lancet* 1983;1:786–790.

80. Heywood DM, Mansfield MW, Grant PJ. Factor VII gene polymorphisms, factor VII:C levels and features of insulin resistance in non-insulin-dependent diabetes mellitus. *Thromb Haemost* 1996;75:401–406.

81. Ceriello A, Giugliano D, Quatraro A, et al. Evidence for a hyperglycaemia-dependent decrease of antithrombin III-thrombin complex formation in humans. *Diabetologia* 1990;33:163–167.

82. Ceriello A, Giugliano D, Quatraro A, et al. Induced hyperglycemia alters antithrombin III activity but not its plasma concentration in healthy normal subjects. *Diabetes* 1987;36:320–323.

83. Brownlee M, Vlassara H, Cerami A. Inhibition of heparin-catalyzed human antithrombin III activity by nonenzymatic glycosylation. Possible role in fibrin deposition in diabetes. *Diabetes* 1984;33:532–535.

84. Ceriello A, Giugliano D, Quatraro A, et al. Daily rapid blood glucose variations may condition antithrombin III biologic activity but not its plasma concentration in insulin-dependent diabetes: a possible role for labile non-enzymatic glycation. *Diabetes Metab* 1987;13:16–19.

85. Vukovich TC, Schernthaner G. Decreased protein C levels in patients with insulin-dependent type I diabetes mellitus. *Diabetes* 1986;35:617–619.

86. Ceriello A, Quatraro A, Dello RP, et al. Protein C deficiency in insulin-dependent diabetes: a hyperglycemia-related phenomenon. *Thromb Haemost* 1990;64:104–107.

87. Carmassi F, Morale M, Puccetti R, et al. Coagulation and fibrinolytic system impairment in insulin dependent diabetes mellitus. *Thromb Res* 1992;67:643–654.

88. Zeitler P, Thiede A, Muller HL. Prospective study on plasma clotting parameters in diabetic children. no evidence for specific changes in coagulation system. *Exp Clin Endocrinol Diabetes* 2001;109:146–150.

89. Veglio M, Gruden G, Mormile A, et al. Anticoagulant protein C activity in non-insulin dependent diabetic patients with normoalbuminuria and microalbuminuria. *Acta Diabetol* 1995;32:106–109.

90. Gabazza EC, Takeya H, Deguchi H, et al. Protein C activation in NIDDM patients. *Diabetologia* 1996;39:1455–1461.

91. Aso Y, Fujiwara Y, Tayama K, et al. Relationship between soluble thrombomodulin in plasma and coagulation or fibrinolysis in type 2 diabetes. *Clin Chim Acta* 2000;301:135–145.

92. Lee P, Jenkins A, Bourke C, et al. Prothrombotic and antithrombotic factors are elevated in patients with type 1 diabetes complicated by microalbuminuria. *Diabet Med* 1993;10:122–128.

93. Knobl P, Schernthaner G, Schnack C, et al. Haemostatic abnormalities persist despite glycaemic improvement by insulin therapy in lean type 2 diabetic patients. *Thromb Haemost* 1994;71.692–697.

94. McLaren M, Elhadd TA, Greene SA, et al. Elevated plasma vascular endothelial cell growth factor and thrombomodulin in juvenile diabetic patients. *Clin Appl Thromb Hemost* 1999;5:21–24.

95. Mormile A, Veglio M, Gruden G, et al. Physiological inhibitors of blood coagulation and prothrombin fragment F 1 + 2 in type 2 diabetic patients with normoalbuminuria and incipient nephropathy. *Acta Diabetol* 1996;33:241–245.

96. Leurs PB, van Oerle R, Wolffenbuttel BH, et al. Increased tissue factor pathway inhibitor (TFPI) and coagulation in patients with insulin-dependent diabetes mellitus. *Thromb Haemost* 1997;77:472–476.

97. Huvers FC, De Leeuw PW, Houben AJ, et al. Endothelium-dependent vasodilatation, plasma markers of endothelial function, and adrenergic vasoconstrictor responses in type 1 diabetes under near-normoglycemic conditions. *Diabetes* 1999;48:1300–1307.

98. Rao AK, Chouhan V, Chen X, et al. Activation of the

tissue factor pathway of blood coagulation during prolonged hyperglycemia in young healthy men. *Diabetes* 1999;48:1156–1161.

99. Auwerx J, Bouillon R, Collen D, et al. Tissue-type plasminogen activator antigen and plasminogen activator inhibitor in diabetes mellitus. *Arteriosclerosis* 1988;8:68–72.

100. Lowe GD, Yarnell JW, Sweetnam PM, et al. Fibrin D-dimer, tissue plasminogen activator, plasminogen activator inhibitor, and the risk of major ischaemic heart disease in the Caerphilly Study. *Thromb Haemost* 1998;79:129–133.

101. Ridker PM, Vaughan DE, Stampfer MJ, et al. Endogenous tissue-type plasminogen activator and risk of myocardial infarction. *Lancet* 1993;341:1165–1168.

102. Vicari AM, Vigano DS, Testa S, et al. Normal tissue plasminogen activator and plasminogen activator inhibitor activity in plasma from patients with type 1 diabetes mellitus. *Horm Metab Res* 1992;24:516–519.

103. Skrha J, Hodinar A, Kvasnicka J, et al. Early changes of serum N-acetyl-beta-glucosaminidase, tissue plasminogen activator and erythrocyte superoxide dismutase in relation to retinopathy in type 1 diabetes mellitus. *Clin Chim Acta* 1994;229:5–14.

104. Ceriello A, Quatraro A, Marchi E, et al. Impaired fibrinolytic response to increased thrombin activation in type 1 diabetes mellitus: effects of the glycosaminoglycan sulodexide. *Diabetes Metab* 1993;19:225–229.

105. McGill JB, Schneider DJ, Arfken CL, et al. Factors responsible for impaired fibrinolysis in obese subjects and NIDDM patients. *Diabetes* 1994;43:104–109.

106. Takanashi K, Inukai T. Insulin resistance and changes in the blood coagulation-fibrinolysis system after a glucose clamp technique in patients with type 2 diabetes mellitus. *J Med* 2000;31:45–62.

107. Mansfield MW, Heywood DM, Grant PJ. Sex differences in coagulation and fibrinolysis in white subjects with non-insulin-dependent diabetes mellitus. *Arterioscler Thromb Vasc Biol* 1996;16:160–164.

108. Pandolfi A, Iacoviello L, Capani F, et al. Glucose and insulin independently reduce the fibrinolytic potential of human vascular smooth muscle cells in culture. *Diabetologia* 1996;39:1425–1431.

109. Chen YQ, Su M, Walia RR, et al. Sp1 sites mediate activation of the plasminogen activator inhibitor-1 promoter by glucose in vascular smooth muscle cells. *J Biol Chem* 1998;273:8225–8231.

110. Maiello M, Boeri D, Podesta F, et al. Increased expression of tissue plasminogen activator and its inhibitor and reduced fibrinolytic potential of human endothelial cells cultured in elevated glucose. *Diabetes* 1992;41:1009–1015.

111. Nordt TK, Klassen KJ, Schneider DJ, et al. Augmentation of synthesis of plasminogen activator inhibitor type-1 in arterial endothelial cells by glucose and its implications for local fibrinolysis. *Arterioscler Thromb* 1993;13:1822–1828.

112. Sampson M, Kong C, Patel A, et al. Ambulatory blood pressure profiles and plasminogen activator inhibitor (PAI-1) activity in lean women with and without the polycystic ovary syndrome. *Clin Endocrinol* 1996;45:623–629.

113. Vague P, Juhan-Vague I, Aillaud MF, et al. Correlation between blood fibrinolytic activity, plasminogen activator inhibitor level, plasma insulin level, and relative body weight in normal and obese subjects. *Metabolism* 1986;35:250–253.

114. Juhan-Vague I, Vague P, Alessi MC, et al. Relationships between plasma insulin triglyceride, body mass index, and plasminogen activator inhibitor 1. *Diabetes Metab* 1987;13:331–336.

115. Alessi MC, Juhan-Vague I, Kooistra T, et al. Insulin stimulates the synthesis of plasminogen activator inhibitor 1 by the human hepatocellular cell line Hep G2. *Thromb Haemost* 1988;60:491–494.

116. Melidonis A, Stefanidis A, Tournis S, et al. The role of strict metabolic control by insulin infusion on fibrinolytic profile during an acute coronary event in diabetic patients. *Clin Cardiol* 2000;23:160–164.

117. Jain SK, Nagi DK, Slavin BM, et al. Insulin therapy in type 2 diabetic subjects suppresses plasminogen activator inhibitor (PAI-1) activity and proinsulin-like molecules independently of glycaemic control. *Diabet Med* 1993;10:27–32.

118. Schneider DJ, Nordt TK, Sobel BE. Stimulation by proinsulin of expression of plasminogen activator inhibitor type-I in endothelial cells. *Diabetes* 1992;41:890–895.

119. Panahloo A, Mohamed-Ali V, Andres C, et al. Effect of insulin versus sulfonylurea therapy on cardiovascular risk factors and fibrinolysis in type II diabetes. *Metabolism* 1998;47:637–643.

120. Schneider DJ, Sobel BE. Synergistic augmentation of expression of plasminogen activator inhibitor type-1 induced by insulin, very-low-density lipoproteins, and fatty acids. *Coron Artery Dis* 1996;7:813–817.

121. Grant PJ, Kruithof EK, Felley CP, et al. Short-term infusions of insulin, triacylglycerol and glucose do not cause acute increases in plasminogen activator inhibitor-1 concentrations in man. *Clin Sci* 1990;79:513–516.

122. Vuorinen-Markkola H, Puhakainen I, Yki-Jarvinen H. No evidence for short-term regulation of plasminogen activator inhibitor activity by insulin in man. *Thromb Haemost* 1992;67:117–120.

123. Calles-Escandon J, Mirza SA, Sobel BE. Induction of hyperinsulinemia combined with hyperglycemia and hypertriglyceridemia increases plasminogen activator inhibitor 1 in blood in normal human subjects. *Diabetes* 1998;47:290–293.

124. Calles-Escandon J, Ballor D, Harvey-Berino J, et al. Amelioration of the inhibition of fibrinolysis in elderly, obese subjects by moderate energy intake restriction. *Am J Clin Nutr* 1996;64:7–11.

125. Samad F, Loskutoff DJ. Tissue distribution and regulation of plasminogen activator inhibitor-1 in obese mice. *Mol Med* 1996;2:568–582.

126. Cigolini M, Tonoli M, Borgato L, et al. Expression of plasminogen activator inhibitor-1 in human adipose tissue: a role for TNF-alpha? *Atherosclerosis* 1999;143:81–90.

127. Morange PE, Alessi MC, Verdier M, et al. PAI-1 produced ex vivo by human adipose tissue is relevant to PAI-1 blood level. *Arterioscler Thromb Vasc Biol* 1999;19:1361–1365.

128. Lundgren CH, Brown SL, Nordt TK, et al. Elaboration of type-1 plasminogen activator inhibitor from adipocytes: a potential pathogenetic link between obesity and cardiovascular disease. *Circulation* 1996;93:106–110.

129. He G, Pedersen SB, Bruun JM, et al. Regulation of

plasminogen activitor inhibitor-1 in human adipose tissue: interaction between cytokines, cortisol and estrogen. *Horm Metab Res* 2000;32:515–520.

130. Mawatari M, Okamura K, Matsuda T, et al. Tumor necrosis factor and epidermal growth factor modulate migration of human microvascular endothelial cells and production of tissue-type plasminogen activator and its inhibitor. *Exp Cell Res* 1991;192:574–580.

131. Morimoto A, Okamura K, Hamanaka R. Hepatocyte growth factor modulates migration and proliferation of human microvascular endothelial cells in culture. *Biochem Biophys Res Commun* 1991;179: 1042–1049.

132. Sawdey M, Podor TJ, Loskutoff DJ. Regulation of type 1 plasminogen activator inhibitor gene expression in cultured bovine aortic endothelial cells: induction by transforming growth factor-beta, lipopolysaccharide, and tumor necrosis factor-alpha. *J Biol Chem* 1989;264:10396–10401.

133. Mitchell BD, Kammerer CM, Blangero J, et al. Genetic and environmental contributions to cardiovascular risk factors in Mexican Americans: the San Antonio Family Heart Study. *Circulation* 1996;94:2159–2170.

134. de Lange M, Snieder H, Ariens RA. The genetics of haemostasis: a twin study. *Lancet* 2001;357:101–105.

135. Hamsten A, Iselius L, de Faire U, Blomback M. Genetic and cultural inheritance of plasma fibrinogen concentration. *Lancet* 1987;2:988–991.

136. Friedlander Y, Elkana Y, Sinnreich R, et al. Genetic and environmental sources of fibrinogen variability in Israeli families: the Kibbutzim Family Study. *Am J Hum Genet* 1995;56:1194–1206.

137. Orstavik KH, Magnus P, Reisner H, et al. Factor VIII and factor IX in a twin population: evidence for a major effect of ABO locus on factor VIII level. *Am J Hum Genet* 1985;37:89–101.

138. Freeman MS, Mansfield MW, Barrett JH, et al. Genetic contribution to circulating levels of hemostatic factors in healthy families with effects of known genetic polymorphisms on heritability. *Arterioscler Thromb Vasc Biol* 2002;22:506–510.

139. Behague I, Poirier O, Nicaud V, et al. Beta fibrinogen gene polymorphisms are associated with plasma fibrinogen and coronary artery disease in patients with myocardial infarction. The ECTIM study: Etude Cas-Temoins sur l'Infarctus du Myocarde. *Circulation* 1996;93:440–449.

140. Gardemann A, Schwartz O, Haberbosch W, et al. Positive association of the beta fibrinogen H1/H2 gene variation to basal fibrinogen levels and to the increase in fibrinogen concentration during acute phase reaction but not to coronary artery disease and myocardial infarction. *Thromb Haemost* 1997;77:1120–1126.

141. Tybjaerg-Hansen A, Agerholm-Larsen B, Humphries SE, et al. A common mutation (G-455→A) in the beta-fibrinogen promoter is an independent predictor of plasma fibrinogen, but not of ischemic heart disease: a study of 9,127 individuals based on the Copenhagen City Heart Study. *J Clin Invest* 1997;99:3034–3039.

142. Carter AM, Mansfield MW, Stickland MH, et al. Beta-fibrinogen gene-455 G/A polymorphism and fibrinogen levels: risk factors for coronary artery disease in subjects with NIDDM. *Diabetes Care* 1996;19:1265–1268.

143. Ossei-Gerning N, Mansfield MW, Stickland MH, et al. Plasminogen activator inhibitor-1 promoter 4G/5G genotype and plasma levels in relation to a history of myocardial infarction in patients characterized by coronary angiography. *Arterioscler Thromb Vasc Biol* 1997;17:33–37.

144. Ye S, Green FR, Scarabin PY, et al. The 4G/5G genetic polymorphism in the promoter of the plasminogen activator inhibitor-1 (PAI-1) gene is associated with differences in plasma PAI-1 activity but not with risk of myocardial infarction in the ECTIM study. Etude CasTemoins de I'nfarctus du Mycocarde. *Thromb Haemost* 1995;74:837–841.

145. Cesari M, Sartori MT, Patrassi GM, et al. Determinants of plasma levels of plasminogen activator inhibitor-1: a study of normotensive twins. *Arterioscler Thromb Vasc Biol* 1999;19:316–320.

146. Henry M, Chomiki N, Scarabin PY, et al. Five frequent polymorphisms of the PAI-1 gene: lack of association between genotypes, PAI activity, and triglyceride levels in a healthy population. *Arterioscler Thromb Vasc Biol* 1997;17:851–858.

147. Henry M, Tregouet DA, Alessi MC, et al. Metabolic determinants are much more important than genetic polymorphisms in determining the PAI-1 activity and antigen plasma concentrations. a family study with part of the Stanislas Cohort. *Arterioscler Thromb Vasc Biol* 1998;18:84–91.

148. Mansfield MW, Stickland MH, Grant PJ. Environmental and genetic factors in relation to elevated circulating levels of plasminogen activator inhibitor-1 in Caucasian patients with non-insulin-dependent diabetes mellitus. *Thromb Haemost* 1995;74:842–847.

149. Eriksson P, Nilsson L, Karpe F, et al. Very-low-density lipoprotein response element in the promoter region of the human plasminogen activator inhibitor-1 gene implicated in the impaired fibrinolysis of hypertriglyceridemia. *Arterioscler Thromb Vasc Biol* 1998;18:20–26.

150. Sironi L, Mussoni L, Prati L, et al. Plasminogen activator inhibitor type-1 synthesis and mRNA expression in HepG2 cells are regulated by VLDL. *Arterioscler Thromb Vasc Biol* 1996;16:89–96.

151. Keightley AM, Lam YM, Brady JN, et al. Variation at the von Willebrand factor (vWF) gene locus is associated with plasma vWF:Ag levels: identification of three novel single nucleotide polymorphisms in the vWF gene promoter. *Blood* 1999;93:4277–4283.

152. Heywood DM, Mansfield MW, Grant PJ. Factor VII gene polymorphisms, factor VII:C levels and features of insulin resistance in non-insulin-dependent diabetes mellitus. *Thromb Haemost* 1996;75:401–406.

153. Lacquemant C, Gaucher C, Delorme C, et al. Association between high von willebrand factor levels and the Thr789Ala vWF gene polymorphism but not with nephropathy in type I diabetes. The GENEDIAB Study Group and the DESIR Study Group. *Kidney Int* 2000;57:1437–1443.

154. Humphries S, Temple A, Lane A, et al. Low plasma levels of factor VIIc and antigen are more strongly associated with the 10 base pair promoter (−323) than the glutamine 353 variant. *Thromb Haemost* 1996;75:567–572.

155. Heywood DM, Ossei-Gerning N, Grant PJ. Association of factor VII:c levels with environmental and

genetic factors in patients with ischaemic heart disease and coronary atheroma characterised by angiography. *Thromb Haemost* 1996;76:161–165.

156. Lane A, Green F, Scarabin PY, et al. Factor VII Arg/Gln 353 polymorphism determines factor VII coagulant activity in patients with myocardial infarction (MI) and control subjects in Belfast and in France but is not a strong indicator of MI risk in the ECTIM study. *Atherosclerosis* 1996;119:119–127.

157. Mansfield MW, Kohler HP, Ariens RA, et al. Circulating levels of coagulation factor XIII in subjects with type 2 diabetes and in their first-degree relatives. *Diabetes Care* 2000;23:703–705.

158. Mavri A, Stegnar M, Sentocnik JT, et al. Impact of weight reduction on early carotid atherosclerosis in obese premenopausal women. *Obes Res* 2001;9:511–516.

159. Rissanen P, Vahtera E, Krusius T, et al. Weight change and blood coagulability and fibrinolysis in healthy obese women. *Int J Obes Relat Metab Disord* 2001;25:212–218.

160. Primrose JN, Davies JA, Prentice CR, et al. Reduction in factor VII, fibrinogen and plasminogen activator inhibitor-1 activity after surgical treatment of morbid obesity. *Thromb Haemost* 1992;68:396–399.

161. Suzuki T, Yamauchi K, Yamada Y, et al. Blood coagulability and fibrinolytic activity before and after physical training during the recovery phase of acute myocardial infarction. *Clin Cardiol* 1992;15:358–364.

162. Eliasson M, Asplund K, Evrin PE. Regular leisure time physical activity predicts high activity of tissue plasminogen activator: the Northern Sweden MONICA Study. *Int J Epidemiol* 1996;25:1182–1188.

163. Meade TW, Chakrabarti R, Haines AP, et al. Characteristics affecting fibrinolytic activity and plasma fibrinogen concentrations. *Br Med J* 1979;1:153–156.

164. United Kingdom Prospective Diabetes Study Group. Intensive blood-glucose control with sulphonylureas or insulin compared with conventional treatment and risk of complications in patients with type 2 diabetes (UKPDS 33). *Lancet* 1998;352:837–853.

165. Standeven KF, Ariens RA, Whitaker P, et al. The effect of dimethylbiguanide on thrombin activity, FXIII activation, fibrin polymerization, and fibrin clot formation. *Diabetes* 2002;51:189–197.

166. Grant PJ. The effects of high- and medium-dose metformin therapy on cardiovascular risk factors in patients with type II diabetes. *Diabetes Care* 1996;19:64–66.

167. Gottschling-Zeller H, Rohrig K, Hauner H. Troglitazone reduces plasminogen activator inhibitor-1 expression and secretion in cultured human adipocytes. *Diabetologia* 2000;43:377–383.

168. Nordt TK, Peter K, Bode C, et al. Differential regulation by troglitazone of plasminogen activator inhibitor type 1 in human hepatic and vascular cells. *J Clin Endocrinol Metab* 2000;85:1563–1568.

169. Ehrmann DA, Schneider DJ, Sobel BE, et al. Troglitazone improves defects in insulin action, insulin secretion, ovarian steroidogenesis, and fibrinolysis in women with polycystic ovary syndrome. *J Clin Endocrinol Metab* 1997;82:2108–2116.

170. Fonseca VA, Reynolds T, Hemphill D, et al. Effect of troglitazone on fibrinolysis and activated coagulation in patients with non-insulin-dependent diabetes mellitus. *J Diabetes Complications* 1998;12:181–186.

171. Kato K, Yamada D, Midorikawa S, et al. Improvement by the insulin-sensitizing agent, troglitazone, of abnormal fibrinolysis in type 2 diabetes mellitus. *Metabolism* 2000;49:662–665.

172. Gomez-Perez FJ, Aguilar-Salinas CA, Vazquez-Chavez C, et al. Further insight on the hypoglycemic and nonhypoglycemic effects of troglitazone 400 or 600 mg/d: effects on the very-low-density and high-density lipoprotein particle distribution. *Metabolism* 2002;51:44–51.

173. Branchi A, Rovellini A, Sommariva D, et al. Effect of three fibrate derivatives and of two HMG-CoA reductase inhibitors on plasma fibrinogen level in patients with primary hypercholesterolemia. *Thromb Haemost* 1993;70:241–243.

174. Frost RJ, Otto C, Geiss HC, et al. Effects of atorvastatin versus fenofibrate on lipoprotein profiles, low-density lipoprotein subfraction distribution, and hemorheologic parameters in type 2 diabetes mellitus with mixed hyperlipoproteinemia. *Am J Cardiol* 2001;87:44–48.

175. Jastrzebska M, Torbus-Lisiecka B, Pieczul-Mroz J, et al. Etofibrate decreases factor VII and fibrinogen levels in patients with polymetabolic syndrome. *Int J Clin Pharmacol Res* 1999;19:19–25.

176. Kockx M, Princen HM, Kooistra T. Fibrate-modulated expression of fibrinogen, plasminogen activator inhibitor-1 and apolipoprotein A-I in cultured cynomolgus monkey hepatocytes: role of the peroxisome proliferator-activated receptor-alpha. *Thromb Haemost* 1998;80:942–948.

177. Kockx M, Gervois PP, Poulain P, et al. Fibrates suppress fibrinogen gene expression in rodents via activation of the peroxisome proliferator-activated receptor-alpha. *Blood* 1999;93:2991–2998.

178. Kockx M, de Maat MP, Knipscheer HC, et al. Effects of gemfibrozil and ciprofibrate on plasma levels of tissue-type plasminogen activator, plasminogen activator inhibitor-1 and fibrinogen in hyperlipidaemic patients. *Thromb Haemost* 1997;78:1167–1172.

179. Effect of fenofibrate on progression of coronary-artery disease in type 2 diabetes: the Diabetes Atherosclerosis Intervention Study, a randomised study. *Lancet* 2001;357:905–910.

180. Maison P, Mennen L, Sapinho D, et al. A pharmacoepidemiological assessment of the effect of statins and fibrates on fibrinogen concentration. *Atherosclerosis* 2002;160:155–160.

181. Gentile S, Turco S, Guarino G, et al. Comparative efficacy study of atorvastatin vs simvastatin, pravastatin, lovastatin and placebo in type 2 diabetic patients with hypercholesterolaemia. *Diabetes Obes Metab* 2000;2:355–362.

182. Farrer M, Winocour PH, Evans K, et al. Simvastatin in non-insulin-dependent diabetes mellitus: effect on serum lipids, lipoproteins and haemostatic measures. *Diabetes Res Clin Pract* 1994;23:111–119.

183. Wiesbauer F, Kaun C, Zorn G, et al. HMG CoA reductase inhibitors affect the fibrinolytic system of human vascular cells in vitro: a comparative study using different statins. *Br J Pharmacol* 2002;135:284–292.

184. Dangas G, Smith DA, Badimon JJ, et al. Gender differences in blood thrombogenicity in hyperlipidemic patients and response to pravastatin. *Am J Cardiol* 1999;84:639–643.

185. Dangas G, Badimon JJ, Smith DA, et al. Pravastatin therapy in hyperlipidemia: effects on thrombus formation and the systemic hemostatic profile. *J Am Coll Cardiol* 1999;33:1294–1304.

186. Wada H, Mori Y, Kaneko T, et al. Elevated plasma levels of vascular endothelial cell markers in patients with hypercholesterolemia. *Am J Hematol* 1993;44:112–116.

187. Pyorala K, Pedersen TR, Kjekshus J, et al. Cholesterol lowering with simvastatin improves prognosis of diabetic patients with coronary heart disease: a subgroup analysis of the Scandinavian Simvastatin Survival Study (4S). *Diabetes Care* 1997;20:614–620.

188. Baseline risk factors and their association with outcome in the West of Scotland Coronary Prevention Study. The West of Scotland Coronary Prevention Study Group. *Am J Cardiol* 1997;79:756–762.

189. Winocour PD, Kinlough-Rathbone RL, Mustard JF. Pathways responsible for platelet hypersensitivity in rats with diabetes: II. Spontaneous diabetes in BB Wistar rats. *J Lab Clin Med* 1986;107:154–158.

190. Mousa SA, Forsythe MS, Bozarth JM, et al. Effect of single oral dose of aspirin on human platelet functions and plasma plasminogen activator inhibitor-1. *Cardiology* 1993;83:367–373.

191. Tohgi H, Takahashi H, Chiba K, et al. Coagulation-fibrinolysis system in poststroke patients receiving antiplatelet medication. *Stroke* 1993;24:801–804.

192. Roffi M, Chew DP, Mukherjee D, et al. Platelet glycoprotein IIb/IIIa inhibitors reduce mortality in diabetic patients with non-ST-segment elevation acute coronary syndromes. *Circulation* 2001;104:2767–2771.

193. Effects of ramipril on cardiovascular and microvascular outcomes in people with diabetes mellitus: results of the HOPE study and MICRO-HOPE substudy. Heart Outcomes Prevention Evaluation study investigators. *Lancet* 2000;355:253–259.

194. Vaughan DE, Rouleau JL, Ridker PM, et al. Effects of ramipril on plasma fibrinolytic balance in patients with acute anterior myocardial infarction. HEART Study Investigators. *Circulation* 1997;96:442–447.

195. Uehara Y, Hirawa N, Numabe A, et al. Angiotensin-converting enzyme inhibition delays onset of glucosuria with regression of renal injuries in genetic rat model of non-insulin-dependent diabetes mellitus. *J Cardiovasc Pharmacol Ther* 1998;3:327–336.

196. Pedersen OD, Gram J, Jeunemaitre X, et al. Does long-term angiotensin converting enzyme inhibition affect the concentration of tissue-type plasminogen activator-plasminogen activator inhibitor-1 in the blood of patients with a previous myocardial infarction. *Coron Artery Dis* 1997;8:283–291.

197. Schalkwijk CG, Smulders RA, Lambert J, et al. ACE-inhibition modulates some endothelial functions in healthy subjects and in normotensive type 1 diabetic patients. *Eur J Clin Invest* 2000;30:853–860.

198. Fogari R, Zoppi A, Lazzari P, et al. ACE inhibition but not angiotensin II antagonism reduces plasma fibrinogen and insulin resistance in overweight hypertensive patients. *J Cardiovasc Pharmacol* 1998;32:616–620.

199. Remkova A, Kratochvilova H. Effect of the angiotensin-converting enzyme inhibitor perindopril on haemostasis in essential hypertension. *Blood Coagul Fibrinolysis* 2000;11:641–644.

200. Islim IF, Bareford D, Beevers DG. A single (investigator)-blind randomised control trial comparing the effects of quinapril and nifedipine on platelet function in patients with mild to moderate hypertension. *Platelets* 2001;12:274–278.

201. Makris TK, Stavroulakis GA, Krespi PG, et al. Fibrinolytic/hemostatic variables in arterial hypertension: response to treatment with irbesartan or atenolol. *Am J Hypertens* 2000;13:783–788.

202. Mehta JL, Li DY, Yang H, et al. Angiotensin II and IV stimulate expression and release of plasminogen activator inhibitor-1 in cultured human coronary artery endothelial cells. *J Cardiovasc Pharmacol* 2002;39:789–794.

203. Sironi L, Calvio AM, Arnaboldi L, et al. Effect of valsartan on angiotensin II-induced plasminogen activator inhibitor-1 biosynthesis in arterial smooth muscle cells. *Hypertension* 2001;37:961–966.

204. Skurk T, Lee YM, Hauner H. Angiotensin II and its metabolites stimulate PAI-1 protein release from human adipocytes in primary culture. *Hypertension* 2001;37:1336–1340.

205. Erdem Y, Usalan C, Haznedaroglu IC, et al. Effects of angiotensin converting enzyme and angiotensin II receptor inhibition on impaired fibrinolysis in systemic hypertension. *Am J Hypertens* 1999;12:1071–1076.

206. Goodfield NE, Newby DE, Ludlam CA, et al. Effects of acute angiotensin II type 1 receptor antagonism and angiotensin converting enzyme inhibition on plasma fibrinolytic parameters in patients with heart failure. *Circulation* 1999;99:2983–2985.

207. Brown NJ, Agirbasli M, Vaughan DE. Comparative effect of angiotensin-converting enzyme inhibition and angiotensin II type 1 receptor antagonism on plasma fibrinolytic balance in humans. *Hypertension* 1999;34:285–290.

208. Erlinger TP, Conlin PR, Macko RF, et al. The impact of angiotensin II receptor blockade and the DASH diet on markers of endogenous fibrinolysis. *J Hum Hypertens* 2002;16:391–397.

209. United Kingdom Prospective Diabetes Study Group. Tight blood pressure control and risk of macrovascular and microvascular complications in type 2 diabetes: UKPDS 38. *BMJ* 1998;317:703–713.

210. Jonas M, Reicher-Reiss H, Boyko V, et al. Usefulness of beta-blocker therapy in patients with non-insulin-dependent diabetes mellitus and coronary artery disease. Bezafibrate Infarction Prevention (BIP) Study Group. *Am J Cardiol* 1996;77:1273–1277.

211. Mangano DT, Layug EL, Wallace A, et al. Effect of atenolol on mortality and cardiovascular morbidity after noncardiac surgery. Multicenter Study of Perioperative Ischemia Research Group. *N Engl J Med* 1996;335:1713–1720.

212. Herrmann JM, Mayer EO. A long-term study of the effects of celiprolol on blood pressure and lipid-associated risk factors. *Am Heart J* 1988;116:1416–1421.

213. Wright RA, Perrie AM, Stenhouse F, et al. The long-term effects of metoprolol and epanolol on tissue-type plasminogen activator and plasminogen activator inhibitor 1 in patients with ischaemic heart disease 11. *Eur J Clin Pharmacol* 1994;46:279–282.

214. Fogari R, Zoppi A, Malamani GD, et al. Effects of

different antihypertensive drugs on plasma fibrinogen in hypertensive patients. *Br J Clin Pharmacol* 1995; 39:471–476.

215. Gebara OC, Mittleman MA, Sutherland P, et al. Association between increased estrogen status and increased fibrinolytic potential in the Framingham Offspring Study. *Circulation* 1995;91:1952–1958.

216. Koh KK, Mincemoyer R, Bui MN, et al. Effects of hormone-replacement therapy on fibrinolysis in postmenopausal women. *N Engl J Med* 1997;336:683–690.

217. Nozaki M, Ogata R, Koera K, et al. Changes in coagulation factors and fibrinolytic components of postmenopausal women receiving continuous hormone replacement therapy. *Climacteric* 1999;2:124–130.

218. Haffner SM, Lehto S, Ronnemaa T, et al. Mortality from coronary heart disease in subjects with type 2 diabetes and in nondiabetic subjects with and without prior myocardial infarction. *N Engl J Med* 1998;339:229–234.

219. Valdorf-Hansen F, Jensen T, Borch-Johnsen K, et al. Cardiovascular risk factors in type I (insulin-dependent) diabetic patients with and without proteinuria. *Acta Med Scand* 1987;222:439–434.

Diabetes and Cardiovascular Disease
edited by Steven P. Marso and David M. Stern
Lippincott Williams & Wilkins, Philadelphia © 2004

16

Restenosis

David S. Lee and Marc S. Penn

*Fellow, Department of Cardiovascular Medicine, Cleveland Clinic Foundation; Director,
Experimental Animal Laboratory, Department of Cardiovascular Medicine and Cell Biology,
Cleveland Clinic Foundation, Cleveland, Ohio*

Cardiovascular disease is the leading cause of morbidity and mortality in patients with diabetes (1). The treatment of coronary atherosclerotic disease has been evolving over the past three decades, with percutaneous coronary interventions (PCIs) gaining popularity, most notably over the past 10 years. Currently, more than 1 million interventions are being performed each year worldwide (2), and this number is likely to increase by 10% to 20% with the advent of drug-eluting stents.

PCIs are associated with more adverse events in diabetic patients compared with nondiabetic patients (3,4). Diabetic patients usually have more comorbidities and have an increased risk of cardiovascular events after PCI, including death, myocardial infarction (MI), and the need for revascularization (4). Although the results of the Bypass Angioplasty Revascularization Investigation (BARI) demonstrated a less than ideal outcome for multivessel balloon angioplasty in diabetic patients (5), the number of PCIs, both single-vessel and multivessel, done in this population has grown. Although only a modest number of patients have been enrolled in trials comparing coronary artery bypass grafting (CABG) with PCI, patients randomly assigned to PCI consistently have a greater need for repeat revascularization procedures. In fact, restenosis occurs in up to 40% of all patients within 6 months after PCI, and restenosis is more common in the diabetic population (3,6). Recurrent restenosis at the site of previously

treated stenoses is also more common in diabetic patients.

Gruentzig et al. (7) initially reported a 31% restenosis rate among patients undergoing repeat angiography at 6 months. Since that time, restenosis has been frequently studied in clinical trials and registries; however, these were often limited by small sample sizes, nonrandomized groups, incomplete follow-up, arbitrary definitions of restenosis that differed across trials, incomplete revascularization, and changing and improving interventional techniques including atherectomy, intracoronary stenting, glycoprotein IIb/IIIa inhibitors, radiation therapy, and drug-eluting stents.

DEFINITION

The first challenge is finding a relevant definition for restenosis. A common definition is based on angiography, using a threshold value, usually stenosis equivalent to about 50% or about 70% of the vessel diameter. Using an angiographic definition of restenosis of approximately 50%, pooled data from 15 clinical trials showed a restenosis rate of 40% in 8,314 patients undergoing balloon angioplasty, and a restenosis rate of 25% in 4,139 patients undergoing intracoronary stenting (8). This binary definition may not be relevant clinically, particularly if there are no symptoms and no associated adverse events. For this reason, clinical trials that require angiography at 6 months, regardless of clinical status, overestimate the clinical restenosis rate.

Frequently, restenosis is associated with recurrent angina or an anginal equivalent. A wide incidence of recurrent chest pain has been described in clinical trials, ranging from one quarter of patients to almost all of them. On average, approximately 50% of patients have recurrent symptoms. When these patients undergo cardiac catheterization, however, evidence of restenosis is found in 48% to 92%. Using angiographic restenosis as the gold standard, the average positive predictive value of symptoms is 60% (8).

Stress testing has also been used to improve the diagnostic accuracy over symptoms alone, without the increased risk and cost of repeat angiography. However, exercise electrocardiographic (ECG) stress testing in asymptomatic patients was found to have a low sensitivity for detecting silent restenosis. In a study of 191 patients undergoing routine exercise ECG stress testing 6 months after successful percutaneous transluminal coronary angioplasty (PTCA), the sensitivity for detecting restenotic lesions of about 50% was 21%, the specificity was 91%, and the accuracy was 68% (9). Numerous techniques have been employed in attempts to improve on the accuracy of noninvasive testing. In a study from Milan, 150 asymptomatic patients underwent either exercise ECG stress testing or dipyridamole echocardiography 12 months after successful PTCA. Using approximately 70% stenosis as the criterion for restenosis, the sensitivity was 71% with either modality; the specificity was 61% with stress testing versus 90% with echocardiography, and the technical feasibility was 91% with stress testing versus 87% with echocardiography (10). Hecht et al. (11) compared supine bicycle stress echocardiography with exercise ECG stress testing in 80 patients; the sensitivity was 87% versus 55%, the specificity 95% versus 79%, and the accuracy 89% versus 61%, respectively. In 53 patients referred for evaluation of restenosis, Takeuchi et al. (12) used both dobutamine stress echocardiography (DSE) and stress thallium single-photon emission computed tomography (SPECT) imaging at 5 months after PTCA. Restenosis was found in 43% of patients. The sensitivity (DSE versus SPECT) was 78%

versus 74%, specificity 93% and 93%, and accuracy 87% and 85%, respectively. For the most part, stress or dobutamine echocardiography was comparable to stress thallium, although most of these studies were small. Overall, the addition of an imaging modality to stress testing improved its diagnostic accuracy to approximately 80% (8).

The studies evaluating symptoms and noninvasive stress testing still use an angiographic definition of restenosis as the gold standard. Other studies have used adverse clinical events that are likely to be related to restenosis as a more clinically relevant measure. Adverse clinical events include death, nonfatal MI, and target vessel revascularization by either PCI or bypass surgery. None of these definitions of restenosis is ideal, but in clinical trials a composite of clinical end points has been the most commonly used criterion to test new interventional modalities or adjuvant therapies.

Intravascular ultrasound (IVUS) has been frequently used in clinical trials to evaluate restenosis. Although the reasons are multifactorial, there remains no accepted definition for restenosis using IVUS. Additionally, because of both the sensitivity of IVUS measurements and the biologic variability of neointima formation after arterial injury, IVUS probably will not evolve as the gold standard for defining restenosis, given sample size considerations.

Based on the aforementioned limitations for the definition and measurement of restenosis, most recent clinical trials evaluating restenosis have used both quantitative coronary angiography and the clinical end points of target vessel failure, which includes the composite of cardiac death, nonfatal MI, or need for repeat revascularization within 9 months after the index revascularization procedure.

CLINICAL RISK FACTORS FOR RESTENOSIS

Multiple studies have identified predictors for restenosis, and most of them have used an angiographic definition of restenosis (greater than 50% luminal narrowing). Multivariate analyses have repeatedly shown that a combination of

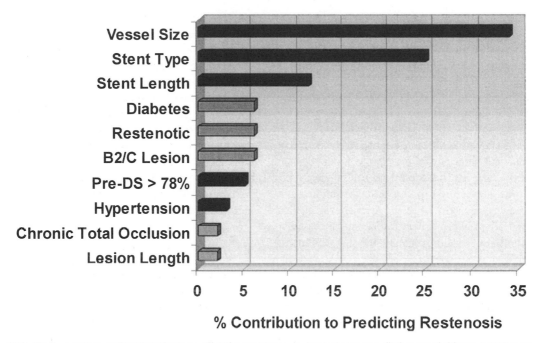

FIG. 16-1. Lesion and patient factors affecting restenosis, based on a predictive model from 4,510 consecutive patients treated with intracoronary stenting. The percentages reflect the amount of the model accounted for by each of the individual factors. (Data adapted from Kastrati A, Mehilli J, Dirschinger J, et al. Restenosis after coronary placement of various stent types. *Am J Cardiol* 2001;87:34–39.)

patient factors and lesion factors predict restenosis (13–15). Patient factors include older age, the presence of diabetes mellitus, unstable angina, and the duration or severity of angina. Of these, the presence of diabetes mellitus and unstable angina appear to be the key clinical drivers of restenosis. Lesion-specific factors include the absence of intimal dissection immediately after PTCA, residual stenosis or significant gradient across the lesion, preintervention minimal luminal diameter, lesion length, thrombus after intervention, and intervention on a bypass graft (16–22). Kastrati et al. (14) developed a multivariate model of restenosis after stenting; vessel size, stent type, and stent length together accounted for 71% of the risk of stenosis (Fig. 16-1). IVUS studies showed that reference vessel size, preintervention quantitative coronary angiographic assessment of lesion severity, and postintervention IVUS cross-sectional measurements predicted late angiographic results. Postinterventional cross-sectional narrow-

ing was the best predictor, overall, in IVUS studies (23). However, no model yet has sufficient discrimination to be applicable to individual patients.

PATHOPHYSIOLOGY

Balloon angioplasty causes acute vascular injury. Initially, it was thought that inflation of the balloon flattened the arteriosclerotic plaque against the vessel wall. Now, it is better understood that balloon inflation causes plaque and vessel fracture, with possible downstream embolism of particulate matter and platelet thrombi and subsequent cell death (24). It is these downstream events that most likely account for postprocedural elevation of creatine kinase-MB (25).

Restenosis, however, is predominantly affected by local conditions at the site of the intervention (14,15,26). After balloon angioplasty, the intima and media of the vessel dissect and fracture. Autopsy specimens in patients who died after PTCA reveal intimal disruption and early focal denudation of the endothelium, microdissections in the intima and media, focal intimal necrosis, and adventitial hemorrhage. Fibrin is deposited on the surface of the intima, within the microdissections, and in areas of necrosis (27). Additionally, balloon angioplasty results in circumferential stretching of the vessel wall, which often leads to a variable degree of elastic recoil that takes place over minutes to hours. Elastic recoil may lead to acute lumen loss shortly after the intervention. Aneurysmal dilatation of the plaque-free segment of the arterial wall is also seen, most likely as the result of an uneven distribution of circumferential stress at the time of dilation.

The pathobiology of restenosis has been actively investigated in many animal models. At best, animal models only approximate the biologic response to arterial injury in humans (28–31). Typically, arterial injury is caused by balloon inflation. In certain models, injury is carried out in the setting of hypercholesterolemia or diabetes (32). The time of maximal arterial narrowing after injury varies according to the animal model. Restenosis in humans is rarely seen after 6 to 9 months (8,33–36).

Coronary restenosis is a reparative response to arterial injury. The endothelial cells, circulating leukocytes, platelets, and smooth muscle cells interact in a complex fashion, not completely understood, that usually results in an early inflammatory response followed by intimal hyperplasia that, in some cases, causes restenosis (Fig. 16-2). In an experimental porcine model, three stages of restenosis were identified: thrombotic, cellular recruitment, and proliferative. The thrombotic stage occurs early and consists of the accumulation of platelets, fibrin, and red blood cells at the vessel injury site. In the recruitment stage, the mural thrombus develops an endothelium, followed by a mononuclear leukocytic infiltrate. In the proliferative stage, a cap of cells forms on the luminal surface, as a result of migration and replication of medial smooth muscle cells, and progressively thickens, forming an obstructive neointima. Extracellular matrix secretion and additional recruitment add to the neointima. The thrombus also provides an absorbable matrix into which smooth muscle cells can proliferate (37).

Overall, in humans, there are four important factors in restenosis: acute recoil, thrombus organization, arterial remodeling, and neointimal hyperplasia. Acute recoil occurs within minutes to days, whereas arterial remodeling and neointimal hyperplasia take weeks to months. Acute recoil and, to a great extent, arterial remodeling are directly reduced by arterial stenting. Neointimal hyperplasia is actually increased in response to arterial stenting.

Endothelium

The endothelial cell layer regulates vascular tone, is antithrombotic, inhibits platelet activation and aggregation, and inhibits smooth muscle cell proliferation (38). In part, the endothelium performs these functions through the production of endothelial-derived relaxing factor (EDRF), nitric oxide (NO), and tissue plasminogen activator (tPA) (39–41). When the endothelium is disrupted, endothelial dysfunction may result from the loss of NO production, with resultant vasoconstriction. In a rabbit balloon arterial injury model, administration of L-arginine for 2 days before and 2 weeks after balloon injury decreased the amount of neointimal hyperplasia by 39%, compared with control rabbits. This effect was inhibited by a nitric oxide synthase inhibitor and suggested that the effect of L-arginine is accomplished primarily through conversion to NO (42), implying an effect beyond vasodilation alone. Moreover, *in vitro,* NO inhibits smooth muscle cell mitogenesis and proliferation (43).

After denudation and balloon injury of the arterial wall, endothelial cells attempt to restore continuity of the endothelium through replication at the edges of the disrupted areas. The loss of contact inhibition in these areas, as well as the mechanical deformation caused by stretching of the vessel wall, induces endothelial replication. There is also evidence that circulating progenitor endothelial cells may contribute to re-endothelialization. Endothelial progenitor cells

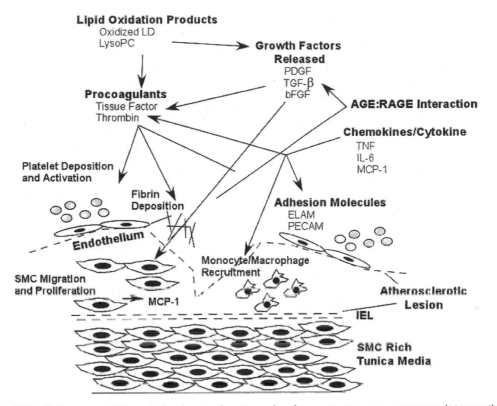

FIG. 16-2. Pathophysiologic mechanisms of restenosis after percutaneous coronary intervention. Balloon angioplasty and stenting result in activation of growth factors and cytokines and smooth muscle cell migration, proliferation, and activation, leading to arterial remodeling and neointimal hyperplasia. LD, low density; LysoPC, lysophosphatidylcholine; PDGF, platelet-derived growth factor; TGF-β, transforming growth factor-β; bFGF, basic fibroblast growth factor; TNF, tumor necrosis factor; IL-6, interleukin-6; MCP-1, monocyte chemotactic protein-1; ELAM, endothelial/leukocyte adhesion molecule-1; PECAM, platelet endothelial cell adhesion molecule; SMC, smooth muscle cell; IEL, internal elastic lamina.

have been isolated from human peripheral blood. *In vitro,* they differentiate into endothelial cells. In animal models, these progenitor cells are incorporated into sites of active angiogenesis (44). When large areas of endothelium are denuded in experimental rat and rabbit models of arterial injury, the reendothelialization process may be incomplete, with endothelial cell replication halting before complete healing is accomplished (31,45). These persistent deendothelialized areas in the intima also exhibit persistent smooth muscle cell proliferation (28), suggesting that the endothelium plays a regulatory role in arterial remodeling. Endothelial cell replacement over these damaged/denuded areas also proceeds more slowly than over normal media (46).

The endothelial cells that regenerate are morphologically different, with irregular sizes and polygonal shapes, and are misaligned with blood flow. These cells have decreased endothelial responsiveness and demonstrate endothelial dysfunction (47,48), with decreased prostacyclin and EDRF production, but with some eventual recovery in function (49). Denuded areas of the vessel wall not covered by endothelium are covered by cells of smooth muscle cell origin (50) that resemble endothelium. These cells actively proliferate and are weakly thrombogenic, but their proliferation is matched by cell death and does not increase neointimal formation (51). In addition, these smooth muscle cells do not seem to retard endothelial regrowth (52).

Activated leukocytes that infiltrate the disrupted area and endothelial cells also release numerous growth factors and cytokines, including basic fibroblast growth factor (bFGF), transforming growth factor-β (TGF-β), and insulin-like growth factor-1 (IGF-1), which enhance proliferation of the smooth muscle cells and their migration into the intima. Platelet-derived growth factor (PDGF), vascular endothelial growth factor (VEGF), and bFGF also act as mitogens for endothelial cells, inducing their replication. These growth factors are also secreted by smooth muscle cells. Interestingly, if bFGF is given exogenously, it will act as a mitogen (53), but it also can improve the responsiveness of the artery to endothelium-dependent vasodilators after balloon injury (54). Therefore, angiogenic growth factors, at least in part, help to reestablish normal endothelial cell function after angioplasty.

Thrombus and Platelet Interactions

The loss of endothelium results in adherence and activation of platelets and leads to thrombus formation with significant platelet deposition. A mural thrombus was found in 70% of animals after balloon angioplasty, even in the presence of heparin, especially in those arteries with a medial tear (55). Interestingly, larger platelet thrombi were seen in less traumatic injury, but only a platelet monolayer was observed in arteries after significant balloon injury (56). When platelets adhere to the disrupted vessel wall and aggregate, they release α-granules that contain, among other things, PDGF, which can act as a chemoattractant and mitogen for smooth muscle cells. In a balloon injury carotid artery rat model, a polyclonal antibody to PDGF inhibited neointimal hyperplasia (57). In addition, in human atherosclerotic plaques, mesenchymal-appearing intimal cells and endothelial cells express PDGF messenger RNA (mRNA) (58). Moreover, IGF-1 is a mitogen that mediates the proliferative effects

of PDGF in mesenchymal cells. After denudation, IGF-1 mRNA is induced early and precedes smooth muscle cell proliferation in the vascular wall (59). In rats made thrombocytopenic, smooth muscle cell proliferation after balloon injury was not decreased, but neointimal thickening was significantly reduced. These results suggest that platelets may play a role in the migration of smooth muscle cells into the intima, but they do not seem to initiate proliferation (60). In other animal models of balloon arterial injury, heparin seems to inhibit both smooth muscle cell migration and proliferation (61,62).

There is also evidence that the thrombus, when organized, may be able to act as a scaffold for the ingrowth of activated smooth muscle cells (37). Moreover, thrombin itself is a potent mitogen for smooth muscle cells (63). However, in some animal models, early thrombus formation accounts for only a small portion of subsequent neointimal formation (64).

Smooth Muscle Cells

Smooth muscle cells play an important role in restenosis (29,65,66). Intimal smooth muscle cell proliferation and thrombus formation are the primary causes of restenoses observed in rabbit, rat, and pig models of intimal hyperplasia after balloon arterial injury. The smooth muscle cells undergoing proliferative activity are predominantly confined to the intima (67) and are usually first seen in the neointima, before the media (27). The disruption of the media in plaque-free segments and the resulting changes in geometry also cause increased proliferation of smooth muscle cells in the media (68). When a gentle denudation technique that does not disrupt the internal elastic lamina is used, medial smooth muscle cell proliferation is markedly reduced (69). These results suggest that acute distention can contribute to smooth muscle cell proliferation after endothelial denudation (70).

Replicating cells at the site of injury, especially smooth muscle cells, express bFGF mRNA. bFGF is a mitogen for vascular smooth muscle cells in the denuded artery. When given exogenously, bFGF leads to increased smooth muscle cell proliferation and intimal thickening. An antibody to bFGF decreases smooth muscle cell proliferation significantly (71,72).

Extracellular Matrix Formation

After arterial injury, smooth muscle cells also change their phenotype. Smooth muscle cells usually are contractile in nature. When activated by growth factors and neurohormones (e.g., angiotensin II), they change to a synthetic phenotype and begin to secrete components of extracellular matrix. In animal models, restenotic lesions are predominantly noncellular, with cellular components making up only a small proportion of the total volume (8,73–75). The rest is made up of extracellular matrix (ECM), secreted primarily by these smooth muscle cells. In a porcine aortic balloon injury model, mRNA levels of elastin and procollagen were significantly elevated after vascular distention and injury. This increase correlated with the increase of cell mass seen in the intima (76). In other animal models, neointimal hyperplasia was noted, with significant increases in collagen and elastin content, consistent with increased ECM formation (77).

Fibronectin, a component of ECM, can influence cellular migration and differentiation. In a rabbit model, fibronectin was upregulated after arterial injury (64). This smooth muscle cell proliferation and secretion of ECM results in increased neointimal hyperplasia. Additionally, TGF-β is expressed and causes the increased expression of proteoglycans in the ECM (78). Human atheroma specimens from restenotic lesions obtained by atherectomy or at the time of bypass surgery demonstrated significant TGF-β mRNA expression, compared with control specimens. This is consistent with the concept that TGF-β plays an important role in modulating repair of vascular injury (79,80). TGF-β can also induce angiogenesis and increase production of collagen by fibroblasts, suggesting that it is an important mediator of tissue repair (81).

Adventitia

Vascular injury triggers differentiation of activated adventitial fibroblasts into myofibroblasts, with increased synthetic ability. Balloon-induced medial layer damage is accompanied by significant adventitial cell proliferation (46). In a pig model, activated adventitial fibroblasts migrate to the neointima and cause increased ECM formation and the accumulation of type I collagen. There is also increased type I collagen in the adventitia and fibrosis with focal adventitial thickening (82). It appears that these adventitial fibroblasts are involved during coronary repair and remodeling (75). In a porcine model of balloon injury, a large number of proliferating cells were initially located in the adventitia, with fewer positive replicating cells in the media or lumen. Later, approximately 7 days after injury, proliferating cells were found primarily in the neointima. PDGF mRNA expression was correlated to sites of proliferation. Overall, adventitial myofibroblasts seem to contribute to vascular stenosis through proliferation, synthesis of growth factors, and possibly migration into the neointima. Increased synthesis of smooth muscle actin in these cells may constrict the injured vessel and contribute to the process of arterial remodeling and late lumen loss after angioplasty (83).

Apoptosis

Apoptosis may modulate the cellularity of lesions. In directional atherectomy specimens, restenotic lesions have more foci of apoptosis than primary lesions do. Total smooth muscle cell content remains constant with continuing neointimal proliferative activity, suggesting some component of cell death or apoptosis to maintain these cell numbers (84). After re-endothelialization is complete, a decrease in the cellularity of the neointima is observed, which is achieved primarily through apoptosis of smooth muscle cells. Apoptosis may be significant in regulating neointimal formation and maintenance (85).

Hemodynamic Factors

Regional flow characteristics and dynamics may also influence restenosis (86). Early neointimal hyperplasia is increased when blood flow is reduced (87). Increased blood flow results in marked decrease in neointimal hyperplasia formation, primarily through reduction in the number of smooth muscle cells in the neointima (88). Reduction in blood flow through arteries can cause a decrease in lumen size related to structural remodeling. This response was abolished when the endothelium was removed, suggesting that the endothelium is essential for compensatory arterial responses to blood flow (89). Moreover, the frequency and severity of cyclic coronary blood flow variations correlate with neointimal proliferation, possibly due to recurrent platelet aggregation and dislodgement. Therapy to block platelet aggregation and activation inhibits the neointimal proliferation and abolishes the response to cyclical blood flow (90).

Neurohormonal Influences

There is an intrinsic renin-angiotensin system in the vascular wall. Smooth muscle cells can form angiotensin. This neurohormonal axis, in smooth muscle cells, may exert a local effect on vascular function and tone (91). Angiotensin II enhances neointimal growth after vascular injury and results in increased protein synthesis and smooth muscle cell hypertrophy (92,93). Angiotensin II and arginine vasopressin are also potent hypertrophic agents for aortic smooth muscle cells (94). In addition, endothelin, an endothelium-derived vasoconstrictive peptide, is a potent mitogen and vasoconstrictor for vascular smooth muscle cells (95) and is associated with neointimal hyperplasia (96).

Arterial Remodeling

Constrictive remodeling and contraction of the external and internal elastic lamina or membrane has also been observed and is one of the most important determinants of restenosis after balloon angioplasty (97). This arterial remodeling is different from the elastic recoil seen acutely after angioplasty. In a rabbit model, there was a discrepancy between the late loss seen with angiography and the result explained by acute recoil or neointimal hyperplasia alone. The primary reason was a reduction in the area circumscribed by the internal elastic membrane, which was described as "arterial remodeling" (32). The artery (internal elastic lamina) enlarges to compensate for neointima formation after angioplasty or constricts and causes further reductions in lumen size.

In atherosclerotic rabbits and other animal models, restenosis after balloon angioplasty is due primarily to this arterial constriction and remodeling (30,98). This finding has also been confirmed in human studies. In IVUS studies after PTCA and atherectomy, 73% of the decrease of the luminal area was found to result from a contraction of the area circumscribed by the external elastic membrane, and 27% from increased intimal and medial thickening. Overall, 78% of lesions had negative remodeling and 22% had positive remodeling. Lesions with positive remodeling had a decreased restenosis rate, 26%, compared with 62% at follow-up. Arterial remodeling is a more important component of restenosis than intimal or medial hyperplasia (99,100).

EFFECT OF INTRACORONARY STENTING

The first stents were placed by Sigwart in the late 1980's, using self-expandable stainless steel mesh. Complete intimal coverage was noted within weeks, and there was no late thrombosis (101). Stenting did not solve the problem of restenosis, however; it only changed the predominant mechanism.

Intracoronary stenting prevents the elastic recoil and arterial remodeling that occur after balloon angioplasty. Instead, the stent causes continued mechanical deformation and stretch of the vessel wall, a localized foreign body reaction at the stent struts, and reendothelialization of the exposed stent on the vessel wall. The primary mechanism of restenosis in stenting is neointimal hyperplasia, through the proliferation and activation of smooth muscle cells.

In a pig model, stenting led to greater intimal smooth muscle cell proliferation than did balloon injury. There was also a marked inflammatory reaction around the stent wires (102). Smooth muscle cell content and proliferation were higher in in-stent restenosis as opposed to post-balloon angioplasty restenosis, in which macrophage, tissue factor, and collagen content were higher. This suggests a more cellular and proliferative response, with less thrombogenic potential, in restenosis after stenting (103). Tissue from 10 atherectomy specimens in 10 patients who had in-stent restenosis in peripheral arteries also revealed histopathologic evidence of hypercellularity, smooth muscle cell proliferation, and apoptosis (104).

DIABETES AND PERCUTANEOUS CORONARY INTERVENTION

Patients with diabetes mellitus comprise almost 25% of individuals undergoing revascularization procedures in the United States (105). Associated comorbidities include hypertension, hyperlipidemia, heart failure, autonomic dysfunction, peripheral vascular disease, cerebrovascular disease, microvascular disease, and nephropathy. The procedural success rate for PTCA with stenting in diabetic patients is 85% to 95%. Decreased endothelial function, prothrombotic state, increased intimal hyperplasia, increased negative remodeling, increased protein glycosylation, and increased vascular matrix deposition have been postulated to account for the heightened vascular response and poorer outcome after PCI among diabetic patients.

According to the National Heart, Lung, and Blood Institute (NHLBI) PTCA Registry, diabetic patients undergoing PCI were more likely to be older, to be female, to have more comorbid conditions, and to have triple-vessel disease. Diabetic patients experienced more in-hospital death and nonfatal MIs. The 9-year mortality rate was twice as high in diabetic patients, with higher rates of nonfatal MI, CABG, and repeat PTCA (106). In another registry by Van Belle et al. (107), diabetic patients were more than 65% more likely to have some restenosis in long-term follow-up; 32% had no restenosis, 50% had nonocclusive restenosis, and 18% had coronary occlusion after 6.5 years. Overall mortality at 10 years was correlated with patency status, with mortality rates of 24%, 35%, and 59% for no restenosis, nonocclusive restenosis, and occlusive restenosis, respectively. Diabetic patients also have a higher incidence of restenosis after balloon angioplasty than do nondiabetic patients (63% versus 36%, $p = .002$) (107).

Lambert et al. (21) studied 119 patients undergoing repeat coronary angiography after successful PTCA of multiple lesions. Using multivariate logistic regression analysis, they determined that diabetes mellitus was the only patient characteristic predictive of restenosis. In addition, patients with restenosis at all sites of intervention were more likely to have diabetes. Kastrati et al. (14) formulated a multivariate model of restenosis after stenting. Diabetes mellitus was associated with an increased risk of stenosis (odds ratio $= 1.21$), with an increase from 31% to 35% (14). Overall, the approximate relative risk of restenosis in patients with diabetes mellitus, compared with nondiabetic patients, is 1.3 (21,108,109).

DIABETES AND RESTENOSIS

Whereas angiographic measures of restenosis are improved with intracoronary stenting, stenting has had limited impact on clinical outcomes in diabetic patients, particularly in patients treated with insulin. Joseph et al. (109a) studied 272 diabetic patients undergoing stenting. Although in-hospital complications were comparable between diabetic and nondiabetic patients, diabetic patients had higher rates of mortality, nonfatal MI, target vessel revascularization, and angiographic restenosis. Diabetes, and especially insulin-dependent diabetes, was an independent predictor by multivariate analysis. Elezi et al. (110) studied 715 diabetic patients and 2,839 nondiabetic patients undergoing stent placement, using 6-month angiographic and 1-year clinical (death, MI, and target lesion revascularization) end points. The event-free survival rate at 1 year was worse in diabetic patients, 73.1% versus 78.5% ($p < .001$); restenosis was higher, 37.5% versus 28.3% ($p < .001$); and stent vessel occlusion was higher, 5.3% versus 3.4% ($p = .037$). In multivariate analyses, diabetes was an independent risk factor for adverse clinical events and restenosis.

In another study, in-hospital complications, including death and MI, tended higher among insulin-requiring diabetic patients compared with nondiabetic patients. Five-year survival and freedom from infarction were lower, and the rates of CABG and repeat PTCA were higher in diabetic patients (111). Among diabetic patients with multivessel coronary disease, those undergoing stenting had a lower event-free survival rate than did those undergoing CABG, because of a higher incidence of repeat revascularization. Overall, however, the total cost at 1 year was less for stenting than for CABG (112). Diabetic patients also were found to have worse survival with multivessel angioplasty than with CABG in the BARI trial (5).

PATHOPHYSIOLOGY OF RESTENOSIS IN DIABETES MELLITUS

Diabetes mellitus is associated with greater restenosis rates after successful angioplasty. Patients with diabetes mellitus also have higher adverse clinical event rates after PCI. Hyperglycemia and hyperinsulinemia potentiate the mechanisms for worsened outcomes after PCI in diabetic patients (3). Diabetes mellitus results in increased inflammation, increased platelet activation, decreased endothelial function, altered blood viscosity, impaired fibrinolysis, and abnormal coagulation (113–129). Decreased EDRF and prostacyclin and increased PDGF, thromboxane A_2, and fibrinogen are observed (115–118,123,124,127,129). Elevated growth factors and cytokines, including bFGF, TGF-β, and IGF-1, have also been found in animal models (114–116,120,128). Impairment of endothelial cell replication after disruption of the endothelial cell layer delays and limits the reparative response and may lead to continuing proliferative responses by underlying smooth muscle cells. Increased smooth muscle cell proliferation with exaggerated intimal hyperplasia has also been observed in diabetic patients. IVUS studies showed that a decrease in arterial area was responsible for most of the late lumen loss in nonstented lesions, whereas neointimal hyperplasia is responsible for late lumen loss in stented lesions and tended to be uniformly distributed over the length of the stent (130,131). Accelerated restenosis may be caused by both a heightened proliferative response and increased vascular matrix deposition (130,132). In addition, advanced glycosylation of proteins on the vascular wall promotes inflammatory cell recruitment and smooth muscle cell proliferation. Many but not all of these mechanisms may be ameliorated by improved metabolic control (3).

Hyperglycemia

Elevated glucose concentrations may have proliferative effects on smooth muscle cells. Hyperglycemia is associated with increased levels of several growth factors that contribute to restenosis. In addition, advanced glycosylation end products (AGEs), especially of proteins on the vascular wall, are increased with increasing levels of hyperglycemia and contribute to increased vascular inflammation, leukocyte recruitment, and smooth muscle cell proliferation (3). Over time, the vascular matrix accumulates AGEs. Macrophages/monocytes have AGE-specific receptors (RAGEs) associated with the expression of several growth factors. AGEs are chemotactic for monocytes and can induce monocyte migration across an intact endothelial cell monolayer. The subsequent monocyte interaction with the AGE-containing matrix results in expression of PDGF (133). AGE-triggered macrophage activation and consequent elaboration of proliferative factors may not only coordinate remodeling but may also lead to diverse pathogenic changes (133). High glucose concentrations can also induce matrix metalloproteinase-9 (MMP-9) expression and activity in endothelial cells in culture, which may be important for both atherosclerosis and restenosis (134). Finally, upregulation of glucose metabolism during intimal lesion formation promotes an antiapoptotic signaling pathway that may lead to accelerated neointima formation (135).

Hyperinsulinemia

Although the elevated glucose levels themselves, together with the presence of AGEs, may be the cause of many of the abnormalities that result in worsened restenosis, hyperinsulinemia is also very significant. The Diabetes

Complications and Control Trial (DCCT) demonstrated that tight control of blood glucose levels and low concentrations of hemoglobin A_{1C} levels did not result in significant decreases in macrovascular complications (136). Concordant with this, in some *in vitro* studies, glucose did not increase, but insulin significantly increased vascular smooth muscle cell proliferation and migration (137). In obese Zucker rats, a typical model for insulin resistance, neointimal hyperplasia was significantly increased after balloon injury, compared with control rats (138,139). Insulin therapy itself also significantly increased neointimal hyperplasia in rats (139). Even in nondiabetic patients, with only impaired glucose tolerance and hyperinsulinemia, coronary stenting resulted in increased neointimal hyperplasia when assessed by IVUS (140).

Endothelial Cells

The endothelial cell layer is dysfunctional in diabetic patients. Johnstone (129) found that patients with insulin-dependent (type 1) diabetes mellitus have abnormal endothelium-dependent vasodilation in their forearms (129). Moreover, after balloon injury and denudation, there is slower reendothelialization, with increased neointimal formation. Platelets also have a longer interaction with the deendothelialized surface than would be observed in nondiabetic patients (126). Elevated glucose concentrations also delayed endothelial cell replication and increased cell death in an *in vitro* system of human endothelial cells obtained from umbilical veins (119).

Coagulopathy and Platelet Reactivity

Many alterations of the fibrinolytic system and platelet reactivity have been found in diabetic patients. These include a state of slightly activated coagulation, increased platelet reactivity, and decreased fibrinolysis (141). In addition, there are abnormalities of blood rheology (142) and metabolic abnormalities that predispose diabetic patients to plaque rupture and intraluminal thrombosis. Angioscopy in patients who presented with unstable angina revealed an ul-

cerated plaque in 94% of diabetic patients, compared with 60% of nondiabetic patients. Intracoronary thrombi were also seen in 94% of diabetic patients, compared with 55% of nondiabetic patients (143).

The platelets of diabetic patients show increased reactivity and aggregability (125). Tschoepe et al. (122) found that there was an increased number of activated, large platelets in the circulation of patients with diabetes mellitus who had vasculopathy (122). Moreover, both in streptozotocin-induced diabetic rats and in humans with non-insulin-dependent (type 2) diabetes mellitus, the prostacyclin stimulatory activity measured in plasma was significantly decreased, possibly correlating with a reduction in prostacyclin synthesis by the vascular endothelium, with resultant platelet hyperaggregability (118). Diabetic patients also had significant reductions in the amount of inducible prostacyclin production (123). Patients with type 2 diabetes who had normal renal function and evidence of macrovascular disease also had higher urinary excretion of thromboxane metabolites from increased platelet production of thromboxane, which may correlate with platelet hyperreactivity and aggregability. Tight metabolic control decreased these levels, and aspirin decreased the metabolites by approximately 80% (124).

Smooth Muscle Cell Proliferation

Walker et al. (127) found that smooth muscle cells derived from the intima of injured rat arteries secreted significantly greater amounts of PDGF-like activity and were different from smooth muscle cells isolated from the media. Scott-Burden et al. (115) found that smooth muscle cell proliferation may be inhibited by NO and concluded that mitogens such as PDGF may act, in part, through reducing the production of NO. In addition, insulin and IGF-1 were found to be additive with PDGF in simulating DNA synthesis by bovine aortic smooth muscle cells. PDGF, insulin, and IGF-1 also increased transcription of the protooncogene c-myc (116). Merimee et al. (120) found that IGF-1 was increased in patients with type 1 diabetes and was higher in those with severe retinopathy. Hyperglycemia also was found to cause increased transcription of bFGF and TGF-α mRNA in vascular smooth muscle cells, possibly through stimulation of the transcription factor Sp1. Interestingly, insulin did not affect this response, in either hyperglycemic or normoglycemic states (114).

Extracellular Matrix Formation

The amount of collagen-rich stenotic tissue was larger in restenotic specimens from patients with diabetes, and there was decreased hypercellular tissue, suggesting an accelerated fibrotic rather than proliferative response in diabetic lesions (132). Yamamato et al. (128) found that TGF-β may be responsible for the excess accumulation of ECM in diabetic nephropathy. This same pathophysiologic process may also be happening in the accumulation of ECM in the neointima. Insulin deficiency is also associated with an increased synthesis of fibrinogen in rats (117).

TREATMENT OF RESTENOSIS

Diabetic patients have a higher likelihood of restenosis after PCI, and they usually have a higher incidence of adverse clinical events. Treatment of restenosis requires consideration of patient-related factors, procedure-related factors, and lesion characteristics. Optimization of medical management for diabetes, improved diabetic control, and aggressive risk factor modification of comorbidities, including hypertension and hyperlipidemia, are likely to reduce the overall incidence of death, MI, and revascularization. As described in the following paragraphs, intracoronary stenting is usually preferred to balloon angioplasty, especially since the advent of adjuvant glycoprotein IIb/IIIa receptor blockers. The roles of intracoronary irradiation and drug-eluting stents are yet to be fully elucidated, but these therapies provide hope that the rate of restenosis can be further reduced in this high-risk population.

Stent Versus Angioplasty

Clinically, stents inhibit acute recoil and chronic remodeling and limit restenosis. IVUS studies allow the differentiation of restenosis into tissue proliferation and arterial remodeling. In nonstented lesions, 73% of late lumen loss was due to arterial remodeling and 27% to tissue proliferation. Stenting resulted in a larger final lumen cross-sectional area and almost abolished arterial remodeling, offsetting a stent-related increase in neointimal tissue accumulation (144). The Benestent trial, Serruys et al. (145), compared stenting versus balloon angioplasty in 520 patients with stable angina. Primary end points were death, cerebrovascular accident, MI, or need for bypass or a second PCI involving the target lesion within 7 months of follow-up. Stenting was associated with improved vessel patency (RR = 0.68 [0.50–0.92], $p = .02$), primarily driven by the decreased need for a second PCI in the stented group (22% versus 32%, $p = .02$). Peripheral vascular complications necessitating surgery, blood transfusions, or both were more frequent after stenting (13.5% versus 3.1%, $p < .001$) (145). Other trials have shown similar results, with stenting having a higher procedural success rate, a higher event-free survival rate, a lower rate of restenosis, and less frequent target lesion revascularization (146).

Studies have consistently demonstrated the benefit of stenting versus PTCA in diabetic patients. Van Belle et al. (147) observed the effect of diabetes on restenosis in 600 patients treated with either PTCA or stenting. Conventional balloon angioplasty was associated with a twofold higher (63% versus 36%) restenosis rate, with greater later loss (0.79 versus 0.41 mm) and a higher rate (14% versus 3%) of late vessel occlusion in diabetic patients, compared with stenting. In the stented group, diabetic patients and nondiabetic patients had a similar restenosis rate (25% versus 27%), late loss (0.77 versus 0.79 mm) and late vessel occlusion rate (2% versus 1%). Subanalysis of the STRESS (stent restenosis study) trial, comparing stenting with PTCA, also showed lower restenosis rates with stenting (24% versus 60%). Other studies have reported higher rates of restenosis in diabetic patients versus nondiabetic patients after intracoronary stenting (148). Carrozza et al. (108) studied 220 consecutive patients with coronary artery disease who underwent intracoronary stenting. Follow-up angiography revealed smaller minimal lumen diameter (1.66 versus 2.24 mm,

$p = .004$), greater percent stenosis (49% versus 32%, $p = .002$), and a higher rate of angiographic restenosis (55% versus 20%, $p = .001$) at follow-up in diabetic patients compared with nondiabetic patients (108). There is no question that stenting results in greater acute gain and improved vessel patency compared with balloon angioplasty. Unfortunately, diabetic patients continue to have higher rates of restenosis than nondiabetic patients in the stent era.

Antiplatelet Therapies for the Treatment of Restenosis in Diabetic Patients

Whereas most clinical trial and registry data show an increased risk of restenosis associated with diabetes mellitus, in the Evaluation of Platelet IIb/IIIa Inhibitor for Stenting Trial (EPISTENT) the combination of abciximab, a humanized murine antibody to the glycoprotein IIb/IIIa receptor, and intracoronary stenting in diabetic patients led to restenosis rates comparable to those of nondiabetic patients (Fig. 16-3). In the diabetic substudy of EPISTENT, 491 patients

underwent PCI with either balloon angioplasty plus abciximab, stenting plus placebo, or stenting plus abciximab. The composite end point for this substudy was death, MI, or target vessel revascularization at 6 months. Abciximab resulted in significant reduction in death or MI at 6 months. Stenting plus abciximab was associated with a significant increase in angiographic net gain and a decrease in late loss. The 1-year target vessel revascularization rate was 22.4% for the diabetic patients treated with stenting plus placebo, versus 13.7% for those treated with stenting plus abciximab ($p = .35$). The rate of target vessel revascularization at 6 months was 8.1% among patients with diabetes and 8.8% among patients without diabetes in the stenting plus abciximab group (4). The use of abciximab at the time of PCI in diabetic patients was also studied by examination of pooled data from the EPIC, EPILOG, and EPISTENT trials. In 1,462 diabetic patients, abciximab decreased the mortality rate from 4.5% to 2.5% ($p = .031$). In patients with insulin resistance, mortality was decreased from 5.1% to 2.3% ($p = .044$). The risk ratio was 0.6 for

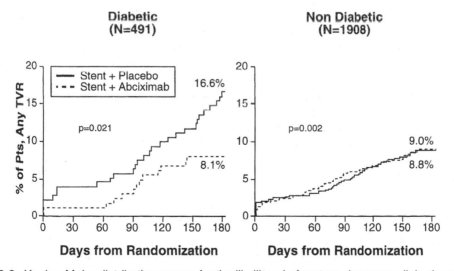

FIG. 16-3. Kaplan-Meier distribution curves for the likelihood of restenosis among diabetic and nondiabetic patients in the Evaluation of Platelet IIB/IIIa Inhibitor for Stenting Trial (EPISTENT). As in previous stent trials, diabetic patients had a higher rate of target vessel revascularization (TVR) than did nondiabetic patients. In contrast, diabetic patients receiving abciximab during intracoronary stent placement had a low 6-month rate of target vessel revascularization, similar to that of nondiabetic patients. (From Moliterno DJ, Topol EJ. Restenosis: epidemiology and treatment. In: Topol EJ, ed. *Textbook of cardiovascular medicine,* 2nd ed. Philadelphia: Lippincott Williams & Wilkins, 2002, with permission.)

mortality (0.5–0.9, $p = .10$). Improvement in multivessel intervention and a trend for improvement in patients with type 1 diabetes were also seen (149). Thus, the use of abciximab seems particularly beneficial in diabetic patients undergoing PCI (150).

Treatment of Hyperinsulinemia

Beyond just diabetic control itself, treatment of insulin resistance may be of benefit in reducing restenosis. Peroxisome proliferator-activated receptor-gamma (PPAR-γ) is a member of the nuclear receptor superfamily that, when activated by thiazolidinedione (TZD) insulin sensitizers, regulates a host of target genes in multiple cell types, including macrophages, vascular smooth muscle cells, and endothelial cells. In animal models of vascular injury, PPAR-γ levels are substantially elevated in the neointima after mechanical injury in the endothelium. There is evidence that PPAR-γ may function to protect the vasculature from injury. PPAR-γ ligands may also protect the vasculature indirectly, by normalizing metabolic abnormalities of the diabetic milieu (151). In 52 patients with abnormal glucose tolerance tests, treatment with troglitazone after stenting improved glucose levels and decreased insulin levels after an oral glucose load and was associated with decreased neointimal hyperplasia (152), suggesting that improvement in insulin resistance in the absence of frank diabetes may still be beneficial. While troglitazone has been withdrawn due to concerns about hepatic injury, further studies are currently underway to evaluate the effects of TZDs in PCI and to determine whether there are any beneficial effects of PPAR-α, and PPAR-δ on restenosis.

Other Pharmacologic Therapies

Vascular angiotensin-converting enzyme (ACE) activity is increased after vascular injury, primarily in neointimal smooth muscle cells. ACE inhibitors may be able to attenuate this process (153,154). ACE inhibitors reduce intimal hyperplasia after balloon injury in some animal models. In a rabbit model, ACE inhibitor-treated animals had improved vascular reactivity and de-

creased neointimal thickening that was almost abolished by inhibitors of NO synthesis (155). However, it is not clear that ACE inhibitors reduce restenosis in humans. Treatment with an ACE inhibitor also decreased neointima formation in guinea pigs but not in rabbits (156).

Radiation Therapy for Restenosis

Because the primary mechanism of in-stent restenosis is accelerated neointimal tissue proliferation, caused primarily by smooth muscle cell migration and proliferation, antiproliferative therapies may be beneficial to reduce the incidence of restenosis. Endovascular irradiation is one method that is now clinically accepted as an antiproliferative treatment for in-stent restenosis. In animal models, radioactive stents suppressed neointimal formation in a dose-dependent fashion. Histopathologic examination revealed decreased smooth muscle cell cellularity and increased ECM formation in the neointima. There was also a dose-related delay in endothelialization (157). Low-dose irradiation from a β-particle-emitting stent resulted in a significant reduction of neointimal area and restenosis without significant inhibition of re-endothelialization (158). Use of a catheter to deliver endovascular radiation also yielded similar results (159).

In human clinical trials, intracoronary irradiation has been shown to be efficacious in the treatment of restenosis, reducing both angiographic restenosis and composite clinical events (160–162). One concerning finding has been the incidence of late thrombosis. Leon et al. (160) reported a 5.3% rate of late thrombosis in the γ-irradiation-treated arm versus 0.8% for placebo ($p = .07$), resulting in a trend for more late MIs (9.9% versus 4.1%, $p = .09$). Late thrombosis was found only in patients who had received new stents along with irradiation and who had discontinued oral antiplatelet medications. In another study, long-term follow-up was reported for the use of γ-irradiation to treat restenotic lesions, using an iridium-192 source, in humans. At 5 years, target lesion revascularization was 23.1% in the radiation-treated group versus 48.3% in the placebo group ($p = .05$). The 5-year event-free survival rate (freedom from death, MI, and target lesion revascularization) was 61.5% in the treated group versus 34.5% in the control ($p = .02$) (163). β-Irradiation using a phosphorus-32 emitter also resulted in improved clinical and angiographic outcomes when used to treat in-stent restenosis (162,164).

In patients with diabetes mellitus, intracoronary irradiation seems to be particularly effective especially in treating patients with recurrent in-stent restenosis. A substudy of the GAMMA I trial assessed the diabetic subgroup. At 6 months of follow-up, the reduction in in-lesion restenosis was greater for the diabetic group than for the nondiabetic group (40% versus 16%) (165). Gruberg et al. (166) analyzed the effect of intracoronary irradiation using both γ- and β-emitters in diabetic patients and found a reduction in binary restenosis rates, target lesion revascularization, and target vessel revascularization, compared with placebo. Patients treated with intracoronary irradiation had similar restenosis and revascularization rates, regardless of their diabetic status (166).

Drug-eluting Stents

In pig and rabbit models, drug-eluting antiproliferative stents implanted *de novo* have been shown to reduce neointima formation. Histopathologic studies, however, show incomplete reendothelialization, evidence of continued fibrin on the neointimal surface, and delayed healing. Long-term follow-up has not consistently shown continued benefit in animal models (167).

The most promising of the antiproliferative drugs for use in stent coatings is rapamycin. Rapamycin has been demonstrated to inhibit the proliferation of smooth muscle cells by blocking cell cycle progression. It is also a potent inducer of inducible nitric oxide synthase (iNOS) (168). In animal models, rapamycin decreases neointima formation by approximately 50%, compared with standard stents (169). In the RAVEL study, in which a rapamycin-eluting stent was compared with an uncoated stent, the rapamycin group at 6-month follow-up had significantly less late luminal loss (-0.01 ± 0.33 mm versus 0.80 ± 0.53 mm, $p < .001$) and a 0% angio-

graphic restenosis rate compared with 26.6% in the control group. During 1 year of follow-up, there was also a reduction in major cardiac events, 5.8% in the rapamycin group versus 28.8% in the standard stent group ($p < .001$), which was due entirely to a lower rate of target vessel revascularization (170).

Diabetic subgroup analysis in the RAVEL study revealed similar results in diabetic and nondiabetic patients. At 6-month follow-up, diabetic patients receiving rapamycin-coated stents had 0.07 mm late lumen loss and a 0% restenosis rate, compared with 0.82 mm late lumen loss and 41.7% restenosis rate with standard stents (170). More experience is needed with drug-eluting stents, especially in diabetic patients. However, these stents hold significant promise for alleviating the problem of restenosis in diabetic patients.

The largest study completed to date is that of a sirolimus eluting stent in *de novo* coronary lesions (known as the *sirolimus*, or SIRIUS, trial) (171). A total of 1,101 patients were randomly assigned to either the sirolimus-eluting Bx velocity stent ($N = 533$) or the control Bx velocity stent ($N = 525$). There were 279 diabetic patients in this trial. Overall, there was a significant reduction in the rate of target vessel failure for the sirolimus-coated stent arm (6.4% versus 19.6%, $p < .001$). With respect to the diabetic subgroup, there was a significant reduction in the in-segment restenosis rate for the sirolimus-coated stent group (17.6% versus 50.5%, $p < .001$). This translated to a significant reduction in the rate of target lesion revascularization in the sirolimus cohort (6.9% versus 22.3%, $p < .001$). It should be noted that the lesion length was 14.0 mm and the reference vessel size was 2.73 mm in the diabetic cohort of SIRIUS.

FUTURE STRATEGIES FOR TREATMENT OF RESTENOSIS: AGONISTS TO RAGE

As discussed earlier, one consequence of long-term hyperglycemia is the formation and accumulation of AGEs, the products of multiple pathways associated with glucose modification of protein backbone components. The accumulation of AGEs in the vessel wall has been implicated in the pathogenesis of diabetic complications (172,173), and the receptor for AGEs, RAGE, is enhanced in diabetic tissue. Agonist binding to RAGE causes cellular activation and enhanced proinflammatory pathways in diabetic tissues (174), and blockade of RAGE with a soluble form of the extracellular domain of RAGE (sRAGE) was shown to suppress accelerated atherosclerotic lesion development in diabetic apo E null mice (175). In parallel with these observations, indices of endothelial cell activation and macrophage migration and function were suppressed in the presence of RAGE blockade (174). Similarly, sRAGE has been shown to decrease neointimal hyperplasia in rodent models of arterial injury (174,176). It is hoped that future clinical trials will demonstrate that RAGE blockade leads to decreased restenosis in diabetic patients.

REFERENCES

1. Haffner SM, Lehto S, Ronnemaa T, et al. Mortality from coronary heart disease in subjects with type 2 diabetes and in nondiabetic subjects with and without prior myocardial infarction. *N Engl J Med* 1998;339:229–234.
2. Bittl JA. Advances in coronary angioplasty. *N Engl J Med* 1996;335:1290–1302.
3. Aronson D, Bloomgarden Z, Rayfield EJ. Potential mechanisms promoting restenosis in diabetic patients. *J Am Coll Cardiol* 1996;27:528–535.
4. Marso SP, Lincoff AM, Ellis SG, et al. Optimizing the percutaneous interventional outcomes for patients with diabetes mellitus: results of the EPISTENT (Evaluation of Platelet IIb/IIIa Inhibitor for Stenting Trial) diabetic substudy. *Circulation* 1999;100:2477–2484.
5. The Bypass Angioplasty Revascularization Investigation (BARI) Investigators. Comparison of coronary bypass surgery with angioplasty in patients with multivessel disease. *N Engl J Med* 1996;335:217–225.
6. Abizaid A, Kornowski R, Mintz GS, et al. The influence of diabetes mellitus on acute and late clinical outcomes following coronary stent implantation. *J Am Coll Cardiol* 1998;32:584–589.
7. Gruentzig AR, King SB 3rd, Schlumpf M, et al. Long-term follow-up after percutaneous transluminal coronary angioplasty: the early Zurich experience. *N Engl J Med* 1987;316:1127–1132.
8. Topol EJ, ed. *Textbook of cardiovascular medicine,* 2002 ed. Philadelphia: Lippincott Williams & Wilkins, 2002.
9. Desmet W, De Scheerder I, Piessens J. Limited value of exercise testing in the detection of silent restenosis after successful coronary angioplasty. *Am Heart J* 1995;129:452–459.
10. Pirelli S, Danzi GB, Alberti A, et al. Comparison of usefulness of high-dose dipyridamole echocardiography and exercise electrocardiography for detection of asymptomatic restenosis after coronary angioplasty. *Am J Cardiol* 1991;67:1335–1338.
11. Hecht HS, DeBord L, Shaw R, et al. Usefulness of supine bicycle stress echocardiography for detection of restenosis after percutaneous transluminal coronary angioplasty. *Am J Cardiol* 1993;71:293–296.
12. Takeuchi M, Miura Y, Toyokawa T, et al. The comparative diagnostic value of dobutamine stress echocardiography and thallium stress tomography for detecting restenosis after coronary angioplasty. *J Am Soc Echocardiogr* 1995;8:696–702.
13. Macdonald RG, Henderson MA, Hirshfeld JW Jr, et al. Patient-related variables and restenosis after percutaneous transluminal coronary angioplasty: a report from the M-HEART Group. *Am J Cardiol* 1990;66:926–931.
14. Kastrati A, Mehilli J, Dirschinger J, et al. Restenosis after coronary placement of various stent types. *Am J Cardiol* 2001;87:34–39.
15. Hirshfeld JW Jr, Schwartz JS, Jugo R, et al. Restenosis after coronary angioplasty: a multivariate statistical model to relate lesion and procedure variables to restenosis. The M-HEART Investigators. *J Am Coll Cardiol* 1991;18:647–656.
16. Leimgruber PP, Roubin GS, Hollman J, et al. Restenosis after successful coronary angioplasty in patients with single-vessel disease. *Circulation* 1986;73:710–717.
17. Rensing BJ, Hermans WR, Vos J, et al. Luminal narrowing after percutaneous transluminal coronary angioplasty: a study of clinical, procedural, and lesional factors related to long-term angiographic outcome. Coronary Artery Restenosis Prevention on Repeated Thromboxane Antagonism (CARPORT) Study Group. *Circulation* 1993;88:975–985.
18. Holmes DR Jr, Vlietstra RE, Smith HC, et al. Restenosis after percutaneous transluminal coronary angioplasty (PTCA): a report from the PTCA Registry of the National Heart, Lung, and Blood Institute. *Am J Cardiol* 1984;53:77C–81C.
19. Weintraub WS, Kosinski AS, Brown CL 3rd, et al. Can restenosis after coronary angioplasty be predicted from clinical variables? *J Am Coll Cardiol* 1993;21:6–14.
20. Quigley PJ, Hlatky MA, Hinohara T, et al. Repeat percutaneous transluminal coronary angioplasty and predictors of recurrent restenosis. *Am J Cardiol* 1989;63:409–413.
21. Lambert M, Bonan R, Cote G, et al. Multiple coronary angioplasty: a model to discriminate systemic and procedural factors related to restenosis. *J Am Coll Cardiol* 1988;12:310–314.
22. Violaris AG, Melkert R, Herrman JP, et al. Role of angiographically identifiable thrombus on long-term luminal renarrowing after coronary angioplasty: a quantitative angiographic analysis. *Circulation* 1996;93:889–897.
23. Mintz GS, Popma JJ, Pichard AD, et al. Intravascular ultrasound predictors of restenosis after percutaneous transcatheter coronary revascularization. *J Am Coll Cardiol* 1996;27:1678–1687.
24. Saber RS, Edwards WD, Bailey KR, et al. Coronary embolization after balloon angioplasty or thrombolytic

therapy: an autopsy study of 32 cases. *J Am Coll Cardiol* 1993;22:1283–1288.

25. Ricciardi MJ, Wu E, Davidson CJ, et al. Visualization of discrete microinfarction after percutaneous coronary intervention associated with mild creatine kinase-MB elevation. *Circulation* 2001;103:2780–2783.

26. Bourassa MG, Lesperance J, Eastwood C, et al. Clinical, physiologic, anatomic and procedural factors predictive of restenosis after percutaneous transluminal coronary angioplasty. *J Am Coll Cardiol* 1991;18:368–376.

27. Austin GE, Ratliff NB, Hollman J, et al. Intimal proliferation of smooth muscle cells as an explanation for recurrent coronary artery stenosis after percutaneous transluminal coronary angioplasty. *J Am Coll Cardiol* 1985;6:369–375.

28. Clowes AW, Reidy MA, Clowes MM. Kinetics of cellular proliferation after arterial injury: I. Smooth muscle growth in the absence of endothelium. *Lab Invest* 1983;49:327–333.

29. Casscells W. Migration of smooth muscle and endothelial cells: critical events in restenosis. *Circulation* 1992;86:723–729.

30. Lafont A, Guzman LA, Whitlow PL, et al. Restenosis after experimental angioplasty: intimal, medial, and adventitial changes associated with constrictive remodeling. *Circ Res* 1995;76:996–1002.

31. Reidy MA, Standaert D, Schwartz SM. Inhibition of endothelial cell regrowth: cessation of aortic endothelial cell replication after balloon catheter denudation. *Arteriosclerosis* 1982;2:216–220.

32. Kakuta T, Currier JW, Haudenschild CC, et al. Differences in compensatory vessel enlargement, not intimal formation, account for restenosis after angioplasty in the hypercholesterolemic rabbit model. *Circulation* 1994;89:2809–2815.

33. Kuntz RE, Gibson CM, Nobuyoshi M, et al. Generalized model of restenosis after conventional balloon angioplasty, stenting and directional atherectomy. *J Am Coll Cardiol* 1993;21:15–25.

34. Kuntz RE, Safian RD, Levine MJ, et al. Novel approach to the analysis of restenosis after the use of three new coronary devices. *J Am Coll Cardiol* 1992;19:1493–1499.

35. Serruys PW, Luijten HE, Beatt KJ, et al. Incidence of restenosis after successful coronary angioplasty: a time-related phenomenon. A quantitative angiographic study in 342 consecutive patients at 1, 2, 3, and 4 months. *Circulation* 1988;77:361–371.

36. Nobuyoshi M, Kimura T, Nosaka H, et al. Restenosis after successful percutaneous transluminal coronary angioplasty: serial angiographic follow-up of 229 patients. *J Am Coll Cardiol* 1988;12:616–623.

37. Schwartz RS, Holmes DR Jr, Topol EJ. The restenosis paradigm revisited: an alternative proposal for cellular mechanisms. *J Am Coll Cardiol* 1992;20:1284–1293.

38. Rubanyi GM. The role of endothelium in cardiovascular homeostasis and diseases. *J Cardiovasc Pharmacol* 1993;22[Suppl 4]:S1–S14.

39. Furchgott RF, Zawadzki JV. The obligatory role of endothelial cells in the relaxation of arterial smooth muscle by acetylcholine. *Nature* 1980;288:373–376.

40. Palmer RM, Ferrige AG, Moncada S. Nitric oxide release accounts for the biological activity of endothelium-derived relaxing factor. *Nature* 1987;327:524–526.

41. Radomski MW, Palmer RM, Moncada S. The anti-aggregating properties of vascular endothelium: interactions between prostacyclin and nitric oxide. *Br J Pharmacol* 1987;92:639–646.

42. McNamara DB, Bedi B, Aurora H, et al. L-Arginine inhibits balloon catheter-induced intimal hyperplasia. *Biochem Biophys Res Commun* 1993;193:291–296.

43. Garg UC, Hassid A. Nitric oxide-generating vasodilators and 8-bromo-cyclic guanosine monophosphate inhibit mitogenesis and proliferation of cultured rat vascular smooth muscle cells. *J Clin Invest* 1989;83:1774–1777.

44. Asahara T, Murohara T, Sullivan A, et al. Isolation of putative progenitor endothelial cells for angiogenesis. *Science* 1997;275:964–967.

45. Reidy MA, Clowes AW, Schwartz SM. Endothelial regeneration: V. Inhibition of endothelial regrowth in arteries of rat and rabbit. *Lab Invest* 1983;49:569–575.

46. Doornekamp FN, Borst C, Post MJ. Endothelial cell recoverage and intimal hyperplasia after endothelium removal with or without smooth muscle cell necrosis in the rabbit carotid artery. *J Vasc Res* 1996;33:146–155.

47. Weidinger FF, McLenachan JM, Cybulsky MI, et al. Persistent dysfunction of regenerated endothelium after balloon angioplasty of rabbit iliac artery. *Circulation* 1990;81:1667–1679.

48. Shimokawa H, Aarhus LL, Vanhoutte PM. Porcine coronary arteries with regenerated endothelium have a reduced endothelium-dependent responsiveness to aggregating platelets and serotonin. *Circ Res* 1987;61:256–270.

49. Saroyan RM, Roberts MP, Light JT Jr, et al. Differential recovery of prostacyclin and endothelium-derived relaxing factor after vascular injury. *Am J Physiol* 1992;262:H1449–H1457.

50. Stemerman MB, Spaet TH, Pitlick F, et al. Intimal healing: the pattern of reendothelialization and intimal thickening. *Am J Pathol* 1977;87:125–142.

51. Clowes AW, Clowes MM, Reidy MA. Kinetics of cellular proliferation after arterial injury: III. Endothelial and smooth muscle growth in chronically denuded vessels. *Lab Invest* 1986;54:295–303.

52. Reidy MA. Endothelial regeneration: VIII. Interaction of smooth muscle cells with endothelial regrowth. *Lab Invest* 1988;59:36–43.

53. Lindner V, Majack RA, Reidy MA. Basic fibroblast growth factor stimulates endothelial regrowth and proliferation in denuded arteries. *J Clin Invest* 1990;85:2004–2008.

54. Meurice T, Bauters C, Auffray JL, et al. Basic fibroblast growth factor restores endothelium-dependent responses after balloon injury of rabbit arteries. *Circulation* 1996;93:18–22.

55. Steele PM, Chesebro JH, Stanson AW, et al. Balloon angioplasty: natural history of the pathophysiological response to injury in a pig model. *Circ Res* 1985;57:105–112.

56. Lindner V, Reidy MA, Fingerle J. Regrowth of arterial endothelium: denudation with minimal trauma leads to complete endothelial cell regrowth. *Lab Invest* 1989;61:556–563.

57. Ferns GA, Raines EW, Sprugel KH, et al. Inhibition of neointimal smooth muscle accumulation

after angioplasty by an antibody to PDGF. *Science* 1991;253:1129–1132.

58. Wilcox JN, Smith KM, Williams LT, et al. Platelet-derived growth factor mRNA detection in human atherosclerotic plaques by in situ hybridization. *J Clin Invest* 1988;82:1134–1143.

59. Cercek B, Fishbein MC, Forrester JS, et al. Induction of insulin-like growth factor I messenger RNA in rat aorta after balloon denudation. *Circ Res* 1990;66:1755–1760.

60. Fingerle J, Johnson R, Clowes AW, et al. Role of platelets in smooth muscle cell proliferation and migration after vascular injury in rat carotid artery. *Proc Natl Acad Sci U S A* 1989;86:8412–8416.

61. Clowes AW, Clowes MM. Kinetics of cellular proliferation after arterial injury: II. Inhibition of smooth muscle growth by heparin. *Lab Invest* 1985;52:611–616.

62. Majesky MW, Schwartz SM, Clowes MM, et al. Heparin regulates smooth muscle S phase entry in the injured rat carotid artery. *Circ Res* 1987;61:296–300.

63. McNamara CA, Sarembock IJ, Gimple LW, et al. Thrombin stimulates proliferation of cultured rat aortic smooth muscle cells by a proteolytically activated receptor. *J Clin Invest* 1993;91:94–98.

64. Bauters C, Marotte F, Hamon M, et al. Accumulation of fetal fibronectin mRNAs after balloon denudation of rabbit arteries. *Circulation* 1995;92:904–911.

65. Thyberg J, Hedin U, Sjolund M, et al. Regulation of differentiated properties and proliferation of arterial smooth muscle cells. *Arteriosclerosis* 1990;10:966–990.

66. Schwartz SM, Campbell GR, Campbell JH. Replication of smooth muscle cells in vascular disease. *Circ Res* 1986;58:427–444.

67. Hanke H, Strohschneider T, Oberhoff M, et al. Time course of smooth muscle cell proliferation in the intima and media of arteries following experimental angioplasty. *Circ Res* 1990;67:651–659.

68. Gravanis MB, Roubin GS. Histopathologic phenomena at the site of percutaneous transluminal coronary angioplasty: the problem of restenosis. *Hum Pathol* 1989;20:477–485.

69. Fingerle J, Au YP, Clowes AW, et al. Intimal lesion formation in rat carotid arteries after endothelial denudation in absence of medial injury. *Arteriosclerosis* 1990;10:1082–1087.

70. Clowes AW, Clowes MM, Fingerle J, et al. Kinetics of cellular proliferation after arterial injury: V. Role of acute distention in the induction of smooth muscle proliferation. *Lab Invest* 1989;60:360–364.

71. Lindner V, Lappi DA, Baird A, et al. Role of basic fibroblast growth factor in vascular lesion formation. *Circ Res* 1991;68:106–113.

72. Lindner V, Reidy MA. Proliferation of smooth muscle cells after vascular injury is inhibited by an antibody against basic fibroblast growth factor. *Proc Natl Acad Sci U S A* 1991;88:3739–3743.

73. Riessen R, Wight TN, Pastore C, et al. Distribution of hyaluronan during extracellular matrix remodeling in human restenotic arteries and balloon-injured rat carotid arteries. *Circulation* 1996;93:1141–1147.

74. Riessen R, Isner JM, Blessing E, et al. Regional differences in the distribution of the proteoglycans biglycan and decorin in the extracellular matrix of atherosclerotic and restenotic human coronary arteries. *Am J Pathol* 1994;144:962–974.

75. Shi Y, O'Brien JE Jr, Ala-Kokko L, et al. Origin of extracellular matrix synthesis during coronary repair. *Circulation* 1997;95:997–1006.

76. Boyd CD, Kniep AC, Pierce RA, et al. Increased elastin mRNA levels associated with surgically induced intimal injury. *Connect Tissue Res* 1988;18:65–78.

77. Strauss BH, Chisholm RJ, Keeley FW, et al. Extracellular matrix remodeling after balloon angioplasty injury in a rabbit model of restenosis. *Circ Res* 1994;75:650–658.

78. Bassols A, Massague J. Transforming growth factor beta regulates the expression and structure of extracellular matrix chondroitin/dermatan sulfate proteoglycans. *J Biol Chem* 1988;263:3039–3045.

79. Border WA, Ruoslahti E. Transforming growth factor-beta in disease: the dark side of tissue repair. *J Clin Invest* 1992;90:1–7.

80. Nikol S, Isner JM, Pickering JG, et al. Expression of transforming growth factor-beta 1 is increased in human vascular restenosis lesions. *J Clin Invest* 1992;90:1582–1592.

81. Roberts AB, Sporn MB, Assoian RK, et al. Transforming growth factor type beta: rapid induction of fibrosis and angiogenesis in vivo and stimulation of collagen formation in vitro. *Proc Natl Acad Sci U S A* 1986;83:4167–4171.

82. Shi Y, Pieniek M, Fard A, et al. Adventitial remodeling after coronary arterial injury. *Circulation* 1996;93:340–348.

83. Scott NA, Cipolla GD, Ross CE, et al. Identification of a potential role for the adventitia in vascular lesion formation after balloon overstretch injury of porcine coronary arteries. *Circulation* 1996;93:2178–2187.

84. Isner JM, Kearney M, Bortman S, et al. Apoptosis in human atherosclerosis and restenosis. *Circulation* 1995;91:2703–2711.

85. Bochaton-Piallat ML, Gabbiani F, Redard M, et al. Apoptosis participates in cellularity regulation during rat aortic intimal thickening. *Am J Pathol* 1995;146:1059–1064.

86. Liu MW, Roubin GS, King SB 3rd. Restenosis after coronary angioplasty: potential biologic determinants and role of intimal hyperplasia. *Circulation* 1989;79:1374–1387.

87. Kohler TR, Jawien A. Flow affects development of intimal hyperplasia after arterial injury in rats. *Arterioscler Thromb* 1992;12:963–971.

88. Kohler TR, Kirkman TR, Kraiss LW, et al. Increased blood flow inhibits neointimal hyperplasia in endothelialized vascular grafts. *Circ Res* 1991;69:1557–1565.

89. Langille BL, O'Donnell F. Reductions in arterial diameter produced by chronic decreases in blood flow are endothelium-dependent. *Science* 1986;231:405–407.

90. Willerson JT, Yao SK, McNatt J, et al. Frequency and severity of cyclic flow alternations and platelet aggregation predict the severity of neointimal proliferation following experimental coronary stenosis and endothelial injury. *Proc Natl Acad Sci U S A* 1991;88:10624–10628.

91. Dzau VJ. Vascular renin-angiotensin: a possible autocrine or paracrine system in control of vascular

function. *J Cardiovasc Pharmacol* 1984;6[Suppl 2]:S377–S382.

92. Berk BC, Vekshtein V, Gordon HM, et al. Angiotensin II-stimulated protein synthesis in cultured vascular smooth muscle cells. *Hypertension* 1989;13:305–314.

93. Daemen MJ, Lombardi DM, Bosman FT, et al. Angiotensin II induces smooth muscle cell proliferation in the normal and injured rat arterial wall. *Circ Res* 1991;68:450–456.

94. Turla MB, Thompson MM, Corjay MH, et al. Mechanisms of angiotensin II- and arginine vasopressin-induced increases in protein synthesis and content in cultured rat aortic smooth muscle cells: evidence for selective increases in smooth muscle isoactin expression. *Circ Res* 1991;68:288–299.

95. Hirata Y, Takagi Y, Fukuda Y, et al. Endothelin is a potent mitogen for rat vascular smooth muscle cells. *Atherosclerosis* 1989;78:225–228.

96. Azuma H, Hamasaki H, Niimi Y, et al. Role of endothelin-1 in neointima formation after endothelial removal in rabbit carotid arteries. *Am J Physiol* 1994;267:H2259 H2267.

97. Gibbons GH, Dzau VJ. The emerging concept of vascular remodeling. *N Engl J Med* 1994;330:1431–1438.

98. Post MJ, Borst C, Kuntz RE. The relative importance of arterial remodeling compared with intimal hyperplasia in lumen renarrowing after balloon angioplasty: a study in the normal rabbit and the hypercholesterolemic Yucatan micropig. *Circulation* 1994;89:2816–2821.

99. Mintz GS, Popma JJ, Pichard AD, et al. Arterial remodeling after coronary angioplasty: a serial intravascular ultrasound study. *Circulation* 1996;94:35–43.

100. Glagov S. Intimal hyperplasia, vascular modeling, and the restenosis problem. *Circulation* 1994;89:2888–2891.

101. Sigwart U, Puel J, Mirkovitch V, et al. Intravascular stents to prevent occlusion and restenosis after transluminal angioplasty. *N Engl J Med* 1987;316:701–706.

102. Karas SP, Gravanis MB, Santoian EC, et al. Coronary intimal proliferation after balloon injury and stenting in swine: an animal model of restenosis. *J Am Coll Cardiol* 1992;20:467–474.

103. Moreno PR, Palacios IF, Leon MN, et al. Histopathologic comparison of human coronary in-stent and post-balloon angioplasty restenotic tissue. *Am J Cardiol* 1999;84:462–466, A9.

104. Kearney M, Pieczek A, Haley L, et al. Histopathology of in-stent restenosis in patients with peripheral artery disease. *Circulation* 1997;95:1998–2002.

105. Smith SC Jr, Faxon D, Cascio W, et al. Prevention Conference VI: Diabetes and Cardiovascular Disease. Writing Group VI: revascularization in diabetic patients. *Circulation* 2002;105:e165–e169.

106. Kip KE, Faxon DP, Detre KM, et al. Coronary angioplasty in diabetic patients: the National Heart, Lung, and Blood Institute Percutaneous Transluminal Coronary Angioplasty Registry. *Circulation* 1996;94:1818–1825.

107. Van Belle E, Ketelers R, Bauters C, et al. Patency of percutaneous transluminal coronary angioplasty sites at 6-month angiographic follow-up: a key determinant of survival in diabetics after coronary balloon angioplasty. *Circulation* 2001;103:1218–1224.

108. Carrozza JP Jr, Kuntz RE, Fishman RF, et al. Restenosis after arterial injury caused by coronary stenting in patients with diabetes mellitus. *Ann Intern Med* 1993;118:344–349.

109. Myler RK, Shaw RE, Stertzer SH, et al. Recurrence after coronary angioplasty. *Cathet Cardiovasc Diagn* 1987;13:77–86.

109a. Joseph T, Fadadet J, Jordan C, et al. Coronary stenting in diabetics: immediate and mid-term clinical outcome. *Catheter Cardiovasc Interv* 1999;47:279–284.

110. Elezi S, Kastrati A, Pache J, et al. Diabetes mellitus and the clinical and angiographic outcome after coronary stent placement. *J Am Coll Cardiol* 1998;32:1866–1873.

111. Stein B, Weintraub WS, Gebhart SP, et al. Influence of diabetes mellitus on early and late outcome after percutaneous transluminal coronary angioplasty. *Circulation* 1995;91:979–989.

112. Abizaid A, Costa MA, Centemero M, et al. Clinical and economic impact of diabetes mellitus on percutaneous and surgical treatment of multivessel coronary disease patients: insights from the Arterial Revascularization Therapy Study (ARTS) trial. *Circulation* 2001;104:533–538.

113. Takahashi K, Ghatei MA, Lam HC, et al. Elevated plasma endothelin in patients with diabetes mellitus. *Diabetologia* 1990;33:306 310.

114. McClain DA, Paterson AJ, Roos MD, et al. Glucose and glucosamine regulate growth factor gene expression in vascular smooth muscle cells. *Proc Natl Acad Sci U S A* 1992;89:8150–8154.

115. Scott-Burden T, Schini VB, Elizondo E, et al. Platelet-derived growth factor suppresses and fibroblast growth factor enhances cytokine-induced production of nitric oxide by cultured smooth muscle cells: effects on cell proliferation. *Circ Res* 1992;71:1088–1100.

116. Banskota NK, Taub R, Zellner K, et al. Insulin, insulin-like growth factor I and platelet-derived growth factor interact additively in the induction of the protooncogene c-myc and cellular proliferation in cultured bovine aortic smooth muscle cells. *Mol Endocrinol* 1989;3:1183–1190.

117. De Feo P, Gaisano MG, Haymond MW. Differential effects of insulin deficiency on albumin and fibrinogen synthesis in humans. *J Clin Invest* 1991;88:833–840.

118. Inoguchi T, Umeda F, Ono H, et al. Abnormality in prostacyclin-stimulatory activity in sera from diabetics. *Metabolism* 1989;38:837–842.

119. Lorenzi M, Cagliero E, Toledo S. Glucose toxicity for human endothelial cells in culture: delayed replication, disturbed cell cycle, and accelerated death. *Diabetes* 1985;34:621–627.

120. Merimee TJ, Zapf J, Froesch ER. Insulin-like growth factors: studies in diabetics with and without retinopathy. *N Engl J Med* 1983;309:527–530.

121. Oliver FJ, de la Rubia G, Feener EP, et al. Stimulation of endothelin-1 gene expression by insulin in endothelial cells. *J Biol Chem* 1991;266:23251–23256.

122. Tschoepe D, Roesen P, Esser J, et al. Large platelets circulate in an activated state in diabetes mellitus. *Semin Thromb Hemost* 1991;17:433–438.

123. Umeda F, Inoguchi T, Nawata H. Reduced stimulatory activity on prostacyclin production by cultured

endothelial cells in serum from aged and diabetic patients. *Atherosclerosis* 1989;75:61–66.

124. Davi G, Catalano I, Averna M, et al. Thromboxane biosynthesis and platelet function in type II diabetes mellitus. *N Engl J Med* 1990;322:1769–1774.

125. Winocour PD. Platelet abnormalities in diabetes mellitus. *Diabetes* 1992;41[Suppl 2]:26–31.

126. Winocour PD, Richardson M, Kinlough-Rathbone RL. Continued platelet interaction with de-endothelialized aortae associated with slower re-endothelialization and more extensive intimal hyperplasia in spontaneously diabetic BB Wistar rats. *Int J Exp Pathol* 1993;74:603–613.

127. Walker LN, Bowen-Pope DF, Ross R, et al. Production of platelet-derived growth factor-like molecules by cultured arterial smooth muscle cells accompanies proliferation after arterial injury. *Proc Natl Acad Sci U S A* 1986;83:7311–7315.

128. Yamamoto T, Nakamura T, Noble NA, et al. Expression of transforming growth factor beta is elevated in human and experimental diabetic nephropathy. *Proc Natl Acad Sci U S A* 1993;90:1814–1818.

129. Johnstone MT, Creager SJ, Scales KM, et al. Impaired endothelium-dependent vasodilation in patients with insulin-dependent diabetes mellitus. *Circulation* 1993;88:2510–2516.

130. Kornowski R, Mintz GS, Kent KM, et al. Increased restenosis in diabetes mellitus after coronary interventions is due to exaggerated intimal hyperplasia: a serial intravascular ultrasound study. *Circulation* 1997;95:1366–1369.

131. Hoffmann R, Mintz GS, Dussaillant GR, et al. Patterns and mechanisms of in-stent restenosis: a serial intravascular ultrasound study. *Circulation* 1996;94:1247–1254.

132. Moreno PR, Fallon JT, Murcia AM, et al. Tissue characteristics of restenosis after percutaneous transluminal coronary angioplasty in diabetic patients. *J Am Coll Cardiol* 1999;34:1045–1049.

133. Kirstein M, Brett J, Radoff S, et al. Advanced protein glycosylation induces transendothelial human monocyte chemotaxis and secretion of platelet-derived growth factor: role in vascular disease of diabetes and aging. *Proc Natl Acad Sci U S A* 1990;87:9010–9014.

134. Uemura S, Matsushita H, Li W, et al. Diabetes mellitus enhances vascular matrix metalloproteinase activity: role of oxidative stress. *Circ Res* 2001;88:1291–1298.

135. Hall JL, Chatham JC, Eldar-Finkelman H, et al. Upregulation of glucose metabolism during intimal lesion formation is coupled to the inhibition of vascular smooth muscle cell apoptosis: role of GSK3beta. *Diabetes* 2001;50:1171–1179.

136. Granger CB, Califf RM, Young S, et al. Outcome of patients with diabetes mellitus and acute myocardial infarction treated with thrombolytic agents: the Thrombolysis and Angioplasty in Myocardial Infarction (TAMI) Study Group. *J Am Coll Cardiol* 1993;21:920–925.

137. Stout RW, Bierman EL, Ross R. Effect of insulin on the proliferation of cultured primate arterial smooth muscle cells. *Circ Res* 1975;36:319–327.

138. Park SH, Marso SP, Zhou Z, et al. Neointimal hyperplasia after arterial injury is increased in a rat model

of non-insulin-dependent diabetes mellitus. *Circulation* 2001;104:815–819.

139. Indolfi C, Torella D, Cavuto L, et al. Effects of balloon injury on neointimal hyperplasia in streptozotocin-induced diabetes and in hyperinsulinemic nondiabetic pancreatic islet-transplanted rats. *Circulation* 2001;103:2980–2986.

140. Takagi T, Yoshida K, Akasaka T, et al. Hyperinsulinemia during oral glucose tolerance test is associated with increased neointimal tissue proliferation after coronary stent implantation in nondiabetic patients: a serial intravascular ultrasound study. *J Am Coll Cardiol* 2000;36:731–738.

141. Ostermann H, van de Loo J. Factors of the hemostatic system in diabetic patients: a survey of controlled studies. *Haemostasis* 1986;16:386–416.

142. MacRury SM, Lowe GD. Blood rheology in diabetes mellitus. *Diabet Med* 1990;7:285–291.

143. Silva JA, Escobar A, Collins TJ, et al. Unstable angina: a comparison of angioscopic findings between diabetic and nondiabetic patients. *Circulation* 1995;92:1731–1736.

144. Mintz GS, Popma JJ, Hong MK, et al. Intravascular ultrasound to discern device-specific effects and mechanisms of restenosis. *Am J Cardiol* 1996;78:18–22.

145. Serruys PW, de Jaegere P, Kiemeneij F, et al. A comparison of balloon-expandable-stent implantation with balloon angioplasty in patients with coronary artery disease: Benestent Study Group. *N Engl J Med* 1994;331:489–495.

146. Fischman DL, Leon MB, Baim DS, et al. A randomized comparison of coronary-stent placement and balloon angioplasty in the treatment of coronary artery disease: Stent Restenosis Study Investigators. *N Engl J Med* 1994;331:496–501.

147. Van Belle E, Bauters C, Hubert E, et al. Restenosis rates in diabetic patients: a comparison of coronary stenting and balloon angioplasty in native coronary vessels. *Circulation* 1997;96:1454–1460.

148. Schofer J, Schluter M, Rau T, et al. Influence of treatment modality on angiographic outcome after coronary stenting in diabetic patients: a controlled study. *J Am Coll Cardiol* 2000;35:1554–1559.

149. Bhatt DL, Marso SP, Lincoff AM, et al. Abciximab reduces mortality in diabetics following percutaneous coronary intervention. *J Am Coll Cardiol* 2000;35:922–928.

150. King SB 3rd, Mahmud E. Will blocking the platelet save the diabetic? *Circulation* 1999;100:2466–2468.

151. Hsueh WA, Jackson S, Law RE. Control of vascular cell proliferation and migration by PPAR-gamma: a new approach to the macrovascular complications of diabetes. *Diabetes Care* 2001;24:392–397.

152. Takagi T, Akasaka T, Yamamuro A, et al. Troglitazone reduces neointimal tissue proliferation after coronary stent implantation in patients with non-insulin dependent diabetes mellitus: a serial intravascular ultrasound study. *J Am Coll Cardiol* 2000;36:1529–1535.

153. Rakugi H, Kim DK, Krieger JE, et al. Induction of angiotensin converting enzyme in the neointima after vascular injury: possible role in restenosis. *J Clin Invest* 1994;93:339–346.

154. Powell JS, Clozel JP, Muller RK, et al. Inhibitors of angiotensin-converting enzyme prevent

myointimal proliferation after vascular injury. *Science* 1989;245:186–188.

155. Van Belle E, Vallet B, Auffray JL, et al. NO synthesis is involved in structural and functional effects of ACE inhibitors in injured arteries. *Am J Physiol* 1996;270:H298–H305.

156. Clozel JP, Hess P, Michael C, et al. Inhibition of converting enzyme and neointima formation after vascular injury in rabbits and guinea pigs. *Hypertension* 1991;18:II55–II59.

157. Hehrlein C, Gollan C, Donges K, et al. Low-dose radioactive endovascular stents prevent smooth muscle cell proliferation and neointimal hyperplasia in rabbits. *Circulation* 1995;92:1570–1575.

158. Laird JR, Carter AJ, Kufs WM, et al. Inhibition of neointimal proliferation with low-dose irradiation from a beta-particle-emitting stent. *Circulation* 1996;93:529–536.

159. Waksman R, Robinson KA, Crocker IR, et al. Intracoronary radiation before stent implantation inhibits neointima formation in stented porcine coronary arteries. *Circulation* 1995;92:1383–1386.

160. Leon MB, Teirstein PS, Moses JW, et al. Localized intracoronary gamma-radiation therapy to inhibit the recurrence of restenosis after stenting. *N Engl J Med* 2001;344:250–256.

161. Waksman R, White RL, Chan RC, et al. Intracoronary gamma-radiation therapy after angioplasty inhibits recurrence in patients with in-stent restenosis. *Circulation* 2000;101:2165–2171.

162. Raizner AE, Oesterle SN, Waksman R, et al. Inhibition of restenosis with beta-emitting radiotherapy: report of the Proliferation Reduction with Vascular Energy Trial (PREVENT). *Circulation* 2000;102:951–958.

163. Grise MA, Massullo V, Jani S, et al. Five-year clinical follow up after intracoronary radiation: results of a randomized clinical trial. *Circulation* 2002;105:2737–2740.

164. Waksman R, Raizner AE, Yeung AC, et al. Use of localised intracoronary beta radiation in treatment of in-stent restenosis: the INHIBIT randomised controlled trial. *Lancet* 2002;359:551–557.

165. Moses JW, Moussa I, Leon MB, et al. Effect of catheter-based iridium-192 gamma brachytherapy on the added risk of restenosis from diabetes mellitus after intervention for in-stent restenosis (subanalysis of the GAMMA I Randomized Trial). *Am J Cardiol* 2002;90:243–247.

166. Gruberg L, Waksman R, Ajani AE, et al. The effect of intracoronary radiation for the treatment of recurrent in-stent restenosis in patients with diabetes mellitus. *J Am Coll Cardiol* 2002;39:1930–1936.

167. Virmani R, Farb A, Kolodgie FD. Histopathologic alterations after endovascular radiation and antiproliferative stents: similarities and differences. *Herz* 2002;27:1–6.

168. Pham SM, Shears LL, Kawaharada N, et al. High local production of nitric oxide as a possible mechanism by which rapamycin prevents transplant arteriosclerosis. *Transplant Proc* 1998;30:953–954.

169. Suzuki T, Kopia G, Hayashi S, et al. Stent-based delivery of sirolimus reduces neointimal formation in a porcine coronary model. *Circulation* 2001;104:1188–1193.

170. Morice MC, Serruys PW, Sousa JE, et al. A randomized comparison of a sirolimus eluting stent with a standard stent for coronary revascularization. *N Engl J Med* 2002;346:1773–1780.

171. SIRIUS Trial Presentation.

172. Vlassara H, Palace MR. Diabetes and advanced glycation endproducts. *J Intern Med* 2002;251:87–101.

173. Stern DM, Yan SD, Yan SF, et al. Receptor for advanced glycation endproducts (RAGE) and the complications of diabetes. *Ageing Res Rev* 2002;1:1–15.

174. Schmidt AM, Yan SD, Yan SF, et al. The multiligand receptor RAGE as a progression factor amplifying immune and inflammatory responses. *J Clin Invest* 2001;108:949–955.

175. Park L, Raman KG, Lee KJ, et al. Suppression of accelerated diabetic atherosclerosis by the soluble receptor for advanced glycation endproducts. *Nat Med* 1998;4:1025–1031.

176. Zhou Z, Marso SP, Schmidt AM, et al. Blockage of receptor for advanced glycation end-products (RAGE) suppresses neointimal formation in diabetic rat carotid artery injury model. *Circulation* 2000;102:II–246.

Diabetes and Cardiovascular Disease
edited by Steven P. Marso and David M. Stern
Lippincott Williams & Wilkins, Philadelphia © 2004

17

The Renin-Angiotensin System, Nephropathy, and Hypertension

Roberto Trevisan and Giancarlo Viberti

Honorary Professor of Diabetology, Department of Clinical and Experimental Medicine, University of Padua, Padua, Italy, Consultant, Diabetes Section, Department of Transplantation, Riuniti Hospital of Bergamo, Bergamo, Italy; Professor, Department of Diabetes, Endocrinology, and Internal Medicine, King's College, London, Honorary Consultant Physician, Department of Endocrinology and Diabetes, Guy's Hospital, London, United Kingdom

THE BURDEN OF DIABETIC NEPHROPATHY

Diabetic nephropathy is the most frequent cause of end-stage renal disease (ESRD) in the United States, Europe, and Japan. In the United States, the incidence of diabetic nephropathy has increased by 150% in the past 10 years, a trend also seen in Europe (1,2) (Fig. 17-1). In North America, 42% of patients starting dialysis in 1998 had diabetic nephropathy. Because the prevalence of non-insulin-dependent (type 2) diabetes mellitus is at least fivefold to sixfold higher than that of insulin-dependent (type 1) diabetes mellitus, type 2 diabetes now accounts for at least 50% of all diabetic patients with ESRD. Among patients requiring dialysis, those with diabetes have a 22% higher mortality rate at 1 year and a 15% higher rate at 5 years than patients without diabetes. In 1998, the estimated cost of care for a diabetic patient undergoing dialysis was $51,000 per year, which was about $12,000 more than the cost for a nondiabetic patient (1).

Clinical diabetic nephropathy is defined by the presence of persistent proteinuria (urine albumin excretion rate [AER] greater than 300 mg/day) in sterile urine of diabetic patients, but without other renal disease or heart failure (3). Once manifest, diabetic nephropathy is characterized by a progressive decline in renal function, resulting in ESRD. Histologic changes of diabetic glomerulopathy are present in more than 96% of patients with type 1 diabetes who have clinical proteinuria and in approximately 85% of those with type 2 diabetes who develop proteinuria with concomitant retinopathy. In the absence of retinopathy, about 30% of proteinuric type 2 patients may have a nondiabetic renal lesion (4).

Between 25% and 50% of diabetic patients develop kidney disease, although a smaller percentage require dialysis or kidney transplantation. In patients with type 1 diabetes, the mortality rate from all causes in patients with nephropathy is 20 to 40 times higher than that of patients without nephropathy (5). In patients with type 2 diabetes with proteinuria, the cardiovascular (CV) mortality rate is approximately eightfold greater than in the general population, compared with a twofold to fourfold increase for type 2 diabetes in general (6).

NEPHROPATHY IN TYPE 1 DIABETES

The evolution of diabetic nephropathy proceeds through several distinct but interconnected phases: an early phase of physiologic abnormalities of renal function, a "microalbuminuria phase," and a clinical phase with persistent clinical proteinuria progressing to ESRD (1,2).

Incidence of ESRD Due to Diabetes in Europe

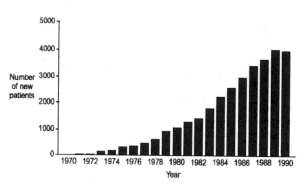

FIG. 17-1. Incidence of end-stage renal disease (ESRD) due to diabetes in Europe.

Early Renal Abnormalities

Soon after the diagnosis of type 1 diabetes, supranormal values of renal plasma flow (RPF) and glomerular filtration rate (GFR; greater than 135 mL/min/1.73 m^2) are found in approximately 20% to 40% of patients (7). Hyperfiltration is partially related to the degree of metabolic control (8), and intensified insulin therapy with improvement of blood glucose control reduces GFR toward normal values (9). These hemodynamic abnormalities are associated with an increase in kidney size. Nephromegaly is a prerequisite for the occurrence of glomerular hyperfiltration (10). However, the prognostic significance of nephromegaly remains unclear.

There is a good correlation between GFR and RPF increases in diabetic patients, but increases in RPF can account for only about 60% of the increase in GFR. The remainder of the GFR increase is accounted for by a rise in intraglomerular pressure, resulting from a diabetes-induced reduction in vascular resistance that is more marked in afferent than in efferent arteriolar vessels (11).

Microalbuminuria

A proportion of diabetic patients exhibit elevated rates of urine albumin excretion well before clinically persistent proteinuria develops. An increase in AER ranging between 20 to 200 μg/min is defined as microalbuminuria (3). Microalbumin-

uria is a predictor for the development of clinical diabetic nephropathy. It is associated with an approximately 20-fold higher risk of progression to overt renal disease, compared with normoalbuminuria (12–15). AERs in healthy individuals range between 1.5 and 20 μg/min, with a median of about 6.5 μg/min. The average day-to-day variation in the AER is about 40% and is similar in normal and diabetic subjects (16). For this reason, an accurate classification of AER requires multiple measurements (usually three urine collections) over a period of a few weeks (3).

Persistent microalbuminuria may be found after 1 year of type 1 diabetes (17). Although the significance of microalbuminuria in patients with short-term diabetes is still unclear, in individuals who have had diabetes for 5 or more years, microalbuminuria is the consequence of definite, albeit early, renal damage (18). Structural lesions, such as increased mesangial fractional volume and decreased filtration surface area are, on average, found at this stage, confirming that microalbuminuria is a sign of renal disease. Once microalbuminuria is established, the AER tends to rise with time, at an average rate of about 14% per year (19).

The excessive AER in diabetic patients with persistent microalbuminuria is most likely the result of an increased transglomerular flux caused by an increase in the transglomerular pressure gradient.

Microalbuminuria is consistently associated with higher levels of blood pressure, independent of age, sex, duration of diabetes, body mass index, and blood glucose control (20). The magnitude of this blood pressure rise is approximately 10% to 15% greater than that of diabetic patients with normal albumin excretion, and it often occurs within the so-called normal blood pressure range (20). At this stage of microalbuminuria, there is no hint of renal failure, and the GFR can even be supranormal.

Overt Nephropathy

In diabetic patients who progress to overt, persistent albuminuria (AER greater than 300 mg/24 hours), GFR gradually declines if left untreated, in a linear fashion, at a rate ranging from 1.2 to 22 mL/min per year (average 10 mL/min per year) (21). The reason for the different rates of progression are not entirely known, but blood pressure, blood glucose control, degree of proteinuria, and degree of hypercholesterolemia are likely contributors (22,23). In several studies, the increase in urinary protein excretion correlated with the progression of renal disease (24). Data suggest that proteins filtered by the glomerulus cause injury to the tubulointerstitium, leading to parenchymal damage and, ultimately, renal scarring and insufficiency (25). Before the introduction of early, intensive treatment for hypertension in diabetic patients, ESRD occurred an average of 7 years after the onset of proteinuria. Today, the period between onset of overt proteinuria and renal replacement therapy is more than double what it once was. Elevation of blood pressure is a feature in about 85% of patients with proteinuria, and blood pressure increases by about 7% per year in association with progressive renal failure (26). The excess of arterial hypertension in type 1 diabetes seems to be largely accounted for by patients with overt clinical nephropathy, whereas patients with long-term uncomplicated diabetes tend to have lower blood pressure levels than those of age-matched normal controls.

Diabetic retinopathy and hyperlipidemia (characterized by increased total cholesterol, low-density lipoprotein [LDL] cholesterol, and triglycerides and lower high-density lipoprotein [HDL] cholesterol) are present in most patients with nephropathy.

NEPHROPATHY IN TYPE 2 DIABETES

Renal failure in type 2 diabetes develops in a smaller percentage of patients of Caucasian origin, but, because the incidence of type 2 diabetes is much greater, about one-half of the patients in ESRD belong to this group (27).

The prevalence of clinical proteinuria ranges between 10% and 40% in patients with type 2 diabetes, with large ethnic variations. Diabetes duration and hypertension are related to the presence of proteinuria. Incidence data show that the cumulative risk of persistent proteinuria varies between 25% and 50% after diabetes duration of 20 years or longer (28). Observational studies of type 2 diabetic patients with nephropathy have demonstrated that the rate of fall in GFR varies considerably from one patient to another, but the increase in blood pressure to a hypertensive level is an early feature and accelerates the progression of renal disease (29). ESRD is about 20 times less frequent in European subjects with type 2 diabetes compared with type 1 diabetes, because other competing causes of death, especially CV disease, in the older type 2 diabetic group prevent progression to end-stage failure (30,31). In ethnic groups in which ischemic heart disease is less common and type 2 diabetes develops at a younger age (e.g., Japanese, Asian, American Indian), the frequency of ESRD is similar to, if not higher than, that in type 1 diabetic patients.

Microalbuminuria in type 2 diabetes appears to be not only a predictor of renal disease but also a powerful marker of CV mortality (32,33). Increased albuminuria is associated with coronary heart disease, cardiac failure, and peripheral vascular disease (34). Several CV risk factors have been linked with microalbuminuria in patients with type 2 diabetes, including lipoprotein abnormalities, hypertension, central obesity, hyperuricemia, and markers of endothelial dysfunction (35,36). None of these factors, however, can entirely explain the increased CV mortality in patients with abnormal AER.

With the euglycemic insulin clamp technique, diabetic patients with microalbuminuria were found to be more insulin resistant than patients with normoalbuminuria (37). This altered insulin sensitivity may explain why patients with microalbuminuria tend to have poorer metabolic control than do patients with normoalbuminuria. It is of particular interest that insulin resistance, an independent risk factor for coronary artery disease in the nondiabetic population, has also been associated with sodium sensitivity of blood pressure in both type 1 and type 2 diabetics with microalbuminuria (38,39).

NEPHROPATHY AND HYPERTENSION IN DIABETES

That the hypertension associated with diabetic nephropathy is not merely a consequence of the renal disease was confirmed by several studies indicating that elevations of arterial pressure develop at very early stages in both type 1 and type 2 diabetics with normoalbuminuria who subsequently progress to microalbuminuria (40,41), and these elevations persist at the microalbuminuria stage (20,28). If the Joint National Committee on Detection, Evaluation, and Treatment of Hypertension (JNC) criterion for the definition of increased blood pressure in diabetes is applied (i.e., values greater than 130/80 mmHg), the prevalence of hypertension in type 1 diabetic patients with microalbuminuria is greater than 70% (42). Subtle changes in blood pressure (e.g., diminished day-to-night variation) in young patients with type 1 diabetes seems to predict the subsequent development of microalbuminuria (43). Studies of transition from normoalbuminuria to microalbuminuria have documented that the diabetic patients who progress show increases in blood pressure as the AER rises within the normal range (40). This raises the possibility that elevated blood pressure levels may be one factor contributing to the initiation of renal damage or, alternatively, that high blood pressure and an increase in urine albumin excretion may represent concomitant manifestations of a common process responsible for the development of diabetic nephropathy.

A genetic predisposition to develop hypertension may confer increased risk for renal disease. Higher arterial pressure was measured in parents of diabetic patients with proteinuria than in parents of patients without proteinuria (44). A higher prevalence of arterial hypertension among the parents of type 1 diabetics with nephropathy was also found in a later study (45). The relative risk of developing overt nephropathy was found to be approximately 3.3 if at least one parent had hypertension. All of these studies suggest that hypertension or a predisposition to hypertension may be an important component in determining the susceptibility to renal disease in diabetes. The suggestion that diabetic nephropathy may, in part, be heritable has stimulated the search for cell and genetic markers that would allow early diagnosis and identification of patients at risk and help to clarify the molecular mechanisms of this complication.

An increase in red blood cell sodium-lithium countertransport activity, a cell membrane cation transport system consistently associated with essential hypertension and its vascular complications, has been reported by several, although not all, authors both in type 1 and type 2 diabetic patients with microalbuminuria or macroalbuminuria (46–48). The significant correlation between the activity of this transport system in diabetic probands with nephropathy and their parents (49), coupled with the close association of sodium-lithium countertransport activities found in diabetic identical twins (50), strongly suggests heritability of elevated activities in diabetic nephropathy. That an increased sodium-lithium countertransport activity may confer an increased risk for nephropathy and its vascular complications is supported by a clustering of metabolic, hemodynamic, and morphologic abnormalities (e.g., poor metabolic control, reduced insulin sensitivity, a more atherogenic lipid profile, greater proximal tubular reabsorption of sodium, higher GFR, increased left ventricular thickness, larger size of kidneys) in those patients who have high sodium-lithium countertransport activity but no overt proteinuria (51).

An increased sodium-hydrogen antiport activity (another membrane cation transport abnormality associated with hypertension) has also been reported in leukocytes and red blood cells of type 1 diabetic patients with nephropathy (52,53). More recently, it was shown that this abnormal phenotype is also conserved in skin fibroblasts after several passages and in Epstein-Barr-immortalized lymphoblasts (54,55), suggesting that the overactivity of the antiport is intrinsically determined. The importance of genetic factors was confirmed by the close association of maximal velocities of antiport activities in fibroblasts of type 1 diabetic sibling pairs (56). Of great relevance was the observation in these same siblings that there was close concordance of degree of glomerular lesions.

In patients with type 2 diabetes, the prevalence of hypertension is approximately 70% or higher if the recent JNC-VI criteria are used (28,34). This high prevalence is partly explained by associated obesity, older age, and insulin resistance. Hypertension often precedes diabetes in patients with type 2 disease; this probably reflects a familial clustering related to the metabolic syndrome, in which insulin resistance is believed to play a pathogenetic role (57). There is now substantial evidence that insulin resistance plays a role in the development of hypertension. Insulin resistance exists in normotensive, first degree relatives of patients with high blood pressure (58). In addition to being insulin resistant, individuals with a family history of hypertension are also dyslipidemic. Furthermore, prospective studies have shown that hyperinsulinemia at baseline (a marker of insulin resistance) predicts the subsequent development of hypertension (59). Finally, all of the maneuvers that enhance insulin sensitivity in both diabetic and nondiabetic individuals also decrease blood pressure levels (60).

It is of note that, although insulin resistance is a typical feature of type 2 diabetes, there is a large interindividual variability among patients in the level of insulin resistance, and microalbuminuria is associated with a more severe reduction in insulin sensitivity (37). Reduced insulin sensitivity has also been found to be associated with sodium-sensitivity of blood pressure and with endothelial dysfunction, both of which are implicated in the target organ complications of diabetes (39,61).

MICROALBUMINURIA AND HYPERTENSION AS CARDIOVASCULAR RISK FACTORS

The presence of hypertension further increases the already high risk of CV disease associated with type 2 diabetes. The higher the systolic blood pressure (SBP), the greater the absolute excess risk, indicating a greater potential for prevention of CV death among patients with diabetes by control of elevated blood pressure (Fig. 17-2). There is an approximately twofold increased risk of CV disease in hypertensive compared with normotensive patients with diabetes; similarly, patients with diabetes have a twofold increased risk for cardiovascular disease, compared with patients without diabetes. The combination of diabetes and hypertension gives

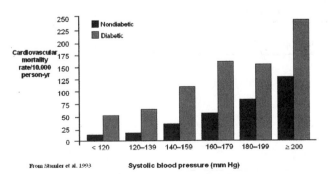

Association of Systolic BP and Cardiovascular Death in Type 2 Diabetes

From Stamler et al. 1993

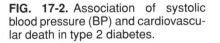

FIG. 17-2. Association of systolic blood pressure (BP) and cardiovascular death in type 2 diabetes.

an approximate fourfold increase in CV risk over the nondiabetic, normotensive population.

In a large cohort screened for the Multiple Risk Factor Intervention Trial (MRFIT), the relationships of SBP and other CV risk factors to CV mortality were compared in men with diabetes ($n = 5,163$) and men without diabetes ($n = 342,815$). The absolute risk of CV death was three times higher for men with diabetes than for those without diabetes, after adjustment for age, race, income, serum cholesterol concentration, SBP, and cigarette smoking ($p < .0001$). SBP was positively correlated with CV death in both nondiabetic and diabetic subjects ($p < .001$). At every level of SBP, CV death was much greater for men with diabetes than for men without diabetes. Moreover, with higher SBP levels, the CV mortality rate increased more steeply among those with diabetes than among those without diabetes (62) (Fig. 17-2). Therefore, the higher the SBP, the greater the absolute excess risk for patients with diabetes, indicating a greater potential for prevention of CV death among patients with diabetes by control of elevated blood pressure.

The simultaneous presence of hypertension and renal disease, as manifested by proteinuria, potentiates the mortality risk in patients with type 2 diabetes. Excess mortality, compared with the background population, was assessed from a 12-year follow-up of 4,714 patients with diabetes participating in the World Health Organization Multinational Study of Vascular Disease in Diabetes. Proteinuria and hypertension were the most important risk factors for mortality. Patients with both hypertension and proteinuria had a strikingly higher mortality risk: fivefold greater for men and eightfold greater for women with type 2 diabetes, compared with type 2 diabetic patients with normal BP and protein excretion (6).

This relationship between renal and CV complications of diabetes is also present at lower levels of urinary albumin excretion. Microalbuminuria is associated with a substantially increased risk of CV disease in diabetes. Several cross-sectional, retrospective and prospective studies have shown the predictive value of microalbuminuria for mortality, an association that is, at least in part, independent of other conventional risk factors. In all of these studies, the predominant cause of death was CV disease (Table 17-1) (63).

In type 1 diabetes, microalbuminuria is not only strongly predictive of the development of nephropathy, but it is also associated with a significant excess of coronary, cerebrovascular, and peripheral arterial disease. In prospective studies, type 1 diabetic patients with microalbuminuria have a significantly higher risk of dying from a CV cause (relative risk, 2.94; 95% confidence interval [CI], 1.18 to 7.34) (64). Coronary heart disease is likely at the stage of microalbuminuria, as evidenced by a reduction in aerobic work capacity and significant coronary lesions (65).

Although the conventional risk factors cannot entirely explain the reason for the interaction between microalbuminuria and CV disease, there is evidence that microalbuminuria is a marker of a generalized endothelial dysfunction. In diabetic patients with microalbuminuria, a variety of markers indicate endothelial dysfunction, including poor endothelial cell-dependent vasodilation

TABLE 17-1. *Microalbuminuria as a predictor of mortality in type 2 diabetes*

Study design	Follow-up (yr)	Outome (relative risk of death [95% confidence interval])
Retrospective		
Jarret et al., 1984	14	2.72 (1.3–5.74)
Mogensen, 1984	9	1.57 (1.2–2.03)
Schmitz and Vaeth, 1988	10	2.28 (unavailable)
Prospective		
Mattock et al., 1992	7	2.73 (81.3–5.73)
Damsgaard et al., 1986	8	1.57 (1.17–2.11)
MacLeod et al., 1995	8	1.7 (1.34–2.16)
Neil et al., 1993	6	2.15 (1.27–3.65)

and increased levels of von Willebrand factor, plasminogen activator inhibitor-1 (PAI-1), selectin, and fibrinogen (66). This suggests that microalbuminuria is associated with an impaired fibrinolytic and hypercoagulable state. There is evidence that the increase in Von Willebrand factor may precede the onset of microalbuminuria in diabetes (67). Many studies have also shown that there is a generalized increase in vascular permeability in subjects with microalbuminuria, as indicated by an increased transcapillary escape of albumin.

A growing body of evidence demonstrates, in microalbuminuria, the coexistence of insulin resistance and endothelial dysfunction. That the metabolic abnormalities of insulin resistance may lead to endothelial dysfunction is now well established (61).

The lipid abnormalities associated with insulin resistance may also contribute to the higher than expected CV risk in microalbuminuric patients. The concentrations of total cholesterol, very-low-density lipoprotein (VLDL) cholesterol, LDL cholesterol, and triglycerides rise with increasing AER in patients with type 1 diabetes. Additionally, there is an increase in LDL mass and atherogenic small, dense LDL particles (68), which correlates with plasma triglyceride concentrations and insulin resistance. Lower levels of HDL cholesterol are also commonly seen in patients with insulin resistance.

Left ventricular hypertrophy, a predictor of CV mortality, is also associated with microalbuminuria in diabetic subjects (51,69). The striking association between microalbuminuria and all these CV risk factors, typical of the insulin resistance syndrome, suggests the possibility of a common pathogenetic factor. A familial predisposition to development of microalbuminuria has been demonstrated, confirming the important role of genetic factors (70).

THE RENIN-ANGIOTENSIN SYSTEM AND DIABETIC NEPHROPATHY

There is no doubt that the diabetic milieu is necessary for diabetic glomerular lesions to develop. Both retrospective and prospective studies have suggested a relationship between blood glucose control and the risk of diabetic nephropathy. The Diabetes Control and Complications Trial (DCCT) (71) and the United Kingdom Prospective Diabetes Study (UKPDS) (72) have now precisely documented that the rate of development and progression of diabetic nephropathy is closely associated with glycemic control both in type 1 and type 2 diabetes. Nevertheless, in many patients, despite several years of poor diabetes control, no renal disease develops, as assessed by levels of urinary AER and level of GFR. It therefore appears, in humans, that hyperglycemia is necessary, but not sufficient, to cause renal damage and that other factors are needed for the manifestation of the clinical syndrome.

Early glomerular hemodynamic disturbances may directly participate in the development of glomerulosclerosis and its attendant proteinuria. In diabetes, transmission of systemic blood pressure to the glomerular capillaries is facilitated by a proportionally greater reduction in afferent versus efferent arteriolar resistance, with a consequent rise of the glomerular capillary hydraulic pressure (11). This increase in intraglomerular pressure was considered to play a pivotal role in mediating progressive glomerular injury in a range of renal diseases including diabetes (73). This hypothesis was partly based on findings in which reduction of intraglomerular pressure by a range of treatments, including angiotensin-converting enzyme (ACE) inhibitors and low-protein diet, was associated with reduced renal injury (74).

Elevated intraglomerular pressure via increased mechanical stress and shear forces may damage the endothelial surface and disrupt the normal structure of the glomerular barrier, eventually leading to mesangial proliferation, increased extracellular matrix production, and thickening of the glomerular basement membrane (75). These hemodynamic abnormalities usually are associated with hypertrophic changes in the glomerulus. Marked renal hypertrophy is a very early event in diabetes, and hyperplastic and hypertrophic changes in the diabetic kidney may precede the hemodynamic abnormalities. Distinct sequential molecular steps translate the mechanical stimuli of altered hemodynamics into metabolic and hypertrophic events. These steps include a sensing mechanism and translation of the signal to evoke changes in protein expression and enzymatic activity. Laminar shear stress results in generation of active transforming growth factor-β1 (TGF-β1) and platelet-derived growth factor (PDGF) and altered extracellular matrix deposition. Application of mechanical stretch induces not only matrix and TGF-β1 production in human mesangial cells, but also production of vascular endothelial growth factor (VEGF), one of the most powerful promoters of vascular permeability (76).

There is evidence that angiotensin II (Ang II) and growth factors play a role in mediating the hemodynamic and structural manifestations of diabetic nephropathy (77). In humans and experimental animals with diabetic nephropathy, ACE inhibitors and angiotensin receptor blockers (ARBs) decrease glomerular injury, by decreasing systemic blood pressure and glomerular capillary pressure. In glomerular, tubular, and interstitial cells, Ang II induces protein synthesis, hypertrophy, proliferation, and matrix expansion, suggesting nonhemodynamic mechanisms of Ang II-induced injury (78). Because diabetic nephropathy is characterized by low or normal circulating renin, activation of local renal renin-angiotensin system (RAS) has been incriminated in renal injury (79). Additionally, the biologic effects of Ang II may be mediated directly or through generation of other mediators, including growth factors.

Renin secretion by juxtaglomerular cells is the rate-limiting step for the generation of circulating Ang II. However, components of RAS also are expressed in many tissues where Ang II is generated locally. Non-ACE pathways of Ang II generation exist and include chymostatin angiotensin II-generating enzyme (CAGE), serine proteinase chymases, tissue plasminogen activator, cathepsin O, and tonin (80). In the human kidney, virtually all Ang I generation is renin dependent, but almost 40% of Ang I may be converted to Ang II by pathways other than ACE. The contribution of non-ACE pathways to angiotensin I and Ang II generation may be substantially augmented in diabetes mellitus. Hyperglycemia, elevated free fatty acids, and insulin resistance may regulate

RAS in the kidney. The status of the RAS in diabetes remains controversial. In general, plasma measurements of various components of the RAS are low or normal in diabetes. However, it is now clear that the RAS also acts locally within the kidney, with all components including enzymes and receptors present within the kidney. In vitro studies in proximal tubular cells have described increased angiotensinogen expression in response to glucose (81). In mesangial cells, hyperglycemia has also been reported to increase Ang II production in association with increased TGF-β production (82).

It is possible that, rather than a uniform change in these components within the kidney, there is primarily a change in the distribution of these proteins within its various compartments. For example, in experimental diabetes a redistribution of ACE to vascular and glomerular sites was reported (83). In the model of subtotal nephrectomy, which has functional and structural similarities to diabetic nephropathy, an increased proximal tubular renin expression was observed, which was attenuated by ACE inhibitor treatment (84). More recently, a similar phenomenon was reported in diabetic Ren 2 rats (a model in which the murine renin gene is introduced into the rat genome), with renin expression particularly in damaged tubules, which was reduced at this site by an Ang II receptor antagonist in the context of an increase in renin expression at the major site of synthesis, the juxtaglomerular apparatus (85). This increase in proximal tubular renin was associated with increased expression of Ang II.

Further evidence for the local activation of the RAS in the tubular compartment was suggested in studies measuring tubular renin by reverse transcription polymerase chain reaction. In those studies, there was an early increase in proximal tubular renin in experimental diabetes (86). This could contribute to a local increase in Ang II, resulting in tubulointerstitial fibrosis in this model. These findings emphasize changes in the distribution of the RAS in the diabetic kidney, which could be important in mediating progressive renal injury. Another important explanation for the disparity in the various measurements of both systemic and intrarenal RAS in diabetes and the responsiveness of the diabetic kidney to blockade of the RAS could be related to increased sensitivity of the diabetic kidney to Ang II (39,87).

Although Ang II has hemodynamic actions both systemically and within the kidney, it is becoming increasingly evident that Ang II has a range of nonhemodynamic effects relevant to progressive renal injury (78). It has been difficult to separate the hemodynamic from the nonhemodynamic effects *in vivo,* but the use of cultured cells has allowed investigators to explore these additional effects of Ang II. Ang II induces extracellular matrix accumulation, a hallmark of diabetic nephropathy, primarily through stimulation of the prosclerotic cytokine, TGF β (88). Several studies have shown that inhibition of the RAS in both nondiabetic and diabetic models of renal injury is associated with reduced renal expression of TGF-β, particularly in the tubulointerstitium (89).

Ang II may also influence a range of other cytokines, including protein kinase C (90) and the nuclear transcription factor, nuclear factor κB (NFκB) (91), which has been implicated in progressive renal injury.

Ang II also influences cell growth, proliferation, and apoptosis via a range of pathways not yet fully defined. In particular, Ang II-induced effects on cell cycle regulation could be relevant to various changes in the diabetic kidney, including renal hypertrophy (92). The reduction in glomerular hypertrophy, which is often observed with blockade of the RAS, may partly relate to effects on cell cycle regulation. For example, treatment of diabetic rats with ACE inhibitors was associated not only with reduced glomerular volume but also with abolition of glomerular expression of cyclin-dependent kinase inhibitors (93). These actions of Ang II may be central to how hemodynamic pathways interact with metabolic and glucose-dependent factors in accelerating diabetic nephropathy.

ACE inhibitors have clearly been shown to confer renoprotective effects, initially in experimental models of diabetic nephropathy, and ultimately in humans. These beneficial effects relate to the capacity of these agents to reduce blood pressure and to block Ang II formation. Although

ACE inhibitors have other effects, including inhibition of degradation of kinins, experimental studies using bradykinin and Ang II receptor antagonists indicate that the long-term renal protection given by these agents mostly occurs via the inhibition of Ang II-dependent pathways (94). The advent of selective Ang II receptor antagonists has allowed examination of the specific role of Ang II in mediating renal injury and provides a new approach for conferring renal protection in diabetic patients.

Ang II interacts with two specific receptors, known as the angiotensin type 1 (AT$_1$) and type 2 (AT$_2$) receptor subtypes. It is generally believed that most of the actions of Ang II occur via the AT$_1$ receptor, including its hemodynamic and prosclerotic effects. AT$_1$ receptors in mesangial cells mediate cell contraction, increased production and decreased degradation of extracellular matrix (ECM), hypertrophy, and increased production of growth factors. In podocytes, AT$_1$ receptors may induce contraction of foot processes and regulate glomerular filtration (87). In proximal tubular epithelial cells, activation of AT$_1$ receptors promotes protein synthesis, contributing to hypertrophy and interstitial matrix expansion.

Although the functional significance of the AT$_2$ receptor in the diabetic kidney remains to be elucidated, selective blockers of both receptor subtypes have been developed; however, long-term studies have reported only on blockers of the AT$_1$ receptor subtype. These studies demonstrated that AT$_1$ receptor blockade is renoprotective in both experimental and human diabetic nephropathy (see later discussion).

Further information about a possible role of RAS in the pathogenesis of diabetic nephropathy was provided by studies on genetic polymorphisms of the components of this system. Initially the insertion/deletion (I/D) polymorphism of the ACE gene, responsible for a large proportion of the genetic variation in serum ACE levels, was found to be associated with diabetic nephropathy in two small studies (95,96), but other case-control studies were unable to confirm this finding, although they did show a relationship with the CV complications of diabetic nephropathy (97,98). A recent multicenter study in type 1 diabetics with nephropathy and proliferative retinopathy showed that the severity of renal involvement was dependent on ACE I/D polymorphism, with a dominant effect of the ACE D allele (adjusted odds ratio for renal involvement attributable to the D allele, 1.9) (99). Although in this study there was no independent effect of angiotensin or AT_1 R polymorphisms on the risk for nephropathy, a significant interaction between ACE I/D and angiotensin AGT M235T polymorphisms was observed, suggesting the possibility that genetically determined angiotensin levels can affect risk for diabetic nephropathy through Ang I generation. Recent metaanalyses of published data from patients with type 2 diabetes have suggested a weak association of the D allele with nephropathy; the association seems to be stronger in Japanese populations, with a much smaller effect of the D allele in Caucasian patients (100). Therefore, within the limitations of available data, the ACE I/D polymorphism does not appear to play a major role in the initiation of diabetic nephropathy in Caucasian diabetic patients. Interestingly, ACE I/D polymorphism seems to affect the rate of GFR decline, once diabetic nephropathy is established (101,102). It has been suggested that ACE inhibition is less effective in preventing the GFR decline or in decreasing microalbuminuria in type 1 diabetic patients with the DD genotype.

TREATMENT OF HYPERTENSION IN DIABETES: END-ORGAN PROTECTION

The Kidney and the Eye

Using data from observational studies, it has been possible to derive in type 1 diabetic patients a threshold of mean arterial pressure at which no progression of microalbuminuria would be expected. This value corresponds to approximately 92 mm Hg. It is remarkable that, in patients with either type 1 or type 2 diabetes who remain persistently normoalbuminuric, the mean arterial pressure is constant at values of approximately 90 mm Hg. There is therefore a theoretical argument to aim for a blood pressure target of 125/75 mm Hg or less in patients with microalbuminuria (3). Treatment of hypertension and the use

of antihypertensive drugs have become central to the management of diabetes in patients at risk for renal disease.

Levels of Intervention

Three levels of intervention can be identified. In *primary prevention studies,* the use of antihypertensive agents has been found to reduce significantly the risk of developing raised AERs. In the UKPDS, newly diagnosed type 2 diabetics with hypertension were randomly assigned to tight versus less tight blood pressure control. Lowering of blood pressure to a mean value of 144/82 mm Hg significantly reduced the risk of developing albuminuria by approximately 33%. This result was obtained independently of the agents used, which in this study were captopril and atenolol (103). The Appropriate Blood Pressure Control in Diabetes (ABCD) trial evaluated the efficacy of intensive blood pressure control on normotensive and hypertensive patients with type 2 diabetes. Patients in the intensive therapy cohort were randomly assigned to receive either the calcium channel blocker nisoldipine or the ACE inhibitor enalapril. Because of a higher rate of fatal and nonfatal myocardial infarction, therapy with nisoldipine was terminated in the hypertensive cohort, following the recommendation of the Data and Safety Monitoring Committee (104). In this study, patients receiving intensive therapy achieved a mean blood pressure of 132/78 mm Hg, resulting in a lower all-cause mortality rate (5.5% versus 10.7%, $p = .037$) compared with patients receiving moderate therapy, who achieved a mean of 138/86 mm Hg. Further, hypertensive patients demonstrated stabilized renal function without overt albuminuria regardless of the therapy received (105). In the normotensive population, randomization to intensive blood pressure control resulted in a blood pressure of 128/75 mm Hg, compared with 137/81 mm Hg in the moderate control group. This resulted in a reduction in the rate of diabetic nephropathy, as measured by urinary albumin concentration, and a significant reduction in the rate of diabetic retinopathy or stroke (106).

In type 1 diabetic patients with normoalbuminuria and arterial blood pressure in the upper reaches of the normal distribution, the Eurodiab Controlled Trial of Lisinopril in Insulin Dependent Diabetes (EUCLID) study demonstrated that lisinopril (20 mg/day) significantly delayed the rise in AER over a period of 2 years. The lisinopril-treated group attained significantly lower blood pressure values (diastolic blood pressure, 74 versus 77 mm Hg) than did the control group, which received "true" placebo treatment (107).

Secondary prevention studies have addressed the question of preventing the transition from microalbuminuria to persistent clinical albuminuria and of reversal of microalbuminuria. A recent metaanalysis of several trials showed that the use of ACE inhibitors reduced the risk of progression from microalbuminuria to macroalbuminuria in type 1 diabetic patients by 62% and increased the likelihood of regression to normoalbuminuria threefold. The estimated treatment effect of ACE inhibition varied by baseline AER, inducing reductions that ranged from 74.1% in patients with an AER of 200 μg/min to 17.8% in patients with an AER of 20 μg/min. These effects were independent of other baseline risk factors (108).

Recently these issues were examined in patients with type 2 diabetes who had microalbuminuria with or without hypertension by a series of new studies. Parving et al. (109) demonstrated that use of the AT_1 receptor blocker irbesartan reduced the risk of progression to persistent clinical proteinuria by 70%. In their study, the control group had equivalent diastolic blood pressure control at 83 mm Hg, but the final SBP remained slightly higher than in the irbesartan-treated group (144 versus 141 mm Hg). Statistical adjustment for this difference did not alter the superiority of the ARB in its antialbuminuric effect (109).

The Microalbuminuria Reduction with Valsartan (MARVAL) study compared the effect of the ARB valsartan with the calcium channel blocker amlodipine on AER in type 2 diabetics with microalbuminuria. Although the reduction in blood pressure between the two groups was indistinguishable, valsartan had reduced AER by 44% after 6 months, compared with 8% for amlodipine ($p < .001$). The frequency of reversal to normoalbuminuria was 29.9% for valsartan versus 14.5% for amlodipine ($p = .001$), suggesting that the effect on albuminuria of this class of drugs is most likely blood pressure independent (110) (Fig. 17-1). It was also found, in the NESTOR study, that the diuretic indapamide SR was as effective as the ACE inhibitor enalapril in reducing blood pressure and AER in type 2 diabetics with hypertension and microalbuminuria (111).

Combination therapy with ACE inhibitors and ARBs may also contribute to further reduction of albuminuria, but this is likely to be an effect of greater blood pressure lowering (112). All of these studies employed the maximal recommended doses of inhibitors of the RAS to lower blood pressure. Preliminary data have been reported of a comparison between two treatment strategies, one based on a very low dose of perindopril and indapamide and the other on conventional doses of enalapril, in type 2 diabetic patients with hypertension and elevated AER, treated for 1 year. In the Preteraxin Albuminuria Regression (PREMIER) study, it was found that perindopril/indapamide reduced blood pressure and AER more effectively than enalapril did. The significant difference in the antialbuminuric effect (-42% versus -27%, $p = .002$) persisted even after adjustment for the small difference in blood pressure between the two treatment strategies (113).

Therefore, convincing evidence indicates that blockade of the RAS by either ACE inhibitors or ARBs is the most effective strategy to treat microalbuminuria and prevent its progression. The use as first-line treatment of a combination of ACE inhibition and a diuretic may be effective at lower drug doses and achieve antialbuminuric effects more promptly.

The use of ACE inhibitors also seems to benefit type 2 diabetic patients with microalbuminuria in terms of protection against CV events. In the Heart Outcomes Prevention Evaluation (HOPE) study, ramipril (10 mg/day) reduced significantly the risk of primary CV end points in type 2 diabetic patients with microalbuminuria, by approximately 30%. This risk reduction was limited to 15% in diabetic subjects with normoalbuminuria (114).

Additionally, studies have examined the effects of ACE inhibitors or ARBs on the

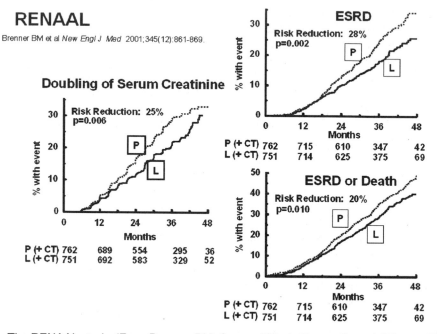

FIG. 17-3. The RENAAL study. (From Brenner BM, Cooper ME, de Zeeuw D, et al. Effects of losartan on renal and mortality outcomes in patients with type 2 diabetes and nephropathy. *N Engl J Med* 2001;345:861–869, with permission.) P, placebo; L, losartan.

progression of renal disease, the incidence of ESRD, and mortality in both type 1 and type 2 diabetics with established nephropathy. The Captopril Collaborative Study, which used the ACE inhibitor captopril in type 1 diabetic patients (115); the Reduction of Endpoints in NIDDM with the Angiotensin II Antagonist Losartan (RENAAL) study, which used losartan in type 2 patients (Fig. 17-3) (116); and the Irbesartan Diabetic Nephropathy Trial (IDNT) study, which used irbesartan in type 2 patients (117) all consistently showed that progression of renal failure, as measured by a doubling of the serum creatinine concentration, was significantly reduced by inhibition of the RAS. The risk reduction ranged from approximately 25% in patients with type 2 diabetes to 50% in those with type 1 diabetes. These trials also showed that the risk of ESRD and death was significantly reduced. Small but significant differences in blood pressure existed in these trials between the control group receiving conventional antihypertensive therapy and the experimental group receiving either ACE inhibitors or ARBs. Statistical adjustments for the blood pressure differences did not alter the significance of the results. Importantly, in the IDNT trial the irbesartan-treated group was also compared with an amlodipine-treated group. Blood pressure was reduced equally in these two groups with treatment, to 140/77 and 141/77 mm Hg, respectively, yet the relative risk of reaching the primary composite end point of doubling of serum creatinine, ESRD, or death from any cause was 23% lower in the irbesartan group ($p = .006$).

Cardiovascular Risk

Major studies in type 2 diabetes, or in "at risk" populations with type 2 diabetes mellitus as a subgroup, have addressed the question of the CV-protective effect of blood pressure-lowering maneuvers.

The UKPDS randomly assigned newly diagnosed type 2 diabetic subjects to tight versus less tight blood pressure control. The intensively treated group achieved an average blood pressure of 144/82 mm Hg, compared with 154/87 mm Hg in the group with less tight control. Better control of blood pressure resulted in a 24% reduction for

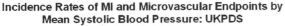

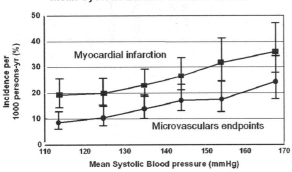

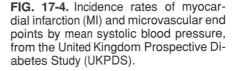

FIG. 17-4. Incidence rates of myocardial infarction (MI) and microvascular end points by mean systolic blood pressure, from the United Kingdom Prospective Diabetes Study (UKPDS).

any end point related to diabetes, a 32% reduction for diabetes-related death, 44% for stroke, 21% for myocardial infarction, and 39% for microvascular complications. As for the development of albuminuria, the risk reduction was independent of the antihypertensive agent used (captopril or atenolol) (104). In a further epidemiologic analysis of its prospective data, the UKPDS determined the relation between SBP and the risk of vascular complications. Among the 3,642 patients analyzed, the incidence of CV events was reduced by between 11% and 15% for each 10 mm Hg reduction in SBP. The lowest risk was observed in those patients with SBPs lower than 120 mm Hg (Fig. 17-4) (118).

Several other randomized, controlled trials (Table 17-2) have provided convincing evidence that reduction of blood pressure in diabetes reduces the risk of CV mortality and morbidity, including coronary heart disease, stroke, and congestive heart failure (114,119–126). These trials differed substantially in population studied, baseline risk status, degree of blood pressure reduction, drugs used at randomization, administration of other antihypertensive drugs during the study, and ascertainment of events. However, all showed that a reduction in arterial pressure is key for protection of the CV system in diabetes and indicated that even seemingly trivial reductions in arterial pressure can translate into a meaningful CV benefit. The results of most of the trials (with some notable exceptions; see Table 17-1) suggest that, given equivalent blood pressure reductions, the overall mortality and CV mortality effect of one class of drugs is similar to that

of the other. However, organ-specific protective effects appeared to differ among drugs (see later discussion).

HYPERTENSION MANAGEMENT GUIDELINES: MEETING THE TARGETS

Several national and international agencies have published new guidelines for the management of hypertension in diabetes. Table 17-3 shows some of the most often quoted international recommendations for clinical practice guidance (127 131). The guidelines outlined in the sixth report of the JNC recommended an aggressive program of blood pressure reduction, aiming for a target of less than 130/85 mm Hg in all diabetic patients and 125/75 mm Hg in those patients with proteinuria greater than 1 g/day. The objective of these recommendations is to contribute to the improvement in the treatment and control of hypertension over time. The recommendations mainly refer to type 2 diabetes, and proper guidelines for type 1 diabetes are absent.

Observational studies in nondiabetic subjects, both cross-sectional and prospective, confirm that there has been an improvement in the treatment and control of blood pressure but that optimal levels are still not achieved. For instance, among patients with coronary heart disease in Europe, who were studied in 1995–1996 and then again in 1999–2000, the proportion achieving a target blood pressure lower than 140/90 mm Hg with blood pressure-lowering drugs was low or did not change over time (44% versus 45%), even though there was an increase in the use of ACE

TABLE 17-2. *Cardiovascular outcome trials that included substantial numbers of patients with diabetes mellitus (DM)*

Trial	No. patients with DM	Entry criteria	Study design drug	% of patients receiving other drugs	Blood pressure basal (mm Hg)	Blood pressure attained (mm Hg)	Outcome
SHEP	583	Age >60 yr SBP ≥160 mm Hg DBP <90 mm Hg	Chlorthalidone + atenolol or reserpine	24	170/77	147/69	Chlortalidone reduced CVD events by 34%
SYST-EUR	492	Age ≥60 yr SBP 160–219 mm Hg DBP <95 mm Hg	Placebo *vs* Nitrendipine *vs* Placebo	54 / 43 / 62	170/75 / 175/85 / 175/85	157/71 / 153/78 / 162/82	Nitrendipine reduced total mortality by 55%, CVD mortality by 76%, all CVD events by 69%, stroke by 73%, CHD events by 63%
NORDIL	727	Age 50–74 yr DBP ≥100 mm Hg	Diltiazem *vs* β-blocker/diuretic	25 / 28	174/106 / 173/106	152/88 / 149/87	Both treatments equally effective in preventing the primary combined end points of all stroke, MI, and CVD deaths
INSIGHT	1302	Age 55–80 yr BP ≥ 150/95 mm Hg or SBP ≥160 mm Hg	Nifedipine GITS *vs* Diuretic	45 / 51	173/99 / 173/99	138/82 / 138/82	Both treatments equally effective in preventing CVD complications
HOT	1501	Age 50–80 yr DBP 110–115 mm Hg	Felodipine to all patients: 1. DBP = 80 mm Hg *vs* 2. DBP = 85 mm Hg *vs* 3. DBP = 95 mm Hg	100 / 92 / 79	170/105 / 166/105 / 170/105	140/81 / 141/83 / 143/85	51% reduction in major CVD events in target group 1 *vs* target group 3
HOPE	3577	Age > 55 yr Previous CVD event or one other CVD risk factor	Ramipril *vs* Placebo		142/80 / 142/79	140/77 / 143/77	Ramipril reduced risk of combined CVD events by 25%, MI by 22%, stroke by 33%, CVD death by 37%

328

Study	N	Inclusion criteria	Treatment		Baseline BP	Achieved BP	Results
CAPPP	572	Age 25–66 yr DBP ≥100 mm Hg	Captopril vs β-blocker/diuretic		164/97 163/97	152/90 150/88	Both treatments equally effective in preventing CVD mortality and morbidity; risk of stroke, fatal and nonfatal, was 43% higher in the captopril group
STOP-2	721	Age 70–84 yr SBP ≥180 mm Hg and/or DBP ≥105 mm Hg	Angiotensin-converting enzyme inhibitors vs Calcium channel blocker vs β-blocker/diuretic		194/98 194/98	159/81 159/80 158/81	All treatments effective in prevention of CVD mortality and morbidity
LIFE	1195	Age 55–80 yr SBP 160–200 mm Hg DBP 95/115 mm Hg and LVH	Losartan vs Atenolol	50 46	194/98 176/97 177/96	158/81 146/79 148/79	Losartan reduced risk of primary composite CVD events by 24.5%, CVD mortality by 36.6%, total mortality by 38%, MI by 17.1% n.s., stroke by 21.1% n.s.
ALLHAT	12063	Age ≥55 yr Stage 1 or 2 hypertension with at least one additional CVD risk factor	Chlorthalidone vs Amlodipine vs Lisinopril	41 40 43	156/89 157/90 156/89	134/75 135/75 136/75	No difference between treatments for the primary outcome (combined fatal and nonfatal CHD) and all-cause mortality

CVD, cardiovascular disease; DBP, diastolic blood pressure; MI, myocardial infarction; SBP, systolic blood pressure.
Data obtained from original publications; missing values were not available. Actual blood pressure values for diabetic patients were used whenever available or derived from graphs if not reported in text.

TABLE 17-3. *Target blood pressure (BP) values for management of hypertension in diabetes*

Recommending body	Year of recommendation	Target systolic BP	Target diastolic BP
Joint National Committee VI	1997	< 130	< 85
In patients with proteinuria		= 125	= 75
American Diabetes Association	2002	<130	<80
European NIDDM Policy Group	1999	<140	<80
European Diabetes Policy Group for type 1 DM with proteinuria	1999	<130	<80
WHO/ISH	1999	<130	<85

inhibitors from 30% to 43% and in β-blockers from 54% to 66% (132). In the United States, data from the National Health and Nutrition Examination Survey comparing the period 1976–1980 with 1991–1994 showed that the proportion of hypertensive patients treated with blood pressure-lowering drugs increased from 31% to 53% and the percentage of subjects obtaining blood pressures lower than 140/90 mm Hg rose from 10% to 27% between the two time periods (127).

Cross-sectional data available for type 2 diabetes in Europe indicate that only 35% of subjects reach the recommended SBP target of 140 mm Hg and 53% reach the diastolic BP target of 85 mm Hg. Across Europe, the average attained blood pressure values in type 2 diabetic patients with hypertension were 146/82 mm Hg (133).

In type 1 diabetes, the Pittsburgh Epidemiology of Diabetes Complications study showed an increase in control of hypertension from 38% to 49.5% between 1986–1988 and 1996–1999 (134). Another report on type 1 diabetes, from the EURODIAB Prospective Complications Study, compared the periods 1989–1990 and 1997–1999 (135). In the later period, a greater proportion of hypertensive patients were receiving treatment (69% versus 40%), and there was a modest increase (from 36% to 41%) in the proportion achieving control of hypertension (blood pressure lower than 140/90 mm Hg). The largest increase in the proportion treated was seen in the hypertensive patients with microalbuminuria (from 35% to 76%) or macroalbuminuria (from 64% to 95%). This suggests a heightened awareness among physicians of the added risk in patients who develop albuminuria. Regrettably, however, control of hypertension in albuminuric

patients was less than 50% and had not changed between the two time periods.

These figures indicate that there is ample scope for improvement in the control of blood pressure. Multiple factors are likely to be involved. It has been suggested that age, duration of diabetes, male sex, alcohol intake, obesity, and patient education may partly explain the reason for poor control. The cost and side effects of drugs, the complexity of treatment regimens, patients' compliance, and lifestyle may also contribute. From the physician's standpoint, factors such as knowledge and acceptance of guidelines, a reluctance to use multiple drug therapy, costs of drugs, dosing of drugs, and side effects have been implicated as explanations for poor management of elevated blood pressure.

DRUG CHOICE: THE NEED FOR POLYPHARMACY

Some clear indications have emerged from the several comparative clinical trials to indicate that, beyond reduction of blood pressure, protective effects differ among drugs and are likely to be organ specific.

ACE inhibitors and ARBs seem to be the unequivocal choice for renal protection. There is evidence that their effect extends beyond the reduction of blood pressure and that reduction of proteinuria is an important goal in its own right to reduce progression of renal failure (136). ACE inhibitors (and to a lesser degree ARBs) have also proved very effective in lowering rates of coronary heart disease, heart failure, and CV mortality. This conclusion was also suggested in trials in which coronary events and congestive heart failure were not the primary outcome measures (137,138). Calcium channel blockers, both dihydropyridine and nondihydropyridine compounds, have proved particularly efficacious in reducing the rates of stroke. β-Blockers and diuretics have confirmed efficacy in reducing coronary heart disease events.

A note of caution is required for the use of doxazosin. In the Anti-hypertensive and Lipid-lowering Therapy to Reduce Heart Attack (ALLHAT) study, the doxazosin monotherapy arm was stopped because, compared with the chlorthalidone group, patients receiving doxazosin had a 19% higher risk of stroke, a 25% higher risk of CV disease, a doubling of congestive heart failure, and a 16% higher risk of angina (139). Whether doxazosin as part of a multidrug regimen results in these untoward effects and detracts from the benefits of other antihypertensive agents is not known.

In clinical practice, it is a common experience that several antihypertensive agents are required to achieve the desired reduction in blood pressure in diabetic patients. Moreover, diuretics are almost invariably needed to achieve goals of therapy, because they enhance the efficacy of all other classes of antihypertensive drugs and because excess fluid retention is a common feature of hypertension in diabetes, more prominently in diabetic patients who develop renal disease. It is important to note that in the recent published results of the ALLHAT study, the thiazide diuretic, chlortalidone, reduced CV events as much as did ACE inhibitors and calcium channel blockers in diabetic patients with hypertension (140). Because this study also demonstrated that a large proportion of patients required more than one drug to control their blood pressure, it is reasonable to infer that a diuretic should be included in all multidrug regimens.

An additional consideration is that diabetic patients with hypertension often have multiple risk factors for vascular complications including dyslipidemia, insulin resistance, and coagulation disorders. A multifaceted, intensive therapy to correct all risk factors must be considered in these patients.

In a randomized, controlled trial of intensive therapy that included lifestyle modifications, smoking cessation, antihypertensive drugs, lipid-lowering drugs, aspirin, and tight control of blood pressure and blood glucose, compared with conventional care by general practitioners in type 2 diabetic patients with microalbuminuria observed for 7.8 years, those patients receiving intensive therapy showed a significantly lower risk of CV disease (hazard ratio [HR], 0.47), nephropathy (HR, 0.39), retinopathy (HR, 0.42), and autonomic neuropathy (HR, 0.37) (141). This trial highlights the need for an aggressive strategy to affect in a positive way the outcomes of persons with type 2 diabetes mellitus.

In conclusion, physicians and patients together have now the means to manage blood pressure elevation and to target treatments to protection against end organ damage. Multifactorial treatment regimens are often needed in diabetic patients to prevent, delay, arrest, and perhaps reverse vascular complications.

REFERENCES

1. Renal Data System. *USRDS 2000 annual data report* Bethesda, MD: National Institute of Diabetes and Digestive and Kidney Diseases, 2001.
2. European Dialysis and Transplant Association. Report on management of renal failure in Europe, XXVI, 1995. *Nephrol Dial Transplant* 1996;11[Suppl 7]:1–32.
3. Mogensen CE, Kerne WF, Bennett PH, et al. Prevention of diabetic renal disease with special reference to microalbuminuria. *Lancet* 1995;346:1080–1084.
4. Parving HH, Gall MA, Skott P, et al. Prevalence and causes of albuminuria in non-insulin-dependent diabetic patients. *Kidney Int* 1992;41:758–762.
5. Andersen AR, Christiansen JS, Andersen JK, et al. Diabetic nephropathy in type I diabetes: an epidemiological study. *Diabetologia* 1983;25:496–501.
6. Colhoun HM, Lee ET, Bennett PH, et al. Risk factor for renal failure: the WHO multinational study of vascular disease in diabetes. *Diabetologia* 2001;44[Suppl 2]:S46–S53.
7. Mogensen CE. Glomerular filtration rate and renal plasma flow in short-term and long-term juvenile diabetes mellitus. *Scand J Clin Lab Invest* 1971;28:91–100.
8. Wiseman MJ, Viberti GC, Keen H. Threshold effect of plasma glucose in the glomerular hyperfiltration in diabetics. *Nephron* 1984;48:257–260.
9. Wiseman MJ, Saunders AJ, Keen H, et al. Effect of blood glucose on increased glomerular filtration rate and kidney size in insulin-dependent diabetes. *N Engl J Med* 1985;312:617–621.
10. Wiseman MJ, Viberti GC. Kidney size and GFR in type 1 insulin-dependent diabetes mellitus revisited. *Diabetologia* 1983;25:530.
11. Hostetter TH, Troy JC, Brenner BM. Glomerular

hemodynamics in experimental diabetes mellitus. *Kidney Int* 1981;19:410–415.

12. Viberti CG, Jarrett RJ, Mahmud U, et al. Microalbuminuria as a predictor of clinical nephropathy in insulin-dependent diabetes mellitus. *Lancet* 1982;1:1430–1432.

13. Parving HH, Oxenboll B, Svendsen PA, et al. Early detection of patients at risk of developing diabetic nephropathy: a longitudinal study of urinary albumin excretion. *Acta Endocrinol* 1982;100:550–555.

14. Mathiesen ER, Oxenboll B, Johansen K, et al. Incipient nephropathy in type 1 (insulin-dependent) diabetes. *Diabetologia* 1984;26:406–410.

15. Mogensen CE, Christensen CK. Predicting diabetic nephropathy in insulin-dependent diabetic patients. *N Engl J Med* 1984;311:89–93.

16. Cohen DL, Close CF, Viberti GC. The variability of overnight urinary albumin excretion in insulin-dependent diabetic and normal subjects. *Diabet Med* 1987;4:437–440.

17. EURODIAB IDDM Complications Study Group. Microvascular and acute complications in IDDM patients: the EURODIAB IDDM Complications Study. *Diabetologia* 1994;37:278–285.

18. Fioretto P, Steffes MW, Mauer M. Glomerular structure in nonproteinuric IDDM patients with various levels of albuminuria. *Diabetes* 1994;48:1358–1364.

19. Feldt-Rasmussen B, Mathiesen E, Deckert T. Effect of two years of strict metabolic control on the progression of incipient nephropathy in insulin-dependent diabetes. *Lancet* 1986;2:1300–1304.

20. Wiseman M, Viberti GC, Mackintosh D, et al. Glycaemia, arterial pressure and microalbuminuria in type I (insulin-dependent) diabetes mellitus. *Diabetologia* 1984;26:401–405.

21. Viberti GC, Bilous RW, Mackintosh D, et al. Monitoring glomerular function in diabetic nephropathy. *Am J Med* 1983;74:256–264.

22. Alaveras AE, Thomas SM, Sagriotis A, et al. Promoters of progression of diabetic nephropathy: the relative roles of blood glucose and blood pressure control. *Nephrol Dial Transplant* 1997;2:71–74.

23. Remuzzi A, Bertani T. Is glomerulosclerosis a consequence of altered glomerular permeability to macromolecules? *Kidney Int* 1990;4:384–394.

24. Rossing P, Hommel E, Smidt UM, et al. Impact of arterial blood pressure and albuminuria on the progression of diabetic nephropathy in IDDM patients. *Diabetes* 1993;42:715–719.

25. Remuzzi G, Bertani T. Pathophysiology of progressive nephropathies. *N Engl J Med* 1998;339:1448–1456.

26. Breyer JA, Bain P, Evans JK, et al. Predictors of the progression of renal insufficiency in patients with insulin-dependent diabetes and overt nephropathy. *Kidney Int* 1996;50:1651–1658.

27. Ritz E, Stefanski A. Diabetic nephropathy in type 2 diabetes. *Am J Kidney Dis* 1996;27:167–194.

28. Gall MA, Rossing P, Skott P, et al. Prevalence of micro- and macroalbuminuria, arterial hypertension, retinopathy and large vessel disease in European type 2 (non-insulin-dependent) diabetic patients. *Diabetologia* 1991;34:655–661.

29. Gall MA, Nielsen FS, Smidt UM, et al. The course of kidney function in type 2 (non-insulin-dependent) dia-

betic patients with diabetic nephropathy. *Diabetologia* 1993;36:1071–1078.

30. Lippert J, Ritz E, Schwarzbeck A, et al. The rising tide of endstage renal failure from diabetic nephropathy type II: an epidemiological analysis. *Nephrol Dial Transplant* 1995;10:462–467.

31. Adler AI, Stevens RJ, Manley SE, et al. Development and progression of nephropathy in type 2 diabetes: the United Kingdom Prospective Diabetes Study (UKPDS 64). *Kidney Int* 2003;63:225–232.

32. Mattock MB, Morrish NJ, Viberti GC, et al. Prospective study of microalbuminuria as predictor of mortality in NIDDM. *Diabetes* 1992;41:736–741.

33. Valmadrid CT, Klein R, Moss SE, et al. The risk of cardiovascular mortality associated with microalbuminuria and gross proteinuria in persons with older-onset diabetes mellitus. *Arch Intern Med* 2000;160:1093–1100.

34. Tiengo A, Briani G, Fedele D, et al. Prevalence of micro- and macro-albuminuria in Italian type II (non-insulin dependent) diabetic patients. *Diab Nutr Metab* 1996;9:59–66.

35. Mogensen CE. Microalbuminuria, blood pressure and diabetic renal disease: origin and development of ideas. *Diabetologia* 1999;42:263–285.

36. Stehouwer CD, Gall MA, Twisk JW, et al. Increased urinary albumin excretion, endothelial dysfunction, and chronic low-grade inflammation in type 2 diabetes: progressive, interrelated, and independently associated with risk of death. *Diabetes* 2002;51:1157–1165.

37. Yip J, Mattock M, Morocutti A, et al. Insulin resistance in insulin-dependent diabetic patients with microalbuminuria. *Lancet* 1993;342:883–887.

38. Imanishi M, Yoshioka K, Okumura M, et al. Sodium sensitivity related to albuminuria appearing before hypertension in type 2 diabetic patients. *Diabetes Care* 2001;24:111–116.

39. Trevisan R, Bruttomesso D, Vedovato M, et al. Enhanced responsiveness of blood pressure to sodium intake and to angiotensin II is associated with insulin resistance in IDDM patients with microalbuminuria. *Diabetes* 1998;47:1347–1353.

40. Microalbuminuria Collaborative Study Group. Risk factors for development of microalbuminuria in insulin-dependent diabetic patients: a cohort study. *B Med J* 1993;306:1235–1239.

41. Nelson RG, Pettitt DJ, Baird HR, et al. Prediabetic blood pressure predicts urinary albumin excretion after the onset of type 2 (noninsulin-dependent) diabetes mellitus in Pima Indians. *Diabetologia* 1993;36:998–1001.

42. Mangili R, Deferrari G, Di Mario U, et al. Arterial hypertension and microalbuminuria in IDDM: the Italian Microalbuminuria Study. *Diabetologia* 1994;3710:1015–1024.

43. Lurbe E, Redon J, Kesani A, et al. Increase in nocturnal blood pressure and progression to microalbuminuria in type 1 diabetes. *N Engl J Med* 2002;347:797–805.

44. Viberti GC, Keen H, Wiseman MJ. Raised arterial pressure in parents of proteinuric insulin-dependent diabetic. *BMJ* 1987;295:515–517.

45. Krolewski AS, Canessa M, Warram J, et al. Predisposition to hypertension and susceptibility to renal disease in insulin-dependent diabetes mellitus. *N Engl J Med* 1988;318:140–145.

46. Mangili R, Bending JJ, Scott G, et al. Increased sodium-lithium countertransport activity in red cells of patients with insulin-dependent diabetes and nephropathy. *N Engl J Med* 1988;318:146–150.

47. Jones SL, Trevisan R, Tariq T, et al. Sodium-lithium countertransport in microalbuminuric insulin-dependent diabetic patients. *Hypertension* 1990;15:570–575.

48. Morocutti A, Barzon I, Solini A, et al. Poor metabolic control and predisposition to hypertension, rather than hypertension itself, are risk factors for nephropathy in type 2 diabetes. *Acta Diabet* 1992;29:123–126.

49. Walker JD, Tariq T, Viberti GC. Sodium-lithium countertransport activity in red cells of patients with insulin-dependent diabetes and nephropathy and their parents. *BMJ* 1990;301:635–638.

50. Hardman TC, Dubrey SW, Leslie RD, et al. Erythrocyte sodium-lithium countertransport and blood pressure in identical twin pairs discordant for insulin-dependent diabetes. *BMJ* 1992;305:215–219.

51. Trevisan R, Nosadini R, Fioretto P, et al. Clustering of risk factors in hypertensive insulin-dependent diabetics with high sodium-lithium countertransport *Kidney Int* 1992;41:855–861.

52. Ng LL, Simmons D, Frighi V, et al. Leukocyte sodium-hydrogen antiport activity in type 1 (insulin-dependent) diabetic patients with nephropathy. *Diabetologia* 1990;33:371–377.

53. Semplicini A, Mozzato MG, Sama B, et al. Sodium-hydrogen and lithium-sodium exchange in red cells of normotensive and hypertensive patients with insulin-dependent diabetes mellitus. *Am J Hypertens* 1989;2:174–177.

54. Trevisan R, Li LK, Messent J, et al. Na/H antiport activity and cell growth in cultured skin fibroblasts of IDDM patients with nephropathy. *Diabetes* 1992;41:1239–1246.

55. Ng LL, Davies JE, Siczkowski M, et al. Abnormal sodium-hydrogen antiporter phenotype and turnover of immortalized lymphoblasts from type 1 diabetic patients with nephropathy. *J Clin Invest* 1994;93:2750–2757.

56. Trevisan R, Fioretto P, Barbosa J, et al. Insulin-dependent diabetic sibling pairs are concordant for sodium-hydrogen antiport activity. *Kidney Int* 1999;55:2383–2389.

57. Reaven G. Metabolic syndrome. *Circulation* 2002;106:286–288.

58. Facchini F, Chen YD, Clinkingbeard C, et al. Insulin resistance, hyperinsulinemia, and dyslipidemia in nonobese individuals with a family history of hypertension. *Am J Hypertens* 1992;5:694–699.

59. Skafors ET, Lithell HO, Selinus I. Risk factors for the development of hypertension: a 10-year longitudinal study in middle-aged men. *J Hypertens* 1991;9:217–223.

60. Reisin E, Abel R, Modan M, et al. Effect of weight loss without salt restriction on the reduction of blood pressure in overweight hypertensive patients. *N Engl J Med* 1978;298:1–6.

61. Calles-Escandon J, Cipolla M. Diabetes and endothelial dysfunction: a clinical perspective. *Endocr Rev* 2001;22:36–52.

62. Stamler J, Vaccaro O, Neaton JD, et al. Diabetes, other risk factors, and 12-yr cardiovascular mortality for men screened in the Multiple Risk Factor Intervention Trial. *Diabetes Care* 1993;16:434–444.

63. Dinneen SF, Gerstein HC. The association of microalbuminuria and mortality in non-insulin-dependent diabetes mellitus: a systematic overview of the literature. *Arch Intern Med* 1997;157:1413–1418.

64. Messent JW, Elliott TG, Hill RD, et al. Prognostic significance of microalbuminuria in insulin dependent diabetes mellitus: a 23-year follow-up study. *Kidney Int* 1992;41:836–839.

65. Earle KA, Mishra A, Morocutti A, et al. Microalbuminuria as a marker of silent myocardial ischemia in IDDM patients. *Diabetologia* 1996;39:854–856.

66. Thomas SM, Viberti GC. Microalbuminuria and cardiovascular disease. In: CE Mogensen, ed. *The kidney and hypertension in diabetes,* 4th ed. Boston: Kluwer Academic Publishers, 1998;39–50.

67. Stehouwer CD, Fisher HR, van Kuijk AW, et al. Endothelial dysfunction precedes development of microalbuminuria in IDDM. *Diabetes* 1995;44:561–564.

68. Sniderman AD, Scantlebury T, Cianflone K. Hypertriglyceridemic hyperapoB: the unappreciated atherogenic dyslipoproteinemia in type 2 diabetes mellitus. *Ann Intern Med* 2001;135:447–459.

69. Redon J, Gomez-Sanchez MA, Baldo E, et al. Microalbuminuria is correlated with left ventricular hypertrophy in male hypertensive patients. *J Hypertens* 1991;9[Suppl 1]:48–49.

70. Forsblom CM, Kanninen T, Lehtovirta M, et al. Heritability of albumin excretion rate in families of patients with type II diabetes. *Diabetologia* 1999;42:1359–1366.

71. The Diabetes Control and Complications Trial Research Group. The effect of intensive treatment on the development and progression of long-term complications in insulin-dependent diabetes mellitus. *N Engl J Med* 1993;329:977–986.

72. United Kingdom Prospective Diabetes Study Group. Intensive blood-glucose control with sulphonylureas or insulin compared with conventional treatment and risk of complications in patients with type 2 diabetes (UKPDS 33). *Lancet* 1998;352:837–853.

73. Hostetter T, Rennke H, Brenner B. The case for intrarenal hypertension in the initiation and progression of diabetic and other glomerulopathies. *Am J Med* 1982;72:375–380.

74. Zatz R, Dunn BR, Meyer MV, et al. Prevention of diabetic glomerulopathy by pharmacological amelioration of glomerular capillary hypertension. *J Clin Invest* 1986;77:1925–1930.

75. Cortes P, Riser BL. The nature of the diabetic glomerulus: pressure induced and metabolic aberrations. In: CE Mogensen, ed. *The kidney and hypertension in diabetes,* 4th ed. Boston: Kluwer Academic Publishers, 1998;7–16.

76. Gruden G, Thomas S, Burt D, et al. Mechanical stretch induces vascular permeability factor in human mesangial cells: mechanisms of signal transduction. *Proc Natl Acad Sci U S A* 1997;94:12112–12116.

77. Cooper ME. Interaction of metabolic and haemodynamic factors in mediating experimental diabetic nephropathy. *Diabetologia* 2001;44:1957–1972.

78. Wolf G, Ziyadeh FN. The role of angiotensin II in diabetic nephropathy: emphasis on non-hemodynamic mechanisms. *Am J Kidney Dis* 1997;29:153–163.

79. Leehey DJ, Singh AK, Alavi N, et al. Role of angiotensin II in diabetic nephropathy. *Kidney Int* 2000; 58:S93–S98.

80. Williams B. The renin angiotensin system in the pathogenesis of diabetic complications. In: CE Mogensen, ed. *The kidney and hypertension in diabetes*, 5th ed. Boston: Kluwer Academic Publishers, 2000;645–654.

81. Zhang SL, Filep JG, Hohman TC, et al. Molecular mechanisms of glucose action on angiotensinogen gene expression in rat proximal tubular cells. *Kidney Int* 1999;55:454–464.

82. Singh R, Alavi N, Singh AK, et al. Role of angiotensin II in glucose-induced inhibition of mesangial matrix degradation. *Diabetes* 1999;48:2066–2073.

83. Anderson S, Jung FF, Ingelfinger JR. Renal renin-angiotensin system in diabetes: functional, immunohistochemical, and molecular biological correlations. *Am J Physiol* 1993;265:F477–F486.

84. Gilbert RE, Wu LL, Kelly DJ, et al. Pathological expression of renin and angiotensin II in the renal tubule after subtotal nephrectomy: implications for the pathologenesis of tubulointerstitial fibrosis. *Am J Pathol* 1999;155:429–440.

85. Kelly DJ, Skinner SL, Gilbert RE, et al. Effects of endothelin or angiotensin Il receptor blockade on diabetes in the transgenic (mRen-2)27 rat. *Kidney Int* 2000;57:1882–1894.

86. Zimpelmann J, Kumar D, Levine DZ, et al. Early diabetes mellitus stimulates proximal tubule renin mRNA expression in the rat. *Kidney Int* 2000;58:2320–2330.

87. Burns KD. Angiotensin II and its receptors in the diabetic kidney. *Am J Kidney Dis* 2000;36:449–467.

88. Kagami S, Border WA, Miller DE, et al. Angiotensin II stimulates extracellular matrix protein synthesis through induction of transforming growth factor-beta expression in rat glomerular mesangial cells. *J Clin Invest* 1994;93:2431–2437.

89. Gilbert RE, Cox A, Wu LL, et al. Expression of transforming growth factor-beta1 and type IV collagen in the renal tubulointerstitium in experimental diabetes: effect of ACE inhibition. *Diabetes* 1998;47:414–422.

90. Nagahama T, Hayashi K, Ozawa Y, et al. Role of PKC in angiotensin II-induced constriction of renal microvessels. *Kidney Int* 2000;57:215–223.

91. Ruiz-Ortega M, Lorenzo O, Ruperez M, et al. Angiotensin II activates nuclear transcription factor kappa B through AT(1) and AT(2) in vascular muscle cells: molecular mechanisms. *Circ Res* 2000;86:1266–1272.

92. Shankland SJ, Wolf G. Cell cycle regulatory proteins in renal disease: role in hypertrophy, proliferation, and apoptosis. *Am J Physiol* 2000;278:F515–F529.

93. Wolf G. Cell cycle regulation in diabetic nephropathy. *Kidney Int* 2000;58:S59–S66.

94. Allen TJ, Cao Z, Youssef S, et al. The role of angiotensin II and bradykinin in experimental diabetic nephropathy: functional and structural studies. *Diabetes* 1997;46:1612–1618.

95. Doria A, Warram JH, Krowlewski AS. Genetic predisposition to diabetic nephropathy: evidence for a role of the angiotensin I-converting enzyme gene. *Diabetes* 1994;43:690–695.

96. Marre M, Bernadet P, Gallois Y, et al. Relationships between angiotensin I converting enzyme gene poly-

morphism, plasma levels, and diabetic retinal and renal complications. *Diabetes* 1994;43:384–388.

97. Tarnow L, Gluud C, Parving HH. Diabetic nephropathy and the insertion/deletion polymorphism of the angiotensin-converting enzyme gene. *Nephrol Dial Transplant* 1998;13:1125–1130.

98. Tarnow L, Cambien F, Rossing P, et al. Insertion/ deletion polymorphism in the angiotensin-I-converting enzyme gene is associated with coronary heart disease in IDDM patients with diabetic nephropathy. *Diabetologia* 1995;38:798–803.

99. Marre M, Jeunemaitre X, Gallois Y, et al. Contribution of genetic polymorphism in the renin-angiotensin system to the development of renal complications in insulin-dependent diabetes. *J Clin Invest* 1997;99:1585–1595.

100. Fujisawa T, Ikegami H, Kawaguchi Y, et al. Meta-analysis of association of insertion/deletion polymorphism of angiotensin I-converting enzyme gene with diabetic nephropathy and retinopathy. *Diabetologia* 1998;41:47–53.

101. Parving HH, Jacobsen P, Tarnow L, et al. Effect of deletion polymorphism of angiotensin converting enzyme gene on progression of diabetic nephropathy during inhibition of angiotensin converting enzyme, observational follow-up study. *BMJ* 1996;313:591–594.

102. Penno G, Chaturvedi N, Talmud PJ, et al. Effect of angiotensin-converting enzyme gene polymorphism on progression of renal disease and the influence of ACE inhibition in IDDM patients. *Diabetes* 1998;47:1507–1511.

103. United Kingdom Prospective Diabetes Study Group. Tight blood pressure control and risk of macrovascular and microvascular complications in type 2 diabetes (UKPDS 35). *BMJ* 1998;317:703–713.

104. Estacio RO, Jeffers BW, Hiatt WR, et al. The effect of nisoldipine as compared with enalapril on cardiovascular outcomes in patients with non-insulin-dependent diabetes and hypertension. *N Engl J Med* 1998;338:645–652.

105. Estacio RO, Gifford N, Jaffers BW, et al. Effect of blood pressure control on diabetic microvascular complications in patients with hypertension and type 2 diabetes. *Diabetes Care* 2000;23[Suppl 2]:B54–B64.

106. Schrier RW, Estacio RO, Esler A, et al. Effects of aggressive blood pressure control in normotensive type 2 diabetic patients on albuminuria, retinopathy and stroke. *Kidney Int* 2002;61:1086–1097.

107. The EUCLID Study Group. Randomised placebo-controlled trial of lisinopril in normotensive patients with insulin-dependent diabetes and normoalbuminuria or microalbuminuria. *Lancet* 1997;349:1787–1792.

108. The ACE Inhibitors in Diabetic Nephropathy Trialist Group. Should all type 1 diabetic patients with microalbuminuria receive ACE inhibitor treatment? A meta regression analysis. *Ann Intern Med* 2001;134:370–379.

109. Parving HH, Lehnert H, Brochner-Mortensen J, et al., for the Irbesartan in Patients with Type 2 Diabetes and Microalbuminuria Study Group. The effect of irbesartan on the development of diabetic nephropathy in patients with type 2 diabetes. *N Engl J Med* 2001;345:870–878.

110. Viberti GC, Wheeldon NM, for the MARVAL Study Investigators. Microalbuminuria reduction with

valasartan in patients with type 2 diabetes mellitus: a blood pressure independent effect. *Circulation* 2002;106:672–678.

111. Marre M, Fernandez M, Garcia Ruig J, et al. Indapamide SR is as efficient as enalapril in reducing microalbuminuria in type 2 diabetic hypertensive patients. *J Hypertens* 2002;20[Suppl 4]:S163.

112. Mogensen CE, Neldam S, Tikkanen I, et al. Randomised controlled trial of dual blockade of renin-angiotensin system in patients with hypertension, microalbuminuria, and non-insulin dependent diabetes: the Candesartan and Lisinopril Microalbuminuria (CALM) study. *BMJ* 2000;321:1440–1444.

113. Mogensen CE, Viberti G. Halimi S, et al. Effect of low-dose Perindopril/Indapamide on albuminuria in diabetes. (Preterax in albuminuria regression-PREMIER *Hypertension* 2003;41:1063–1071.

114. Heart Outcomes Prevention Evaluation (HOPE) Study Investigators. Effects of ramipril on cardiovascular and microvascular outcomes in people with diabetes mellitus: results of the HOPE study and MICRO HOPE substudy. *Lancet* 2000;355:253–259.

115. Lewis EJ, Hunsicker LG, Bain RP, et al., for the Collaborative Study Group. The effect of angiotensin-converting-enzyme inhibition on diabetic nephropathy. *N Engl J Med* 1993;329:1456–1462.

116. Brenner BM, Cooper ME, De Zeeuw D, et al., for the RENAAL Study Investigators. Effects of losartan on renal and cardiovascular outcomes in patients with type 2 diabetes and nephropathy. *N Engl J Med* 2001;345:861–869.

117. Lewis EJ, Hunsicker LG, Clarke WR, et al., for the Collaborative Study Group. Renoprotective effect of the angiotensin-receptor antagonist irbesartan in patients with nephropathy due to type 2 diabetes. *N Engl J Med* 2001;345:851–860.

118. Adler AI, Stratton IM, Nell HA, et al. Association of systolic blood pressure with macrovascular and microvascular complications of type 2 diabetes: prospective observational study. *BMJ* 2000;321:412–419.

119. Curb JD, Pressel SL, Cutler JA, et al., for the Systolic Hypertension in the Elderly Program Cooperative Research Group. Effect of diuretic-based antihypertensive treatment on cardiovascular disease risk in older diabetic patients with isolated systolic hypertension. *JAMA* 1996;276:1886–1892.

120. Tuomilehto J, Rastenyte D, Birkenhäger WH, et al., for the Systolic Hypertension in Europe Trial Investigators. Effects of calcium-channel blockade in older patients with diabetes and systolic hypertension. *N Engl J Med* 1999;340:677–684.

121. Hansson L, Hedner I, Lund-Johansen P, et al., for the NORDIL Study Group. Randomised trial of effect of calcium antagonists compared with diuretics and beta-blockers on cardiovascular morbidity and mortality in hypertension: the Nordic Diltiazem (NORDIL) study. *Lancet* 2000;356:359–365.

122. Brown MJ, Palmer CR, Castaigne A, et al. Morbidity and mortality in patients randomised to double-blind treatment with a long-acting calcium-channel blocker or diuretic in the International Nifedipine GITS study: Intervention as a Goal in Hypertension Treatment (INSIGHT). *Lancet* 2000;356:366–372.

123. Hansson L, Zanchetti A, Carruthers SG, et al., for the HOT Study Group. Effects of intensive blood pressure lowering and low-dose aspirin in patients with hypertension: principal results of the Hypertension Optimal Treatment (HOT) randomised trial. *Lancet* 1998;351:1755–1762.

124. Hansson L, Hedner T, Lindholm L, et al. The Captopril Prevention Project (CAPP) in hypertension: baseline data and current status. *Blood Press* 1997;6:365–367.

125. Hansson L, Lindholm LH, Ekbom T, et al., for the STOP-Hypertension-2 Study Group. Randomised trial of old and new antihypertensive drugs in elderly patients: cardiovascular mortality and morbidity. The Swedish Trial in Old Patients with Hypertension-2 study. *Lancet* 1999;354:1751–1756.

126. Lindholm LH, Ibsen H, Dahlöf B, et al., for the LIFE Study Group. Cardiovascular morbidity and mortality in patients with diabetes in the Losartan Intervention For Endpoint reduction in hypertension study (LIFE): a randomised trial against atenolol. *Lancet* 2002;359: 1004–1010.

127. Joint National Committee. The sixth report of the Joint National Committee on prevention, detection, evaluation and treatment of high blood pressure. *Arch Intern Med* 1997;157:2413–2446.

128. European Diabetes Policy Group. A desktop guide to type 1 (insulin-dependent) diabetes mellitus. European Diabetes Policy Group 1998. *Diabet Med* 1999;16:253–266.

129. European Diabetes Policy Group. A desktop guide to type 2 (insulin-dependent) diabetes mellitus. European Diabetes Policy Group 1999. *Diabet Med* 1999;16:718–730.

130. 1999 World Health Organization-International Society of Hypertension. Guidelines for the Management of Hypertension. Guidelines Subcommittee. *J Hypertens* 1999;17:151–183.

131. American Diabetes Association. Treatment of hypertension in adults with diabetes. *Diabetes Care* 2002;25:199–201.

132. EUROASPIRE I and II Group. Clinical reality of coronary prevention guidelines: a comparison of EUROASPIRE I and II in nine countries. European Action on Secondary Prevention by Intervention to Reduce Events. *Lancet* 2001;357:995–1001.

133. Liebl A, Mata M, Eschwege E. Evaluation of risk factors for development of complications in type 2 diabetes in Europe. *Diabetologia* 2002;45:S23–S28.

134. Zgibor J, Orchard T. Has control of hyperlipidemia and hypertension in patients with type 1 diabetes improved over time? *Diabetes* 2001;50:A255, 1049-P (Abstract).

135. Soedamah-Muthu SS, Colhoun HM, Abrahamian H, et al., for the EURODIAB Prospective Complications Study Group. Trends in hypertension management in type 1 diabetes across Europe, 1989/1990–1997/1999. *Diabetologia* 2002;45:1362–1371.

136. Ruggenenti P, Schieppati A, Remuzzi G. Progression, remission, regression of chronic renal disease. *Lancet* 2001;357:1601–1608.

137. Estacio RO, Jeffers BW, Hiatt WR, et al. The effect of nisoldipine as compared with enalapril on cardiovascular outcomes in patients with non-insulin-dependent diabetes and hypertension. *N Engl J Med* 1998;338:645–652.

138. Tatti P, Pahor M, Byington RP, et al. Outcome results

of the Fosinopril Versus Amlodipine Cardiovascular
Events Randomized Trial (FACET) in patients with hypertension and NIDDM. *Diabetes Care* 1998;21:597–
603.

139. Major cardiovascular events in hypertensive patients
     randomised to doxazosin vs chlorthalidone: the Anti-
     hypertensive and Lipid-lowering Treatment to Prevent
     Heart Attack Trial (ALLHAT). ALLHAT Collaborative
     Research Group. *JAMA* 2000;283:1967–1975.

140. The Antihypertensive and Lipid-lowering Therapy to
     Prevent Heart Attack Trial (ALLHAT). Major out-
     comes in high-risk hypertensive patients randomised
     to angiotensin-converting enzyme inhibitor or calcium
     channel blocker vs diuretic. *JAMA* 2002;288:2981–
     2997.

141. Gaede P, Vedel P, Larsen N, et al. Multifactorial inter-
     vention and cardiovascular disease in patients with type
     2 diabetes. *N Engl J Med* 2003;348:383–393.

Diabetes and Cardiovascular Disease
edited by Steven P. Marso and David M. Stern
Lippincott Williams & Wilkins, Philadelphia © 2004

18

Lipoprotein Abnormalities

William L. Isley and William S. Harris

*Associate Professor, Department of Medicine, University of Missouri–Kansas City, Medical Director,
Lipid and Diabetes Research Center, Saint Luke's Hospital; Professor, Department of Medicine,
University of Missouri–Kansas City, Lipid and Diabetes Research Center, Saint Luke's Hospital,
Kansas City, Missouri*

Coronary heart disease (CHD) is the leading cause of death in Western societies. Diabetic patients are at twofold to fourfold increased risk for CHD events, compared with their nondiabetic counterparts. Despite the reductions in CHD seen in the nondiabetic population over the last 30 years, diabetic CHD death rates are stable or increasing. This is partially due to increased numbers of diabetic patients, as Americans become more obese and as diabetes-prone minority groups account for a larger proportion of the population. This trend is especially disturbing considering that there continue to be advances in the treatments for hyperglycemia, dyslipidemia, and hypertension, as well as improved revascularization procedures and intensive acute coronary care. Clearly, one of the reasons for increased CHD in diabetic patients is dyslipidemia. The statin interventional trials, which targeted elevated low-density lipoprotein cholesterol (LDL-C), showed that diabetic patients have equal, if not greater, benefit with therapy than their nondiabetic peers. This chapter reviews salient aspects of normal and diabetic lipoprotein metabolism and discusses relevant clinical trials and their application to clinical practice.

LIPOPROTEIN METABOLISM

Lipoproteins are particles in plasma that are made up of lipids and proteins. (See Table 18-1 for a glossary of terms). They enter the blood via two routes, the liver or the intestine. There is only one intestinally derived particle, the chylomicron. Chylomicrons appear in the circulation after the consumption of fat and are very rich in triglycerides. They also carry cholesterol, derived both from the diet and from biliary sources. Normally, each chylomicron particle stays in circulation for no more than about 10 minutes, but because fat is gradually absorbed after a meal, chylomicrons may be found in the blood for 2 to 8 hours after eating. Therefore, in the United States, where fat is often consumed at every meal, chylomicrons may be circulating for most of the day. By the action of lipoprotein lipase (LpL), chylomicrons deposit their load of triglycerides, either in muscle (for energy) or in adipose tissue (for storage); in the process, they become chylomicron remnants.

Most of the other lipoproteins are made in the liver. These include very-low-density lipoproteins (VLDL), LDL, and, to some extent, high-density lipoproteins (HDL). VLDL particles carry 90% of the triglycerides found in blood in the fasting state, but only about 10% of the cholesterol. The liver packages VLDL with triglycerides and ships these moieties to peripheral tissues in order to provide fatty acids (energy) to muscles or, when more fat is present than can be burned, to adipose tissue for storage. Once VLDL particles have delivered fatty acids, they become "VLDL remnants" or intermediate-density lipoproteins (IDL). These particles can be irreversibly removed from the circulation by the hepatic apo B/E receptor, or they can be

TABLE 18-1. *Plasma lipid and lipoprotein metabolism: a glossary*

LIPIDS

Cholesterol	30% present as free (i.e., unesterified to fatty acids) cholesterol, a surface component of lipoproteins; 70% present as esterified cholesterol, a core component of lipoproteins
Triglycerides (TG)	Fats; glycerol esterified with a wide variety of fatty acids (three per molecule)
Fatty acids (FA)	Hydrocarbon chains 12–22 carbons long with 0–6 double bonds
Saturated	FA with no double bonds (e.g., palmitate, stearate)
Monounsaturated	FA with 1 double bond (e.g., oleate)
Polyunsaturated	FA with 2–6 double bonds (e.g., linoleate)
n-6	Polyunsaturated FA derived from linoleate (e.g., arachidonate)
n-3	Polyunsaturated FA derived from linolenate (e.g., eicosapentaenoate [EPA], docosahexaenoate [DHA])
trans	In most unsaturated FA, the double bonds are in the *cis* configuration, but in hydrogenated fats, many assume the *trans* configuration, increasing the atherogenicity of the fat
Nonesterified	Free FA (FFA); released into the bloodstream from adipose tissue and the action of LpL; circulate bound to albumin
Phospholipids	Surface components of lipoproteins; 90% are lecithin (phosphatidyl choline)
Other	Fat-soluble vitamins such as vitamin E, β-carotene
LIPOPROTEINS	Blood-borne particles made up of lipids and (apo)proteins that are secreted by liver and intestine, transformed by enzymes, and removed by cellular receptors
Chylomicrons	Intestinally derived particles that carry dietary fat; 90% TG
VLDL	Very-low-density lipoproteins made in the liver; primary carriers of TG in fasting state
IDL	Intermediate-density lipoproteins; produced from VLDL by LpL; also known as VLDL remnants
LDL	Low-density lipoproteins derived from IDL; principal carriers of cholesterol in plasma; LDL-cholesterol is known as the "bad" cholesterol
Lp(a)	"Lipoprotein little a" is a subfraction of LDL in which apo(a) is attached to apoB-100
HDL	High-density lipoproteins; they mediate "reverse cholesterol transport"; HDL-cholesterol is known as the "good" cholesterol
HDL_2	Larger HDL particles, thought to be antiatherogenic
HDL_3	Smaller HDL particles, thought to be atherogenic neutral
APOPROTEINS	The proteins found on the surface of lipoprotein particles
A-I	60% of HDL protein; activates LCAT
A-II	30% of HDL protein; structural
B-100	25% of VLDL and >90% of LDL protein; ligand for LDL receptor
B-48	Chylomicrons; structural; first 48% of apoB-100
C-I, -II, -III	50% of VLDL protein; modulate LpL activity (apoC-II activates; apoC-III inhibits)
E	20% of VLDL protein; ligand for remnant removal
(a)	"apo little a" bound to some B-100 particles in LDL, creating Lp(a); similar in structure to plasminogen and therefore may inhibit thrombolysis
ENZYMES	These either circulate free in blood or are bound to lipoproteins or the endothelium
LpL	Lipoprotein lipase; bound to capillary endothelium in muscle and adipose tissue; converts TG to FFA, and creates IDL from VLDL
HL	Hepatic lipase; converts IDL to LDL and HDL_2 to HDL_3
LCAT	Lecithin-cholesterol acyltransferase; esterifies free cholesterol on the surface of HDL, causing it to move into the core; this contributes to the conversion of HDL_3 into HDL_2
CETP	Cholesterol ester transfer protein; exchanges cholesterol in HDL for triglyceride in VLDL and LDL; a component of the reverse cholesterol transport system
PON-1	Paraoxonase; an antioxidant enzyme associated with HDL that may help prevent LDL oxidation
HSL	Hormone-sensitive lipase; adipose tissue enzyme that hydrolyzes stored triglycerides and releases FFA into the circulation; HSL activity is suppressed by insulin
RECEPTORS	Found on cell membranes; remove lipoproteins from circulation
Chylomicron	An uncharacterized hepatic receptor that removes chylomicron remnants; may be the "LDL receptor-related protein" (LRP)
VLDL	Recognizes apoE but not apoB-100
LDL	Also called the B/E receptor because both apoproteins are recognized; functions to remove IDL and LDL from circulation; 70% of whole-body activity in the liver
HDL	High-density lipoproteins
Scavenger receptor-B1	Hepatic receptor that removes HDL-cholesterol and diverts it to bile for excretion
ABCA1	Adenosine triphosphate (ATP)-binding cassette A-1; receptor on peripheral cells that facilitates the transfer of free cholesterol to the maturing HDL particle

converted by hepatic lipase (HL) and re-released into the circulation as LDL particles.

LDL particles are rich in cholesterol, accounting for about 70% of the total plasma cholesterol. The primary purpose of LDL is to deliver cholesterol to peripheral tissues. LDL particles can infiltrate into the artery wall, become deposited, and decompose, leaving their load of cholesterol to irritate tissues and attract inflammatory cells. LDL deposition plays an instrumental role in early plaque formation and rupture leading to myocardial infarction (MI) or stroke or both (1). LDL lowering, by either diet or drugs, has been shown to reduce the incidence of CHD.

The last major lipoprotein in the blood is HDL. These particles are present in the greatest numbers, but because they are much smaller than LDL and on a per-particle basis contain less than half as much cholesterol, they carry only about 20% of the total plasma cholesterol. HDL particles are more complex than VLDL or LDL. They are constantly being reformed in the plasma: exchanging cholesterol esters for triglycerides in other lipoproteins, picking up cholesterol from the peripheral tissues, growing bigger and smaller under the influence of several enzymes, and serving as a reservoir for exchangeable apoproteins. This varied activity occurs in part because these particles are assembled from components originally made in the liver and in the intestine. HDL particles are the central mediators of a process called "reverse cholesterol transport," which is the transport of cholesterol from peripheral tissues back to the liver, where it is excreted via the bile. The adenosine triphosphate (ATP)-binding cassette A-1 (ABCA1) receptor on peripheral cells shuttles excess free cholesterol from the cell membrane to an immature apoprotein A-I (apoA-I)-rich HDL particle. That particle grows larger as the HDL-associated enzyme, lecithin cholesterol acyl transferase (LCAT), converts free cholesterol on the surface to cholesterol esters that migrate into the core of the particle. HDL cholesterol (HDL-C) is ultimately unloaded via the hepatic scavenger receptor B-l.

Unlike the situation with LDL noted previously, direct evidence to show that increasing the HDL level reduces the risk for CHD is still lacking, although the circumstantial evidence is strong. Until an intervention is developed that specifically and uniquely alters HDL levels without at the same time affecting other risk factors, proving a causal link between HDL and CHD risk will remain elusive.

HYPERLIPIDEMIAS

If serum lipoprotein levels are abnormal, atherosclerosis may develop. Lipoproteins rise, or fall, in concentration depending on two simple processes, secretion and clearance. They may either enter the bloodstream too fast or be removed too slowly. Both processes appear to play a role in the dyslipidemias common in Western societies. The liver, which is the major sink for LDL, slowly loses its capacity to remove LDL from the blood as LDL receptors become either less active or less abundant. Most interventions to lower cholesterol levels focus on stimulating the LDL receptors. This alteration causes LDL to be removed more rapidly, resulting in a falling LDL-C. On the other hand, increased levels of triglycerides (VLDL) are often caused by excessive synthesis and secretion from the liver.

DIABETIC DYSLIPIDEMIA

Both insulin-dependent (type 1) and non-insulin-dependent (type 2) diabetes mellitus have associated lipid abnormalities, and in both conditions patients with poorly controlled disease have greater abnormalities than those with well-controlled disease (2). For example, the patient with well-controlled type 1 diabetes may have a virtually normal lipid profile, whereas in the patient with poorly controlled disease, total cholesterol and LDL-C may be elevated, HDL-C reduced, and triglycerides increased. In contrast, even with good control the type 2 patient often has elevated triglycerides and depressed HDL-C, and with poor glycemic control, the triglycerides are likely to be further increased. Because more than 90% of the diabetic patients in the United States have type 2 diabetes (3), the discussion here focuses predominantly on type 2 disease (Table 18-2).

TABLE 18-2. Simplified approach to abnormalities of lipoprotein metabolism in type 2 diabetes mellitus

Particle	Serum surrogate	Production defect	Composition defect	Removal defect	Drugs to correct defects
VLDL	Fasting triglycerides (TG)	Increased due to increased FFA		Decreased LPL activity	Fibrates > niacin ~ fish oil > statins > glitazones > metformin
Chylomicron	Postprandial TG	Diet induced		Competition with VLDL for LPL; decreased LPL activity	Fibrates > niacin ≈ fish oil > glitazones > metformin
Remnants	IDL-C			Decreased due to apo E2 allele or to protein glycosylation	?
LDL	LDL-C	Diet-induced*	Small dense (reduced in size due to CETP-mediated exchange of VLDL-TG for cholesterol followed by TG hydrolysis by HL)	Possible decrease due to protein glycosylation	Statins (decreased LDL particle number) > niacin ~ fibrates (abnormal LDL particle composition)
All atherogenic particles	Non-HDL-C; Apo B-100	Increased due to insulin resistance			Statins > fibrates ≈ niacin > glitazones ~ metformin
HDL	HDL-C	Decreased due to increased VLDL-TG		Increased	Niacin > fibrates ≈ statins ~ glitazones > metformin

Apo, apoprotein; CETP, cholesterol ester transfer protein; FFA, free fatty acids; HDL-C, high-density lipoprotein cholesterol; IDL-C, intermediate-density lipoprotein cholesterol; LDL-C, low-density lipoprotein cholesterol; VLDL, very-low-density lipoprotein.
*LDL-C levels may not be more elevated in patients with type 2 diabetes compared with nondiabetic subjects.

Free Fatty Acids and Atherogenic Dyslipidemia in Diabetes

The classic dyslipidemia of type 2 diabetes mellitus is so-called atherogenic dyslipidemia. This is a constellation of lipid abnormalities also known as the "lipid triad" (4). It includes increased serum triglycerides, decreased HDL-C, and the presence of small, dense LDL particles. Concentrations of total cholesterol and LDL-C are not typically increased in diabetic dyslipidemia.

All of the components of the lipid triad may be the result of increased free fatty acid (FFA) levels characteristic of the insulin-resistant state (5). The increase in triglycerides is secondary to the increased flux of FFA from adipose tissue to the liver and the decreased ability of muscle to oxidize fatty acids. Both of these abnormalities are caused by a loss of cellular sensitivity to insulin. In the adipocyte, insulin resistance results in an impairment in insulin-mediated suppression of lipolysis. Normally, insulin is a powerful suppressor of hormone-sensitive lipase (HSL), such that the flux of FFA from adipose tissue is markedly reduced after each meal (6). If adipocytes are insulin resistant, then HSL does not receive the inhibitory signal, even though insulin is present, and it continues to inappropriately release FFA. Insulin resistance in visceral adipose tissue may be particularly egregious, because FFA in these stores are released directly to the liver (via the portal vein), where they are synthesized into triglycerides and secreted in VLDL particles.

FFA dysregulation begins a cascade of interwoven events that can ultimately disrupt the entire lipid profile. Increased triglyceride concentrations contribute to a reduction in HDL-C via the cholesterol ester transfer protein (CETP) reaction. This enzyme exchanges cholesterol in LDL and HDL for triglycerides in VLDL. As these particles take on more triglyceride, they become better substrate for HL. This enzyme removes the triglycerides from both particles, resulting in not only smaller HDL particles (HDL$_3$) but also in the formation of small, dense LDL particles. As a result of the former

effect, HDL-C levels are lowered; in addition, apoA-I, the principal HDL-associated apoprotein, binds less well to smaller HDL particles. The disassociated apoA-I is filtered by the kidney and degraded, ultimately lowering plasma apoA-I levels (7). Finally, normal HDL particles contain natural antioxidant enzymes (e.g., paraoxonase) that are able to slow the peroxidation of LDL particles (8); lowering of HDL moieties results in a reduction of the antioxidant potential.

The effect of high triglycerides on LDL results in the generation of smaller, denser, more atherogenic LDL particles. Such particles are more susceptible to oxidation than larger LDL, and they more readily enter the subendothelial space. They also have a longer plasma residence time (9).

The insulin-resistant state not only changes LDL and HDL size, but also alters the chemical composition of VLDL in a proatherogenic manner. Diabetic VLDL particles can more easily penetrate the subendothelial space and, in a hyperglycemic milieu, are more tenaciously retained (10), initiating inflammatory responses that ultimately lead to atherosclerotic plaque growth. Diabetic patients also have increased levels of IDL. These particles arise from VLDL after LpL has extracted most of the triglyceride. IDL particles are known to be at least as atherogenic as LDL particles, by virtue of the fact that patients with type III hyperlipidemia (so-called remnant disease, involving accumulation of high levels of IDL secondary to a genetic defect in the structure of apoE) often develop rampant atherosclerosis (11). The other remnant lipoprotein particles that may be atherogenic are chylomicron remnants (12). These are more likely to accumulate in the plasma of subjects with fasting hypertriglyceridemia (as in patients with type 2 diabetes), because VLDL particles compete with chylomicrons for clearance by LpL.

In summary, driven largely by insulin resistance at the level of the adipocyte, the diabetic dyslipidemic syndrome emerges as a natural consequence of increased FFA flux. Because diabetic (or atherogenic) dyslipidemia has many proatherogenic features, interventions to help normalize these lipid abnormalities would be expected to reduce CHD risk.

DIETARY RECOMMENDATIONS

Remarkably, there remains significant controversy regarding the "proper" diet for diabetic patients. The current recommendation from the American Diabetes Association states, "Carbohydrate and monounsaturated fat together should provide 60% to 70% of energy intake. However, the metabolic profile and need for weight loss should be considered when determining the monounsaturated fat content of the diet. Sucrose and sucrose-containing foods should be eaten in the context of a healthy diet" (13).

Contained within this recommendation are the two clashing perspectives: higher complex carbohydrates and lower fat ("low fat") versus higher fat and lower carbohydrates ("low carb"). There is unanimity regarding the need to reduce saturated fat intake to less than 7% to 10% of energy, as also endorsed by the Adult Treatment Panel III (ATP-III) of the National Cholesterol Education Program (NCEP) (14). The question is with what to replace it: carbohydrates or unsaturated fats? Both approaches are designed to reduce the risk for CHD, the low-fat diet by focusing on reducing LDL-C and the low-carb diet by aiming to reduce serum triglycerides and raise HDL-C. Proponents of the low-fat approach criticize the low-carb advocates (15) by pointing out that recommending higher-fat diets to diabetic patients will simply increase total caloric intake, thereby fostering additional weight gain, a clearly undesirable outcome in this population. Those supporting the low-carb diet (16) point to well-controlled trials that clearly show that this diet produces a more favorable lipid profile than the higher carbohydrate diet does. However, such studies involved the isocaloric substitution of oils for carbohydrates, thereby automatically preventing weight gain. Whether diabetic patients can, in an unsupervised setting, eat a high-fat diet and maintain weight is an open question.

Our practice is to recommend that saturated fats be replaced by monounsaturated fats (instead of carbohydrates) and only in patients with high triglycerides (e.g., greater than 400 mg/dL),

especially if triglycerides exceed 1,000 mg/dL. For those patients with more normal triglyceride levels, we emphasize carbohydrates more than oils. Another strategy is to recommend oily fish, which contain high levels of long-chain omega-3 (n-3) fatty acids. These oils have a unique effect in lowering serum triglycerides and, when substituted for saturated fats, lower cholesterol as well (17).

EFFICACY OF LIPID DRUGS IN DIABETES PATIENTS

Over the last decade, we have witnessed the so-called cholesterol revolution, as randomized, controlled trials have finally proved that LDL-C reductions, anticipated by epidemiologic studies and animal models, actually produce clinical benefits. Event and mortality reductions have been achieved largely through the use of statin drugs (hydroxymethylglutaryl coenzyme A [HMG-CoA] reductase inhibitors). The following discussion focuses on the proven benefits attributed to these drugs and includes other dyslipidemic treatment issues as well.

Statin Trials

Large, randomized, controlled trials with "hard" clinical end points are considered the best evidence of efficacy, safety, and tolerability of drug therapy. The last 10 years have seen the publication of a number of landmark trials that have paved the way for the cholesterol revolution. Most of these studies have used statins, but not all have included patients with diabetes mellitus; our analysis here is limited to investigations that included diabetic patients (Table 18-3).

The Scandinavian Simvastatin Survival Study (4S) was the trial that solidified the cholesterol hypothesis, because it was the first study to show not only decreased CHD events in patients treated with a statin, but also that statin therapy was associated with improved overall survival (18). Simvastatin (20 to 40 mg/day; mean dose, 27 mg/day) was given for a mean of 5.4 years and was well tolerated by both nondiabetic and diabetic patients. Of the 4,444 enrolled patients with known heart disease (previous MI

TABLE 18-3. *Major statin trials with diabetic subgroup analyses*

Trial (ref. no.)	Other conditions	N	No. of diabetic subjects	Drug and dose	Mean entry LDL (mg/dL)	LDL reduction (%)	CHD event reduction (%)
4S (20)	Previous MI or angina	4,444	483*	Simvastatin, 20–40 mg/day	187	36	42
CARE (21)	Previous MI	4,159	586	Pravastatin, 40 mg/day	137	27	25
LIPID (22)	MI or ischemia	9,014	782	Pravastatin, 40 mg/day	150	25	19
HPS (25)	CVD or high risk	20,536	5,963	Simvastatin, 40 mg/day	132	29	22

CHD, coronary heart disease; CVD, cardiovascular disease; LDL, low-density lipoprotein; MI, myocardial infarction.

*The original report from this trial (19) defined diabetes as a fasting glucose $\geq$140 mg/dL, not $\geq$126 mg/dL as defined here; 202 patients met that stricter criterion, and the overall event reduction for those treated with simvastatin was 55%.

or angina), 202 subjects were known at baseline to have a diagnosis of diabetes mellitus (19). *Post hoc* analysis showed that, compared with the 32% reduction ($p < .0001$) in major coronary events among the nondiabetic subjects, diabetic subjects experienced a remarkable 55% decrease ($p = .002$) in major CHD events. Mortality was reduced by 30% in the total population and by 43% in diabetic patients, but the latter was not a statistically significant difference. In 1997, after the American Diabetes Association revised the diagnostic criteria for diabetes mellitus (fasting plasma glucose $\geq$126 mg/dL), the 4S data set was reanalyzed using the new diagnostic criteria (20). This led to classification of 483 subjects as diabetic, more than double the previous number. Major CHD events were reduced in the simvastatin-treated group by 42% ($p = .001$) and revascularizations by 48% ($p = .005$), compared with placebo treatment in diabetic patients. Total and CHD mortality reductions (31% and 38%, respectively) still did not reach statistical significance.

In the Cholesterol and Recurrent Events (CARE) Trial, 586 of the 4,159 patients with CHD (history of MI in the previous 3 to 20 months) were known to have diabetes at baseline (21). The active treatment group received pravastatin 40 mg/day for 5 years, which reduced the CHD event rate by 23% ($p < .001$) in the nondiabetic group and 25% ($p = .05$) in the diabetic group. Total mortality was not significantly reduced in either group, but revascularizations were reduced by 32% ($p = .04$) in the diabetic patients.

Pravastatin was also used in the Long-term Intervention with Pravastatin in Ischaemic Disease (LIPID) trial (22). Doses of 40 mg/day were given for 6.1 years to subjects with known myocardial ischemia. Whereas about one fifth of the 9,014 patients had diabetes, the reduction in CHD events in this subgroup was less than that seen in nondiabetic subjects (19% versus 25%) and was not statistically significant. It has been hypothesized that the lack of greater effect may have been due to the fact that a large portion of the placebo-designated subjects were actually receiving statins from their personal physicians.

The two major primary prevention trials have been the West of Scotland Coronary Prevention Study (WOSCOPS) (23) and the Air Force/Texas Coronary Atherosclerosis Prevention Study (AFCAPS/TexCAPS) (24). They involved subjects without known CHD and contained only a small number of diabetic subjects (approximately 1% of 6,595 subjects and approximately 2% of 6,605 subjects, respectively). Although the reduction in CHD events was 43% in the diabetic subgroup of the latter study (which used lovastatin 20 to 40 mg/day for a mean of 5.2 years), the number of events was too small to reach statistical significance.

Finally, the Heart Protection Study (HPS) provided the clearest evidence of benefit from statin therapy for patients with diabetes (25). This study was carried out in approximately

20,000 subjects with known cardiovascular disease or diabetes mellitus, whose serum cholesterol concentrations were higher than 135 mg/dL. The active treatment group received simvastatin 40 mg/day for 5 years. Mortality rates were reduced by 12.9% with active therapy ($p = .0003$), and coronary event rates were decreased by 25% ($p < .0001$). Most interestingly, all patient subgroups, including those patients with low baseline LDL-C concentrations (lower than 100 mg/dL), noted similar reductions in CHD events. Almost 6,000 of the subjects had diabetes mellitus (90% type 2). Simvastatin therapy was associated with a statistically significant 22% reduction in these patients. The results of this study have caused some authorities to suggest initiation of statin therapy, based on other risk factors rather than solely on LDL-C values.

Fibrate Trials

The Helsinki Heart Study (HHS) was a primary prevention study carried out in hypercholesterolemic men in Finland. Of 4,081 subjects, 135 had diabetes mellitus (26). The HHS used gemfibrozil, an agent whose primary effect is to lower triglycerides, which produces a slight increase in HDL-C. Although the result was not statistically significant, gemfibrozil therapy was associated with a 57% reduction in CHD events among the diabetic patients, compared with placebo.

In the Veterans Affairs HDL-C Intervention Trial (VA-HIT), 2,531 men with CHD, isolated low HDL-C (approximately 32 mg/dL), and a mean LDL-C of approximately 112 mg/dL were treated with gemfibrozil, 1200 mg/day for 5 years (27). Approximately one quarter of the subjects had diabetes. Similar reductions (24%) in CHD events were seen in the nondiabetic group ($p = .009$) and in the diabetic group ($p = .05$). *Post hoc* analyses suggested that the bulk of the treatment effect could be explained by a rather meager 2.5 mg/dL rise in HDL-C in the treated group (28).

The Diabetes Atherosclerosis Intervention Study (DAIS) (29) was an angiographic endpoint trial that included 731 men and women with type 2 diabetes mellitus. Active therapy was with micronized fenofibrate 200 mg/day. As was also seen in statin angiographic trials, fenofibrate therapy was associated with reduced progression of angiographic disease, compared with placebo. Clinical events were reduced, but the difference was not statistically significant, because the study was not powered to show a reduction in clinical events.

Prediabetes

Patients with elevated blood glucose concentrations that are not yet in the diabetic range are at increased risk for the development of diabetes (usually type 2 diabetes mellitus) and are probably at increased risk for CHD. In the United States, this scenario is usually identified by a fasting plasma glucose concentration greater than 110 and less than 126 mg/dL (impaired fasting glucose, or IFG). In Europe, a 2-hour post-glucose load value is frequently used (greater than 140 and less than 200 mg/dL); this is known as impaired glucose tolerance (IGT). The latter values are more predictive of CHD risk, but they usually are not measured in the United States, because of the practical limitations of glucose tolerance testing.

Investigators have reanalyzed the data from two of the major statin trials, looking specifically at subjects with IFG. In the 4S trial, 678 of the subjects had IFG. CHD events, revascularizations, coronary mortality, and total mortality were markedly reduced: by 38% ($p = .003$), 43% ($p = .009$), 55% ($p = .007$), and 43% ($p = .02$), respectively. In the CARE trial, 342 of the participants had IFG, and the reduction in recurrent nonfatal MIs was 50% ($p = .05$) with pravastatin therapy. Both of these analyses underscore the fact that these patients appear to be at increased CHD risk before the development of type 2 diabetes, and that LDL-C lowering may be particularly efficacious in this group.

AREAS OF CONTROVERSY REGARDING TREATMENT OF DYSLIPIDEMIAS

Despite the dramatic reductions in CHD events seen with statin therapy, most patients with diabetes ultimately die from CHD. This has led many clinicians to wonder what lipid factors besides LDL-C, if any, may be modifiable in such a way that CHD risk can be further decreased. Several possible targets are addressed here.

Low-density Lipoprotein Particle Size

The pioneering work of Krauss and Austen (30) has raised the possibility that not only LDL particle number, but LDL particle size may be an important determinant of risk. Some (31,32) but not all (33,34) epidemiologic studies have found LDL particle size to be an independent predictor of CHD risk. There are no clear results from intervention trials to support this hypothesis. A recent case-control analysis of a subset of the CARE study failed to identify small LDL particle size as a risk factor (35). Furthermore, statins usually do not change the LDL particle size, despite their very positive effects on CHD risk (36). Fibrates (37) and niacin (38), on the other hand, often do increase particle size, because they lower triglyceride levels (see previous discussion). Clearly, for patients with elevated LDL-C, the effect of fibrates on CHD risk is less than that of statins, and it is unknown whether adding a fibrate (or niacin) to a statin would further reduce CHD risk. In short, although reducing LDL concentrations is clearly beneficial, increasing LDL particle size remains an unproved strategy for reducing CHD risk.

ApoproteinB-100

ApoproteinB-100 is the major protein in all of the atherogenic lipoproteins (LDL, IDL, and VLDL). Whole-plasma apoB-100 can be used as a surrogate for atherogenic particle number, as can the non-HDL cholesterol, as recommended by the NCEP ATP-III guidelines as a secondary treatment goal (39). Statins are excellent reducers of apoB-100; however, no compelling epidemiologic or interventional data have yet shown apoB-100 to be a better risk predictor than traditional lipoprotein analysis.

High-density Lipoprotein-C

The serum HDL-C concentration is clearly a potent risk predictor in nondiabetic and diabetic subjects. In the United Kingdom Prospective Diabetes Study (UKPDS), a purely glycemic intervention, HDL-C was second only to LDL-C as a risk factor for CHD events (40). As noted earlier, genetics and several lifestyle factors affect HDL-C. Central obesity and the resultant metabolic syndrome are probably the most common adverse effectors of HDL-C. Weight loss, aerobic exercise, moderate alcohol intake, and smoking cessation increase HDL-C, whereas insulin resistance and high-carbohydrate, low-fat diets reduce HDL-C (41). Although diabetes control has little effect on HDL-C, metformin may raise it slightly, and thiazolidinediones may increase HDL-C by 5% to 20%; however, the latter drugs may also increase LDL-C, particularly large, buoyant LDL. Fibrates increase HDL-C moderately, and niacin has a pronounced HDL-C raising effect. Extended-release niacin preparations may be particularly effective in this regard (42).

As noted earlier, minimal increases in HDL-C in the HHS and VA-HIT were associated with reductions in CHD events. Several factors make translation of these findings into clinical practice difficult. First, it is unclear whether treatment of patients with a fibrate, after statin treatment has lowered the LDL-C, will give the same risk benefit as seen in the patients in VA-HIT, in which LDL-C was relatively low before any treatment. Certainly, the addition of fibrate to statin increases costs and risks. Second, in the light of HPS, it is hard to withhold statin therapy from high-risk patients, even with low LDL-C at baseline. Whether use of combination therapy would result in additive benefit is clearly speculative. A prospective clinical endpoint trial in diabetic patients, comparing therapy with statin plus fibrate to statin alone, was recently initiated. Third, despite analyses attributing the bulk of the benefit seen in HHS and VA-HIT to modest rises in HDL-C, we still consider that other mechanisms (triglyceride lowering, changes in LDL particle size, improvement in clotting parameters) may have contributed significantly to the observed benefit. The addition of niacin (particularly sustained-release niacin) to statin is advocated by many clinicians for patients who have low HDL-C levels after appropriate LDL-C lowering with statin. This strategy was given theoretical impetus by the angiographic studies of Brown and colleagues (43,44). Although addition of niacin to very low doses of statins may add benefit, this strategy has not been tested against doses of statins commonly used in trials or clinical practice. Furthermore, analyses of the major statin trials have shown partial elimination of excess CHD risk in patients with low HDL-C by statin treatment alone (45). This effect may be due to the HDL-C raising effect seen with most statins, to nonlipid effects of statins, or to effects of statins on other lipoprotein fractions, including LDL.

Lipid treatment guidelines generally have not targeted raising HDL-C by pharmacologic measures as a major priority. Certainly, the lipid profile can be improved with combination therapy, but whether such therapy is actually efficacious is unknown. The recent publication of the Women's Health Initiative (46) and Heart and Estrogen/progestin Replacement Study (HERS) (47) trials and the antioxidant studies (25,48,49) have underscored the need for caution before relying on epidemiologic data in choosing therapies. Controlled clinical trials with "hard" clinical end points are the gold standard for determining practice.

Triglycerides

The serum triglyceride concentration has often been shown by univariate analysis to be a predictor of CHD risk (50). However, it often ceases to be so in multivariate analyses, probably because of the relationship of serum triglycerides to other factors (i.e., directly related to central obesity and insulin resistance, inversely proportional to HDL-C and LDL particle size). Therefore, serum triglycerides may be just a risk marker, rather than a risk factor. Surprisingly, *post hoc* analyses of major fibrate trials (HHS and VA- HIT) failed to reveal triglyceride changes as predictive of changes in risk, despite 20% to 40% reductions (51,52). Serum triglycerides increase with poor diabetes control and high-carbohydrate diets (36). Assuming the patient does not have extreme chylomicronemia (triglycerides greater than 1,000 mg/dL), in which the major concern

is risk for pancreatitis, an elevated serum triglyceride concentration is a marker for an increased number of atherogenic particles. Because non-HDL cholesterol is a surrogate for these particles *in toto*, we would endorse the NCEP ATP-III recommendation to use non-HDL cholesterol as a goal when serum triglycerides remain higher than 200 mg/dL after statin therapy has brought LDL-C to goal. This concept is attractive because it is simple, it approximates known physiology, and it will probably keep the majority of patients on statin monotherapy, avoiding the increased costs and elevated risks of combination therapy. In fact, we predict that future guidelines will switch to non-HDL cholesterol as the primary target for therapy.

INDIVIDUAL LIPID-ALTERING AGENTS

Statins

The cholesterol revolution has been fueled largely by the remarkable efficacy, safety, and tolerability of the statins (53). As noted earlier, some of these agents have been shown to reduce CHD events and mortality and increase overall survival. Their use in diabetic patients is deemed highly cost-effective (54).

The statins can be classified by origin (natural or synthetic), by relative lipophilicity, or by metabolism. These classifications are rarely clinically relevant, except for the notation that statins that are not metabolized by cytochrome P450 enzymes (e.g., pravastatin) carry a theoretically lower risk for drug interactions when other drugs metabolized by these pathways are coadministered. However, even this potential interaction is only rarely clinically significant. All statins may be associated with muscle damage when given with fibrates. The mechanism has recently been elucidated (55). The risk for drug interactions is reduced when statins are given at relatively low doses.

As is clear from the earlier discussion, the efficacy of statins in diabetic patients is similar to that in nondiabetic subjects (56). We categorize the efficacy of LDL-C lowering at maximal doses of statins as moderate (pravastatin and fluvastatin) or high (lovastatin, simvastatin, ator-vastatin, and rosuvastatin) (57). Because the highest dose of the latter statins is not often used outside of lipid specialty clinics, this differentiation is not important for most patients. The highest doses of the high-efficacy statins are associated with increased risk for liver function abnormalities and rhabdomyolysis.

If triglycerides are significantly elevated, all statins will lower them and raise HDL-C (58). The magnitude of triglyceride lowering depends on the baseline level. In some studies, high-dose atorvastatin was associated with less HDL-C raising than that seen with high-dose simvastatin (59).

Although all of the statins currently on the market have been used in some end-point trial (angiographic or clinical end point), the major statin end-point trials, including substantial numbers of diabetic patients, have used simvastatin, pravastatin, or lovastatin (18,21–25). However, trials are in progress using some of the other marketed statins, and positive results are anticipated.

Because all statins can be associated with liver function test abnormalities, liver function monitoring is recommended by the U. S. Food and Drug Administration. However, most of the liver function abnormalities are mild, and they rarely necessitate discontinuation of therapy (60). Muscle pain without creatine kinase (CK) elevations is common in patients taking statins (61). Routine monitoring of CK is not recommended; clinical monitoring is the most practical approach. We instruct all patients prescribed a statin, regardless of dose, to immediately report diffuse muscle aches. CK levels are then checked, although most tests will be normal. Clinical vigilance is particularly important when potentially interacting drugs are administered with statins.

Cholesterol and Bile Acid Absorption Inhibitors

Plant sterol and stanol esters, cholesterol absorption inhibitors, and bile acid sequestrants interfere with the intestinal absorption of cholesterol or bile acids (which are made from cholesterol).

Bile acid sequestrants, also known as resins because they are ion exchange resins, bind bile acids in the gut, disrupting their normal enterohepatic circulation and forcing the liver to divert large amounts of cholesterol into *de novo* bile acid synthesis. This has the ultimate effect of reducing serum LDL-C by 15% to 25%. These agents slightly increase HDL-C and, in patients with hypertriglyceridemia, may markedly raise triglycerides. Their poor gastrointestinal tolerability and interference with absorption of other medications limit their use to patients who are intolerant to statins or are unable to reach their LDL-C goal with statin monotherapy. Patients with heterozygous familial hypercholesterolemia constitute the latter category. Resins alone (62) or in combination with niacin (63) have been shown to reduce CHD events in non-diabetic patients.

Plant sterol and stanol esters are available over the counter as margarine products (64). These agents interfere with micellar dissolution of cholesterol in the gut and thereby reduce cholesterol absorption. They can reduce LDL-C by approximately 10%. Pharmacologic approaches to the inhibition of cholesterol absorption may be accomplished with a new drug called ezetimibe. It is well tolerated and has none of the troublesome side effects of resins but lowers LDL-C by 15% to 20% (65). The addition of this agent to starting doses of statins allows most patients to achieve their LDL-C goal.

Fibrates

Fibrates primarily reduce triglycerides and modestly raise HDL-C, an effect that probably is related to the magnitude of triglyceride-lowering. Fenofibrate lowers LDL-C significantly in some patients (66). These drugs have been shown to reduce CHD risk, although the magnitude and duration of effect may be less than that seen with statins. The dose of gemfibrozil is 600 mg twice daily, whereas micronized fenofibrate is dosed at 160 mg daily. The dose should be reduced in renal insufficiency and also, perhaps, when these drugs are used in combination with statins. The risk for gallstone formation is increased with fibrates.

Niacin (Nicotinic Acid)

Niacin is a B vitamin which, when given in high doses, can improve the entire lipid profile (LDL-C ↓10% to 20%, HDL-C ↑10% to 20%, triglycerides ↓20% to 35%) (67). Its widespread use has been lessened by its troublesome side effects, particularly flushing. Sustained-release preparations may reduce the flushing, but liver toxicity is increased. Niacin therapy has been associated with increased insulin resistance and worsening glycemia in some diabetic patients (68), but this is not seen in the majority of patients given moderate doses of extended-release preparations (42). A combination product containing extended-release niacin plus lovastatin is now available (69).

When niacin is used for increasing HDL-C, we prefer extended-release preparations such as Niaspan (1 to 2 g after starting with a lower dose) taken at night. If triglyceride lowering is the primary aim, we prefer immediate-release niacin and titrate to effect. In this scenario, the drug must be started at a low dose with meals (100 mg t.i.d.) and increased slowly as tolerated. Pretreatment with aspirin may be used, if needed, to reduce flushing. Some degree of tachyphylaxis to the flushing occurs over time. We regularly use 3 g crystalline niacin per day (given t.i.d.) and have used 6 to 8 g/day in severely hypertriglyceridemic patients. In terms of changes in the lipid profile, the patient and clinician will be amply rewarded if patience is exercised in initiating therapy. Routine liver function monitoring is recommended when using niacin. Peptic ulcer disease and gout may rarely be precipitated. The risk for rhabdomyolysis may be increased when niacin is given in combination with a statin.

Fish Oil

The administration of low-dose (850 mg/day) n-3 fatty acids, eicosapentaenoic acid (EPA) and docosahexaenoic acid (DHA), in patients with known CHD has been associated with decreased incidence of sudden death (49). The effect was similar in diabetic subjects. This dose of n-3 fatty acids has little effect on lipids except for a modest decrease in triglycerides. Larger doses (about 3 to 4 g/day) of DHA and EPA markedly reduce triglycerides in most patients (17). This therapy is attractive from a side effect standpoint, because the only adverse effects are a fish taste with posttherapy belching (common) and a fishy odor (uncommon). Very-high-dose fish oil (more than 5 g/day) has been associated with deteriorations in glucose tolerance in poorly controlled type 2 diabetes mellitus (70), probably due to an effect on insulin secretion. Lower doses appear to have no effect on glycemic control (71). When purchasing this over-the-counter "nutraceutical," the consumer may be bewildered by the array of preparations available. Low-potency fish oil is one-third to one-half EPA/DHA. We prefer very-high-potency preparations (approximately 80% EPA/DHA). When prescribing fish oil, make clear to the patient that EPA/DHA is the active component and that enough capsules should be taken to achieve the EPA/DHA dose prescribed (i.e., take six 50%-potent, 1-g capsules to get 3 g of EPA/DHA daily). The vegetable oil n-3 fatty acid linolenic acid (found in flaxseed oil) does not lower plasma triglycerides, and its effect on CHD risk has not been documented.

PRACTICAL ASPECTS OF DYSLIPIDEMIA TREATMENT

Recommended treatment goals for lipids in diabetic patients are given in Table 18-4 (14,72). The effects of the various drugs for diabetes and dyslipidemia on lipid fractions are listed in Table 18-5. Our approach to treatment of lipid disorders in diabetic patients is outlined in Figure 18-1.

Before initiation of dyslipidemic therapy, the practitioner must always be aware of secondary causes of dyslipidemia (14). Some causes of high LDL-C include liver disease, nephrotic syndrome, renal disease, and hypothyroidism. Secondary causes of hypertriglyceridemia include excess alcohol intake, high doses of β-blockers or thiazides, unopposed oral

TABLE 18-4. *National recommendations for lipid treatment goals for diabetic patients*

Source (ref. no.)	First goal	Second goal	Third goal
National Cholesterol Education Program Adult Treatment Panel III 2001 (14)	LDL-C <100 mg/dL	Non-HDL-C <130 mg/dL if TG ≥200 mg/dL	—
American Diabetes Association 2002 (72)	LDL-C <100 mg/dL	HDL-C >45 mg/dL	TG <200 mg/dL

HDL-C, high-density lipoprotein cholesterol; LDL-C, low-density lipoprotein cholesterol; TG, triglycerides.

estrogen therapy, and poorly controlled diabetes mellitus.

Although statin therapy is clearly indicated in the overwhelming majority of patients, we have seen numerous diabetic patients inappropriately treated with statins who had chylomicronemia and high risk for pancreatitis. Such patients often have eruptive xanthomas. No statin monotherapy in any dose is effective for these patients. In patients with marked hypertriglyceridemia, we usually start with a fibrate, a very-low-fat diet, and diabetes control. Glycemic agents that affect triglycerides (glitazones and metformin), fish oils, and niacin prove effective add-on therapies in most such patients. In acute chylomicronemia syndromes (especially serum triglycerides 2,000 to 20,000 mg/dL), we have extensive experience using insulin infusions to rapidly reduce triglycerides, presumably by an effect on LpL. (In nondiabetic patients, intravenous glucose is concomitantly administered to prevent hypoglycemia.)

For the vast majority of diabetic patients with LDL-C concentrations of ≥ 100 mg/dL, statin therapy is now universally advocated (73). The recently published HPS suggests that all diabetic patients, regardless of LDL-C level, are likely to benefit from statin therapy. We consider this finding as a provisional recommendation at this time. If the LDL-C concentration is indeed too high, in virtually all patients with diabetes, it is unclear what target, if any, should be reached to achieve maximum efficacy without undue side effects. Studies are presently underway assessing lower LDL-C treatment goals than those currently advocated. In light of VA-HIT, a minority of clinicians would consider fibrate therapy in patients with low baseline LDL-C. However, due to the impressive efficacy and safety record of statins, including the massive

TABLE 18-5. *Effects of drugs on serum lipid levels*

Agent	Low-density lipoprotein cholesterol (LDL-C)	High-density lipoprotein cholesterol (HDL-C)	Triglycerides
Antidiabetic drugs			
Insulin secretagogues	Minimal	Minimal	↓ if glycemic control previously poor
Metformin	Minimal	Minimal	↓
Glitazones	↑[a]	↑	↓ to ↓↓
α-Glucosidase inhibitors	Minimal	Minimal	Minimal
Insulin	Minimal	Minimal	↓ if glycemic control previously poor
Antilipidemic drugs			
Statins	↓↓	↑	↓
Absorption inhibitors	↓	Minimal	↑ (resins)
Niacin	↓	↑↑	↓ to ↓↓
Fibrates	Variable[b]	↑	↓↓
Fish oils	Low dose, →; High dose, ↑	→↑	↓↓

[a]LDL particle size increased.
[b]LDL-C often increases if serum triglycerides are markedly increased; fenofibrate lowers LDL-C more than gemfibrozil does.

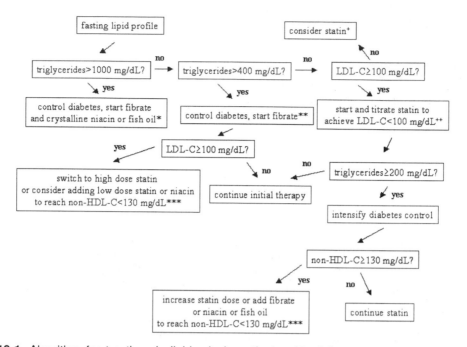

FIG. 18-1. Algorithm for treating dyslipidemia in patients with diabetes mellitus. * Major risk is pancreatitis—do not stop triglyceride-lowering drugs; insulin, metformin, or glitazones may be useful adjuncts for triglyceride control. ** Some authorities use a higher triglyceride cut point, such as 500 mg/dL for initial fibrate therapy, and use statins below this threshold. *** The practitioner must weigh the risks and costs of high-dose statin therapy versus combination therapy. + In light of the Heart Protection Study, all diabetic patients may benefit from statin therapy; in light of the Veterans Affairs HDL-C Intervention Trial, the practitioner might consider fibrate therapy, particularly if baseline HDL-C is less than 35 mg/dL. ++ May add absorption inhibitor or niacin to reach LDL-C goal if needed. HDL-C, high-density lipoprotein cholesterol; LDL-C, low-density lipoprotein cholesterol.

numbers of patients who have completed clinical trials, we stress a strong preference for statin therapy in these patients, whenever pharmacologic therapy is to be administered. The treatment algorithm we have advocated avoids combination therapy in most patients. Clearly, some lipid specialists disagree with this approach, preferring to add niacin or fibrates to "tweak" the HDL-C or triglycerides or both. However, as was emphasized earlier, hard clinical end-point trials using such a strategy have not been completed. Clinical end-point trials have almost uniformly enrolled patients with type 2 diabetes mellitus. It is doubtful that an end-point trial for lipid therapy will ever be carried out in patients with type 1 diabetes mellitus. However, recent epidemiologic

data from a large group of such patients suggest similar lipid goals for patients with either type 1 or type 2 diabetes mellitus (74).

REFERENCES

1. Libby P, Ridker PM, Maseri A. Inflammation and atherosclerosis. *Circulation* 2002;105:1135–1143.
2. O'Brien T, Nguyen TT, Zimmerman BR. Hyperlipidemia and diabetes mellitus. *Mayo Clin Proc* 1998;73:969–976.
3. Grundy SM, Benjamin IJ, Burke GL, et al. Diabetes and cardiovascular disease: a statement for healthcare professionals from the American Heart Association. *Circulation* 1999;100:1134–1146.
4. Grundy SM. Hypertriglyceridemia, atherogenic dyslipidemia, and the metabolic syndrome. *Am J Cardiol* 1998;81:18B–25B.

5. McGarry JD. Dysregulation of fatty acid metabolism in the etiology of type 2 diabetes: the Banting Lecture 2001. *Diabetes* 2002;51:7–18.

6. Coppack SW, Jensen MD, Miles JM. In vivo regulation of lipolysis in humans. *J Lipid Res* 1994;35:177–193.

7. Ginsberg HN. Diabetic dyslipidemia: basic mechanisms underlying the common hypertriglyceridemia and low HDL cholesterol levels. *Diabetes* 1996;45[Suppl3]:S27–S30.

8. Durrington PN, Mackness B, Mackness MI. Paraoxonase and atherosclerosis. *Arterioscler Thromb Vasc Biol* 2001;21:473–480.

9. Sniderman AD, Scantlebury T, Cianflone K. Hypertriglyceridemic hyperapoB: the unappreciated atherogenic dyslipoproteinemia in type 2 diabetes mellitus. *Ann Intern Med* 2001;135:447–459.

10. Proctor SD, Pabla CK, Mamo JC. Arterial intimal retention of pro-atherogenic lipoproteins in insulin deficient rabbits and rats. *Atherosclerosis* 2000;149:315–322.

11. Mahley RW, Huang Y, Rall SC Jr. Pathogenesis of type III hyperlipoproteinemia (dysbetalipoproteinemia): questions, quandaries, and paradoxes. *J Lipid Res* 1999;40:1933–1949.

12. Roche HM, Gibney MJ. The impact of postprandial lipemia in accelerating atherothrombosis. *J Cardiovasc Risk* 2000;7:317–324.

13. American Diabetes Association. Evidence-based nutrition principles and recommendations for the treatment and prevention of diabetes and related complications. *Diabetes Care* 2002;25:S50–S60.

14. Executive Summary of the Third Report of the National Cholesterol Education Program (NCEP) Expert Panel on Detection, Evaluation, and Treatment of High Blood Cholesterol in Adults (Adult Treatment Panel III). *JAMA* 2001;285:2486–2497.

15. Purnell JQ, Brunzell JD. The central role of dietary fat, not carbohydrate, in the insulin resistance syndrome. *Curr Opin Lipidol* 1997;8:17–22.

16. Reaven GM. Do high carbohydrate diets prevent the development or attenuate the manifestations (or both) of syndrome X? A viewpoint strongly against. *Curr Opin Lipidol* 1997;8:23–27.

17. Harris WS. n-3 Fatty acids and serum lipoproteins: human studies. *Am J Clin Nutr* 1997;65[Suppl]:1645S–1654S.

18. The Scandinavian Simvastatin Survival Study (4S). Randomised trial of cholesterol lowering in 4444 patients with coronary heart disease. *Lancet* 1994;344:1383–1389.

19. Pyorala K, Pedersen TR, Kjekshus J, et al. Cholesterol lowering with simvastatin improves prognosis of diabetic patients with coronary heart disease: a subgroup analysis of the Scandinavian Simvastatin Survival Study (4S). *Diabetes Care* 1997;20:614–620.

20. Haffner SM, Alexander CM, Cook TJ, et al. Reduced coronary events in simvastatin-treated patients with coronary heart disease and diabetes or impaired fasting glucose levels: subgroup analyses in the Scandinavian Simvastatin Survival Study. *Arch Intern Med* 1999;159:2661–2667.

21. Goldberg RB, Mellies MJ, Sacks PM, et al. Cardiovascular events and their reduction with pravastatin in diabetic and glucose-intolerant myocardial infarction survivors with average cholesterol levels: subgroup analyses in the Cholesterol and Recurrent Events (CARE) trial. The Care Investigators. *Circulation* 1998;98:2513–2519.

22. The Long-Term Intervention with Pravastatin in Ischaemic Disease (LIPID) Study Group. Prevention of cardiovascular events and death with pravastatin in patients with coronary heart disease and a broad range of initial cholesterol levels. *N Engl J Med* 1998;339:1349–1357.

23. Shepherd J, Cobbe SM, Ford I, et al. Prevention of coronary heart disease with pravastatin in men with hypercholesterolemia. West of Scotland Coronary Prevention Study Group. *N Engl J Med* 1995;333:1301–1307.

24. Downs JR, Clearfield M, Weis S, et al. Primary prevention of acute coronary events with lovastatin in men and women with average cholesterol levels: results of AFCAPS/TexCAPS. Air Force/Texas Coronary Atherosclerosis Prevention Study. *JAMA* 1998;279:1615–1622.

25. Heart Protection Study Collaborative Group. MRC/BHF Heart Protection Study of cholesterol lowering with simvastatin in 20,536 high-risk individuals: a randomised placebo-controlled trial. *Lancet* 2002;360:7–22.

26. Koskinen P, Manttari M, Manninen V, et al. Coronary heart disease incidence in NIDDM patients in the Helsinki Heart Study. *Diabetes Care* 1992;15:820–825.

27. Rubins HB, Robins SJ, Collins D, et al., for the Veterans Affairs High-Density Lipoprotein Cholesterol Intervention Trial Study Group. Gemfibrozil for the secondary prevention of coronary heart disease in men with low levels of high-density lipoprotein cholesterol. *N Engl J Med* 1999;341:410–418.

28. Robins SJ, Collins D, Wittes JT, et al., and the VA-HIT Study Group. Relation of gemfibrozil treatment and lipid levels with major coronary events. Veterans Affairs High-Density Lipoprotein Intervention Trial. a randomized controlled trial. *JAMA* 2001;285:1585–1591.

29. Effect of fenofibrate on progression of coronary-artery disease in type 2 diabetes: the Diabetes Atherosclerosis Intervention Study, a randomised study. *Lancet* 2001;357:905–910.

30. Austin MA, Breslow JL, Hennekens CH, et al. Low-density lipoprotein subclass patterns and risk of myocardial infarction. *JAMA* 1988;260:1917–1921.

31. Lamarche B, Tchemof A, Moorjani S, et al. Small, dense low-density lipoprotein particles as a predictor of the risk of ischemic heart disease in men. *Circulation* 1997;95:69–75.

32. Gardner CD, Fortmann SP, Krauss RM. Association of small low-density lipoprotein particles with the incidence of coronary artery disease in men and women. *JAMA* 1996;276:875–881.

33. Stampfer MJ, Krauss RM, Ma J, et al. A prospective study of triglyceride level, low-density lipoprotein particle diameter, and risk of myocardial infarction. *JAMA* 1996;276:882–888.

34. Coresh J, Kwiterovich PO, Smith HH, et al. Association of plasma triglyceride concentration and LDL

particle diameter, density, and chemical composition with premature coronary artery disease in men and women. *J Lipid Res* 1993;34:1687–1697.

35. Campos H, Moye LA, Glasser SP, et al. Low-density lipoprotein size, pravastatin treatment, and coronary events. *JAMA* 2001;286:1468–1474.

36. Garber AJ, Karlsson FO. Treatment of dyslipidemia in diabetes. *Endocrinol Metab Clin North Am* 2001;30:999–1010.

37. Lemieux I, Laperriere L, Dzavik V, et al. A 16-week fenofibrate treatment increases LDL particle size in type IIA dyslipidemic patients. *Atherosclerosis* 2002;162:363–371.

38. Pan J, Lin M, Kesala R, et al. Niacin treatment of the atherogenic lipid profile and Lp(a) in diabetes. *Diabetes Obes Metab* 2002;4:255–261.

39. Expert Panel on Detection, Evaluation, and Treatment of High Blood Cholesterol in Adults. Executive summary of the Third Report of the National Cholesterol Education Program (NCEP) Expert Panel on Detection, Evaluation, and Treatment of High Blood Cholesterol in Adults (Adult Treatment Panel III). *JAMA* 2001;285:2486–2509.

40. Turner RC, Millns H, Neil HA, et al. Risk factors for coronary artery disease in non-insulin dependent diabetes mellitus: United Kingdom Prospective Diabetes Study (UKPDS 23). *BMJ* 1998;316:823–828.

41. Tonkin A. High-density lipoprotein cholesterol and treatment guidelines. *Am J Cardiol* 2001;88[12A]:41N–44N.

42. Grundy SM, Vega GL, McGovern ME, et al. Efficacy, safety, and tolerability of once-daily niacin for the treatment of dyslipidemia associated with type 2 diabetes: results of the Assessment of Diabetes Control and Evaluation of the Efficacy of Niaspan Trial. *Arch Intern Med* 2002;162:1568–1576.

43. Brown G, Albers JJ, Fisher LD, et al. Regression of coronary artery disease as a result of intensive lipid-lowering therapy in men with high levels of apolipoprotein B. *N Engl J Med* 1990;323:1289–1298.

44. Brown BG, Zhao X-Q, Chait A, et al. Simvastatin and niacin, antioxidant vitamins, or the combination for the prevention of coronary disease. *N Engl J Med* 2001;345:1583–1592.

45. Ballantyne CM, Herd JA, Ferlic LL, et al. Influence of low HDL on progression of coronary artery disease and response to fluvastatin therapy. *Circulation* 1999;99:736–743.

46. Writing Group for the Women's Health Initiative Investigators. Risks and benefits of estrogen plus progestin in healthy postmenopausal women: principal results from the Women's Health Initiative randomized controlled trial. *JAMA* 2002;288:321–333.

47. Grady D, Herrington D, Bittner V, et al. Cardiovascular disease outcomes during 6.8 years of hormone therapy: Heart and Estrogen/progestin Replacement Study follow-up (HERS II). *JAMA* 2002;288:49–57.

48. Heart Outcomes Prevention Evaluation (HOPE) Study Investigators. Effects of ramipril on cardiovascular and microvascular outcomes in people with diabetes mellitus: results of the HOPE study and MICRO-HOPE sub study. *Lancet* 2000;355:253–259.

49. GISSI-Prevenzione Investigators. Dietary supplementation with n-3 polyunsaturated fatty acids and vitamin E in 11,324 patients with myocardial infarction: results of the GISSI-Prevenzione trial. *Lancet* 1999;354:447–455.

50. Cullen P. Evidence that triglycerides are an independent coronary heart disease risk factor. *Am J Cardiol* 2000;86:943–949.

51. Manninen V, Tenkanen L, Koskinen P, et al. Joint effects of serum triglyceride and LDL cholesterol and HDL cholesterol concentrations on coronary heart disease risk in the Helsinki Heart Study: implications for treatment. *Circulation* 1992;85:37–45.

52. Rubins HB. Triglycerides and coronary heart disease: implications of recent clinical trials. *J Cardiovasc Risk* 2000;7:339–345.

53. Pasternak RC, Smith SC, Bairey-Merz CN, et al. ACC/AHA/NHLBI clinical advisory on the use and safety of statins. *J Am Coll Cardiol* 2002;40:567–572.

54. Grover SA, Coupal L, Zowall H, et al. Cost-effectiveness of treating hyperlipidemia in the presence of diabetes: who should be treated? *Circulation* 2000;102:722–727.

55. Prueksaritanont T, Zhao JJ, Ma B, et al. Mechanistic studies on metabolic interactions between gemfibrozil and statins. *J Pharmacol Exp Ther* 2002;301:1042–1051.

56. Marcus A. Current lipid-lowering strategies for the treatment of diabetic dyslipidemia: an integrated approach to therapy. *The Endocrinologist* 2001;11:368–383.

57. Davidson M, Ma P, Stein EA, et al. Comparison of effects on low-density lipoprotein cholesterol and high-density lipoprotein cholesterol with rosuvastatin versus atorvastatin in patients with type IIa or IIb hypercholesterolemia. *Am J Cardiol* 2002;89:268–275.

58. Jones P, Kafonek S, Laurora I, et al. Comparative dose efficacy study of atorvastatin versus simvastatin, pravastatin, lovastatin, and fluvastatin in patients with hypercholesterolemia (the CURVES study). *Am J Cardiol* 1998;81:582–587.

59. Crouse JR, Frohlich J, Ose L, et al. Effects of high doses of simvastatin and atorvastatin on high-density lipoprotein cholesterol and apolipoprotein A-I. *Am J Cardiol* 1999;83:1476–1477, A7.

60. Tolman KG. The liver and lovastatin. *Am J Cardiol* 2002;89:1374–1380.

61. Dujovne CA. Side effects of statins: hepatitis versus "transaminitis"-myositis versus "CPKitis." *Am J Cardiol* 2002;89:1411–1413.

62. The Lipid Research Clinics Coronary Primary Prevention Trial results: I. Reduction in incidence of coronary heart disease. *JAMA* 1984;25:351–364.

63. Cashin-Hemphill L, Mack WJ, Pogoda JM, et al. Beneficial effects of colestipol-niacin on coronary atherosclerosis: a 4-year follow-up. *JAMA* 1990;264:3013–3017.

64. Hallikainen MA, Uusitupa MI. Effects of low-fat stanol ester-containing margarines on serum cholesterol concentrations as part of a low-fat diet in hypercholesterolemic subjects. *Am J Clin Nutr* 1999;69:403–410.

65. Gagne C, Gaudet D, Bruckert E. Efficacy and safety of ezetimibe coadministered with atorvastatin or simvastatin in patients with homozygous familial hypercholesterolemia. *Circulation* 2002;105:2469–2475.

66. Fruchart JC, Staels B, Duriez P. The role of fibric acids in atherosclerosis. *Curr Atheroscler Rep* 2001;3:83–92.

67. Elam MB, Hunninghake DB, Davis KB, et al. Effect

of niacin on lipid and lipoprotein levels and glycemic control in patients with diabetes and peripheral arterial disease. The ADMIT Study: a randomized trial. *JAMA* 2000;284:1263–1270.

68. Garg A, Grundy SM. Nicotinic acid as therapy for dyslipidemia in non-insulin-dependent diabetes mellitus. *J Am Med Assoc* 1990;264:723–726.

69. Gupta EK, Ito MK. Lovastatin and extended-release niacin combination product: the first drug combination for the management of hyperlipidemia. *Heart Dis* 2002;4:124–137.

70. Glauber H, Wallace P, Griver K, et al. Adverse metabolic effect of omega-3 fatty acids in non-insulin-dependent diabetes mellitus. *Ann Intern Med* 1988;108:663–668.

71. Montori VM, Farmer A, Wollan PC, et al. Fish oil supplementation in type 2 diabetes: a quantitative systematic review. *Diabetes Care* 2000;23:1407–1415.

72. American Diabetes Association. Management of dyslipidemia in adults with diabetes. *Diabetes Care* 2002;25:S74–S77.

73. Haffner SM, Goldberg RB. New strategies for the treatment of diabetic dyslipidemia. *Diabetes Care* 2002;25:1237–1239.

74. Orchard TJ, Forrest KY, Kuller LH, et al. Lipid and blood pressure treatment goals for type 1 diabetes: 10-year incidence data from the Pittsburgh Epidemiology of Diabetes Complications Study. *Diabetes Care* 2001;24:1053–1059.

Diabetes and Cardiovascular Disease
edited by Steven P. Marso and David M. Stern
Lippincott Williams & Wilkins, Philadelphia © 2004

19

Diabetes Mellitus and Ischemic Heart Disease

Benjamin H. Trichon and Matthew T. Roe

Fellow, Division of Cardiology, Duke University Medical Center; Assistant Professor of Medicine, Division of Cardiology, Duke University Medical Center, Durham, North Carolina

Cardiovascular complications are the leading cause of morbidity among patients with diabetes, and ischemic heart disease is the most common cause of death (Fig. 19-1) (1,2). A central contributor to the high cardiovascular morbidity and mortality rates among diabetic persons is the premature development and accelerated progression of atherosclerosis. More than 75% of cardiovascular deaths in diabetic patients result from complications of acute myocardial ischemia.

The presence of diabetes mellitus increases the risk of developing coronary artery disease (CAD) by a factor of twofold to fourfold (3). Furthermore, among patients with CAD, diabetes is associated with an increased risk of developing an acute coronary syndrome (ACS) and an increased risk of death after an acute myocardial infarction (MI) (4,5). Patients with diabetes may therefore have a greater proportional benefit from proven therapies for acute ischemic heart disease. This chapter focuses on the pathophysiology, clinical presentation, and treatment of ACS among patients with diabetes, including non-ST-segment elevation acute coronary syndrome (NSTE-ACS) and acute ST-segment elevation myocardial infarction (STEMI).

PATHOPHYSIOLOGY OF ACUTE CORONARY SYNDROME IN PATIENTS WITH DIABETES MELLITUS

Multiple metabolic, vascular, and coagulation abnormalities among patients with diabetes interact and contribute to the high rates of atherosclerosis and ischemic complications in this population. Important abnormalities of endothelial function, plaque stability, and platelet function underlie the higher frequency of ACS.

The single layer of endothelial cells lining all blood vessels provides a metabolically active interface between the intravascular space and the surrounding tissue that modulates blood flow, oxygen and nutrient delivery, coagulation, and thrombosis. Endothelial cells synthesize important bioactive substances, including nitric oxide, prostaglandins, endothelin, and angiotensin II, which regulate vascular function (6). The presence of diabetes affects endothelial function in many ways leading to the accelerated development of atherosclerosis. Hyperglycemia inhibits the activity of endothelial nitric oxide synthase (eNOS), which reduces the production of nitric oxide and thus impairs endothelium-dependent vasodilation. The production of reactive oxygen species (especially superoxide anion O_2^-) is increased, further inhibiting the action of eNOS. Moreover, production of the vasoconstrictive agents, endothelin-1 and angiotensin II, is higher among persons with diabetes, and lymphocytes and other inflammatory cells more commonly infiltrate the intimal layer of the endothelium (6). Therefore, patients with diabetes are more prone to vasoconstriction and disorders in autoregulation of coronary flow.

The atherosclerotic plaque is more prone to instability in patients with diabetes. Endothelial cells release cytokines, which decrease the

Causes of Death in Persons with Diabetes, Based on US Studies

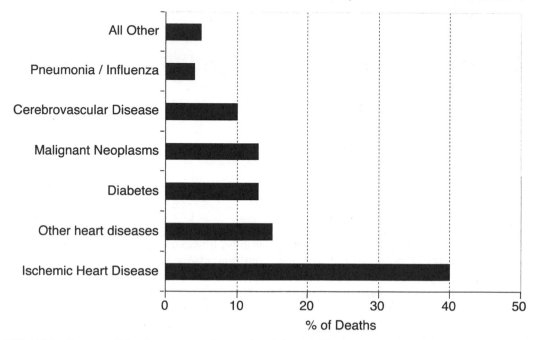

FIG. 19-1. Causes of death among patients with diabetes. (From Geiss LS, Herman WH, Smith PJ, and the National Diabetes Data Group. *Diabetes in America.* Bethesda, MD: National Institutes of Health, National Institute of Diabetes and Digestive and Kidney Diseases; 1995:233–257.)

synthesis of collagen by vascular smooth muscle cells and increase the production of matrix metalloproteinases, which promote collagen breakdown (6). The decreased synthesis and increased breakdown of collagen reduces the mechanical stability of the plaque's fibrous cap, leading to a propensity for plaque rupture and the subsequent formation of an overlying thrombus.

Abnormalities of platelet function are central to the increased risk of thrombotic events among patients with diabetes (Table 19-1). Platelets in patients with diabetes are larger, have a greater concentration of glycoprotein (GP) IIb/IIIa surface receptors (central contributors to platelet aggregation), and are prone to aggregate more commonly when stimulated than platelets of patients without diabetes (7). *In vivo* studies have demonstrated increased shear-induced platelet adhesion and aggregation, augmented synthesis of proaggregating thromboxanes, and a high percentage of platelets circulating in the activated state in

persons with diabetes (8). These abnormalities of platelet function underlie the enhanced thrombotic potential and higher morbidity and mortality rates among diabetic patients in the setting of ACS. The propensity for thrombosis most likely

TABLE 19-1. *Abnormalities of platelet function and coagulation in diabetes mellitus*

↑Fibrinogen
↑Plasminogen activator inhibitor-1
↓Antithrombin III
↓Proteins C and S
↑Factors VII and VIII
↑Vascular cell adhesion molecule-1
↑Platelet adhesiveness
↑Platelet aggregation
↓Platelet nitric oxide production
↓Platelet prostacyclin production
↑Glycation of platelet proteins

From Kirpichnikov D, Sowers JR. Diabetes mellitus and diabetes-associated vascular disease. *Trends Endocrinol Metab* 2001;12:225–230.

affects plaque morphology among diabetic persons presenting with ACS (9). In a cohort of 55 ACS patients, diabetic persons were more likely to have complex lesion morphology and evidence for coronary thrombi when evaluated with angioscopy, compared with nondiabetic patients.

EFFECT OF DIABETES MELLITUS ON THE CLINICAL PRESENTATION OF ACUTE CORONARY SYNDROMES

Patients with diabetes may have mild or atypical symptoms and signs accompanying an ACS, presumably as a consequence of underlying autonomic and sensory neuropathies. As a result, the frequency of silent myocardial ischemia and MI among patients with diabetes is high. In a cohort of patients undergoing treadmill testing, more than 60% of those with silent ischemia had diabetes, and all had underlying autonomic nervous system abnormalities, despite the absence of overt vascular complications of diabetes (10). Additionally, diabetes is often associated with abnormalities of gastric emptying, which causes frequent noncardiac chest pain syndromes in certain patients. This may reduce the degree of urgency accompanying an episode of chest discomfort in the setting of actual myocardial ischemia.

The impaired sensation of chest discomfort among many patients with diabetes also contributes to late presentation for medical attention in the setting of an ACS, with subsequent delayed institution of initial therapies. In the Global Utilization of Streptokinase and Tissue Plasminogen Activator for Occluded Coronary Arteries (GUSTO-I) trial, diabetic patients with STEMI presented, on average, about 15 minutes later for treatment than did nondiabetic patients (11). In a pooled analysis of almost 70,000 patients receiving fibrinolytic therapy, the Fibrinolytic Therapy Trialists Group found that mortality related to STEMI was 1% higher for every hour delay in treatment after presentation (12). A similar decrement in benefit is seen with delays in primary percutaneous coronary intervention (PCI) for STEMI (13). This time-dependent benefit of primary reperfusion therapy, in the setting of STEMI, warrants the continued education of patients with diabetes on the importance of early presentation and the potential atypical clinical manifestations of myocardial ischemia (14).

Vigilance is also needed in interpreting the electrocardiogram (ECG) in diabetic patients presenting with a suspected ACS. The use of certain oral hypoglycemic medications may produce alterations in the ECG, possibly reducing its sensitivity in detecting the characteristic changes of myocardial ischemia. Several animal studies suggest that certain sulfonylurea drugs are associated with reduced amplitude of ST-segment elevation and T-wave peaking during the early phases of acute myocardial ischemia (15). Other, nonspecific repolarization abnormalities may also be associated with the use of these medications (16). Because of these potential confounding effects on the ECG and the high pretest probability of CAD in patients with diabetes, physicians and other health care providers should maintain a high index of suspicion of myocardial ischemia in patients with diabetes who present with typical or atypical chest pain symptoms and equivocal ECG findings.

EPIDEMIOLOGY OF ACUTE CORONARY SYNDROME AMONG PATIENTS WITH DIABETES MELLITUS

Traditionally, it is estimated that approximately 30% of patients hospitalized with a MI will have diabetes, compared with a diabetes prevalence of 6% to 8% in the general population (2). However, recent data suggests that an additional 30% of hospitalized persons may have undiagnosed diabetes in the setting of a MI (17). Further, diabetes mellitus increases the risk of ACS and of complications after presenting with ACS. In a recent population-based study, the 7-year incidence of a first MI or death for patients with diabetes was 20%, compared with 3.5% for patients without diabetes (18). Furthermore, short- and long-term mortality rates after STEMI are twice as high among patients with diabetes, compared with those who do not have diabetes (19). Although the use of fibrinolytic therapy for the treatment of STEMI has led to a considerable improvement in survival, the presence of diabetes still remains a significant predictor of mortality among patients receiving this form of reperfusion therapy (20).

Several factors most likely explain this unfavorable prognosis in diabetic patients after STEMI, including delayed presentation, higher frequency of comorbidities, autonomic neuropathy, and possibly reduced efficacy of certain medical and interventional therapies (21). Additionally, patients with diabetes have a higher frequency of complications after STEMI, including higher rates of reinfarction, postinfarction angina, infarct expansion, and congestive heart failure (22).

The presence of diabetes also adversely affects early and late outcomes in the setting of NSTE-ACS. Boersma et al. (23) investigated the relationship between baseline characteristics and the rate of death and MI in a large, international trial of patients with NSTE-ACS. They demonstrated that those patients with diabetes had a 5.6% rate of death at 30 days, compared with 3.0% for nondiabetic patients, and that diabetes independently predicted the risk of death at 30 days (OR = 1.38; 95% confidence interval [CI], 1.07 to 1.76). The occurrence of death and nonfatal MI was also higher among the subgroup of patients with diabetes, compared with nondiabetic patients (18.5% versus 14.0%). In the Organization to Assess Strategies for Ischemic Syndromes (OASIS) registry, 1,718 (21%) of 8,013 patients had diabetes. After adjusting for other important clinical characteristics, the presence of diabetes was independently related to survival, with diabetics having a 56% higher mortality rate than nondiabetics (24). Interestingly, diabetes was of greater prognostic importance in women than in men; the risk of adverse outcomes in women with diabetes was increased by 98%, compared to 28% in men with diabetes (24).

The increased frequency of adverse outcomes among diabetic patients with ACS probably has several explanations in addition to the pathophysiologic abnormalities mentioned earlier. Patients with diabetes and ACS have a higher prevalence of comorbidities, including dyslipidemia, hypertension, congestive heart failure, and renal insufficiency (11). In addition, the extent of vascular disease is also greater in diabetic patients, with a higher frequency of multivessel CAD, cerebral vascular disease, and peripheral vascular disease compared with nondiabetic patients (19). Therefore, patients with diabetes who present with ACS should be considered to be at high risk for adverse outcomes and deserve aggressive medical interventions to mitigate the risk of subsequent recurrent ischemic events.

REPERFUSION THERAPY FOR ACUTE ST-SEGMENT ELEVATION MYOCARDIAL INFARCTION

Clinical Outcomes After Fibrinolysis

Pooled analyses of the major fibrinolytic trials have provided insight into the influence of diabetes on clinical outcomes of patients with a STEMI and the relative efficacy of fibrinolysis in this population. The GUSTO-I trial enrolled more than 41,000 patients with STEMI, who received one of four fibrinolytic regimens. The 30-day mortality rate among the 5,944 patients with diabetes was 10.5%, compared with 6.2% among patients without diabetes (11). The highest mortality rate occurred among diabetic patients being treated with insulin (12.5%), compared with 9.7% in those not receiving insulin (Fig. 19-2). Mortality rates at 1 year were over 60% higher among diabetics (14.5%) compared with nondiabetics (8.9%).

Similar findings of worse outcomes in patients with diabetes were reported from the Thrombolysis and Angioplasty in Myocardial Infarction (TAMI) experience. The 148 patients (16% of total enrollment) with diabetes had a significantly higher in-hospital mortality rate, compared with subjects without diabetes (11% versus 6%, respectively) (25). In a pooled analysis of data from several large fibrinolytic trials, patients with diabetes who received fibrinolytic therapy had an almost twofold higher rate of mortality at 30 days than did nondiabetic persons similarly treated (13.6% versus 8.7%, respectively). The mortality rate was also highest among those subjects with diabetes who received insulin therapy (1.3 times greater than in those not receiving insulin)

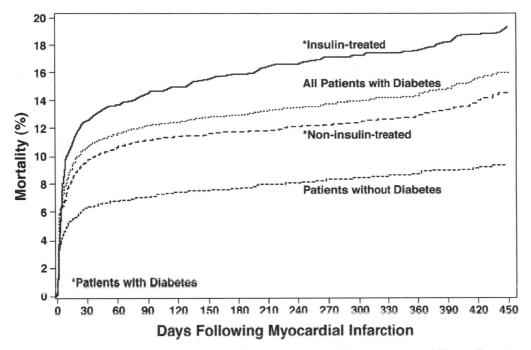

FIG. 19-2. Mortality by diabetic status in the Global Utilization of Streptokinase and Tissue Plasminogen Activator for Occluded Coronary Arteries (GUSTO-I) trial. (From Mak KH, Moliterno DJ, Granger CB, et al. Influence of diabetes mellitus on clinical outcome in the thrombolytic era of acute myocardial infarction. GUSTO-I Investigators. Global Utilization of Streptokinase and Tissue Plasminogen Activator for Occluded Coronary Arteries. *J Am Coll Cardiol* 1997;30:171 179.)

(12). Despite an increased risk of adverse outcomes after reperfusion therapy, patients with diabetes derive a greater absolute benefit from the use of fibrinolysis. The Fibrinolytic Therapy Trialists (FTT) Group demonstrated that the use of fibrinolytics saved 37 lives per 1,000 patients with diabetes who were treated, compared with 15 lives per 1,000 patients without diabetes treated (12).

More recent studies, using new pharmacologic reperfusion strategies with bolus fibrinolytic agents (reteplase and tenecteplase) and combinations of reduced-dose fibrinolytic agents and GP IIb/IIIa inhibitors, have also evaluated the relative treatment effects in patients with diabetes (26–28). In the GUSTO-V trial, patients presenting with STEMI were randomly assigned to receive either full-dose reteplase or combination therapy with half-dose reteplase plus the GP IIb/IIIa inhibitor, abciximab. Among the

16,588 patients studied, 16% had diabetes. Diabetic patients receiving abciximab and low-dose reteplase had a higher 30-day mortality rate than did nondiabetic patients similarly treated (8.2% versus 5.0%). There was a similarly modest relative reduction in 30-day mortality with combination therapy, as was seen in the overall study population.

Use of Fibrinolytics in Patients with Diabetes

Despite receiving a greater absolute benefit with fibrinolytics, patients with diabetes are less likely to receive fibrinolytics for STEMI, compared with patients who do not have diabetes. In the Survival and Ventricular Enlargement (SAVE) study, the use of fibrinolytic therapy was not specified in the trial design and was left to the discretion of the attending physician. More than 67% of patients enrolled with STEMI did not

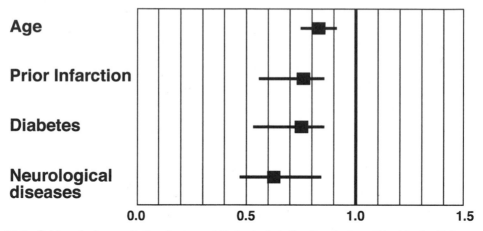

FIG. 19-3. Odds ratio for predicting the use of fibrinolysis in the Survival and Ventricular Enlargement (SAVE) trial. (From Mak KH, Topol EJ. Emerging concepts in the management of acute myocardial infarction in patients with diabetes mellitus. *J Am Coll Cardiol* 2000;35:563–568, with permission.)

receive fibrinolytic therapy, and the presence of diabetes was among the clinical characteristics that independently predicted the *non*-use of fibrinolytics (Fig. 19-3) (29). The underuse of fibrinolytics among patients with diabetes was also found in an observational analysis from the second National Registry of Myocardial Infarction (NRMI-2). Among almost 85,000 patients with STEMI in the registry who were eligible for fibrinolytics, 24% did not receive any form of reperfusion therapy. In a multivariable analysis, the presence of diabetes was an independent predictor for the non-use of reperfusion therapy (OR = 0.67; 95% CI, 0.52 to 0.87) (30). These data from the United States were verified in separate reports of nationwide practices from France and the United Kingdom, where eligible patients with STEMI who had diabetes were significantly less likely to receive primary reperfusion therapy than were nondiabetic patients with STEMI (31,32).

The reasons underlying the lower rate of use of fibrinolytic therapy among patients with diabetes are not clearly understood. Factors such as atypical or late presentation and concern regarding the adverse effects of fibrinolytic agents in patients with diabetes probably play a role. The evidence to date, however, does not suggest that patients with diabetes who receive fibrinolytic therapy have significantly higher complication rates than nondiabetic patients do. In the GUSTO-I trial, patients with diabetes had only a small increase in moderate bleeding complications after fibrinolysis, compared with nondiabetic patients (13% versus 11%, respectively), and they had no increase in the risk of major bleeding events. The risk of intracranial hemorrhage in GUSTO-I was also similar between patients with and without diabetes (0.6% versus 0.7%, respectively) (11). Although there has been a long-standing concern that the risk of intraocular hemorrhage after fibrinolysis is increased in patients with diabetes who have retinopathy, only 12 patients (0.03%) had an ocular hemorrhage in GUSTO-I. Intraocular hemorrhage was confirmed in only one nondiabetic patient. Among the 6,011 patients with diabetes, only one had an eyelid hematoma after a documented fall, and none had an intraocular hemorrhage (33). Therefore, concern about hemorrhagic complications should not preclude the use of fibrinolytic agents in appropriate diabetic patients with STEMI.

Angiographic Results after Fibrinolysis

The underlying mechanisms that may explain the higher mortality rates among patients with diabetes after STEMI remain elusive. The increased risk of adverse outcomes may be related to a lower rate of successful reperfusion with fibrinolysis, a higher rate of reocclusion after successful fibrinolysis, larger infarct size, more extensive angiographic CAD, or a more unfavorable clinical risk factor profile (21). The GUSTO-I angiographic investigators sought to analyze the relative contributions of several of these factors to clinical outcomes among diabetic persons enrolled in the angiographic substudy of the GUSTO-I trial (34). Patients with diabetes represented 12.8% of the total angiographic substudy population. They were older, more often female, presented later for medical attention, and had more signs of heart failure than did patients without diabetes in the substudy. Interestingly, 90-minute patency rates (Thrombolysis in Myocardial Infarction [TIMI] flow grades II and III) after treatment with fibrinolytics were similar in both diabetic and nondiabetic patients (70.1% versus 66.6%, respectively). Therefore, fibrinolytic therapy seems to achieve equivalent coronary artery patency rates in patients both with and without diabetes.

In addition to similar initial patency rates after fibrinolysis, there was no significant difference in the rates of angiographically confirmed infarct artery reocclusion between patients with or without diabetes in the GUSTO angiographic analysis (34). However, not all patients in this study underwent follow-up angiography, and the proportion of patients who died before follow-up study was almost threefold higher among diabetic patients (21). Despite the apparent similarities in angiographic rates of reperfusion, recurrent ischemia occurred more frequently among diabetic subjects (11). This higher rate of recurrent ischemia may be a partial explanation of the poorer outcomes among diabetics after STEMI.

One week after fibrinolysis, regional ventricular function in the area of the infarct was similar in a subgroup of diabetic subjects versus nondiabetic subjects analyzed in GUSTO-I (34). No significant differences in ejection fraction were observed at 90 minutes, 5 days, or 1 week. However, the function of the "noninfarcted" area of myocardium differed: patients with diabetes had significantly less hyperkinesia in noninfarcted zones than did nondiabetic patients at 90 minutes after fibrinolysis. These findings suggest that diabetic persons may have a greater degree of myocardium with reversible dysfunction (stunned myocardium) in noninfarcted territories after fibrinolysis. These findings may result from impaired coronary blood flow in "nonculprit" coronary arteries that could be exaggerated in patients with diabetes, who are more likely to have multivessel CAD and endothelial dysfunction (35).

Primary Percutaneous Coronary Intervention

Primary percutaneous transluminal coronary angioplasty (PTCA) has been shown to improve outcomes among patients with STEMI and to reduce the rates of death, reinfarction, and stroke, compared with fibrinolytic therapy (36). This reperfusion strategy has been rarely studied specifically in patients with diabetes, so data regarding procedural success and long-term outcomes is derived primarily from subanalyses of large clinical trials. The GUSTO-IIb Primary Angioplasty Substudy analyzed the relative benefits of pharmacologic and mechanical reperfusion strategies among the 1,138 patients with STEMI, who were randomly assigned to primary PTCA or accelerated tissue plasminogen activator (tPA) (37). Patients with diabetes (16% of the total population) had higher-risk baseline clinical characteristics and more extensive CAD than did the nondiabetic patients. Procedural success after primary angioplasty (normal infarct artery flow and stenosis less than 50%) was similar between diabetic and nondiabetic subjects (70.4% versus 72.4%, respectively). The rate of the primary end point at 30 days (death, MI, or disabling stroke) was greater among diabetic persons treated with primary PTCA than among nondiabetic persons (11.1% versus 9.3%, respectively). However, both diabetics (OR = 0.70; 95% CI, 0.29 to 1.72) and nondiabetics (OR = 0.62; 95% CI, 0.41 to 0.96) had improved outcomes at 30 days with primary PTCA compared with accelerated tPA.

In a combined analysis of two large primary PTCA trials, GUSTO-IIb and RAPPORT (primary PTCA with GP IIb/IIIa inhibitor versus placebo), the presence of diabetes did not independently predict death or reinfarction at 30 days (38). Similarly, the presence of diabetes mellitus did not independently predict adverse in-hospital or 6-month outcomes in a subgroup analysis of the first Primary Angioplasty in Myocardial Infarction (PAMI) trial comparing primary angioplasty with tPA (22). However, Thomas et al. (39) found a threefold increase in the risk of long-term mortality among diabetic persons participating in a trial comparing streptokinase with primary angioplasty. Therefore, primary angioplasty appears to provide equal benefit to diabetic and nondiabetic persons, and the increased risk of adverse outcomes commonly seen in patients with diabetes after STEMI may be somewhat mitigated by mechanical reperfusion.

The use of stents and platelet GP IIb/IIIa inhibitors, in conjunction with primary PTCA, reduces the risk of recurrent ischemia and late restenosis of the infarct-related artery and improves clinical outcomes (40). Several trials using stents and GP IIb/IIIa inhibitors have included significant numbers of patients with diabetes. The Controlled Abciximab and Device Investigation to Lower Late Angioplasty Complications (CADILLAC) trial randomly assigned eligible patients with STEMI to one of four primary reperfusion strategies: PTCA alone, PTCA plus the GP IIb/IIIa inhibitor abciximab, stenting alone, or stenting plus abciximab. The strategy of primary stenting was superior to PTCA alone, and the rate of the primary end point (composite of death, reinfarction, revascularization, or disabling stroke) at 30 days and at 6 months was lowest among patients receiving the combination of stenting and abciximab (41). Among the 2,082 study participants, 16.6% had diabetes, and they received a magnitude of benefit with stenting and abciximab similar to that of the overall study population (OR = 0.56; 95% CI, 0.32 to 0.97 in diabetics; OR = 0.54; 95% CI, 0.42 to 0.69 in total population). In the ADMIRAL trial, patients with STEMI undergoing primary stenting were randomly assigned to receive either abciximab or placebo. Patients with diabetes had an absolute reduction in the rate of death, MI, or ur-

gent revascularization at 30 days that was greater than that of the total study population (13.9% versus 8.0%, respectively) (42). Therefore, patients with diabetes who present with STEMI appear to derive particular benefit from a reperfusion strategy that includes primary stenting plus GP IIb/IIIa inhibition.

Despite these encouraging results, the presence of diabetes increases the risk of early complications after primary PCI. In a cohort of 104 consecutive patients undergoing primary stenting for STEMI, Silva et al. (43) demonstrated that the only independent predictors of stent thrombosis were diabetes and tobacco use. This finding may reflect the heightened platelet activation and aggregation among patients with diabetes. This preliminary evidence suggests that diabetes may be an important risk factor for stent thrombosis, in addition to its established role in the development of in-stent restenosis after elective PCI (8).

In addition to the data from these trials, important information is provided by several registries regarding the use of catheter-based reperfusion in the setting of STEMI. Twenty-year data from the Mid America Heart Institute confirms that patients with diabetes have an approximately twofold increase in in-hospital mortality after primary PCI (12.7% versus 6.9%, $p < .001$) (44). Furthermore, unlike data from both the elective PCI cohort and the nondiabetic acute MI cohort, there has not been an adjusted improvement in in-hospital mortality for diabetic patients after primary PCI in two decades. The aforementioned data highlight the continuing need to improve the recognition of and reperfusion strategy for diabetic patients in the setting of an acute MI.

Glycemic/Metabolic Therapy for STEMI

During periods of myocardial ischemia, glucose begins to undergo anaerobic metabolism, with less efficient generation of adenosine triphosphate (ATP). In addition, the relative insulin deficiency seen in diabetic persons leads to a reduction in the intracellular translocation of glucose. These processes, when accompanied by increased sympathetic nervous system activity in the setting of myocardial ischemia, lead to a shift toward fatty acid metabolism in the cardiomyocyte. This shift in substrate for ATP generation ultimately results in increased oxygen consumption and the accumulation of free-fatty acids (FFA). FFA accumulation leads to impaired myocardial contractility and the production of free radicals, which may promote membrane instability and increase the risk of arrhythmias (45). Consequently, there is a loss of cell membrane stability that leads to eventual myocardial cellular necrosis.

Approximately 30 years ago, Sodi-Pallares et al (46) reported that the infusion of a solution of glucose-insulin-potassium (GIK) shortened the ECG evolution of an acute MI, reduced the incidence of ventricular ectopy, and improved short-term survival in acute STEMI. With exogenous supplementation of glucose and insulin, the investigators hoped to promote more efficient generation of ATP, lower FFA generation, and thus a lower risk of myocyte injury during ischemia and reperfusion.

In an overview of nine early (prefibrinolytic era), randomized trials enrolling a total of 1,932 acute MI patients with and without diabetes, GIK reduced in-hospital mortality by 28%, with approximately 49 lives saved per 1,000 patients treated (47). Four of the trials used high-dose GIK infusions to more completely suppress FFA generation, and this strategy resulted in a 48% reduction in short-term mortality. Therefore, preliminary studies suggested that GIK could be a useful adjunctive therapy for the treatment of STEMI.

Subsequently, the Diabetes and Insulin-Glucose Infusion in Acute Myocardial Infarction (DIGAMI) study investigators randomly assigned 620 patients with diabetes and STEMI to GIK followed by multidose subcutaneous insulin for at least 3 months or to conventional post-STEMI therapy (48). After 3 months, patients receiving GIK had lower values of glycosylated hemoglobin, and at 1 year they had a 29% reduction in mortality compared with those receiving conventional therapy. However, mortality rates through 3 months were similar between treatment and placebo groups. The benefit of GIK in-

fusion was particularly striking among patients with a low baseline cardiovascular risk profile and no prior insulin therapy (52% mortality reduction with GIK at 1 year). More recently, extended follow-up (mean, 3.4 years) of the study population demonstrated a persistent mortality reduction in the GIK-treated group (relative risk reduction [RRR], 25%; absolute risk reduction [ARR], 11%; $p = .011$) (49).

Despite these results, several perceived limitations of the DIGAMI trial have prevented the incorporation of GIK into routine clinical practice (50). The lower-than-expected overall mortality rate in the trial suggested that the study was not powered to truly demonstrate a difference in survival at 3 months (the primary study end point). Furthermore, the mechanism of benefit of GIK infusion has been questioned. Given that survival was not improved in the GIK group until more than 3 months after randomization, a potential favorable effect of acute GIK infusion cannot be separated from the benefits of the outpatient insulin regimen the treatment group received over the course of the entire study period. Finally, the apparent benefits of GIK and subcutaneous insulin may, in fact, reflect a detrimental effect of oral hypoglycemic agents that were more commonly used in the placebo arm.

Nonetheless, the Estudios Cardiologicos Latinoamerica (ECLA) group subsequently reported the results of another randomized trial of GIK for the treatment of STEMI (51). A total of 477 patients, with and without diabetes, were randomly assigned to either placebo or two doses of GIK. A subgroup of 252 (62%) patients received concomitant fibrinolytic therapy. Among patients treated with fibrinolytics, the use of GIK was associated with a highly significant 66% relative reduction (ARR, 10%) in the rate of in-hospital mortality. This survival benefit persisted for 1 year after treatment in the group receiving the high-dose GIK infusion along with fibrinolytics.

Although the findings of the ECLA study are provocative, a more definitive investigation of GIK therapy is needed before this strategy can be accepted for the treatment of STEMI. The patients in the control arm of the ECLA study who underwent reperfusion therapy had an unusually high mortality rate of 15.2%, approximately twice as high as that reported in the large fibrinolytic trials (52). This could certainly explain the large apparent benefit of GIK in the treatment group. Furthermore, the ECLA trial was not large, and a statistically significant reduction in mortality occurred only in the subgroup that received concomitant reperfusion therapy, not in the entire trial population.

These concerns were further emphasized by the results of the Glucose-Insulin-Potassium Study (GIPS), recently presented at the European Society of Cardiology Meeting in September, 2002 (53). In this trial, 940 patients (with and without diabetes) presenting with STEMI were randomly assigned to receive either an infusion of GIK or placebo. The 30-day mortality rate was 4.8% in the GIK-treated group and 5.8% in the control group ($p = .10$). When stratified by the presence or absence of diabetes or successful reperfusion, no significant differences in 30-day mortality were seen. Interestingly, the 30-day mortality rate among patients without heart failure who were treated with GIK was 1.2%, compared with 4.2% in the control group. The apparent survival benefit of GIK in a subgroup of patients from a relatively small trial confirms the hazards of estimating the benefits of GIK without a definitive, large-scale trial.

Early Invasive Management for Non-ST-segment Elevation Acute Coronary Syndrome

The syndromes of unstable angina and non-ST-segment elevation myocardial infarction (NSTEMI) account for approximately 1.5 million hospital admissions annually in the United States and 2.5 million worldwide (54). Unstable angina or NSTEMI (collectively known as NSTE-ACS) can be managed in hospital with either an "early-conservative" strategy (characterized by medical stabilization, noninvasive risk stratification, and coronary angiography only if high-risk clinical indicators are present) or an "early-invasive" strategy (with routine angiography and revascularization, if needed, within 48 hours after admission, unless contraindications exist). These two approaches have been compared in several randomized, controlled trials, but they have never been studied specifically in patients with diabetes. Evidence of their effectiveness in patients with diabetes is obtained from subgroup analysis of these larger trials (55,56).

Several trials evaluating early-invasive versus early-conservative approaches have been performed in the contemporary era and are characterized by the use of platelet GP IIb/IIIa inhibitors and low-molecular-weight heparin (LMWH) as components of early medical stabilization. The Fragmin and Fast Revascularization during Instability in Coronary Artery Disease (FRISC II) study randomly assigned 2,457 patients with NSTE-ACS to an early-invasive or early-conservative management strategy (55). In the overall study, the rate of death or MI through 3 months was reduced in the group treated with the early-invasive strategy (RR = 0.78; 95% CI, 0.62 to 0.98). Of those enrolled, 299 (13% of total study population) had diabetes. Patients with diabetes who were randomly assigned to the early-invasive strategy had a substantially higher rate of death and/or MI at 6 months, compared with nondiabetic patients treated in the same fashion (18.3% versus 8.1%). The absolute benefit of the early-invasive strategy was greater among diabetic than nondiabetic patients (ARR, 6.2% versus 2.3%, respectively).

The superiority of the early-invasive approach among patients with diabetes was also seen in the TACTICS-TIMI 18 trial. Diabetic patients (28% of the entire population of 2,220) who were randomly assigned to the early-invasive management strategy had a higher rate of death, MI, or rehospitalization for ACS than did nondiabetic patients (20.1% versus 14.2%). Similar to the FRISC II findings, patients with diabetes derived a greater absolute benefit from the early-invasive strategy (ARR, 7.6% versus 3.5% for the whole study population). The results of these two studies demonstrate that patients with diabetes presenting with NSTE-ACS have a higher risk profile than nondiabetic patients do, but they derive a greater absolute benefit when managed with a deliberate strategy of rapid initiation of intensive medical management and early angiography and revascularization.

ADJUNCTIVE MEDICAL THERAPY FOR PATIENTS WITH DIABETES AND ACUTE CORONARY SYNDROME

Intravenous Glycoprotein IIb/IIIa Receptor Inhibitors for Non-ST-elevation Acute Coronary Syndrome

Since 1993, three intravenous GP IIb/IIIa inhibitors (abciximab, tirofiban, and eptifibatide) have been investigated in more than 50,000 patients with NSTE-ACS. These agents have been shown to reduce the frequency of death, MI, and recurrent ischemia when used as primary therapy (eptifibatide and tirofiban) and when used as an adjunct to PCI (abciximab and eptifibatide) (57,58). The benefit of GP IIb/IIIa inhibitors for the initial medical treatment of NSTE-ACS is especially apparent among patients with high-risk clinical features including ST-segment deviation on the presenting ECG, positive cardiac markers, and diabetes mellitus.

Theroux et al. sought to determine whether diabetic persons derived a particular benefit from the use of tirofiban in addition to standard antithrombotic therapy for NSTE-ACS in the Platelet Receptor Inhibition in Ischemic Syndrome Management in Patients Limited by Unstable Signs and Symptoms (PRISM-PLUS) trial (59). Of the 1,570 patients enrolled in PRISM-PLUS, 362 (23%) had diabetes. The rate of the primary end point (death, MI, or refractory ischemia at 6 months) was higher among diabetics compared with nondiabetics (36.2% versus 28.1%, respectively). The rate of death or MI at 6 months in patients with diabetes was significantly reduced with tirofiban (19.2% versus 11.2%; $p = .03$), and the relative treatment effect of tirofiban was greater among diabetic patients than among nondiabetics ($p = .007$ for interaction).

The GUSTO-IV ACS investigators performed a randomized, multicenter trial to investigate the effect of abciximab on patients presenting with ACS who did not undergo routine early revascularization (60). Patients were randomly assigned to receive either placebo or abciximab for either 24 or 48 hours. Of the 7,800 enrolled patients, 1,677 (21.5%) had diabetes. Although there was no reduction in the rate of death or MI at 30 days among all patients treated with abciximab or placebo, patients with diabetes had a greater treatment benefit with abciximab than did nondiabetic patients (ARR, 1.8% versus 0.7%, respectively).

Further evidence of an enhanced benefit of GP IIb/IIIa inhibitors for the primary treatment of NSTE-ACS among patients with diabetes was provided in two recent metaanalyses (61,62). Roffi et al. (62) pooled outcome data of the diabetic populations enrolled in six large-scale NSTE-ACS trials evaluating the use of GP IIb/IIIa inhibitors. Among 6,458 patients with diabetes, treatment with GP IIb/IIIa inhibitors was associated with a significant reduction in mortality at 30 days (OR = .74; 95% CI, 0.59 to 0.92; $p = .001$) (Fig. 19-4). However, there was no apparent survival benefit with GP IIb/IIIa inhibitors in nondiabetic patients. The interaction between GP IIb/IIIa inhibitor use and diabetes was statistically significant ($p = .036$). The reduction in 30-day mortality with GP IIb/IIIa inhibitors in diabetic patients was especially pronounced among 1,279 patients who underwent PCI during the index hospitalization (OR = 0.30; 95% CI, 0.14 to 0.69; $p = .002$). Boersma et al. (61) pooled individual patient data for all participants in the six large-scale ACS trials to assess the magnitude of benefit of GP IIb/IIIa inhibitors among patients who were not routinely scheduled to undergo coronary revascularization. Diabetic persons (22% of the population) had a higher risk of death or MI at 30 days, compared with nondiabetic persons (13.7% versus 10.6%, respectively, and they seemed to derive a greater benefit with the use of GP IIb/IIIa inhibitors (OR = 0.93 for diabetes; OR = 0.88 for no diabetes; $p = .48$ for interaction). Although these two metaanalyses used different approaches for evaluating the treatment effect of GP IIb/IIIa inhibitors from the same six trials, the results suggest an especially

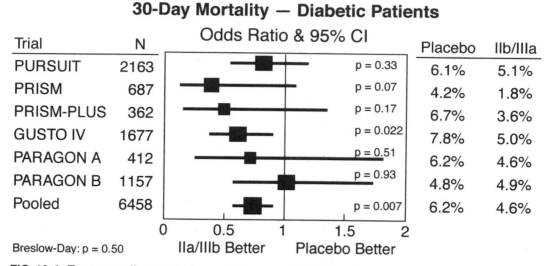

FIG. 19-4. Treatment effect on 30-day mortality among diabetics with acute coronary syndrome. (From Roffi M, Chew DP, Mukherjee D, et al. Platelet glycoprotein IIb/IIIa inhibitors reduce mortality in diabetic patients with non-ST-segment-elevation acute coronary syndromes. *Circulation* 2001;104:2767–2771.)

important benefit of GP IIb/IIIa inhibitors in the diabetic population presenting with NSTE-ACS, particularly in the setting of early angiography and PCI.

Oral Antiplatelet Therapy

Given the important platelet structural and functional abnormalities among patients with diabetes, it is not surprising that they derive substantial benefit from the use of aspirin (ASA) therapy for the treatment of coronary disease. The Anti-Platelet Trialists Collaboration Group sought to determine the effects of prolonged antiplatelet therapy on vascular events by pooling results from more than 140 randomized trials that collectively enrolled about 70,000 patients at risk of or with established vascular disease and 30,000 low-risk subjects. Among diabetic subjects, ASA lowered the combined risk of vascular death, MI, or stroke by 19% ($p < .01$). An estimated 38 vascular events were prevented per 1,000 patients treated (63). The magnitude of benefit of ASA among diabetic patients was similar to that among patients with prior MI (40 events prevented per 1,000 treated). The U. S.

Physicians' Health Study evaluated the efficacy of ASA (325 mg every other day) in the primary prevention of cardiovascular events. The underlying frequency of MI and the absolute risk reduction in the rate of MI with ASA were substantially higher among diabetics versus nondiabetics (ARR, 6.1% versus 0.8%, respectively) (64).

Further evidence of the efficacy of ASA among diabetic patients is found in the results of the Early Treatment Diabetic Retinopathy Study (65). More than 3,700 patients with diabetes (13% with a history of CAD or prior MI) were randomly assigned to ASA (650 mg/day) or placebo with a mean follow-up period of 5 years. Total and cardiovascular mortality rates at 5 years were similar in the two groups. However, patients who received ASA had lower rates of fatal and nonfatal MI (RR = 0.83; $p = .04$) during the follow-up period. Although there are no specific studies evaluating the benefits of ASA in diabetic patients with ACS, the accumulated evidence strongly supports the use of ASA in all diabetic patients with ischemic heart disease.

Treatment with the thienopyridine derivatives, ticlopidine or clopidogrel, either alone or in combination with ASA, may provide additional benefit in reducing ischemic events among patients with diabetes. The Clopidogrel versus Aspirin in Patients at Risk for Ischemic Events (CAPRIE) trial randomly assigned 19,185 patients with previous atherosclerotic vascular disease to treatment with either ASA or clopidogrel. Overall, there was a small reduction in the rate of the composite of ischemic stroke, MI, or vascular death for clopidogrel compared with ASA (5.32% versus 5.83%; $p = .04$) (66). The treatment effect was greater among the 4,000 enrolled diabetic patients, with event rates of 15.6% and 17.7% in the clopidogrel and ASA groups, respectively ($p = .04$)

The Clopidogrel in Unstable Angina to Prevent Recurrent Events (CURE) trial randomly assigned 12,562 patients within 24 hours of an ACS to either clopidogrel plus ASA or placebo plus ASA for 3 to 12 months. The frequency of the primary end point (a composite of death, nonfatal MI, or stroke) was significantly reduced in the group receiving clopidogrel plus ASA (RRR = 0.80; 95% CI, 0.72 to 0.90; $p < .001$) compared with ASA alone (67). Among patients with diabetes (23% of the total study population), those who received clopidogrel plus ASA had higher rates of the primary end point than did nondiabetic patients (14.2% versus 7.9%, respectively). The absolute and relative reductions in the rates of these events were similar among patients with and without diabetes receiving combination antiplatelet therapy (ARR = 2.5% in diabetics versus 2.0% in nondiabetics). These results suggest that combined antiplatelet therapy with ASA and clopidogrel may be preferable for eligible patients with diabetes who present with ACS.

Antithrombin Therapy

Antithrombin therapy with unfractionated heparin (UFH) is commonly used for patients presenting with STEMI. Six trials have compared ASA plus UFH to ASA alone, enrolling more than 68,000 patients (more than 90% of whom received concomitant fibrinolytic therapy). The addition of heparin was associated with a small reduction in in-hospital mortality, compared with ASA alone (approximately 5 fewer deaths per 1,000 treated). This beneficial effect was tempered by a small increase in the rate of major bleeding (approximately 2 instances per 1,000 treated) (68). Although UFH has not been studied specifically among patients with diabetes, there appears to be benefit for all patients with STEMI.

Among patients presenting with NSTE-ACS, there is modest clinical trial evidence to support the use of UFH together with ASA. Individual trials have been too small to provide unequivocal evidence, though a metaanalysis aggregating data from six small trials showed a trend for a reduced rate of death or MI with ASA plus UFH, compared with ASA alone (69). As in the setting of STEMI, the use of UFH for NSTE-ACS has not been specifically studied in patients with diabetes.

The LMWHs have several potential advantages over UFH. They have a more predictable anticoagulant effect without the need for monitoring of the partial thromboplastin time, a higher ratio of antifactor Xa to factor IIa inhibition, an easier route of administration (subcutaneous), and a lower incidence of heparin-induced thrombocytopenia. Several large clinical trials have studied the use of LMWH in the setting of non-ST-elevation ACS (70,71). The Efficacy and Safety of Subcutaneous Enoxaparin in Non-Q-Wave Coronary Events (ESSENCE) study group randomly assigned 3,171 patients with NSTE-ACS to receive LMWH (enoxaparin) or UFH. Overall, the rates of death, MI, or recurrent angina were significantly lower among patients receiving enoxaparin at 14 days (ARR = 3.2%, $p = .019$) and at 30 days (ARR = 3.5%, $p = .016$). The treatment effect of enoxaparin among diabetic patients (22% of the total population) was consistent with that seen in the total patient cohort (70). Similarly, the Thrombolysis in Myocardial Infarction (TIMI) IIB trial found that enoxaparin use was also associated with a significant reduction in the rate of death and serious cardiac ischemic events, when compared with UFH for NSTE-ACS (71). More than 20% of patients enrolled in TIMI IIB had diabetes. Despite the evidence suggesting benefit with the use of LMWHs in diabetic patients, current difficulties with monitoring of the level of anticoagulation with LMWH during PCI have limited the use of these agents in patients with NSTE-ACS who are treated with an early-invasive management strategy.

Despite the apparent benefits of heparins as standard antithrombotic therapy for patients with ACS, certain limitations of heparins have stimulated the search for more effective anticoagulants. Heparins work indirectly (requiring the presence of antithrombin III), are subject to inhibition by certain plasma proteins and platelet factor IV, and are ineffective against clot-bound thrombin. Newer antithrombin agents act directly against both free and clot-bound thrombin and lack most of the qualities that can interfere with the action of heparin. Several direct thrombin inhibitors (lepirudin, hirudin, bivalirudin) have been evaluated in large-scale trials of patients presenting with both STEMI and NSTE-ACS. Although direct thrombin inhibitors have not been specifically studied in patients with diabetes, each of these studies included a subpopulation of diabetic patients.

The GUSTO-IIb investigators randomly assigned 12,142 patients presenting with NSTE-ACS or STEMI to 72 hours of therapy with either UFH or hirudin (72). Patients were stratified by the presence of ST-segment elevation ($n = 4,131$) or ST-segment depression ($n = 8,011$) on the presenting ECG. Almost 18% of the total study population had diabetes, and the diabetic subjects were divided equally among ECG patterns of ST-elevation or ST-depression. The 30-day rate of death or MI (the primary end point) was 8.9% for those receiving hirudin and 9.8% for those receiving heparin (OR = 0.89; 95% CI, 0.79 to 1.00; $p = .06$). The effect of hirudin was not influenced by ST-segment status and was mostly confined to the first 24 hours of treatment. The event rates for patients with diabetes were not reported in the published results, but the authors did not indicate the presence of any unfavorable interaction between hirudin treatment and diabetic status.

Similarly, the Organization to Assess Strategies for Ischemic Syndromes (OASIS-2) investigators randomly assigned 10,141 patients with NSTE-ACS to 72 hours of UFH or hirudin. Approximately 21% of participating patients had diabetes. The rate of the primary end point (cardiovascular death or MI at 7 days) was not significantly different in the two treatment arms (4.2% with UFH versus 3.6% with hirudin; OR = 0.84, 95% CI, 0.69 to 1.02; $p = .078$). In subgroup analyses, there was no evidence of heterogeneity in the relative benefit of hirudin among patients with or without diabetes (73).

The Hirulog and Early Reperfusion or Occlusion (HERO-2) investigators studied the effect of bivalirudin versus UFH in the setting of STEMI (74). More than 17,000 patients were randomly assigned to a 48-hour infusion of either bivalirudin or UFH, together with the standard dose of streptokinase. The primary end point (30-day mortality) occurred in 10.8% of those receiving bivalirudin and 10.9% of those receiving heparin (ARR = 0.1%, $p = .85$). The 30-day mortality rate was substantially greater in diabetic patients receiving bivalirudin than in similarly treated nondiabetic patients (14.9% versus 9.8%, respectively). The use of bivalirudin was associated with a greater absolute risk reduction in death in diabetic than in nondiabetic patients (2.7% versus 0%, respectively), although the interaction between treatment and diabetic status was not significant ($p = .14$) (74).

Based on these results, most diabetic patients will continue to receive UFH as their primary anticoagulant therapy when presenting with an ACS. As evidence supporting the use of LMWHs in the setting of early angiography and PCI accumulates, they will probably become the preferred antithrombin agents in patients presenting with ACS. The direct thrombin inhibitors have been shown to have only modest benefit beyond that of UFH in the setting of STEMI and NSTE-ACS, and they are likely to remain the anticoagulants of choice only in the setting of heparin-induced thrombocytopenia, or when UFH and LMWH are contraindicated.

β-Adrenergic Antagonists

Many practitioners have had reservations regarding the use of β-blockers in diabetic patients because of the perceived risk of masking hypoglycemia and reducing insulin production (6). However, most studies show equal or greater

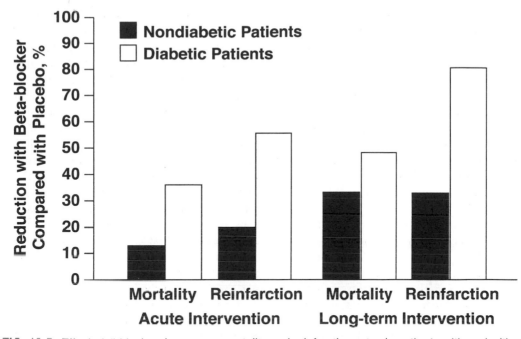

FIG. 19-5. Effect of β-blocker therapy on mortality and reinfarction rates in patients with and without diabetes after myocardial infarction, expressed as percentage reduction compared with patients receiving placebo. (From Kendall MJ, Lynch KP, Hjalmarson A, et al. Beta-blockers and sudden cardiac death. *Ann Intern Med* 1995;123:358–367. Review.)

reductions in mortality and reinfarction with β-blockers in diabetic persons than in those without diabetes. Long-term studies of β-blockers in patients with STEMI revealed mortality reductions of 33% in the general population and 48% in those patients with diabetes (75). The findings are similar for rates of reinfarction: patients without diabetes treated with β-blockers after STEMI had a 21% reduction, and similarly treated patients with diabetes had a 55% reduction (Fig. 19-5) (75,76).

Malmberg et al. (77) conducted a retrospective review of outcomes among diabetic patients participating in two trials that randomly assigned patients with acute MI to metoprolol or placebo: the Göteborg Metoprolol Trial and the MIAMI trial. Among the 120 diabetic subjects (9% of the total population) in the Göteburg trial, mortality at 3 months was reduced from 17.9% to 7.5% with metoprolol (*p* = .16). Among the 413 patients with diabetes in the MIAMI trial, mortality was decreased by metoprolol from 11.3%

to 5.7% (*p* = .06). In both of these trials, the magnitude of benefit with β-blockers in patients with diabetes was substantially greater than in similarly enrolled patients without diabetes. Furthermore, in a subgroup analysis of the Norwegian Multicenter Study, Gundersen and Kjekshus (78) found that patients with diabetes who were randomly assigned to receive timolol after MI, had a reduction in overall mortality, cardiac death, and reinfarction similar to that of the nondiabetic patients.

Additional insight into the use and benefits of β-blockers in patients with diabetes after MI is found in a recent analysis of the National Cooperative Cardiovascular Project (CCP) Database (79). Of the 45,308 Medicare beneficiaries presenting with acute MI who did not have contraindications to β-blocker therapy, almost 26% had diabetes. Patients with diabetes were prescribed β-blockers on discharge after MI in fewer than 50% of cases. After adjusting for other demographic and clinical factors, diabetic patients were less likely to receive β-blockers at discharge than were nondiabetic patients (OR = 0.88; 95% CI, 0.82 to 0.96). b-Blocker use was associated with a lower 1-year mortality rate for both insulin-treated diabetics (hazard ratio [HR] = 0.87; 95% CI, 0.72 to 1.07) and non-insulin-treated diabetics (HR = 0.77; 95% CI, 0.67 to 0.88) after adjustment for potential confounders. Also, the use of β-blockers was not associated with increased readmission rates for diabetic complications among patients with or without diabetes. A similar analysis of patients in the CCP by Gottlieb et al. (80) also demonstrated a significant mortality reduction among diabetic patients receiving β-blockers.

The totality of evidence, to date, confirms the central role of β-blockers for the treatment for patients with ACS. β-Blockers are associated with a greater absolute reduction in the rate of major adverse cardiac events and death in diabetic patients compared with nondiabetic patients. The commonly held belief that β-blockers will increase the rate of diabetic complications and worsen glycemic control has not been demonstrated in clinical studies and should not preclude the use of these important agents in diabetic patients with ACS.

Angiotensin-converting Enzyme Inhibitors

A number of large, randomized, clinical trials (collectively enrolling more than 100,000 patients) have unequivocally demonstrated improved survival with angiotensin-converting enzyme (ACE) inhibitors started during or after an acute STEMI (81). Mortality and morbidity were reduced when ACE inhibitors were given during the early stages (before 24 to 36 hours) of a STEMI in a relatively unselected population of patients (82–84), and also when they were started later (3 to 16 days) in patients with symptoms or signs of left ventricular dysfunction (85–87). Although the benefits of ACE inhibitors in the setting of an ACS have not been studied specifically in diabetic persons, analysis of the aforementioned trial results suggests a particular benefit in this population.

The ACE Inhibitor Myocardial Infarction Collaborative Group published in 1998 a systematic overview of all randomized trials in which ACE inhibitors were started in the early phase of acute MI and continued for 4 to 6 weeks (81). In this large dataset of more than 98,000 patients, 30-day mortality was 7.1% among those allocated to ACE inhibitors and 7.6% among controls, corresponding to a 7% relative reduction in mortality (p < .004), or 5 deaths prevented per 1,000 patients treated. Of the total cohort, 5,014 (5.1%) of the patients had diabetes. In this subgroup, the proportional reduction in mortality was similar to that of the total cohort (approximately 7%). However, because of their higher risk of death after MI, the absolute benefits of ACE inhibitor treatment were greater in patients with diabetes (17.3 lives saved per 1,000 treated, compared with 3.2 lives saved per 1,000 in nondiabetic patients).

A retrospective analysis of the GISSI-3 trial (included in the collaboration just described), which randomly assigned patients with acute MI to lisinopril or placebo within 24 hours after presentation, provided further support (88). Among the 2,790 diabetic patients (15% of the total population), treatment with lisinopril was associated with a decreased mortality at 6 weeks (ARR = 3.7%; 37 lives saved per 1,000 treated), a treatment effect that was significantly greater than that observed in nondiabetic patients (p < .025 for interaction).

These results support the recommendation that diabetic patients with acute MI should receive oral ACE inhibitor therapy early in the course of their presentation. Although ACE inhibitors have not been specifically studied in diabetic persons with NSTE-ACS, they are likely to be beneficial in this setting and should be used routinely, given their established benefit among patients with risk factors for, or clinical manifestations of, vascular disease (89).

The evidence supporting the early routine use of ACE inhibitors in diabetic patients presenting with an ACS was supplemented by a recently reported substudy of the Heart Outcomes Prevention Evaluation (HOPE) study. The HOPE investigators sought to determine whether the ACE inhibitor, ramipril, reduced the risk of cardiovascular and renal disease among 3,577 diabetic patients participating in the overall HOPE trial (termed the MICRO-HOPE substudy) (89). Patients with diabetes included in this study had either a previous cardiovascular event or one other cardiovascular risk factor, and they had no clinical proteinuria or heart failure. Among these diabetic patients in the MICRO-HOPE substudy, ramipril reduced the rate of the composite endpoint of MI, stroke, or death by 25%: MI by 22%, stroke by 33%, and total mortality by 24% (Fig. 19-6). The rate of overt nephropathy was also reduced by 24% with ramipril ($p = .027$). These benefits persisted after adjustment for changes in systolic and diastolic blood pressure (89). These results confirm that diabetic patients with coronary disease derive substantial benefit from ACE inhibitors, in the setting of either an ACS or established vascular disease.

Lipid-lowering Therapy

The benefit of statins for secondary prevention of cardiovascular complications in patients who are at risk for CAD or who have CAD (both with and without diabetes) has been clearly demonstrated (90). However, previous secondary prevention studies excluded patients who had experienced ACS in the 3 to 4 months before study enrollment. Given that the highest risk of death and recurrent ischemic events is early after presentation with an ACS, several groups of investigators have sought to determine whether early initiation of statin therapy (before ACS hospital discharge) can improve outcomes and shorten time to benefit with this strategy.

The Myocardial Ischemia Reduction with Aggressive Lowering (MIRACL) study investigators randomly assigned more than 3,000 patients with NSTE-ACS to receive either atorvastatin (80 mg) or placebo, between 24 and 96 hours after hospital admission. The rate of the composite primary end point (death, nonfatal MI, cardiac arrest, or recurrent ischemia requiring hospitalization) was 14.8% among those receiving atorvastatin and 17.4% among those receiving placebo (RR = 0.84; 95% CI, 0.70 to 1.00; $p = .48$). The difference in event rates was entirely due to lower rates of recurrent ischemia among those receiving atorvastatin. Approximately 23% of enrolled patients had diabetes. Though the event rates in

this subgroup were not reported, there was no significant interaction between treatment assignment and the presence of diabetes (91).

In the Lescol Intervention Prevention (LIPS) Study, 1,600 patients undergoing their initial PCI were randomly assigned to early statin therapy with fluvastatin or placebo. Approximately one half of the enrolled patients were undergoing intervention in the setting of ACS, and the mean time between PCI and randomization was 2.7 days. During the 4-year follow-up, patients receiving statin therapy had a 22% reduction in the risk of major adverse cardiac events (defined as cardiac death, nonfatal MI, coronary artery bypass grafting, or repeat PCI), compared with patients receiving placebo ($p = .013$). The reduction in this end point with statin therapy was especially prominent among enrolled diabetic patients, who experienced a 47% lower rate of adverse cardiac events ($p = .041$) (92).

The association between early statin initiation (7 days or less after ACS) and outcomes was explored by the SYMPHONY and 2nd SYMPHONY investigators (93).They recently reported 90-day and 1-year outcomes in an observational cohort of more than 12,300 patients who were not taking statins before hospitalization for an index ACS. Patients were stratified by the receipt of early (median, 2 days) or no statin therapy during their hospitalization. After adjustment for important covariates, there was no association between the use of early statin therapy and a reduction in death, recurrent MI, or severe recurrent ischemia at 90 days (HR = 1.15; 95% CI, 0.99 to 1.34; $p = .06$) or between early statin therapy and death at 1 year (HR = 0.99; 95% CI, 0.73 to 1.33; $p = .93$). When stratified by lipoprotein profile results, there seemed to be an association between early statin use and higher risk of death among patients with cholesterol levels below treatment guidelines. Approximately 17% of patients in the cohort had diabetes, and no interaction was reported in this subgroup.

The results of the MIRACL and LIPS studies suggest that early initiation of statin therapy after presentation with ACS and/or PCI may reduce the rate of subsequent adverse cardiac events. Diabetic patients participating in these

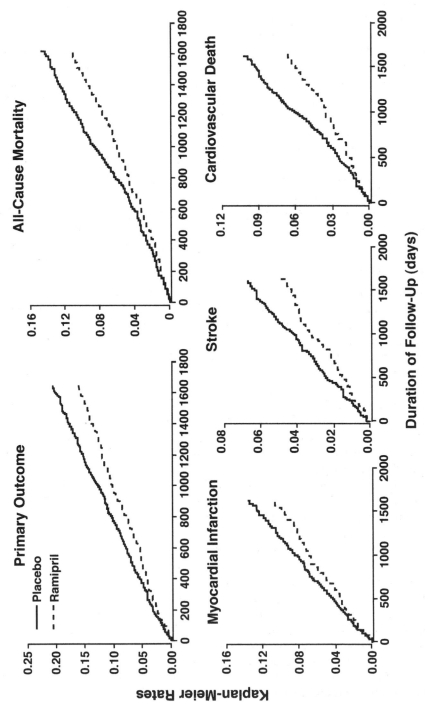

FIG. 19-6. Kaplan–Meier survival curves for participants in Heart Outcomes Prevention Evaluation (HOPE) trial with diabetes mellitus. (From Effects of ramipril on cardiovascular and microvascular outcomes in people with diabetes mellitus: results of the HOPE study and MICRO-HOPE substudy. Heart Outcomes Prevention Evaluation Study Investigators. *Lancet* 2000;355:253–259.)

TABLE 19-2. *Event rates and treatment effects of various therapeutic agents for ischemic heart disease*

Treatment	Outcome		Diabetic patients (%)			Nondiabetic patients			Source (no. of diabetic patients)
	Duration	End points	Plac.	Tx.	ARR	Plac.	Tx.	ARR	
Fibrinolytic therapy (STEMI)	35 days	Mortality	17.3	13.6	3.7	10.2	8.7	1.5	FTT (4,496)
Primary PTCA (STEMI)	30 days	Death Reinfarction CVA	16.7	11.1	5.6	13.2	9.3	3.9	GUSTO-IIb (77)
Early invasive management (NSTE ACS)	6 mo	Death MI ACS hosp.	27.7	20.1	7.6	15.4	14.2	2.2	TACTICS-TIMI 18 (613)
Glycoprotein IIb/IIIa inhibitors (NSTE ACS)	30 days	Mortality	6.2	4.6	1.6	3.0	3.0	0	Roffi, et al (6,458)
Clopidogrel (NSTE ACS)	9 mo	CV death MI, CVA	16.7	14.2	2.5	9.9	7.9	2.0	CURE (2,840)
β-Blockers (STEMI)	3 mo	Mortality	17.9	7.5	10.4	8.9	5.7	3.2[a]	Göteburg (120)
	15 days	Mortality	11.3	5.7	5.6	2.9	4.3	0.6[a]	MIAMI (413)
Angiotensin-converting enzyme (ACE) inhibitors (vascular disease)	3.5 yr	MI CVA CV death	19.8	15.3	4.5	16.5[b]			HOPE/MICRO-HOPE (3,577)

ARR, absolute risk reduction; CV, cardiovascular; CVA, cerebrovascular accident; MI, myocardial infarction; NSTE ACS, non-ST-segment elevation acute coronary syndromes; Plac., placebo; PTCA, percutaneous transluminal coronary angioplasty; STEMI, acute ST-segment elevation myocardial infarction; Tx., treatment.

[a]Includes diabetic and nondiabetic patients.

[b]Event rates for nondiabetic patients not reported.

trials seemed to derive a particular benefit from this strategy. The results of the SYMPHONY cohort study require prospective confirmation and should not be used as an argument against routine statin use among patients with clinical manifestations of vascular disease. The administration of statins before discharge in patients with diabetes, as in all patients presenting with an ACS, may serve to improve the likelihood that these agents will be used in the long term, where their benefits are well established.

CONCLUSION

CAD leads to substantial morbidity and mortality among patients with diabetes. The risk for development of CAD in diabetic persons is increased by twofold to fourfold, and their risk of a first STEMI is equivalent to that of patients who have already experienced an MI (18). Even with the use of reperfusion therapy, the presence of diabetes is associated with a higher risk of reinfarction, heart failure, and death after STEMI (11). Diabetic patients who experience an NSTE-ACS also have a higher risk of death or nonfatal MI (24).

The reasons for the increased risk of CAD and the higher frequency of poor outcomes among patients with diabetes who have ACS are multifactorial. The diabetic state leads to profound alterations in the function of the endothelium and vascular smooth muscle, promoting arterial dysfunction and the accelerated development of atherosclerosis. Abnormal activation of platelets and the coagulation cascade, as well as impairment of the endogenous fibrinolytic systems, all contribute to a heightened risk of adverse outcomes when diabetic persons present with an ACS. The higher risk of death after STEMI in patients with diabetes may also be related to delayed clinical presentation, higher frequencies of multivessel and renal disease, or impaired compensatory function of the noninfarcted myocardium (21).

It is disturbingly obvious that diabetic persons are less likely to receive proven therapies that reduce morbidity and mortality during treatment of an ACS. Diabetic persons are less likely to receive fibrinolytic therapy for STEMI. When

pharmacologic fibrinolysis is administered, it is often given to diabetics later after presentation compared with nondiabetics. Therefore, physicians and other health care providers should maintain vigilance when evaluating diabetics seeking medical care, so that atypical symptoms of myocardial ischemia are not overlooked and left untreated. A summary of the clinical event rates and treatment effects of various therapeutic agents in diabetics, compared with nondiabetics, are listed in Table 19-2.

REFERENCES

1. Wingard DL, Barret-Connor E. Heart disease and diabetes. *Diabetes in America.* Bethesda, MD: U.S. Department of Health and Human Services, 1995:429–448.
2. Grundy SM, Howard B, Smith S Jr, et al. Prevention Conference VI: Diabetes and Cardiovascular Disease. Executive summary: conference proceeding for healthcare professionals from a special writing group of the American Heart Association. *Circulation* 2002;105:2231–2239.
3. Garcia MJ, McNamara PM, Gordon T, et al. Morbidity and mortality in diabetic patients in the Framingham population: sixteen-year follow-up study. *Diabetes* 1974;23:105–111.
4. Aronson D, Rayfield EJ, Chesebro JH. Mechanisms determining course and outcome of diabetic patients who have had acute myocardial infarction. *Ann Intern Med* 1997;126:296–306.
5. Gu K, Cowie CC, Harris MI. Diabetes and decline in heart disease mortality in US adults [see comments.] *JAMA* 1999;281:1291–1297.
6. Beckman JA, Creager MA, Libby P. Diabetes and atherosclerosis: epidemiology, pathophysiology, and management. *JAMA* 2002;287:2570–2581.
7. Tschoepe D, Roesen P, Kaufmann L, et al. Evidence for abnormal platelet glycoprotein expression in diabetes mellitus. *Eur J Clin Invest* 1990;20:166–170.
8. Aronson D, Bloomgarden Z, Rayfield EJ. Potential mechanisms promoting restenosis in diabetic patients. *J Am Coll Cardiol* 1996;27:528–535.
9. Silva JA, Escobar A, Collins TJ, et al. Unstable angina: a comparison of angioscopic findings between diabetic and nondiabetic patients. *Circulation* 1995;92:1731–1736.
10. Marchant B, Umachandran V, Stevenson R, et al. Silent myocardial ischemia: role of subclinical neuropathy in patients with and without diabetes. *J Am Coll Cardiol* 1993;22:1433–1437.
11. Mak KH, Moliterno DJ, Granger CB, et al. Influence of diabetes mellitus on clinical outcome in the thrombolytic era of acute myocardial infarction. GUSTO-I Investigators. Global Utilization of Streptokinase and Tissue Plasminogen Activator for Occluded Coronary Arteries. *J Am Coll Cardiol* 1997;30:171–179.
12. Indications for fibrinolytic therapy in suspected acute myocardial infarction: collaborative overview of early mortality and major morbidity results from all randomised trials of more than 1000 patients. Fibrinolytic

Therapy Trialists' (FTT) Collaborative Group. [Erratum in *Lancet* 1994;343:742.] *Lancet* 1994;343:311–322.

13. Brodie BR, Stuckey TD, Wall TC, et al. Importance of time to reperfusion for 30-days and late survival and recovery of left ventricular function after primary angioplasty for acute myocardial infarction. *J Am Coll Cardiol* 1998;32:1312–1319.

14. Dracup K, Alonzo AA, Atkins JM, et al. The physician's role in minimizing prehospital delay in patients at high risk for acute myocardial infarction: recommendations from the National Heart Attack Alert Program. Working Group on Educational Strategies to Prevent Prehospital Delay in Patients at High Risk for Acute Myocardial Infarction. *Ann Intern Med* 1997;126:645–651.

15. Kondo T, Kubota I, Tachibana H, et al. Glibenclamide attenuates peaked T wave in early phase of myocardial ischemia. *Cardiovasc Res* 1996;31:683–687.

16. Kubota I, Yamaki M, Shibata T, et al. Role of ATP-sensitive K+ channel on ECG ST segment elevation during a bout of myocardial ischemia: a study on epicardial mapping in dogs. *Circulation* 1993;88:1845–1851.

17. Norhammar A, Tenerz A, Nilsson G, et al. Glucose metabolism in patients with acute myocardial infarction and no previous diagnosis of diabetes mellitus: a prospective study. *Lancet* 2002;359:2140–2144.

18. Haffner SM, Lehto S, Ronnemaa T, et al. Mortality from coronary heart disease in subjects with type 2 diabetes and in nondiabetic subjects with and without prior myocardial infarction. *N Engl J Med* 1998;339:229–234.

19. Bonow RO, Mitch WE, Nesto RW, et al. Prevention Conference VI: Diabetes and Cardiovascular Disease. Writing Group V: management of cardiovascular-renal complications. *Circulation* 2002;105:e159–e164.

20. Lee KL, Woodlief LH, Topol EJ, et al. Predictors of 30-day mortality in the era of reperfusion for acute myocardial infarction: results from an international trial of 41,021 patients. GUSTO-I Investigators. *Circulation* 1995;91:1659–1668.

21. Mak KH, Topol EJ. Emerging concepts in the management of acute myocardial infarction in patients with diabetes mellitus. *J Am Coll Cardiol* 2000;35:563–568.

22. Stone GW, Grines CL, Browne KF, et al. Predictors of in-hospital and 6-month outcome after acute myocardial infarction in the reperfusion era: the Primary Angioplasty in Myocardial Infarction (PAMI) trial. *J Am Coll Cardiol* 1995;25:370–377.

23. Boersma E, Pieper KS, Steyerberg EW, et al. Predictors of outcome in patients with acute coronary syndromes without persistent ST-segment elevation. Results from an international trial of 9461 patients. *Circulation* 2000;101:2557–2567.

24. Malmberg K, Yusuf S, Gerstein HC, et al. Impact of diabetes on long-term prognosis in patients with unstable angina and non-Q-wave myocardial infarction: results of the OASIS (Organization to Assess Strategies for Ischemic Syndromes) Registry. *Circulation* 2000;102:1014–1019.

25. Granger CB, Califf RM, Young S, et al. Outcome of patients with diabetes mellitus and acute myocardial infarction treated with thrombolytic agents: the Thrombolysis and Angioplasty in Myocardial Infarction (TAMI) Study Group. *J Am Coll Cardiol* 1993;21:920–925.

26. The GUSTO-III Investigators. A comparison of reteplase with alteplase for acute myocardial infarction. The Global Use of Strategies to Open Occluded Coronary Arteries (GUSTO III) Investigators. *N Engl J Med* 1997;337:1118–1123.

27. ASSENT-2 Investigators. Single-bolus tenecteplase compared with front-loaded alteplase in acute myocardial infarction: the ASSENT-2 double-blind randomised trial. *Lancet* 1999;354:716–722.

28. The GUSTO-V Investigators. Reperfusion therapy for acute myocardial infarction with fibrinolytic therapy or combination reduced fibrinolytic therapy and platelet glycoprotein IIb/IIIa inhibition: the GUSTO V randomised trial. *Lancet* 2001;357:1905–1914.

29. Pfeffer MA, Moye LA, Braunwald E, et al. Selection bias in the use of thrombolytic therapy in acute myocardial infarction. The SAVE Investigators. *JAMA* 1991;266:528–532.

30. Barron HV, Bowlby LJ, Breen T, et al. Use of reperfusion therapy for acute myocardial infarction in the United States: data from the National Registry of Myocardial Infarction 2. *Circulation* 1998;97:1150–1156.

31. Danchin N, Vaur L, Genes N, et al. Treatment of acute myocardial infarction by primary coronary angioplasty or intravenous thrombolysis in the "real world": one-year results from a nationwide French survey. *Circulation* 1999;99:2639–2644.

32. Menown I, Patterson R, McMechan S, et al. Use of thrombolytic therapy in females, diabetic patients and the elderly: trial selection—bias or a real problem? [Abstract]. *J Am Coll Cardiol* 1999;33:325A.

33. Mahaffey KW, Granger CB, Toth CA, et al. Diabetic retinopathy should not be a contraindication to thrombolytic therapy for acute myocardial infarction: review of ocular hemorrhage incidence and location in the GUSTO I trial. Global Utilization of Streptokinase and t-PA for Occluded Coronary Arteries. *J Am Coll Cardiol* 1997;30:1606–1610.

34. Woodfield SL, Lundergan CF, Reiner JS, et al. Angiographic findings and outcome in diabetic patients treated with thrombolytic therapy for acute myocardial infarction: the GUSTO-I experience. *J Am Coll Cardiol* 1996;28:1661–1669.

35. Gibson CM, Ryan KA, Murphy SA, et al. Impaired coronary blood flow in nonculprit arteries in the setting of acute myocardial infarction. The TIMI Study Group. Thrombolysis in Myocardial Infarction. *J Am Coll Cardiol* 1999;34:974–982.

36. Weaver WD, Simes RJ, Betriu A, et al. Comparison of primary coronary angioplasty and intravenous thrombolytic therapy for acute myocardial infarction: a quantitative review. *JAMA* 1997;278:2093–2098.

37. Hasdai D, Granger CB, Srivatsa SS, et al. Diabetes mellitus and outcome after primary coronary angioplasty for acute myocardial infarction: lessons from the GUSTO-IIb Angioplasty Substudy. Global Use of Strategies to Open Occluded Arteries in Acute Coronary Syndromes. *J Am Coll Cardiol* 2000;35:1502–1512.

38. Brener SJ, Ellis SG, Sapp SK, et al. Predictors of death and reinfarction at 30 days after primary angioplasty: the GUSTO IIb and RAPPORT trials. *Am Heart J* 2000;9:476–481.

39. Thomas K, Ottervanger JP, de Boer MJ, et al. Primary angioplasty compared with thrombolysis in acute myocardial infarction in diabetic patients. *Diabetes Care* 1999;22:647–649.

40. Van De Werf F, Baim DS. Reperfusion for ST-segment

elevation myocardial infarction: an overview of current treatment options. *Circulation* 2002;105:2813–2816.

41. Stone GW, Grines CL, Cox DA, et al. Comparison of angioplasty with stenting, with or without abciximab, in acute myocardial infarction. *N Engl J Med* 2002;346:957–966.

42. Montalescot G, Barragan P, Wittenberg O, et al. Platelet glycoprotein IIb/IIIa inhibition with coronary stenting for acute myocardial infarction. *N Engl J Med* 2001;344:1895–1903.

43. Silva JA, Nunez E, White CJ, et al. Predictors of stent thrombosis after primary stenting for acute myocardial infarction. *Catheter Cardiovasc Interv* 1999;47:415–422.

44. Marso SP, Giorgi LV, Johnson WL, et al. Diabetes mellitus is associated with a shift in the temporal risk profile of in hospital death after percutaneous coronary intervention: an analysis of 25,223 patients over 20 years. *Am Heart J* 2003;145:270–277.

45. Malmberg K, McGuire DK. Diabetes and acute myocardial infarction: the role of insulin therapy. *Am Heart J* 1999;138:S381–S386.

46. Sodi-Pallares D, Testelli MR, Fishleder BL, et al. Effects of an intravenous infusion of a potasssium-glucose-insulin solution on the electrocardiographic signs of myocardial infarction. *Am J Cardiol* 1962;9:66–181.

47. Fath-Ordoubadi F, Beatt KJ. Glucose-insulin-potassium therapy for treatment of acute myocardial infarction: an overview of randomized placebo-controlled trials. *Circulation* 1997;96:1152–1156.

48. Malmberg K, Ryden L, Efendic S, et al. Randomized trial of insulin-glucose infusion followed by subcutaneous insulin treatment in diabetic patients with acute myocardial infarction (DIGAMI study): effects on mortality at 1 year. *J Am Coll Cardiol* 1995;26:57–65.

49. Malmberg K, Norhammar A, Wedel H, et al. Glycometabolic state at admission: important risk marker of mortality in conventionally treated patients with diabetes mellitus and acute myocardial infarction. Long-term results from the Diabetes and Insulin-Glucose Infusion in Acute Myocardial Infarction (DIGAMI) study. *Circulation* 1999;99:2626–2632.

50. McGuire DK, Granger CB. Diabetes and ischemic heart disease. *Am Heart J* 1999;138:S366–S375.

51. Diaz R, Paolasso EA, Piegas LS, et al. Metabolic modulation of acute myocardial infarction. The ECLA (Estudios Cardiologicos Latinoamerica) Collaborative Group. *Circulation* 1998;98:2227–2234.

52. Apstein CS. Glucose-insulin-potassium for acute myocardial infarction: remarkable results from a new prospective, randomized trial. *Circulation* 1998;98:2223–2226.

53. Zijlstra F. Effects of glucose-insulin potassium infusion on 30-day mortality in patients with acute myocardial infarction treated with primary angioplasty. European Society of Cardiology Congress, September 2002.

54. Braunwald E, Antman EM, Beasley JW, et al. ACC/AHA guidelines for the management of patients with unstable angina and non-ST-segment elevation myocardial infarction: a report of the American College of Cardiology/American Heart Association Task Force on Practice Guidelines (Committee on the Management of Patients with Unstable Angina). *J Am Coll Cardiol* 2000;36:970–1062.

55. Invasive compared with non-invasive treatment in unstable coronary-artery disease: FRISC II prospective randomised multicentre study. FRagmin and Fast Revascularisation during InStability in Coronary artery disease Investigators. *Lancet* 1999;354:708–715.

56. Cannon CP, Weintraub WS, Demopoulos LA, et al. Comparison of early invasive and conservative strategies in patients with unstable coronary syndromes treated with the glycoprotein IIb/IIIa inhibitor tirofiban. *N Engl J Med* 2001;344:1879–1887.

57. Kong DF, Califf RM. Glycoprotein IIb/IIIa receptor antagonists in non-ST elevation acute coronary syndromes and percutaneous revascularisation: a review of trial reports. *Drugs* 1999;58:609–620.

58. Kong DF, Califf RM, Miller DP, et al. Clinical outcomes of therapeutic agents that block the platelet glycoprotein IIb/IIIa integrin in ischemic heart disease. *Circulation* 1998;98:2829–2835.

59. Theroux P, Alexander J Jr, Pharand C, et al. Glycoprotein IIb/IIIa receptor blockade improves outcomes in presenting with unstable angina/non-ST-elevation myocardial infarction: results from the Platelet Receptor Inhibition in Ischemic Syndrome Management in Patients Limited by Unstable Signs and Symptoms (PRISM-PLUS) study. *Circulation* 2000;102:2466–2472.

60. Simoons ML, GUSTO IA. Effect of glycoprotein IIb/IIIa receptor blocker abciximab on outcome in patients with acute coronary syndromes without early coronary revascularisation: the GUSTO IV-ACS randomised trial. *Lancet* 2000;357:1915–1924.

61. Boersma E, Harrington RA, Moliterno DJ, et al. Platelet glycoprotein IIb/IIIa inhibitors in acute coronary syndromes: a meta-analysis of all major randomised clinical trials. *Lancet* 2002;359:189–198.

62. Roffi M, Chew DP, Mukherjee D, et al. Platelet glycoprotein IIb/IIIa inhibitors reduce mortality in diabetic patients with non-ST-segment-elevation acute coronary syndromes. *Circulation* 2001;104:2767–2771.

63. Collaborative overview of randomised trials of antiplatelet therapy I: prevention of death, myocardial infarction, and stroke by prolonged antiplatelet therapy in various categories of patients. Antiplatelet Trialists' Collaboration. *BMJ* 1994;308:81–106.

64. Final report on the aspirin component of the ongoing Physicians' Health Study. Steering Committee of the Physicians' Health Study Research Group. *N Engl J Med* 1989;321:129–135.

65. Aspirin effects on mortality and morbidity in patients with diabetes mellitus. Early Treatment Diabetic Retinopathy Study report 14. ETDRS Investigators. *JAMA* 1992;268:1292–1300.

66. A randomised, blinded, trial of clopidogrel versus aspirin in patients at risk of ischaemic events (CAPRIE). CAPRIE Steering Committee. *Lancet* 1996;348:1329–1339.

67. Yusuf S, Zhao F, Mehta SR, et al. Effects of clopidogrel in addition to aspirin in patients with acute coronary syndromes without ST-segment elevation. *N Engl J Med* 2001;345:494–502.

68. Collins R, MacMahon S, Flather M, et al. Clinical effects of anticoagulant therapy in suspected acute myocardial infarction: systematic overview of randomised trials. *BMJ* 1996;313:652–659.

69. Oler A, Whooley MA, Oler J, et al. Adding heparin to aspirin reduces the incidence of myocardial infarction and

death in patients with unstable angina: a meta-analysis. *JAMA* 1996;276:811–815.

70. Cohen M, Demers C, Gurfinkel EP, et al. A comparison of low-molecular-weight heparin with unfractionated heparin for unstable coronary artery disease. Efficacy and Safety of Subcutaneous Enoxaparin in Non-Q-Wave Coronary Events Study Group. *N Engl J Med* 1997;337:447–452.

71. Antman EM, McCabe CH, Gurfinkel EP, et al. Enoxaparin prevents death and cardiac ischemic events in unstable angina/non-Q-wave myocardial infarction: results of the thrombolysis in myocardial infarction (TIMI) 11B trial. *Circulation* 1999;100:1593–1601.

72. Metz BK, White HD, Granger CB, et al. Randomized comparison of direct thrombin inhibition versus heparin in conjunction with fibrinolytic therapy for acute myocardial infarction: results from the GUSTO-IIb Trial. Global Use of Strategies to Open Occluded Coronary Arteries in Acute Coronary Syndromes (GUSTO-IIb) Investigators. *J Am Coll Cardiol* 1998;31:1493–1498.

73. Effects of recombinant hirudin (lepirudin) compared with heparin on death, myocardial infarction, refractory angina, and revascularisation procedures in patients with acute myocardial ischaemia without ST elevation: a randomised trial. Organisation to Assess Strategies for Ischemic Syndromes (OASIS-2) Investigators. *Lancet* 1999;353:429–438.

74. White H, and the Hirulog and Early Reperfusion or Occlusion (HERO)-2 Trial Investigators. Thrombin-specific anticoagulation with bivalirudin versus heparin in patients receiving fibrinolytic therapy for acute myocardial infarction: the HERO-2 randomised trial. *Lancet* 2001;358:1855–1863.

75. Gullestad L, Kjekshus J [Myocardial disease in diabetes mellitus]. *Tidsskrift for Den Norske Laegeforening* 1992;112:1016–1019.

76. Kendall MJ, Lynch KP, Hjalmarson A, et al. Beta-blockers and sudden cardiac death. *Ann Intern Med* 1995;123:358–367.

77. Malmberg K, Herlitz J, Hjalmarson A, et al. Effects of metoprolol on mortality and late infarction in diabetic patients with suspected acute myocardial infarction: retrospective data from two large studies. *Eur Heart J* 1989;10.423–428.

78. Gundersen T, Kjekshus J. Timolol treatment after myocardial infarction in diabetic patients. *Diabetes Care* 1983;6:285–290.

79. Chen J, Marciniak TA, Radford MJ, et al. Beta-blocker therapy for secondary prevention of myocardial infarction in elderly: results from the National Cooperative Cardiovascular Project. *J Am Coll Cardiol* 1999;34:1388–1394.

80. Gottlieb SS, McCarter RJ, Vogel RA. Effect of beta-blockade on mortality among high-risk and low-risk patients after myocardial infarction. *N Engl J Med* 1998;339:489–497.

81. Indications for ACE inhibitors in the early treatment of acute myocardial infarction: systematic overview of individual data from 100,000 patients in randomized trials. ACE Inhibitor Myocardial Infarction Collaborative Group. *Circulation* 1998;97:2202–2212.

82. Swedberg K, Held P, Kjekshus J, et al. Effects of the early administration of enalapril on mortality in patients with acute myocardial infarction: results of the Cooperative New Scandinavian Enalapril Survival Study II (CONSENSUS II). *N Engl J Med* 1992;327:678–684.

83. Gruppo Italiano per lo Studio della Sopravvivenza nell'infarto Miocardico. GISSI-3: effects of lisinopril and transdermal glyceryl trinitrate singly and together on 6-week mortality and ventricular function after acute myocardial infarction. *Lancet* 1994;343:1115–1122.

84. ISIS-4 (Fourth International Study of Infarct Survival) Collaborative Group. ISIS-4: a randomised factorial trial assessing early oral captopril, oral mononitrate, and intravenous magnesium sulphate in 58,050 patients with suspected acute myocardial infarction. *Lancet* 1995;345:669–685.

85. Pfeffer MA, Braunwald E, Moye LA, et al. Effect of captopril on mortality and morbidity in patients with left ventricular dysfunction after myocardial infarction: results of the survival and ventricular enlargement trial. The SAVE Investigators [see comments.] *N Engl J Med* 1992;327:669–677.

86. Effect of ramipril on mortality and morbidity of survivors of acute myocardial infarction with clinical evidence of heart failure. The Acute Infarction Ramipril Efficacy (AIRE) Study Investigators. *Lancet* 1993;342:821–828.

87. Gustafsson I, Torp-Pedersen C, Kober L, et al. Effect of the angiotensin converting enzyme inhibitor trandolapril on mortality and morbidity in diabetic patients with left ventricular dysfunction after acute myocardial infarction. Trace Study Group. *J Am Coll Cardiol* 1999;34.83–89.

88. Zuanetti G, Latini R, Maggioni AP, et al. Effect of the ACE inhibitor lisinopril on mortality in diabetic patients with acute myocardial infarction: data from the GISSI-3 study. *Circulation* 1997;96:4239–4245.

89. Effects of ramipril on cardiovascular and microvascular outcomes in people with diabetes mellitus: results of the HOPE study and MICRO-HOPE substudy. Heart Outcomes Prevention Evaluation Study Investigators. *Lancet* 2000;355:253–259.

90. Grundy SM, Garber A, Goldberg R, et al. Prevention Conference VI: Diabetes and Cardiovascular Disease. Writing Group IV: lifestyle and medical management of risk factors. *Circulation* 2002;105:e153–e158.

91. Schwartz GG, Olsson AG, Ezekowitz MD, et al. Effects of atorvastatin on early recurrent ischemic events in acute coronary syndromes: the MIRACL study—a randomized controlled trial. *JAMA* 2001;285:1711–1718.

92. Serruys PW, de Feyter P, Macaya C, et al. Fluvastatin for prevention of cardiac events following successful first percutaneous coronary intervention: a randomized controlled trial. *JAMA* 2002;287:3215–3222.

93. Newby LK, Kristinsson A, Bhapkar MV, et al. Early statin initiation and outcomes in patients with acute coronary syndromes. *JAMA* 2002;287:3087–3095.

Diabetes and Cardiovascular Disease
edited by Steven P. Marso and David M. Stern
Lippincott Williams & Wilkins, Philadelphia © 2004

20

Diabetes and Coronary Revascularization

Deepak P. Vivekananthan and Deepak L. Bhatt

*Fellow, Department of Cardiovascular Medicine, Cleveland Clinic Foundation; Director,
Interventional Cardiology Fellowship, Department of Cardiovascular Medicine, Cleveland Clinic
Foundation, Cleveland, Ohio*

Diabetic patients present difficult management problems for cardiovascular physicians. The increased rates of restenosis after percutaneous coronary intervention (PCI) (1–4) and adverse outcomes after surgical revascularization (5,6) make decision making about the optimal revascularization strategy challenging. The problem of restenosis after coronary stenting in diabetic patients is especially important because a growing number of these patients are being referred for PCI. For example, the initial National Heart, Lung, and Blood Institute (NHLBI) registry from 1977 to 1981 found that only 9% of patients undergoing PCI had diabetes (7). More recent studies from the contemporary era of PCI, using the American College of Cardiology National Cardiovascular Data Registry (ACC-NCDR), have indicated that up to 26% of patients have diabetes (8), and even this figure is probably an underestimate. Although retrospective data from older randomized trials such as Bypass Angioplasty Revascularization Investigation (BARI) (9,10) do suggest that coronary artery bypass grafting (CABG) is the preferred modality of revascularization in diabetic patients with multivessel disease, this notion is being challenged in the contemporary era of coronary stenting, glycoprotein (GP) IIb/IIIa inhibition, and drug-coated stents. Therefore, clinicians must have a working knowledge of the extensive clinical data documenting the benefits and potential hazards of various revascularization options in diabetic patients, in order to refer these patients appropriately to the least invasive, most cost-effective, and most durable revascularization strategy.

This chapter outlines the pathophysiologic mechanisms for adverse outcomes unique to diabetic patients who undergo revascularization, provides insight into optimizing outcomes for diabetic patients undergoing PCI, and makes recommendations regarding revascularization strategies in diabetic patients with coronary artery disease (CAD).

CLINICAL OUTCOMES AFTER PERCUTANEOUS CORONARY INTERVENTION

Early studies suggested that patients with diabetes had initial success rates with PCI that were very similar to those of their nondiabetic counterparts (3,10,11). The initial studies evaluating the early outcome of diabetic patients were rather underpowered to evaluate early outcomes after PCI. Data from the Mid America Heart Institute evaluating more than 25,000 patients from 1980 to 2000 suggest an increased hazard for in-hospital mortality for diabetic patients after PCI (12). In the overall cohort, diabetes was associated with an approximately twofold increase in mortality. This finding persisted after multivariate analysis. The major predictors of mortality in this registry included age (OR = 1.06, $p < .001$), creatinine higher than 1.5 mg/dL (OR = 3.3, $p < .001$), ejection fraction less than 40% (OR = 3.4, $p < .001$), prior myocardial infarction (MI) (OR = 1.3, $p = .007$), multivessel disease

(OR = 2.8, $p < .001$), urgent PCI (OR = 9.0, $p < .001$), female gender (OR = 1.8, $p < .001$), and diabetes mellitus (OR = 1.8, $p < .001$). Specifically, the in-hospital mortality rate in the elective PCI cohort was 0.8% for nondiabetic patients as compared with 1.4% for the diabetic patients. Similarly, there was an almost twofold increase in in-hospital mortality for diabetic patients undergoing PCI in the setting of an acute MI (6.9% for nondiabetics with acute MI compared with 12.7% for diabetics with acute MI, $p < .001$). Numerous other studies have clearly defined the additional risk among diabetic patients. Compared with nondiabetic persons, diabetics have an increased risk of later MI and mortality.

Furthermore, restenosis rates are significantly higher in diabetic patients (2–4). Notably, diabetic patients have trends toward increased rates of stent thrombosis (13) and increased in-hospital complications such as death, MI, and need for emergency CABG (11,14,15). Additional data from the NHLBI-I registry of early angioplasty procedures, before the advent of GP IIb/IIIa inhibition and coronary stenting, show that diabetic patients had a 15% higher absolute restenosis rate, compared with nondiabetic patients (16). In the modern era of PCI including coronary stenting, the risk of restenosis is still approximately 1.5 times that in nondiabetic patients (17–20). These higher rates of restenosis may be responsible for the increased long-term morbidity and mortality after PCI (3,5,10,11,17,21). However, the use of periprocedural GP IIb/IIIa inhibition with abciximab, in diabetic patients treated with coronary stenting in the Evaluation of Platelet IIb/IIIa Inhibition in Stenting (EPI-STENT) study, significantly reduced the incidence of target vessel revascularization (TVR) at 6 months by more than 50% (16.6% for stent plus placebo versus 8.1% for stent plus abciximab, $p = .021$) (22). Despite the salutary effect of GP IIb/IIIa inhibition in reducing the incidence of restenosis, the Do Tirofiban and ReoPro Give Similar Efficacy Outcomes Trial (TARGET) still found that diabetic patients had a higher incidence of need for TVR at 6 months, compared with nondiabetic patients (10.3% versus 7.8%, $p = .008$) (23). Therefore, even though modern interventional techniques and periprocedural antiplatelet therapy have improved outcomes in diabetic patients, restenosis after PCI continues to be a major problem.

The factors involved in restenosis, such as endothelial dysfunction, mural thrombus, growth factor expression, and smooth muscle hyperplasia, are particularly active in diabetic patients and are a direct result of hyperinsulinemia, poor glycemic control, or both.

Influence of Hyperinsulinemia

Several studies have investigated the role of hyperinsulinemia in restenosis after coronary angioplasty. These studies found that diabetic patients treated with insulin have poorer outcomes after PCI in comparison with diabetic patients who do not use insulin (17,24). Therefore, it was proposed that insulin or proinsulin exerts harmful effects on the vessel wall that may predispose to restenosis (24,25). This notion is supported by the clinical evidence, which shows that "prediabetic" patients who are insulin resistant or who have the metabolic syndrome (characterized by glucose intolerance and hyperinsulinemia) are more apt to have higher restenosis rates and adverse clinical events (26–28). Insulin resistance has been associated with increased platelet activation and derangements in the coagulation cascade and the fibrinolytic system (25). Moreover, insulin has been found to enhance the synthesis of plasminogen activator inhibitor type-1 (PAI-1) (29). This protein has been implicated in the inhibition of proteolysis, which allows for increased deposition of lipid and extracellular matrix, important components of restenotic lesions in diabetic patients (30). Elevated plasma levels of PAI-1 also impair fibrinolysis, which predisposes to vessel thrombosis (25). In the clinical setting, a retrospective analysis from the Emory Cardiovascular Registry found that insulin use was an independent marker of long-term mortality in both PCI- and CABG-treated patients (5).

The use of sulfonylureas by diabetic patients may also adversely affect outcomes after PCI. For example, sulfonylureas may reduce the effects of ischemic preconditioning (31), leading to increased periprocedural complications (32–34). Although blockade of myocardial adenosine triphosphate (ATP)-sensitive potassium channels by glibenclamide, an oral hypoglycemic agent, has been implicated as the pathogenic mechanism of inhibition of ischemic preconditioning, sulfonylureas may also exert deleterious effects by attenuating coronary vasodilation (35,36). On the other hand, administration of an insulin-sensitizing agent such as troglitazone has been shown to reduce neointimal proliferation after stent implantation (37,38). Insulin resistance may be associated with similar detrimental outcomes after PCI. As with patients who have overt diabetes (22), there may be enhanced neointimal proliferation after stent placement, compared with nondiabetic patients (38).

The use of insulin-modulating agents such as rosiglitazone is currently being studied in this patient population, as adjunctive therapy in PCI, in the PPARγ agonists for the Prevention of Adverse Events following Percutaneous Coronary Revascularization trial. The antiproliferative (39) and antiinflammatory (40) effects of peroxisome proliferator-activated receptor (PPAR) agonists may prove particularly useful in both prediabetic and diabetic patients after PCI. For instance, the association between the metabolic syndrome of insulin resistance, low high-density lipoproteins (HDL), hyperglycemia, and increased body mass index has been associated with markers of vascular inflammation such as C-reactive protein (CRP) (41). Moreover, inflammatory markers such as CRP, white blood cell count, and fibrinogen have been directly correlated with indices of insulin insensitivity (42). Other subclinical signs of vascular inflammation (e.g., microalbuminuria) have also been associated with increased levels of CRP (43). These associations are particularly relevant because these inflammatory markers have been associated with increased mortality after PCI (44,45), and attenuation of these inflammatory markers through postprocedural treatment with PPAR agonists may be associated with improved outcomes after PCI.

Role of Hyperglycemia

Although there is some evidence to support the role of insulin or proinsulin as a mediator in the process of restenosis, the role of hyperinsulinemia as a culprit in restenosis has been called into question (46). For example, animal models of insulin deficiency (47) have been shown to have a higher rate of intimal thickening after balloon injury, compared with nondiabetic controls. These findings have led other experts to support the notion that restenosis in diabetic patients is primarily a result of hyperglycemia, and therefore improved outcomes can be achieved with better glycemic control (47) (Fig. 20-1). For instance, hyperglycemia promotes endothelial dysfunction by increasing the formation of free radicals (48,49), decreasing the production of prostacyclin (50), and, most importantly, inhibiting the effects of endothelium-derived relaxing factor (EDRF), either by blocking its production or attenuating its vasodilatory effect on the endothelium (51,52). Furthermore, hyperglycemia may impair fibrinolysis (53), promote platelet aggregation (54–56), and enhance a procoagulant state (57).

It is likely that both hyperinsulinemia and hyperglycemia play a role in the pathogenesis of restenosis, although this interesting debate has not been settled. Ongoing clinical trials such as the PPAR trial, which is looking at the use of rosiglitazone in prediabetic patients undergoing PCI, will probably help to answer some of these questions.

Endothelial Dysfunction

Endothelial dysfunction plays an important role in the increased tendency toward restenosis after PCI in diabetic patients, and this process may be mediated through inhibition of EDRF (51,52). Specifically, EDRF plays a vital role in maintaining the functional integrity of the vascular endothelium by promoting vasodilation, inhibiting platelet aggregation, and preventing smooth muscle proliferation. Inhibition of EDRF blocks these salutary effects, thereby predisposing to restenosis. Hyperglycemia, through the formation of advanced glycosylation end products (AGEs), also impairs endothelial regeneration after balloon injury (58). The extended time needed for endothelial regeneration results in pronounced neointimal

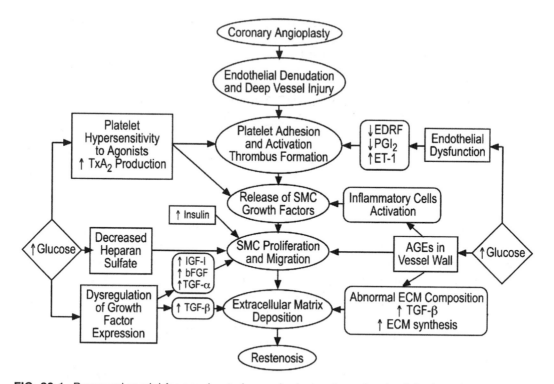

FIG. 20-1. Proposed model for accelerated vascular lesion formation in diabetic patients after percutaneous coronary intervention (PCI). AGEs, advanced glycosylation end products; bFGF, basic fibroblast growth factor; ECM, extracellular matrix; EDRF, endothelium-derived relaxing factor; ET-1, endothelin-1; IGF-1, insulin-like growth factor-1; PGI$_2$, prostacyclin; TGF-α, transforming growth factor-α; TGF-*b*, transforming growth factor-β; TxA$_2$, thromboxane A$_2$. (From Aronson D, et al. Potential mechanisms promoting restenosis in diabetic patients. *J AM Coll Cardiol* 1996;27:528–535, with permission.)

proliferation due to a lengthened interaction between activated platelets and the balloon-injured vessel wall (47,59). Therefore, it has been speculated that hastened endothelialization through the delivery of growth factors may reduce neointimal formation after stent placement (60).

Qualitative Abnormalities in Platelet Function

Several studies have documented qualitative platelet abnormalities in diabetic patients that most likely contribute to the increased tendency toward restenosis and periprocedural complications. For instance, platelets in diabetic patients are larger (61,62), have enhanced fibrinogen binding (63), and are less able to mediate vasodi-lation (64,65). The larger size of platelets in diabetic patients corresponds to a higher number of GP IIb/IIIa receptors (66) and results in enhanced platelet aggregation (47,67), compared with non-diabetic patients, thus providing a mechanism for increased rates of thrombosis and restenosis after PCI. The increased glycation of GP IIb/IIIa receptors (68,69) and the formation of AGEs (70) have also been proposed as mechanisms for enhanced platelet aggregation in diabetic patients. Moreover, platelets in diabetic patients have an increased tendency to circulate in the activated state, resulting in enhanced expression of adhesion molecules such as P-selectin, CD40 ligand, and thrombospondin (71). The expression of P-selectin mediates platelet-leukocyte interactions, thereby affecting leukocyte recruitment and activation patterns (72–74). In fact, platelet-neutrophil interactions occur after balloon angioplasty (75), resulting in the increased tendency for thrombosis (76), but inhibition of this interaction may reduce restenosis (77).

It appears that platelets in particular actively promote vascular inflammation, and this inflammatory response may lead to adverse outcomes after PCI. This point is exemplified by the abundance of recent data correlating elevated markers of inflammation (e.g., CRP, serum amyloid type A) with increased mortality and morbidity after PCI (44,78–81). The reduction in these inflammatory markers with periprocedural abciximab administration (82) may be in part responsible for the dramatic reduction in the 6-month rate of death or MI in diabetic patients treated with abciximab in the EPISTENT trial (22). In addition, Chew et al. (83,84) found that pretreatment with clopidogrel and aspirin before PCI was associated with improved outcomes; this benefit was greatest in patients with elevated baseline CRP levels and was particularly notable in patients who also had diabetes. It is becoming apparent that platelets modulate both the thrombotic and the inflammatory response in acute coronary syndromes (ACS) and after PCI, and this process may be magnified in patients with diabetes. Therefore, periprocedural inhibition of platelet activity is essential for optimizing outcomes for diabetic patients after PCI.

Growth Factors and Maladaptive Remodeling

Glagov pioneered the theory of arterial remodeling as a compensatory mechanism for the increased plaque burden seen in atherosclerosis (85). His model concluded that coronary arteries dilate in order to compensate for luminal narrowing caused by an atherosclerotic plaque. This process, known as positive remodeling, may be attenuated in diabetic patients, and maladaptive or negative remodeling may predispose to the increased incidence of restenosis after coronary angioplasty. In fact, serial intravascular ultrasound studies have found that restenosis is determined by a decrease in the external elastic membrane (86), a surrogate for the magnitude of vessel wall remodeling. In diabetic patients, the significant upregulation of growth factors af-

ter PCI may play a prominent role in negative remodeling of the vessel wall leading to restenosis. For example, platelet-derived growth factor (PDGF) (87) and insulin-like growth factor-1 (IGF-1) (88,89) enhance the replication and development of contractile smooth muscle cells, hastening restenosis. Other growth mediators, such as transforming growth factor-β (90), enhance production of extracellular matrix, another key contributor to restenosis in diabetic patients. In fact, these growth factors have been found to play a role in the pathogenesis of diabetic vasculopathy in other arterial beds, including the kidney and retina, and their expression may be influenced by the state of glycemic control (91). Modulation of these growth factors has been the focus of intense research in the prevention of restenosis. For instance, the use of antiproliferative agents such as paclitaxel and sirolimus embedded in drug-coated stents is currently being studied in large-scale trials to evaluate the effects on restenosis. The low restenosis rates at 6 months for sirolimus-coated stents in the Randomized Study with the Sirolimus-Coated Bx Velocity Balloon-Expandable Stent in the Treatment of Patients with de Novo Native Coronary Artery Lesions (RAVEL) trial (92) provide promise that a cure for restenosis is near. Large-scale trials are needed to specifically test the efficacy of drug-eluting stents in diabetic patients, in smaller-caliber vessels, and in bifurcation lesions, as well as the long-term effects of these agents on hard end points such as MI and death.

Propensity For Embolization During Percutaneous Coronary Intervention

Embolization plays an important role in the pathogenesis of ACS and complications resulting from PCI by causing myocardial necrosis through microvascular obstruction. Diabetic patients in particular are more apt to have significant clinical sequelae from embolic phenomena. For example, studies of coronary angioscopy (93) in patients presenting with unstable angina have shown that diabetic patients have a high incidence of intracoronary thrombus and plaque ulceration, as well as lesion characteristics that have a higher propensity for embolization into the microvasculature. Due to a diffusely diseased microvascular bed and a significant reduction in coronary flow reserve (94–96), the microvasculature of diabetic patients is less able to tolerate an embolic shower. Finally, the diabetic state promotes the interaction between leukocytes and platelets (76), which may lead to more pronounced embolic phenomena. Therefore, abciximab, which acts as a potent antiplatelet and antiinflammatory agent through blockade of GP IIb/IIIa, MAC-1 (CDIIb/CD 18, $\alpha_m\beta_2$) (97), and vitronectin (98) receptors, may be particularly ideal in attenuating the clinical effects of embolization. In fact, abciximab therapy most notably reduces mortality in diabetic patients after PCI (99).

Poor Coronary Collateral Vessel Formation

Attenuated formation of coronary collateral vessels in diabetic patients may also be responsible for the poor outcomes after coronary stenting. Abaci et al. (100) found that diabetic patients had a significantly lower coronary collateral score than nondiabetic patients did. Poor collateral formation in diabetic patients may be related to endothelial dysfunction caused by hyperglycemia and its impairment of the effects of nitric oxide on angiogenesis. Other studies have suggested a reduction in vascular endothelial growth factor (VEGF) as a mechanism for poor collateral development in diabetic patients; this condition can be ameliorated with gene transfer of VEGF via an adenovirus vector (101). Moreover, poor collateral development makes embolization less well tolerated and may increase the likelihood of periprocedural MI, a marker of long-term mortality after PCI (102,103).

SPECIAL CONSIDERATIONS IN DIABETIC PATIENTS WHO UNDERGO CORONARY ARTERY BYPASS GRAFTING

It is clear from the available data that diabetic patients undergoing CABG have higher in-hospital mortality, higher long-term mortality, and increased need for repeat revascularizations, compared with nondiabetic patients (5,6). Thourani et al. (104) found that the in-hospital mortality rate of diabetic patients undergoing CABG

was 3.9%, compared with 1.6% in patients without diabetes. Survival at 10-year follow-up was also significantly lower in diabetic patients than in nondiabetic patients (50% versus 71%, $p <$ .05) (104). This finding was confirmed in the Bypass Angioplasty Revascularization Investigation (BARI) (9,10), a randomized clinical trial comparing the efficacy of CABG versus PCI in patients with multivessel CAD. This trial found that, among patients randomly assigned to CABG, diabetics had a lower survival rate at 7-year follow-up than did nondiabetics (76.4% versus 86.8%, respectively). These findings have now been extended through 10-year follow-up.

Diabetic patients who undergo CABG have an increased risk of perioperative death, higher 30-day and long-term mortality, and increased need for repeat revascularization procedures. In a series of patients who underwent CABG, patients with diabetes were more likely to experience wound infections, postoperative arrhythmias, respiratory failure, and intraaortic balloon pump use (105). Despite the increased periprocedural complications seen in diabetic patients treated with CABG, initial clinical trial data support the use of surgical revascularization in diabetic patients with multivessel disease. For example, several randomized trials found improved long-term survival of diabetic patients treated with CABG, compared with balloon angioplasty (Table 20-1).

The marked benefit of CABG in these patients is probably related to several factors, including the completeness of the revascularization, the protection provided by patent grafts after a subsequent MI, and the placement of an internal mammary artery (IMA). This point was exemplified in a retrospective analysis of the BARI study performed by Detre et al. (106), who evaluated the impact of previous CABG surgery on the prognosis of patients with diabetes who subsequently had an MI. This provocative study found that, despite a similar incidence of Q-wave MIs in patients treated with either CABG or PTCA only, the mortality rate was 17% among those patients who had undergone CABG, as opposed to 80% in the PTCA-only arm (OR = 0.09; 95% confidence interval [CI], 0.03 to 0.29) (Fig. 20-2). Of note, this dramatic risk reduction in CABG-treated diabetic patients

TABLE 20-1. *Randomized trials comparing coronary artery bypass grafting (CABG) versus percutaneous coronary intervention (PCI) in multivessel disease: the diabetic experience*

Trial	N	Follow-up (yr)	Mortality (%)		Relative risk	Probability
			CABG	PCI		
BARI	353	7	23.6	44.3	1.88	.0011
CABRI	125	4	12.5	22.6	1.81	NS
EAST	59	8	24.5	39.9	1.63	.23
ARTS	208	1	3.1	6.3	2.03	.30

ARTS, Arterial Revascularization Therapy Study; BARI, Bypass Angioplasty Revascularization Investigation; CABRI, Coronary Angioplasty Versus Bypass Revascularization Investigation; EAST, Emory Angioplasty Surgery Trial.

was not found in nondiabetic patients treated with CABG.

The retrospective study of the BARI randomized trial emphasized two important points in diabetic patients who undergo surgical revascularization. First, the likely benefit of CABG in these patients is due to protection afforded by patent grafts after MI rather than prevention of MI. Second, graft protection after MI appears to be related to the completeness of revascularization and the reduction in myocardium at jeopardy during an MI (107).

Moreover, the majority of patients evaluated in the aforementioned trials underwent conventional balloon angioplasty. Previous work suggested that diabetic arteries undergo a negative remodeling process, resulting in greater arterial narrowing for any given degree of atherosclerosis

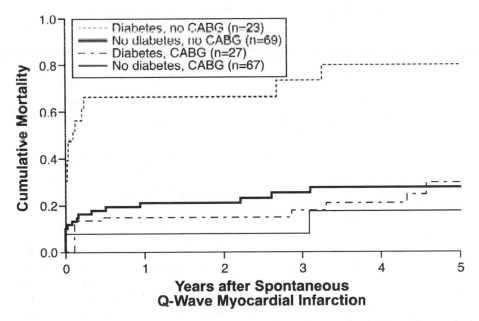

Patients with Q-Wave Myocardial Infarction

FIG. 20-2. Kaplan–Meier mortality estimates of patients in the Bypass Angioplasty Revascularization Investigation (BARI) with a Q-wave myocardial infarction according to diabetic and coronary artery bypass grafting (CABG) status. Patients not treated with CABG were treated only with percutaneous coronary intervention (PCI). (From Detre KM, et al. The effect of previous coronary artery bypass surgery on the prognosis of patients with diabetes who have acute myocardial infarction. *NEJM* 2000;342:989–997, with permission.)

and a resultant smaller reference diameter. This "typical" diabetic arteriopathy after balloon angioplasty results in a higher than expected rate of late-vessel occlusion. Studies conducted by Van Belle et al. (108) showed that patients with diabetes mellitus have late vessel occlusion rates approximating 15% after balloon angioplasty. This number is markedly higher than the 3% to 4% rate of occlusion after angioplasty previously reported. Late vessel occlusion among this cohort of patients resulted in adverse left ventricular remodeling. Furthermore, those patients with occlusive restenosis had a significantly higher risk of cardiovascular mortality at 10 years.

The appropriate choice of vascular conduits is an important surgical decision at the time of CABG that may directly affect the survival of diabetic patients. Retrospective analysis from BARI suggests that the use of the IMA graft conferred a survival benefit in treated diabetic patients, compared with diabetic patients not treated with an IMA graft (106). For example, the dramatic risk reduction in CABG-treated diabetic patients was most noteworthy among those patients who were treated with at least one internal thoracic artery graft. The important role of the use of IMA grafting in diabetic patients was also exemplified in a study by Yamamoto et al. (109), which found that, despite a higher overall mortality rate among diabetic patients, there was no significant mortality difference between the diabetic subgroup revascularized with an IMA graft and the group of nondiabetic patients bypassed with an IMA graft (109). This finding exemplifies the need to use the IMA, if surgically feasible, in all diabetic patients who undergo CABG. Moreover, studies have suggested that the patients who received two IMA grafts had a lower composite end point of death, reoperation, or need for angioplasty, compared with patients who received only one IMA graft (110,111).

Despite the mortality benefits of CABG in diabetic patients with multivessel disease treated with IMA grafting, several important considerations must be addressed. Diabetic patients have a significantly higher risk of sternal wound complications after CABG compared with nondiabetic patients (112), which may be related to the use of two IMA grafts (113), although not all data support this hypothesis (112,114). It does appear, however, that obese diabetic women are particularly prone to this postoperative complication (113,115). Moreover, one study found that diabetes and the use of an IMA graft are associated with persistent elevation of the hemidiaphragm after surgery (116). Diabetes is also a risk factor for perioperative stroke (117,118). Another interesting point to consider in the risk stratification of diabetic patients undergoing CABG is the use of insulin or oral hypoglycemic agents. There may be a dichotomy in outcome of diabetic patients treated with insulin or oral hypoglycemic agents, compared with those who are not treated with these agents. In fact, based on a retrospective analysis from the BARI registry, the 5-year mortality rate in diabetic patients treated with insulin or oral agents was 35% in patients randomly assigned to PCI, compared with 19% in diabetic patients initially randomized to CABG. For those diabetic patients not using insulin or oral hypoglycemics, the mortality rate was only 9% in both the CABG group and PTCA group. An analysis of a series of patients with diabetes treated with CABG (119,120) found that diabetic patients treated with insulin had significantly worse outcome in comparison with patients treated with oral agents or with diet alone (121). Use of insulin or oral agents that enhance insulin secretion may simply be a marker of a more ill diabetic patient population, or this finding may represent unique adverse effects of hyperinsulinemia in patients after CABG.

PERCUTANEOUS CORONARY INTERVENTION VERSUS CORONARY ARTERY BYPASS GRAFTING IN THE PRE-STENT ERA

Many of the clinical trials comparing CABG with PCI were done in the pre-stent era. Focusing on the details of these trials is prudent. The advent and refinement of PCI techniques in patients with CAD has led to the direct comparison of PCI and CABG in several randomized trials (121–123). Although no study has formally assessed the utility of these revascularization strategies in diabetic patients in a randomized fashion, the wealth of clinical data on this topic stems from retrospective analyses of these randomized trials. Over the entire spectrum of patients, those with multivessel coronary disease had no differences between the two strategies in regard to mortality, nonfatal MI, or cerebrovascular accident. However, PCI was associated with a significantly increased need for repeat revascularizations.

Several randomized trials have compared the long-term efficacy of CABG with PCI in patients with multivessel CAD (see Table 20-1). As mentioned, the BARI study demonstrated a 5-year survival rate of 89.3% for those assigned to CABG, compared with 86.3% for those assigned to PTCA ($p = .19$; 95% CI for survival difference, -0.2% to 6.0%) (121). However, an analysis of the diabetic patients treated in this study found a significant survival benefit for those treated with CABG, compared with PCI, at 5 years (80.6% versus 65.5%, $p = .0003$) (10). Moreover, at 7 years, CABG provided a more pronounced survival benefit over PCI in diabetic patients (76.4% versus 55.7%, $p = .0011$) (124). It is important to note, however, that the bulk of the surgical benefit in diabetic patients seen in this study was found in those treated with an IMA graft. For example, patients who were revascularized with at least one IMA graft had improved survival at 7 years (83.2%, $n = 140$), compared with those patients who received saphenous vein grafts (54.5%, $n = 33$) (124). In fact, the mortality rate was similar for diabetic patients who received saphenous vein grafts and diabetic patients who received PCI (55.5%, $n = 170$) in this cohort.

Two smaller randomized trials also compared the efficacy of PCI with CABG in patients with multivessel CAD. The 1,050-patient Coronary Angioplasty Versus Bypass Revascularization Investigation (CABRI) trial (122) found no significant difference in mortality between PCI and CABG at 1 year (2.7% for CABG versus 3.9% for PCI, $p = \text{NS}$). However, there was a strong trend toward improved mortality in diabetic patients treated with CABG after 4 years of follow-up (12.5% for CABG versus 22.6% for PCI) (125). Only 59 of the 393 patients in the Emory Angioplasty versus Surgery Trial (EAST) trial had diabetes (123,126–128). At 3-year follow-up, there were similar survival rates in the two groups (90% for surgery versus 93.1% for angioplasty). The survival curves began to diverge at 5 years, and by 8 years there was a strong trend toward improved survival in patients treated with CABG (24.5% mortality for CABG versus 39.9% mortality for PCI, $p = .23$) (123). Moreover, diabetic patients treated with angioplasty had a significantly lower survival rate than did nondiabetic patients treated with PTCA (60.1% versus 82.6%, respectively; $p = .02$). Because the data from these studies were derived from retrospective analyses of nonprespecified subgroups, caution should be used before these results are applied to the general population.

When evaluating the clinical applicability of these early randomized trials, several caveats must be noted. Most of these trials were carried out in the late 1980's or early 1990's, before the routine use of periprocedural GP IIb/IIIa inhibition and coronary stenting, two modalities that have been shown to effectively improve the safety profile for diabetic patients undergoing PCI (22,99). For example, in this era, the rate of abrupt closure was 10% and the need for emergency CABG was 8%, rates that are significantly higher than those seen in modern clinical practice (129). On the other hand, the increased use of arterial conduits with the goal of complete arterial revascularization has improved graft patency rates in the modern era and may improve long-term outcomes (130,131). These advanced surgical revascularization options were not available at the time of BARI. Moreover, patients enrolled in clinical trials are not always reflective of those patients routinely seen in clinical practice. For example, only 16% of patients eligible for BARI were actually randomly assigned to a treatment arm; most patients were monitored in the BARI registry (132). Notably, in an analysis of the diabetic patients in the BARI registry ($N = 339$), there were no significant differences in all-cause mortality or cardiac mortality between the two revascularization strategies (133). Therefore, it has been speculated that physician selection may be an important factor in achieving comparable outcomes between PCI and CABG in diabetic patients (134).

Additional angiographic data from the BARI randomized study does give insight into why diabetic patients had a higher likelihood of adverse outcomes after PCI in comparison with CABG. Kip et al. (107) found that the amount of jeopardized myocardium in diabetic patients treated with angioplasty was significantly greater than in nondiabetic patients treated with angioplasty, but this finding was not true for diabetic patients treated with CABG. Therefore, a possible explanation for the adverse outcomes in the diabetic patients in BARI was incomplete revascularization in the angioplasty arm. In fact, only 70% of patients randomly assigned to the PCI arm actually underwent multivessel PCI. Of these patients, the angiographic success rate in dilating an average of 1.9 to 3.5 hemodynamically significant lesions was only 54%. On the other hand, 91% of patients in the CABG arm had successful grafting of all intended vessels (average, 3.1 vessels) (10). These findings suggest that complete revascularization, which is now often attainable with modern interventional techniques, may diminish the gap in long-term outcomes between these two strategies in diabetic patients.

Retrospective analyses from BARI have also evaluated other mechanisms as potential reasons for why diabetic patients fared poorly after conventional balloon angioplasty. Van Belle et al. (135) found that occlusive restenosis after PCI was adversely associated with increased long-term mortality (hazard ratio [HR] = 2.16; 95% CI, 1.43 to 3.26, $p = .0003$). On the other hand, there has been speculation that the increased rates of restenosis and increased need for TVR in BARI do not completely explain the adverse outcomes of diabetic patients in this study. For example, Rozenman et al. (136), in a cohort of 248 patients, found that diabetic patients had a significantly higher rate of new narrowings at an angiographic location different from the treated lesion, compared with nondiabetic patients (14.8% versus 9.8%, $p = 0.03$). Because these new narrowings plausibly lead to increased plaque rupture, resulting in ACS, the authors speculated that the increased mortality and morbidity in diabetic patients was due to new lesion progression rather than restenosis of the treated arterial segment. In fact, the dichotomy in mortality between PCI and CABG seen in the BARI study occurred after the first year of enrollment, well beyond the established period of restenosis. This fact adds credence to the notion that disease progression is the main factor for adverse outcomes in diabetic patients treated with PCI. It follows that patients revascularized with CABG have protection from nonobstructive but unstable plaques that may subsequently rupture (106).

GLYCOPROTEIN IIb/IIIa INHIBITION AND PERCUTANEOUS CORONARY INTERVENTION IN THE DIABETIC PATIENT

Abciximab

Several studies have specifically documented the clinical benefit of GP IIb/IIIa inhibition in diabetic patients with ACS (137) and in diabetic patients undergoing PCI (22,99,138). Although all three clinically available GP IIb/IIIa inhibitors (abciximab, tirofiban, and eptifibatide) have been shown to have benefit in diabetic patients undergoing PCI, abciximab has the most robust data for early and sustained benefit in this patient population. For example, a pooled analysis of the Early Postmenopausal Intervention Cohort (EPIC), Evaluation in PTCA to Improve Long-Term Outcome with Abciximab GP IIb/IIIa Blockade (EPILOG), and EPISTENT trials showed that abciximab significantly reduced mortality, from 4.5% to 2.5% ($p = .031$), at 1 year in diabetic patients undergoing PCI (99) (Fig. 20-3). Moreover, abciximab reduced mortality by more than 50% (5.1% versus 2.3%, $p = .044$) in patients with the insulin resistance syndrome (defined as diabetes, hypertension, and obesity) (99). The beneficial effects of abciximab in diabetic patients relate to the consistent level of platelet inhibition (139) in these patients. In addition, earlier studies also found salutary antiinflammatory effects mediated by the Mac-1 (82,97) and vitronectin (98) receptors. The treatment of multivessel disease is an especially important consideration in diabetic patients because of its high prevalence in this population. In this subset of patients, mortality was dramatically reduced, from 7.7% to 0.9% ($p = .018$), with abciximab use (99,138,140) (Fig. 20-4). An analysis of the

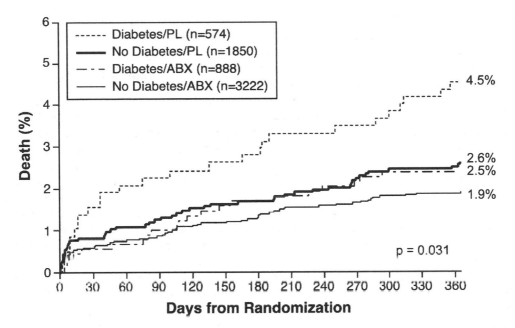

FIG. 20-3. Influence of diabetes on mortality in patients undergoing percutaneous coronary intervention (PCI) and randomly assigned to either abciximab (ABX) or placebo (PL). (From Bhatt DL, Marso SP, Lincoff AM, et al. Abciximab reduces mortality in diabetic patients following percutaneous coronary intervention. *J Am Coll Cardiol* 2000;35:922–928, with permission.)

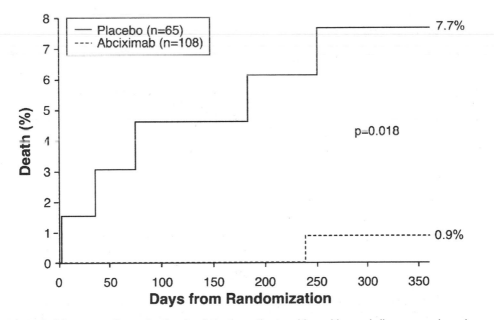

FIG. 20-4. Striking mortality reduction in diabetic patients with multivessel disease undergoing percutaneous coronary intervention (PCI) who were randomly assigned to abciximab or placebo. (From Bhatt D, Chew D, Topol E. The importance of intravenous antiplatelet therapy with abciximab during percutaneous coronary intervention in diabetic patients. *Cardiovasc Rev Rep* 2001;21:161–164, with permission.)

diabetic subgroup in the EPISTENT trial provided data supporting a beneficial interaction between the use of abciximab and coronary stenting in this population (22). Marso et al. (22) also found that abciximab administration resulted in a progressive decrease in the incidence of death or MI at 6 months, depending on revascularization strategy, in comparison to placebo (12.7% for stent plus placebo versus 7.8% for balloon angioplasty plus abciximab versus 6.2% for stent plus abciximab, $p = .029$). The need for TVR at 6 months was significantly reduced by the periprocedural use of abciximab (16.6% for stent plus placebo versus 18.4% for balloon plus abciximab versus 8.1% for stent plus abciximab, $p = .021$) (Fig. 20-5). Most importantly, abciximab reduced mortality at 6 months in diabetic patients treated with coronary stenting: 4.1% for stent plus placebo versus 1.2% for stent plus abciximab, $p = .11$. These data provide strong

evidence for a durable, salutary effect of abciximab in diabetic patients undergoing PCI.

Eptifibatide

The use of eptifibatide in PCI with coronary stenting was evaluated formally in the Enhanced Suppression of the Platelet IIb/IIIa Receptor with Integrilin Therapy (ESPRIT) study (141). This randomized trial of 2,064 patients found that a novel, double-bolus of eptifibatide reduced the 30-day composite end point of death, MI, or urgent TVR from 10.5% in the placebo group to 6.8% ($p = .0034$). Durability of benefit was confirmed: statistically significant reductions in the composite end point were found at 6 months (142) and at 1 year (143). Treatment with eptifibatide improved the outcomes of the subset of diabetic patients as well. For example, at 6 months, eptifibatide reduced the composite end point

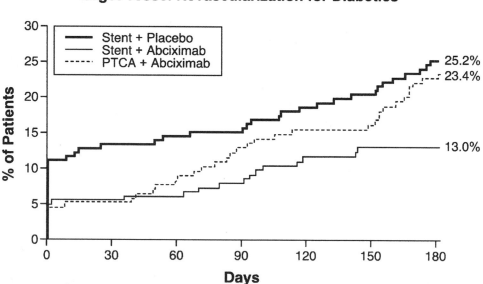

FIG. 20-5. Comparison of 6-month composite outcomes in diabetic patients undergoing percutaneous coronary intervention (PCI) who were randomly assigned to abciximab and/or coronary stenting. (From Marso SP, Lincoff AM, Ellis SG, et al. Optimizing the percutaneous interventional outcomes for patients with diabetes mellitus: results of the EPISTENT (Evaluation of Platelet IIb/IIIa Inhibitor for Stenting Trial) diabetic substudy [see comments]. *Circulation* 1999;100:2477–2484, with permission.)

in both diabetic patients (10.2% versus 6.3%, $p = $ NS) and nondiabetic patients (11.8% versus 7.7%, $p < .05$), compared with placebo. After 6 months, event rates were actually higher in the nondiabetic patients than in the diabetic patients. Moreover, at 1-year follow-up, the event rates of death or MI in placebo-treated diabetic patients were only slightly higher than in placebo treated nondiabetic patients (13.4% versus 12.0%, respectively). This raises speculation that the diabetic patients in ESPRIT were not as ill as those found in other studies of coronary stenting and GP IIb/IIIa inhibition, such as EPISTENT. In any case, at 1-year follow-up, eptifibatide was shown to effectively reduce the end point of death or MI in all subgroups of patients, including diabetic patients (7.8% for stent plus eptifibatide versus 13.4% stent plus placebo). The ESPRIT data, in addition to the results of the Platelet Glycoprotein IIb/IIIa in Unstable Angina Receptor Suppression Using Integrilin Therapy (PURSUIT) trial, which found an almost 50% reduction in 30-day mortality in insulin-treated diabetic patients, provide good evidence that diabetic patients do have substantial benefit with eptifibatide treatment (144).

Tirofiban

Tirofiban is a small-molecule GP IIb/IIIa inhibition agent that has been extensively studied in patients presenting with ACS (145,146), but there are fewer data on its efficacy in patients undergoing PCI with coronary stent placement. The Platelet Receptor Inhibition in Ischemic Syndrome Management in Patients Limited by Unstable Signs and Symptoms (PRISM-PLUS) study (146) evaluated the effect of the addition of tirofiban to heparin and aspirin in patients presenting with unstable angina or non-ST-segment elevation myocardial infarction (NSTEMI). A substudy of the diabetic patients in this trial (147) found that the composite end point of death, MI, or refractory ischemia was reduced at 30 days and at 6 months (20.1% versus 29.0% and 32.0% versus 39.9%, respectively; $p = $ NS), and the incidence of death or MI was significantly reduced at 30 days and at 6 months (4.7%

versus 15.5%, $p = .002$, and 11.2% versus 19.2%, $p = .03$, respectively). A significant interaction was found between tirofiban treatment and diabetic status. At 30-day follow-up, tirofiban was found to have reduced the composite end point in patients treated medically (7.6% versus 11.2%, $p = $ NS), with PCI (1.9% versus 12.7%, $p = $ NS), or with CABG (2.6% versus 26.5%, $p < .05$).

The TARGET study (148) was a head-to-head comparison between tirofiban and abciximab in patients undergoing coronary artery stenting. The initial aim of the study was to assess the noninferiority of tirofiban compared with abciximab at the prespecified time of 30-day follow-up. Compared with the 2,398 patients randomly assigned to tirofiban, the primary end point of death, MI, or need for urgent TVR was significantly reduced in the 2,411 patients randomly assigned to abciximab (7.6% versus 6.1%, $p = .038$). The composite end point was driven by a reduction in MI with abciximab use (6.9% versus 5.4%, $p = .04$). In an analysis of diabetic patients in the TARGET study at 30 days, the incidence of death, MI, or urgent TVR was 6.2% in patients receiving tirofiban and 5.4% in those receiving abciximab (HR = 1.16, $p = .54$) (23). At 6 months, the composite end point in diabetic patients was reached in 15.7% of patients treated with tirofiban and 16.9% of patients treated with abciximab (HR = 0.93, $p = .610$). The mortality rate at 1 year in diabetic patients was 2.1% in the tirofiban group and 2.9% in the abciximab group (HR = 0.74, $p = .44$). Although abciximab and tirofiban provided comparable benefits at 6 months and 1 year in the diabetic cohort of TARGET, caution must be used when interpreting these long-term follow-up data. Specifically, TARGET (148) was only powered to detect a difference in the composite end point of death, MI, or urgent TVR at 30 days in both diabetic patients and nondiabetic patients. Therefore, evaluation limited to the diabetic cohort may have been underpowered to detect a difference in efficacy between abciximab and tirofiban at long-term follow-up. A prospective, randomized trial powered to compare the clinical efficacy and economic impact of abciximab, tirofiban, and eptifibatide in diabetic patients undergoing PCI is needed to provide better answers regarding the most efficacious and cost-effective agent in this cohort of patients.

Based on the available data from randomized clinical trials, all three commercially available GP IIb/IIIa inhibitors have beneficial effects in diabetic patients undergoing PCI. This point was particularly exemplified in a recent metaanalysis by Roffi et al. (137) that analyzed the data from several trials involving abciximab, eptifibatide, and tirofiban. This analysis found that GP IIb/IIIa inhibition significantly reduced 30-day mortality in diabetic patients with ACS (6.2% versus 4.6%; OR = 0.74; 95% CI, 0.59 to 0.92; $p = .007$), whereas nondiabetic patients had no survival benefit (3.0% versus 3.0%). Of note, the majority of survival benefit was found in diabetic patients undergoing PCI (4.0% versus 1.2%; OR = 0.30; 95% CI, 0.14 to 0.69; $p = .002$) (Fig. 20-6). Moreover, there was a significant interaction between diabetic status and platelet GP IIb/IIIa inhibitor treatment, suggesting an inde-

pendent link between the diabetic state and GP IIb/IIIa treatment effect. This interaction translated into an impressive 1 life saved for every 36 patients who underwent PCI (137). These data strongly suggest that GP IIb/IIIa inhibitors should be prescribed to diabetic patients with ACS, especially if early PCI is planned.

COST-EFFECTIVENESS OF CORONARY ARTERY BYPASS GRAFTING VERSUS PERCUTANEOUS TRANSLUMINAL CORONARY ANGIOGRAPHY IN DIABETIC PATIENTS IN THE BARI STUDY

Hlatky et al. (149) performed a formal cost-effectiveness analysis of CABG versus PTCA in the BARI study. In the entire cohort, the 5-year cost of care in patients randomly assigned to initial angioplasty was significantly lower then CABG in patients with two-vessel disease ($52,930 versus $58,498; $p < .05$), but not in patients with three-vessel disease. CABG was

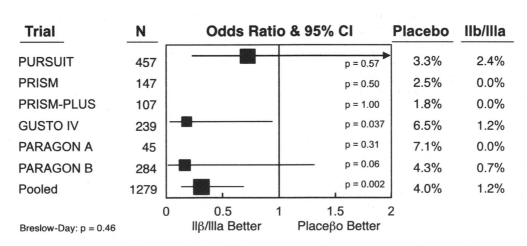

FIG. 20-6. Odds ratios (OR) with 95% confidence intervals (CI) and corresponding probability values (P) for treatment effect on 30-day mortality among diabetic patients with acute coronary syndromes (ACS) undergoing percutaneous coronary intervention (PCI). Values to left of 1.0 indicate a survival benefit of platelet glycoprotein IIb/IIIa inhibition. (From Roffi M, Chew DP, Mukherjee D, et al. Platelet glycoprotein IIb/IIIa inhibitors reduce mortality in diabetic patients with non-ST-segment-elevation acute coronary syndromes. *Circulation* 2001;104:2767–2771, with permission.)

particularly cost-effective in diabetic patients with two- or three-vessel disease because of the improved survival in this group of patients. For instance, in diabetic patients with three-vessel disease, cost at 5 years was $95,376 in patients receiving PTCA and $72,837 in patients receiving CABG ($p =$ NS). CABG added, on average, 4.3 years of life, compared with 3.5 years for PTCA ($p < .01$). Again, it is important to note that this cost analysis was performed in the era before coronary stenting and GP IIb/IIIa inhibition, strategies that have been shown to be cost-effective in more recent analyses (150). Additionally, drug-eluting stents have been shown to markedly reduce restenosis, thereby leading to a decrease in repeat revascularization procedures.

PERCUTANEOUS CORONARY INTERVENTION VERSUS CORONARY ARTERY BYPASS GRAFTING IN THE STENT ERA

The growing data on the importance of coronary stent placement (151) at the time of PCI in decreasing the rate of restenosis, particularly in diabetic patients, has resulted in a head-to-head comparison of CABG with coronary stenting in patients with multivessel coronary disease. The Arterial Revascularization Therapies Study (ARTS) (152) compared the outcomes of CABG with those of multivessel PCI and coronary stenting in 1,205 patients. The study found no significant difference between the two groups in the primary end point of freedom from death, stroke, or MI at 1 year (91.3% for CABG versus 90.6% for PCI; $p =$ NS). However, the 208 diabetic patients in this trial fared poorly, with a higher rate of mortality in the stenting arm than in the CABG arm of the trial (6.3% versus 3.1%, respectively; $p = .294$) (118). Furthermore, patients randomly assigned to the PCI arm had a significantly higher requirement for repeat TVR after PCI (3.1% for CABG versus 25% for PCI; $p < .01$). In a multivariate analysis, diabetes mellitus was found to be an independent correlate for major adverse cardiac events at 1 year in the stenting arm only (OR = 2.1; $p = .002$) (118). However, diabetic patients randomly assigned to CABG had a significantly higher incidence of in-hospital cerebrovascular accidents, compared with those diabetic patients assigned to stenting (4.2% versus 0% PCI, respectively; $p = .041$), and a higher rate of CVAs at 1 year (6.3% versus 1.8%; $p = .096$) (118). Despite the increased need for repeat revascularizations in the stent group, the average total cost was significantly less in the PCI arm than in the CABG arm at 1 year ($12,855 versus $16,585; $p < .001$), but no cost differences were found at 3 years of follow-up (153). The use of abciximab in this trial was extremely low, less than 5%; additional cost-effectiveness with clinical benefit could have been achieved with increased use of periprocedural abciximab (150). The Stent or Surgery (SoS) trial (154) also compared CABG against PCI in patients with multivessel CAD. This study found a lower rate of mortality at 1 year in those patients undergoing CABG compared with PCI (0.8% versus 2.5%, respectively). The overall number of diabetic patients in this study was low, and therefore the increased mortality with PCI observed in this study could not be explained by diabetes alone. Patients in the PCI arm did have an unusually high number of cancer deaths, but this should not lead to dismissal of the concerning findings of increased mortality with PCI in patients with multivessel disease.

On initial review of the results of ARTS and SoS, CABG still appears to be superior to PCI in the era of bare metal stenting without the routine use of a GP IIb/IIIa inhibitor. Of note, the use of GP IIb/IIIa inhibition in both of these studies was astonishingly low. For example, only 3.5% of patients in ARTS received periprocedural abciximab during coronary stent implantation. This point is extremely important, because periprocedural abciximab administration is associated with reduced mortality, compared with placebo, in patients who receive stents (150). In fact, the mortality benefit of GP IIb/IIIa inhibition is more pronounced in patients with diabetes. For example, a pooled analysis of the trials studying the use of abciximab in patients with PCI demonstrated that diabetic patients who received abciximab had a mortality rate similar to that of nondiabetic patients receiving placebo (99). Moreover, this mortality benefit is marked in diabetic patients with multivessel CAD, such as those in the ARTS trial (99,138). The reduction in mortality may be related to the decreased rates of restenosis, a key determinant of mortality in diabetic patients after PCI (135). Therefore, increased use of periprocedural abciximab might have dramatically improved the long-term results of PCI in ARTS and SoS. Finally, it must be noted that the ARTS trial randomly assigned only those patients who were deemed amenable to complete percutaneous revascularization. The characteristics of the ARTS patient population did not necessarily reflect what clinicians see in their daily practice of cardiology. For instance, most patients in ARTS had normal left ventricular systolic function, and about 60% had only two-vessel disease. Therefore, it would be difficult to extrapolate the data from this trial to patients seen in clinical practice with left ventricular systolic dysfunction and three-vessel disease involving the proximal left anterior descending artery.

The optimal management of multivessel disease in diabetic patients is an ever-changing issue. The problem with using randomized clinical trial data to make decisions regarding coronary revascularization in diabetic patients is that the latest advances in modern PCI techniques can never be fully realized in a randomized trial. Surgical techniques and outcomes have improved through the years but, arguably, less than recent PCI advances. By the time data from the large trials are analyzed and presented, interventional techniques and methods have advanced, making the findings of these trials not necessarily applicable to current standards of patient care. A recent example is the issue of drug-coated stents. The RAVEL trial (92) found a 0% restenosis rate at 6-month angiographic follow-up, but the latest randomized studies comparing coronary stenting against CABG in patients with multivessel CAD did not use drug-coated stents.

In summary, data from randomized controlled trials is time sensitive, and current revascularization techniques and adjunctive therapies are rapidly evolving. Additional studies are needed to clearly delineate the optimal revascularization strategy in diabetic patients with multivessel dis-

ease. Until these well-conducted randomized trials are done, no firm guidelines can be put in place regarding the optimal mode of revascularization in diabetic patients with multivessel disease, but general recommendations can be made. The revascularization option of choice for diabetic patients with single-vessel disease should be PCI. Several angiographic factors should be considered in determining the best revascularization strategy in diabetic patients with multivessel disease. For example, lesion characteristics (including vessel diameter, plaque morphology, lesion length and location, and vessel calcification) should play a role in determining whether a vessel is suitable for PCI (155). With the use of appropriate adjunctive therapy including GP IIb/IIIa inhibition, excellent percutaneous revascularization results can be achieved in diabetic patients with discrete, focal, high-grade stenosis in multiple large-caliber vessels. However, patients with long, calcified lesions or chronic total occlusions in diffusely diseased vessels would have suboptimal results with PCI and would be better served by CABG. Because diabetic patients do have a higher incidence of left main coronary artery disease (156) and more severe and diffuse CAD (157) when presenting for coronary angiography, it logically follows that a sizable percentage of diabetic patients would be better candidates for CABG than for multivessel PCI. However, determination of the best mode of revascularization should not be made on the basis of diabetic status alone, but also on angiographic characteristics. If complete revascularization can be achieved with PCI, then this approach would be a viable revascularization option in these patients. As was shown in the BARI registry, good clinical judgment is likely to achieve comparable long-term results with multivessel PCI compared with CABG (133).

UPCOMING CLINICAL TRIALS

BARI-2D and the proposed Future Revascularization Evaluation in Patients with Diabetes Mellitus (FREEDOM) trial will provide further insight into the optimal medical and revascularization treatment for diabetic patients with multivessel CAD. BARI-2D will specifically attempt to identify the optimal timing of revascularization (CABG or PCI) in diabetic patients with stable angina. For example, diabetic patients with severe coronary artery disease involving at least two vessels will be randomly assigned to a revascularization arm (CABG or PCI) versus intensification of medical therapy. The choice of CABG or PCI will not be randomized but will be left to the discretion of the treating physician. The medical therapy arm will consist of either an insulin-providing regimen (insulin and/or sulfonylurea) or an insulin-sensitizing regimen (metformin and/or thiazolidinedione). The primary end point is cardiovascular death; the planned follow-up time is 4 to 7 years. The FREEDOM trial will be a randomized clinical trial comparing CABG with modern PCI techniques (sirolimus-coated stents and periprocedural GP IIb/IIIa inhibition) in diabetic patients with multivessel CAD. The primary end points are major adverse cardiac or cerebrovascular events at 1 year and mortality at 5 years of follow up.

CONCLUSION AND FUTURE DIRECTIONS

Despite advances in both percutaneous and surgical revascularization strategies, diabetic patients continue to have worse periprocedural and long-term outcomes, although the discrepancies in outcomes between diabetic and nondiabetic patients are improving. Tremendous progress has been made, particularly in the realm of percutaneous coronary revascularization, where GP IIb/IIIa inhibition and coronary stenting have significantly reduced rates of periprocedural MI and both urgent and elective TVR in diabetic patients. The recent data from trials of coated stents show promise of significantly improved rates of restenosis. Moreover, the increased use of arterial conduits in CABG procedures has improved rates of graft patency. Off-pump surgical procedures might improve neurocognitive outcomes (158) and reduce lengths of stay after CABG (159). Additional studies are still needed to clarify formally the optimal revascularization strategy in diabetic patients with multivessel disease.

Regardless of which revascularization strategy is chosen, clinicians must understand that diabetes is a chronic metabolic disease that continues to promote atherosclerosis; revascularization alone does not ameliorate the pathophysiology of the disease process. Therefore, aggressive adjunctive medical therapies (e.g., lipid-lowering therapy, aggressive glycemic control, aggressive antiplatelet therapy) are needed to prevent disease progression in both native arteries and vascular conduits after revascularization procedures. Retrospective data from the Scandinavian Simvastatin Survival Study (4S) study (160) found simvastatin to be a particularly cost-effective (161) and beneficial secondary prevention strategy in both diabetic (162) and prediabetic (160) patients by reducing all-cause mortality and the need for repeat revascularizations. These effects may be mediated by its lipid-lowering properties (163) and its pleiotropic effects (164), such as protection from ischemia-reperfusion injury (165). Although tight glycemic control has been shown to improve mortality after MI (166), randomized clinical trials are needed to test this hypothesis in diabetic patients treated with elective PCI or CABG. The comparative efficacy of an insulin-utilizing versus an insulin-sparing medical regimen also needs to be studied. Regarding chronic antiplatelet therapy in diabetic patients, clopidogrel appears superior to aspirin (167), though the combination of clopidogrel plus aspirin may be particularly efficacious in the diabetic patient, a hypothesis that will be examined in the Clopidogrel for High Atherothrombotic Risk and Ischemic Stabilization, Management and Avoidance (CHARISMA) trial. The Clopidogrel for the Reduction of Events During Observation (CREDO) trial (168) will help answer the question of whether routine use of prolonged dual antiplatelet therapy with aspirin and clopidogrel improves outcomes after PCI. Therefore, postrevascularization management in the future will likely involve the use of multiple medications that serve as components of a comprehensive pharmacologic armamentarium designed to attenuate the deleterious metabolic sequelae of diabetes, thereby reducing morbidity and mortality after coronary revascularization.

REFERENCES

1. Halon DA, Merdler A, Flugelman MY, et al. Importance of diabetes mellitus and systemic hypertension rather than completeness of revascularization in determining long-term outcome after coronary balloon angioplasty (the LDCMC registry). Lady Davis Carmel Medical Center. *Am J Cardiol* 1998;82:547–553.
2. Myler RK, Topol EJ, Shaw RE, et al. Multiple vessel coronary angioplasty: classification, results, and patterns of restenosis in 494 consecutive patients. *Cathet Cardiovasc Diagn* 1987;13:1–15.
3. Stein B, Weintraub WS, Gebhart SP, et al. Influence of diabetes mellitus on early and late outcome after percutaneous transluminal coronary angioplasty. *Circulation* 1995;91:979–989.
4. Weintraub WS, Kosinski AS, Brown CL 3rd, et al. Can restenosis after coronary angioplasty be predicted from clinical variables? *J Am Coll Cardiol* 1993;21:6–14.
5. Weintraub WS, Stein B, Kosinski A, et al. Outcome of coronary bypass surgery versus coronary angioplasty in diabetic patients with multivessel coronary artery disease. *J Am Coll Cardiol* 1998;31:10–19.
6. Barsness GW, Peterson ED, Ohman EM, et al. Relationship between diabetes mellitus and long-term survival after coronary bypass and angioplasty. *Circulation* 1997;96:2551–2556.
7. Detre K, Holubkov R, Kelsey S, et al. Percutaneous transluminal coronary angioplasty in 1985–1986 and 1977–1981. The National Heart, Lung, and Blood Institute Registry. *N Engl J Med* 1988;318:265–270.
8. Anderson HV, Shaw RE, Brindis RG, et al. A contemporary overview of percutaneous coronary interventions. The American College of Cardiology-National Cardiovascular Data Registry (ACC-NCDR). *J Am Coll Cardiol* 2002;39:1096–1103.
9. The BARI Investigators. Comparison of coronary bypass surgery with angioplasty in patients with multivessel disease. The Bypass Angioplasty Revascularization Investigation (BARI) Investigators. *N Engl J Med* 1996;335:217–225.
10. The BARI Investigators. Influence of diabetes on 5-year mortality and morbidity in a randomized trial comparing CABG and PTCA in patients with multivessel disease. The Bypass Angioplasty Revascularization Investigation (BARI). *Circulation* 1997;96:1761–1769.
11. Kip KE, Faxon DP, Detre KM, et al. Coronary angioplasty in diabetic patients. The National Heart, Lung, and Blood Institute Percutaneous Transluminal Coronary Angioplasty Registry. *Circulation* 1996;94:1818–1825.
12. Marso SP, Giorgi LV, Johnson WL, et al. Diabetes mellitus is associated with a shift in the temporal risk profile of in-hospital mortality following percutaneous coronary intervention: an analysis of 25,223 patients over 20 years. *Am Heart J* 2003;145:270–277.
13. Elezi S, Kastrati A, Pache J, et al. Diabetes mellitus and the clinical and angiographic outcome after coro-

nary stent placement. *J Am Coll Cardiol* 1998;32:1866–1873.
14. Levine GN, Jacobs AK, Keeler GP, et al. Impact of diabetes mellitus on percutaneous revascularization (CAVEAT-I). Coronary Angioplasty Versus Excisional Atherectomy Trial Investigators. *Am J Cardiol* 1997;79:748–755.
15. Shaw RE, Anderson HV, Brindis RG, et al. Development of a risk adjustment mortality model using the American College of Cardiology-National Cardiovascular Data Registry (ACC-NCDR) experience: 1998–2000. *J Am Coll Cardiol* 2002;39:1104–1112.
16. Holmes DR Jr, Vlietstra RE, Smith HC, et al. Restenosis after percutaneous transluminal coronary angioplasty (PTCA): a report from the PTCA Registry of the National Heart, Lung, and Blood Institute. *Am J Cardiol* 1984;53:77C–81C.
17. Abizaid A, Kornowski R, Mintz GS, et al. The influence of diabetes mellitus on acute and late clinical outcomes following coronary stent implantation. *J Am Coll Cardiol* 1998;32:584–589.
18. Tilli F, Aliabadi D, Bowers T, et al. Optimal coronary stenting in diabetic patients: a viable percutaneous alternative to cardiac surgery. *J Am Coll Cardiol* 1997;29:455A.
19. Yokoi H, Nosaka H, Kimura T, et al. Coronary stenting in diabetic patients: early and follow-up results. *J Am Coll Cardiol* 1997;29:455A.
20. Elezi S, Schulen H, Wehinger A, et al. Stent placement in diabetic versus non-diabetic patients: six-month angiographic follow-up. *J Am Coll Cardiol* 1997:455A.
21. Schofer J, Schluter M, Rau T, et al. Influence of treatment modality on angiographic outcome after coronary stenting in diabetic patients: a controlled study. *J Am Coll Cardiol* 2000;35:1554–1559.
22. Marso SP, Lincoff AM, Ellis SG, et al. Optimizing the percutaneous interventional outcomes for patients with diabetes mellitus: results of the EPISTENT (Evaluation of Platelet IIb/IIIa Inhibitor for Stenting Trial) diabetic substudy [see comments]. *Circulation* 1999;100:2477–2484.
23. Roffi M, Moliterno DJ, Meier B, et al. Impact of different platelet glycoprotein IIb/IIIa receptor inhibitors among diabetic patients undergoing percutaneous coronary intervention: Do Tirofiban and ReoPro Give Similar Efficacy Outcomes Trial (TARGET) 1-year follow-up. *Circulation* 2002;105:2730–2736.
24. Nishimoto Y, Miyazaki Y, Toki Y, et al. Enhanced secretion of insulin plays a role in the development of atherosclerosis and restenosis of coronary arteries: elective percutaneous transluminal coronary angioplasty in patients with effort angina. *J Am Coll Cardiol* 1998;32:1624–1629.
25. Sobel BE. Acceleration of restenosis by diabetes: pathogenetic implications. *Circulation* 2001;103:1185–1187.
26. Lamarche B, Tchernof A, Mauriege P, et al. Fasting insulin and apolipoprotein B levels and low-density lipoprotein particle size as risk factors for ischemic heart disease. *JAMA* 1998;279:1955–1961.
27. Despres JP, Lamarche B, Mauriege P, et al. Hyperinsulinemia as an independent risk factor for ischemic heart disease. *N Engl J Med* 1996;334:952–957.
28. Reaven GM. Role of insulin resistance in human disease. *Diabetes* 1988;37:27–36.

29. Sobel BE. Increased plasminogen activator inhibitor-1 and vasculopathy: a reconcilable paradox. *Circulation* 1999;99:2496–2498.

30. Moreno PR, Fallon JT, Murcia AM, et al. Tissue characteristics of restenosis after percutaneous transluminal coronary angioplasty in diabetic patients. *J Am Coll Cardiol* 1999;34:1045–1049.

31. Cleveland JC Jr, Meldrum DR, Cain BS, et al. Oral sulfonylurea hypoglycemic agents prevent ischemic preconditioning in human myocardium: two paradoxes revisited. *Circulation* 1997;96:29–32.

32. Klepzig H, Kober G, Matter C, et al. Sulfonylureas and ischaemic preconditioning: a double-blind, placebo-controlled evaluation of glimepiride and glibenclamde. *Eur Heart J* 1999;20:439–446.

33. Tomai F, Crea F, Gaspardone A, et al. Ischemic preconditioning during coronary angioplasty is prevented by glibenclamide, a selective ATP-sensitive K+ channel blocker. *Circulation* 1994;90:700–705.

34. Lee TM, Su SF, Chou TF, et al. Loss of preconditioning by attenuated activation of myocardial ATP-sensitive potassium channels in elderly patients undergoing coronary angioplasty. *Circulation* 2002;105:334–340.

35. Katsuda Y, Egashira K, Ueno H, et al. Glibenclamide, a selective inhibitor of ATP-sensitive K+ channels, attenuates metabolic coronary vasodilatation induced by pacing tachycardia in dogs. *Circulation* 1995;92:511–517.

36. Davis CA 3rd, Sherman AJ, Yaroshenko Y, et al. Coronary vascular responsiveness to adenosine is impaired additively by blockade of nitric oxide synthesis and a sulfonylurea. *J Am Coll Cardiol* 1998;31:816–822.

37. Takagi T, Akasaka T, Yamamuro A, et al. Troglitazone reduces neointimal tissue proliferation after coronary stent implantation in patients with non-insulin dependent diabetes mellitus: a serial intravascular ultrasound study. *J Am Coll Cardiol* 2000;36:1529–1535.

38. Takagi T, Akasaka T, Yamamuro A, et al. Impact of insulin resistance on neointimal tissue proliferation after coronary stent implantation. Intravascular ultrasound studies. *J Diabetes Complications* 2002;16:50–55.

39. Marx N, Schonbeck U, Lazar MA, et al. Peroxisome proliferator-activated receptor gamma activators inhibit gene expression and migration in human vascular smooth muscle cells. *Circ Res* 1998;83:1097–1103.

40. Pasceri V, Wu HD, Willerson JT, et al. Modulation of vascular inflammation in vitro and in vivo by peroxisome proliferator-activated receptor-gamma activators. *Circulation* 2000;101:235–238.

41. Yudkin JS, Stehouwer CD, Emeis JJ, et al. C-reactive protein in healthy subjects: associations with obesity, insulin resistance, and endothelial dysfunction: a potential role for cytokines originating from adipose tissue? *Arterioscler Thromb Vasc Biol* 1999;19:972–978.

42. Festa A, D'Agostino R Jr, Howard G, et al. Chronic subclinical inflammation as part of the insulin resistance syndrome: the Insulin Resistance Atherosclerosis Study (IRAS). *Circulation* 2000;102:42–47.

43. Festa A, D'Agostino R, Howard G, et al. Inflammation and microalbuminuria in nondiabetic and type 2 diabetic subjects: the Insulin Resistance Atherosclerosis Study. *Kidney Int* 2000;58:1703–1710.

44. Chew DP, Bhatt DL, Robbins MA, et al. Incremental prognostic value of elevated baseline C-reactive protein among established markers of risk in percutaneous coronary intervention. *Circulation* 2001;104:992–997.

45. Marso SP, Ellis SG, Tuzcu M, et al. The importance of proteinuria as a determinant of mortality following percutaneous coronary revascularization in diabetic patients. *J Am Coll Cardiol* 1999;33:1269–1277.

46. Aronson D. Restenosis in diabetic patients: is hyperinsulinemia the culprit? *Circulation* 1996;94:3003–3035.

47. Aronson D, Bloomgarden Z, Rayfield EJ. Potential mechanisms promoting restenosis in diabetic patients. *J Am Coll Cardiol* 1996;27:528–535.

48. Tesfamariam B. Free radicals in diabetic endothelial cell dysfunction. *Free Radic Biol Med* 1994;16:383–391.

49. Tesfamariam B, Cohen RA. Free radicals mediate endothelial cell dysfunction caused by elevated glucose. *Am J Physiol* 1992;263:H321–H326.

50. Umeda F, Inoguchi T, Nawata H. Reduced stimulatory activity on prostacyclin production by cultured endothelial cells in serum from aged and diabetic patients. *Atherosclerosis* 1989;75:61–66.

51. Williams SB, Cusco JA, Roddy MA, et al. Impaired nitric oxide-mediated vasodilation in patients with non insulin-dependent diabetes mellitus. *J Am Coll Cardiol* 1996;27:567–574.

52. Johnstone MT, Creager SJ, Scales KM, et al. Impaired endothelium-dependent vasodilation in patients with insulin-dependent diabetes mellitus. *Circulation* 1993;88:2510–2516.

53. McGill JB, Schneider DJ, Arfken CL, et al. Factors responsible for impaired fibrinolysis in obese subjects and NIDDM patients. *Diabetes* 1994;43:104–109.

54. Davi G, Rini GB, Averna M, et al. Thromboxane B2 formation and platelet sensitivity to prostacyclin in insulin-dependent and insulin-independent diabetic patients. *Thromb Res* 1982;26:359–370.

55. Davi G, Rini GB, Averna M, et al. Enhanced platelet release reaction in insulin-dependent and insulin-independent diabetic patients. *Haemostasis* 1982;12:275–281.

56. Davi G, Catalano I, Averna M, et al. Thromboxane biosynthesis and platelet function in type II diabetes mellitus. *N Engl J Med* 1990;322:1769–1774.

57. O'Neill W. Multivessel balloon angioplasty should be abandoned in diabetic patients! *J Am Coll Cardiol* 1998;31:20–22.

58. Lorenzi M, Cagliero E, Markey B, et al. Interaction of human endothelial cells with elevated glucose concentrations and native and glycosylated low density lipoproteins. *Diabetologia* 1984;26:218–222.

59. Winocour PD, Richardson M, Kinlough-Rathbone RL. Continued platelet interaction with de-endothelialized aortae associated with slower re-endothelialization and more extensive intimal hyperplasia in spontaneously diabetic BB Wistar rats. *Int J Exp Pathol* 1993;74:603–613.

60. Van Belle E, Maillard L, Tio F, et al. Accelerated endothelialization by local delivery of recombinant human VEGF reduces in-stent intimal formation. *J Am Coll Cardiol* 1997;29:77A.

61. Sharpe P, Trinick T. Mean platelet volume in diabetes mellitus. *Q J Med* 1993;86:739–742.

62. Tschoepe D, Roesen P, Esser J, et al. Large platelets circulate in an activated state in diabetes mellitus. *Semin Thromb Hemost* 1991;17:433–438.

63. Winocour PD, Perry DW, Kinlough-Rathbone RL. Hypersensitivity to ADP of platelets from diabetic rats associated with enhanced fibrinogen binding. *Eur J Clin Invest* 1992;22:19–23.

64. Oskarsson HJ, Hofmeyer TG. Platelets from patients with diabetes mellitus have impaired ability to mediate vasodilation. *J Am Coll Cardiol* 1996;27:1464–1470.

65. Oskarsson HJ, Hofmeyer TG. Diabetic human platelets release a substance that inhibits platelet-mediated vasodilation. *Am J Physiol* 1997;273:H371–H379.

66. Tschoepe D, Roesen P, Kaufmann L, et al. Evidence for abnormal platelet glycoprotein expression in diabetes mellitus. *Eur J Clin Invest* 1990;20:166–170.

67. Davi G, Gresele P, Violi F, et al. Diabetes mellitus, hypercholesterolemia, and hypertension but not vascular disease per se are associated with persistent platelet activation in vivo: evidence derived from the study of peripheral arterial disease. *Circulation* 1997;96:69–75.

68. Sampietro T, Lenzi S, Cecchetti P, et al. Nonenyzmatic glycation of human membrane proteins in vitro and in vivo. *Clin Chem* 1986;32:1328–1331.

69. Cohen I, Burk D, Fullerton R, et al. Nonenzymatic glycation of human blood platelet proteins. *Thromb Res* 1989;55:341–349.

70. Hangaishi M, Taguchi J, Miyata T, et al. Increased aggregation of human platelets produced by advanced glycation end products in vitro. *Biochem Biophys Res Commun* 1998;248:285–292.

71. Jilma B, Fasching P, Ruthner C, et al. Elevated circulating P-selectin in insulin dependent diabetes mellitus. *Thromb Haemost* 1996;76:328–332.

72. Merhi Y, Provost P, Guidoin R, et al. Importance of platelets in neutrophil adhesion and vasoconstriction after deep carotid arterial injury by angioplasty in pigs. *Arterioscler Thromb Vasc Biol* 1997;17:1185–1191.

73. Theilmeier G, Lenaerts T, Remacle C, et al. Circulating activated platelets assist THP-1 monocytoid/endothelial cell interaction under shear stress. *Blood* 1999;94:2725–2734.

74. Neumann FJ, Marx N, Gawaz M, et al. Induction of cytokine expression in leukocytes by binding of thrombin-stimulated platelets. *Circulation* 1997;95:2387–2394.

75. Hayashi S, Watanabe N, Nakazawa K, et al. Roles of P-selectin in inflammation, neointimal formation, and vascular remodeling in balloon-injured rat carotid arteries. *Circulation* 2000;102:1710–1717.

76. Tschoepe D, Rauch U, Schwippert B. Platelet-leukocyte cross-talk in diabetes mellitus. *Horm Metab Res* 1997;29:631–635.

77. Bienvenu JG, Tanguay JF, Theoret JF, et al. Recombinant soluble P-selectin glycoprotein ligand-1-Ig reduces restenosis through inhibition of platelet-neutrophil adhesion after double angioplasty in swine. *Circulation* 2001;103:1128–1134.

78. Buffon A, Liuzzo G, Biasucci LM, et al. Preprocedural serum levels of C-reactive protein predict early complications and late restenosis after coronary angioplasty. *J Am Coll Cardiol* 1999;34:1512–1521.

79. Blum A, Kaplan G, Vardinon N, et al. Serum amyloid type A may be a predictor of restenosis. *Clin Cardiol* 1998;21:655–658.

80. Tashiro H, Shimokawa H, Sadamatsu K, et al. Role of cytokines in the pathogenesis of restenosis after percutaneous transluminal coronary angioplasty. *Coron Artery Dis* 2001;12:107–113.

81. Schillinger M, Haumer M, Schlerka G, et al. Restenosis after percutaneous transluminal angioplasty in the femoropopliteal segment: the role of inflammation. *J Endovasc Ther* 2001;8:477–483.

82. Lincoff AM, Kereiakes DJ, Mascelli MA, et al. Abciximab suppresses the rise in levels of circulating inflammatory markers after percutaneous coronary revascularization. *Circulation* 2001;104:163–167.

83. Chew DP, Bhatt DL, Robbins MA, et al. Effect of clopidogrel added to aspirin before percutaneous coronary intervention on the risk associated with C-reactive protein. *Am J Cardiol* 2001;88:672–674.

84. Bhatt DL, Chew DP, Roffi M, et al. Elevated baseline CRP levels predict death or MI in diabetic patients undergoing percutaneous coronary intervention. *J Am Coll Cardiol* 2001;37:66A.

85. Glagov S, Weisenberg E, Zarins CK, et al. Compensatory enlargement of human atherosclerotic coronary arteries. *N Engl J Med* 1987;316:1371–1375.

86. Mintz GS, Popma JJ, Pichard AD, et al. Intravascular ultrasound assessment of the mechanisms and predictors of restenosis following coronary angioplasty. *J Invasive Cardiol* 1996;8:1–14.

87. Walker L, Bowen Pope D, Ross R, et al. Production of platelet-like growth factor-like molecules by cultured arterial smooth muscle cells accompanies proliferation after arterial injury. *Proc Natl Acad Sci U S A* 1986;83:7311–7315.

88. Merimee TJ, Zapf J, Froesch ER. Insulin-like growth factors. Studies in diabetic patients with and without retinopathy. *N Engl J Med* 1983;309:527–530.

89. Banskota NK, Taub R, Zellner K, et al. Insulin, insulin-like growth factor I and platelet-derived growth factor interact additively in the induction of the protooncogene c-myc and cellular proliferation in cultured bovine aortic smooth muscle cells. *Mol Endocrinol* 1989;3:1183–1190.

90. Yamamoto T, Nakamura T, Noble N, et al. Expression of transforming growth factor beta is elevated in human experimental diabetic nephropathy. *Proc Natl Acad Sci U S A* 1993;90:1814–1818.

91. Koschinsky T, Bunting CE, Schwippert B, et al. Regulation of diabetic serum growth factors for human vascular cells by the metabolic control of diabetes mellitus. *Atherosclerosis* 1981;39:313–319.

92. Morice MC, Serruys PW, Sousa JE, et al. A randomized comparison of a sirolimus-eluting stent with a standard stent for coronary revascularization. *N Engl J Med* 2002;346:1773–1780.

93. Silva JA, Escobar A, Collins TJ, et al. Unstable angina: a comparison of angioscopic findings between diabetic and nondiabetic patients. *Circulation* 1995;92:1731–1736.

94. Yokoyama I, Momomura S, Ohtake T, et al. Reduced myocardial flow reserve in non-insulin-dependent diabetes mellitus. *J Am Coll Cardiol* 1997;30:1472–1477.

95. Yokoyama I, Ohtake T, Momomura S, et al. Hyperglycemia rather than insulin resistance is related to reduced coronary flow reserve in NIDDM. *Diabetes* 1998;47:119–124.

96. Akasaka T, Yoshida K, Hozumi T, et al. Retinopathy identifies marked restriction of coronary flow reserve

in patients with diabetes mellitus. *J Am Coll Cardiol* 1997;30:935–941.

97. Simon DI, Xu H, Ortlepp S, et al. 7E3 monoclonal antibody directed against the platelet glycoprotein IIb/IIIa cross-reacts with the leukocyte integrin Mac-1 and blocks adhesion to fibrinogen and ICAM-1. *Arterioscler Thromb Vasc Biol* 1997;17:528–535.

98. Coller BS. Potential non-glycoprotein IIb/IIIa effects of abciximab. *Am Heart J* 1999;138:S1–S5.

99. Bhatt DL, Marso SP, Lincoff AM, et al. Abciximab reduces mortality in diabetic patients following percutaneous coronary intervention. *J Am Coll Cardiol* 2000;35:922–928.

100. Abaci A, Oguzhan A, Kahraman S, et al. Effect of diabetes mellitus on formation of coronary collateral vessels. *Circulation* 1999;99:2239–2242.

101. Rivard A, Silver M, Chen D, et al. Rescue of diabetes-related impairment of angiogenesis by intramuscular gene therapy with adeno-VEGF. *Am J Pathol* 1999;154:355–363.

102. Abdelmeguid AE, Topol EJ. The myth of the myocardial "infarctlet" during percutaneous coronary revascularization procedures. *Circulation* 1996;94:3369–3375.

103. Abdelmeguid AE, Topol EJ, Whitlow PL, et al. Significance of mild transient release of creatine kinase-MB fraction after percutaneous coronary interventions. *Circulation* 1996;94:1528–1536.

104. Thourani VH, Weintraub WS, Stein B, et al. Influence of diabetes mellitus on early and late outcome after coronary artery bypass grafting. *Ann Thorac Surg* 1999;67:1045–1052.

105. Wilson SH, Kennedy FP, Garratt KN. Optimisation of the management of patients with coronary heart disease and type 2 diabetes mellitus. *Drugs Aging* 2001;18:325–333.

106. Detre KM, Lombardero MS, Brooks MM, et al. The effect of previous coronary-artery bypass surgery on the prognosis of patients with diabetes who have acute myocardial infarction. Bypass Angioplasty Revascularization Investigation Investigators. *N Engl J Med* 2000;342:989–997.

107. Kip KE, Alderman EL, Bourassa MG, et al. Differential influence of diabetes mellitus on increased jeopardized myocardium after initial angioplasty or bypass surgery: bypass angioplasty revascularization investigation. *Circulation* 2002;105:1914–1920.

108. Van Belle E, Abolmaali K, Bauters C, et al. Restenosis, late vessel occlusion and left ventricular function six months after balloon angioplasty in diabetic patients. *J Am Coll Cardiol* 1999;34:476–485.

109. Yamamoto T, Hosoda Y, Takazawa K, et al. Is diabetes mellitus a major risk factor in coronary artery bypass grafting? The influence of internal thoracic artery grafting on late survival in diabetic patients. *Jpn J Thorac Cardiovasc Surg* 2000;48:344–352.

110. Lytle BW, Blackstone EH, Loop FD, et al. Two internal thoracic artery grafts are better than one. *J Thorac Cardiovasc Surg* 1999;117:855–872.

111. Pick AW, Orszulak TA, Anderson BJ, et al. Single versus bilateral internal mammary artery grafts: 10-year outcome analysis. *Ann Thorac Surg* 1997;64:599–605.

112. Wouters R, Wellens F, Vanermen H, et al. Sternitis and mediastinitis after coronary artery bypass grafting:

analysis of risk factors. *Tex Heart Inst J* 1994;21:183–188.

113. Matsa M, Paz Y, Gurevitch J, et al. Bilateral skeletonized internal thoracic artery grafts in patients with diabetes mellitus. *J Thorac Cardiovasc Surg* 2001;121:668–674.

114. Lytle BW, Cosgrove DM, Loop FD, et al. Perioperative risk of bilateral internal mammary artery grafting: analysis of 500 cases from 1971 to 1984. *Circulation* 1986;74:III37–III41.

115. McDonald WS, Brame M, Sharp C, et al. Risk factors for median sternotomy dehiscence in cardiac surgery. *South Med J* 1989;82:1361–1364.

116. Yamazaki K, Kato H, Tsujimoto S, et al. Diabetes mellitus, internal thoracic artery grafting, and risk of an elevated hemidiaphragm after coronary artery bypass surgery. *J Cardiothorac Vasc Anesth* 1994;8:437–440.

117. Nussmeier NA. A review of risk factors for adverse neurologic outcome after cardiac surgery. *J Extra Corpor Technol* 2002;34:4–10.

118. Abizaid A, Costa MA, Centemero M, et al. Clinical and economic impact of diabetes mellitus on percutaneous and surgical treatment of multivessel coronary disease patients: insights from the Arterial Revascularization Therapy Study (ARTS) trial. *Circulation* 2001;104:533–538.

119. Lawrie GM, Morris GC Jr, Glaeser DH. Influence of diabetes mellitus on the results of coronary bypass surgery: follow-up of 212 diabetic patients ten to 15 years after surgery. *JAMA* 1986;256:2967–2971.

120. Yasuura K, Matsuura A, Sawazaki M, et al. [Surgical results in diabetic patients undergoing coronary artery bypass grafting]. *Nippon Kyobu Geka Gakkai Zasshi* 1993;41:363–366.

121. The BARI Investigators. Five-year clinical and functional outcome comparing bypass surgery and angioplasty in patients with multivessel coronary disease: a multicenter randomized trial. Writing Group for the Bypass Angioplasty Revascularization Investigation (BARI) Investigators. *JAMA* 1997;277:715–721.

122. CABRI Trial Participants. First-year results of CABRI (Coronary Angioplasty versus Bypass Revascularization Investigation). *Circulation* 1996;93:847.

123. King SB 3rd, Kosinski AS, Guyton RA, et al. Eight-year mortality in the Emory Angioplasty versus Surgery Trial (EAST). *J Am Coll Cardiol* 2000;35:1116–1121.

124. The BARI Investigators. Seven-year outcome in the Bypass Angioplasty Revascularization Investigation (BARI) by treatment and diabetic status. *J Am Coll Cardiol* 2000;35:1122–1129.

125. Kurbaan AS, Bowker TJ, Ilsley CD, et al. Difference in the mortality of the CABRI diabetic and nondiabetic populations and its relation to coronary artery disease and the revascularization mode. *Am J Cardiol* 2001;87:947–950; A3.

126. King SB 3rd, Barnhart HX, Kosinski AS, et al. Angioplasty or surgery for multivessel coronary artery disease: comparison of eligible registry and randomized patients in the EAST trial and influence of treatment selection on outcomes. Emory Angioplasty versus Surgery Trial Investigators. *Am J Cardiol* 1997;79:1453–1459.

127. King SB 3rd, Lembo NJ, Weintraub WS, et al. Emory Angioplasty Versus Surgery Trial (EAST): design,

recruitment, and baseline description of patients. *Am J Cardiol* 1995;75:42C–59C.

128. King SB 3rd, Lembo NJ, Weintraub WS, et al. A randomized trial comparing coronary angioplasty with coronary bypass surgery: Emory Angioplasty versus Surgery Trial (EAST). *N Engl J Med* 1994;331:1044–1050.

129. Kapur A, Malik IS. Is surgery still the preferred option for coronary revascularisation in diabetic patients with multivessel coronary disease? *Heart* 2002;87:407–409.

130. Tatoulis J, Buxton BF, Fuller JA, et al. Total arterial coronary revascularization: techniques and results in 3,220 patients. *Ann Thorac Surg* 1999;68:2093–2099.

131. Buxton BF, Fuller JA, Tatoulis J. Evolution of complete arterial grafting for coronary artery disease. *Tex Heart Inst J* 1998;25:17–23.

132. Feit F, Brooks MM, Sopko G, et al. Long-term clinical outcome in the Bypass Angioplasty Revascularization Investigation Registry: comparison with the randomized trial. BARI Investigators. *Circulation* 2000;101:2795–2802.

133. Detre KM, Guo P, Holubkov R, et al. Coronary revascularization in diabetic patients: a comparison of the randomized and observational components of the Aypass Angioplasty Revascularization Investigation (BARI). *Circulation* 1999;99:633–640.

134. Smith SC Jr, Faxon D, Cascio W, et al. Prevention Conference VI: Diabetes and Cardiovascular Disease. Writing Group VI: Revascularization in Diabetic Patients. *Circulation* 2002;105:e165–e169.

135. Van Belle E, Ketelers R, Bauters C, et al. Patency of percutaneous transluminal coronary angioplasty sites at 6-month angiographic follow-up: a key determinant of survival in diabetic patients after coronary balloon angioplasty. *Circulation* 2001;103:1218–1224.

136. Rozenman Y, Sapoznikov D, Mosseri M, et al. Long-term angiographic follow-up of coronary balloon angioplasty in patients with diabetes mellitus: a clue to the explanation of the results of the BARI study. Balloon Angioplasty Revascularization Investigation. *J Am Coll Cardiol* 1997;30:1420–1425.

137. Roffi M, Chew DP, Mukherjee D, et al. Platelet glycoprotein IIb/IIIa inhibitors reduce mortality in diabetic patients with non-ST-segment-elevation acute coronary syndromes. *Circulation* 2001;104:2767–2771.

138. Bhatt D, Lincoff A, Tcheng J, et al. The impact of abciximab on mortality after multivessel PCI: a striking effect in diabetic patients [Abstract]. *J Am Coll Cardiol* 2000;35:91A.

139. Steinhubl SR, Kottke-Marchant K, Moliterno DJ, et al. Attainment and maintenance of platelet inhibition through standard dosing of abciximab in diabetic and nondiabetic patients undergoing percutaneous coronary intervention. *Circulation* 1999;100:1977–1982.

140. Bhatt D, Chew D, Topol E. The importance of intravenous antiplatelet therapy with abciximab during percutaneous coronary intervention in diabetic patients. *Cardiovasc Rev Rep* 2001;21:161–164.

141. The ESPRIT Investigators. Novel dosing regimen of eptifibatide in planned coronary stent implantation (ESPRIT): a randomised, placebo-controlled trial. *Lancet* 2000;356:2037–2044.

142. O'Shea JC, Hafley GE, Greenberg S, et al. Platelet glycoprotein IIb/IIIa integrin blockade with eptifibatide in coronary stent intervention: the ESPRIT trial, a randomized controlled trial. *JAMA* 2001;285:2468–2473.

143. O'Shea JC, Buller CE, Cantor WJ, et al. Long-term efficacy of platelet glycoprotein IIb/IIIa integrin blockade with eptifibatide in coronary stent intervention. *JAMA* 2002;287:618–621.

144. Wright R, Kopecky S, Barsness G, et al. Impact of diabetes mellitus on outcome in non-ST elevation myocardial infarction and unstable angina: is there a benefit from treatment with eptifibatide? *Circulation* 1999;100:I-640.

145. The PRISM Study Investigators. A comparison of aspirin plus tirofiban with aspirin plus heparin for unstable angina. Platelet Receptor Inhibition in Ischemic Syndrome Management (PRISM) Study Investigators. *N Engl J Med* 1998;338:1498–1505.

146. The PRISM-PLUS Study Investigators. Inhibition of the platelet glycoprotein IIb/IIIa receptor with tirofiban in unstable angina and non-Q-wave myocardial infarction. Platelet Receptor Inhibition in Ischemic Syndrome Management in Patients Limited by Unstable Signs and Symptoms (PRISM-PLUS) Study Investigators. *N Engl J Med* 1998;338:1488–1497.

147. Theroux P, Alexander J Jr., Pharand C, et al. Glycoprotein IIb/IIIa receptor blockade improves outcomes in diabetic patients presenting with unstable angina/non-ST-elevation myocardial infarction: results from the Platelet Receptor Inhibition in Ischemic Syndrome Management in Patients Limited by Unstable Signs and Symptoms (PRISM-PLUS) study. *Circulation* 2000;102:2466–2472.

148. Topol EJ, Moliterno DJ, Herrmann HC, et al. Comparison of two platelet glycoprotein IIb/IIIa inhibitors, tirofiban and abciximab, for the prevention of ischemic events with percutaneous coronary revascularization. *N Engl J Med* 2001;344:1888–1894.

149. Hlatky MA, Rogers WJ, Johnstone I, et al. Medical care costs and quality of life after randomization to coronary angioplasty or coronary bypass surgery. Bypass Angioplasty Revascularization Investigation (BARI) Investigators. *N Engl J Med* 1997;336:92–99.

150. Topol EJ, Mark DB, Lincoff AM, et al. Outcomes at 1 year and economic implications of platelet glycoprotein IIb/IIIa blockade in patients undergoing coronary stenting: results from a multicentre randomised trial. EPISTENT Investigators. Evaluation of Platelet IIb/IIIa Inhibitor for Stenting. *Lancet* 1999;354:2019–2024.

151. Kiemeneij F, Serruys PW, Macaya C, et al. Continued benefit of coronary stenting versus balloon angioplasty: five-year clinical follow-up of Benestent-I trial. *J Am Coll Cardiol* 2001;37:1598–1603.

152. Serruys PW, Unger F, Sousa JE, et al. Comparison of coronary-artery bypass surgery and stenting for the treatment of multivessel disease. *N Engl J Med* 2001;344:1117–1124.

153. Serruys PW. ARTS: three year follow-up data. Presented at the European Society of Cardiology Meeting, Stockholm, Sweden, 2001.

154. Stables R. Stent or Surgery (SoS) trial results. Presented at the Annual Meeting of the American College of Cardiology, Orlando, Florida, 2001.

155. Kastrati A, Mehilli J, Dirschinger J, et al. Restenosis after coronary placement of various stent types. *Am J Cardiol* 2001;87:34–39.

156. Cariou B, Bonnevie L, Mayaudon H, et al. Angiographic characteristics of coronary artery disease in diabetic patients compared with matched non-diabetic subjects. *Diabetes Nutr Metab* 2000;13:134–141.

157. Natali A, Vichi S, Landi P, et al. Coronary atherosclerosis in type II diabetes: angiographic findings and clinical outcome. *Diabetologia* 2000;43:632–641.

158. Diegeler A, Hirsch R, Schneider F, et al. Neuromonitoring and neurocognitive outcome in off-pump versus conventional coronary bypass operation. *Ann Thorac Surg* 2000;69:1162–1166.

159. Boyd WD, Desai ND, Del Rizzo DF, et al. Off-pump surgery decreases postoperative complications and resource utilization in the elderly. *Ann Thorac Surg* 1999;68:1490–1493.

160. Haffner SM, Alexander CM, Cook TJ, et al. Reduced coronary events in simvastatin-treated patients with coronary heart disease and diabetes or impaired fasting glucose levels: subgroup analyses in the Scandinavian Simvastatin Survival Study. *Arch Intern Med* 1999;159:2661–2667.

161. Jonsson B, Cook JR, Pedersen TR. The cost-effectiveness of lipid lowering in patients with diabetes: results from the 4S trial. *Diabetologia* 1999;42:1293–1301.

162. Haffner SM. The Scandinavian Simvastatin Survival Study (4S) subgroup analysis of diabetic subjects: implications for the prevention of coronary heart disease. *Diabetes Care* 1997;20:469–471.

163. Popma JJ, Sawyer M, Selwyn AP, et al. Lipid-lowering therapy after coronary revascularization. *Am J Cardiol* 2000;86:18H–28H.

164. Bellosta S, Ferri N, Arnaboldi L, et al. Pleiotropic effects of statins in atherosclerosis and diabetes. *Diabetes Care.* 2000;23 Suppl 2:B72–B78.

165. Lefer DJ, Scalia R, Jones SP, et al. HMG-CoA reductase inhibition protects the diabetic myocardium from ischemia-reperfusion injury. *Faseb J* 2001;15:1454–1456.

166. Malmberg K, Ryden L, Efendic S, et al. Randomized trial of insulin-glucose infusion followed by subcutaneous insulin treatment in diabetic patients with acute myocardial infarction (DIGAMI study): effects on mortality at 1 year. *J Am Coll Cardiol* 1995;26:57–65.

167. Bhatt D, Marso S, Hirsch A, et al. Amplified benefit of clopidogrel versus aspirin in patients with a history of diabetes mellitus. *Am J Cardiol* 2002;90:625–628.

168. Moore SA, Steinhubl SR. Clopidogrel and coronary stenting: what is the next question? *J Thromb Thrombolysis* 2000;10:121–126.

Diabetes and Cardiovascular Disease
edited by Steven P. Marso and David M. Stern
Lippincott Williams & Wilkins, Philadelphia © 2004

21

Diabetes and Peripheral Artery Disease

Roberto A. Corpus

Mid America Heart Institute, Saint Luke's Hospital, Kansas City, Misouri

EPIDEMIOLOGY

Peripheral artery disease (PAD) affects as many as 10 million people in the United States (1). The presence of diabetes mellitus markedly increases the risk of developing PAD. Data from the Cardiovascular Health Study demonstrated that diabetes confers a fourfold increase in the risk of developing PAD (2). It is estimated that 8% of diabetics have PAD at the time of diagnosis of diabetes, 15% after 10 years, and 45% after 20 years (3). In diabetic patients, significant independent predictors of incident PAD include age, elevated systolic blood pressure, elevated hemoglobin A_{1C}, low concentration of high-density lipoproteins (HDL), current smoking, and coexisting cardiovascular disease (Table 21-1) (4).

The duration and severity of diabetes correlates significantly with PAD severity, progression, and clinical outcome (4–6). Compared with nondiabetic patients, diabetics have increased atherosclerotic burden, more symptoms of claudication, and poorer outcome in terms of reduced lower-extremity function and quality of life (7,8). The risk of lower-extremity amputation is markedly increased in diabetic patients and is compounded by the presence of peripheral neuropathy and susceptibility to infection (9). Diabetes is implicated in more than half of all nontraumatic amputations (10). Major amputations occur 11 times more frequently in diabetic patients than in nondiabetic patients (11). The presence of PAD in the diabetic patient attests to the underlying systemic atherosclerotic process; as such, it confers an extremely high risk of cardiovascular morbidity and mortality. Patients with lower-extremity vascular disease have a threefold increase in all-cause mortality, a sixfold increase in cardiovascular morbidity, and a sevenfold increase in the risk of death specifically due to coronary artery disease (12). From an economic perspective, diabetic patients with PAD have a significantly longer length of hospital stay, and consume greater than 80% more health care resources compared with nondiabetic patients (13). These data underscore the enormous physiologic, psychological, and economic implications of peripheral atherosclerosis in the diabetic population. For these reasons, accurate diagnosis and effective treatment of PAD is of paramount importance in the management of patients with diabetes.

PATHOPHYSIOLOGY

In the past, the pathophysiology of PAD in diabetic patients was thought to be microvascular in origin. This misconception originated from early retrospective observations by Goldenberg et al. (14) of periodic-acid–Schiff-positive material in the arterioles of amputated limbs from diabetic patients. Initially, such substances were thought to be the obstructive pathologic lesions in diabetic PAD. Subsequent pathologic studies, however, did not confirm the presence of such deposits, thus refuting prior concepts of diabetic peripheral arteriopathy as a microvascular disease (15,16).

Pathologic examination of the diabetic microvasculature does reveal thickening of the

TABLE 21-1. *Predictors of incident peripheral artery disease in diabetic patients*

Factor	Comparison	Odds ratio (95% confidence interval)
Age	Each year older at diagnosis of diabetes	1.10 (1.05–1.15)
Hemoglobin$_{1C}$	Each 1% increase	1.28 (1.12–1.46)
Systolic blood pressure	Each 10 mm Hg increase	1.25 (1.10–1.43)
High-density lipoprotein	Each 0.1 mmol/L decrease	1.22 (1.07–1.39)
Former smoking	Never smoked	0.80 (0.37–1.72)
Current smoking	Never smoked	2.90 (1.46–5.73)
Cardiovascular disease	None	3.00 (1.30–6.70)
Retinopathy	Presence of retinopathy	1.64 (0.97–2.78)
Peripheral sensory neuropathy	Doubling of voltage threshold	1.31 (0.89–1.93)

From Adler AI, Stevens RJ, Neil A, et al. UKPDS 59: hyperglycemia and other potentially modifiable risk factors for peripheral vascular disease in type 2 diabetes. *Diabetes Care* 2002;25:894–899, with permission of American Diabetes Association.

capillary basement membrane. Studies have documented that this microvascular abnormality does not significantly impair gas exchange: transcutaneous oxygen tensions are similar in diabetic and nondiabetic patients with similar degrees of vascular disease (17). Although oxygen diffusion through the capillary membrane in diabetic patients is not impaired, the hyperglycemic state causes glycosylation of the red blood cell, which results in increased affinity for oxygen, decreased deformability, and a propensity for aggregation. These factors contribute significantly to ischemia in affected tissues (18). Thickening of the capillary basement membrane may alter leukocyte migration and thus predispose the diabetic patient to infection of the distal extremities (19).

The vascular endothelium plays a central role in regulating vascular tone, produces substances that modulate thrombosis, and is a principal factor in the development and progression of atherosclerosis. In both diabetic patients and patients with insulin resistance, endothelial function is significantly impaired. Studies have documented increases in circulating adhesion molecules, impaired nitric oxide-mediated vasodilation, enhanced mitogenesis, and enhanced platelet aggregation leading to a propensity for atherosclerotic disease in these patients (20–23).

The role of inflammation in the pathogenesis of atherosclerosis is now recognized to be of paramount importance. Peripheral vascular disease is associated with elevations of various acute phase proteins such as C-reactive protein, inflammatory mediators such as tumor necrosis factor-α (TNF-α) and interleukin-6 (IL-6), and circulating adhesion molecules such as vascular cell adhesion molecules (VCAM) (24). Similarly, evidence now links diabetes, insulin resistance, and obesity with inflammation. These conditions are associated with elevations in inflammatory mediators such as IL-6, TNF-α and plasminogen activator inhibitor-1 (PAI-1) (25–27).

Chronic hyperglycemia results in the glycosylation of proteins to form advanced glycation end products (AGEs). Production of AGEs in combination with oxidative stress induces vascular inflammation via AGE receptors (RAGE) located on the endothelium, smooth muscle cells, and macrophages, thus promoting the atherosclerotic process (24, 28–30). Experimental work in animal models of diabetes has demonstrated that blockade of RAGE may attenuate the progression of atherosclerosis (30).

PATTERN OF DIABETIC PERIPHERAL ARTERY DISEASE

Lower extremity PAD is typically described according to the anatomic location of the obstruction. It is useful to further classify PAD into inflow (aorta, iliac arteries) and outflow disease. Atherosclerotic disease of the outflow vessels can be further described as femoral, popliteal, and infrapopliteal (anterior tibial, posterior tibial, and peroneal arteries) in location.

Both pathologic and clinicopathologic studies performed almost 30 years ago indicated that diabetic atherosclerotic PAD tends to be calcific and diffuse, with primary involvement of the distal arterial segments and relative sparing of more proximal segments (31,32). Recent angiographic studies have demonstrated that diabetic patients tend more commonly to have infrapopliteal arterial disease, whereas nondiabetic patients have a higher incidence of aortoiliac and femoropopliteal disease (33). Other studies have documented an increased prevalence of both femoropopliteal and infrapopliteal disease in diabetic patients (8). Furthermore, in diabetic PAD, although the runoff vessels (i.e., infrainguinal vessels) may be occluded, there is often sparing of the arteries of the foot, thus allowing for surgical bypass or percutaneous arterial reconstruction for relief of claudication and/or limb salvage.

To date, explanations for the pattern of lower-extremity atherosclerosis in diabetes remain elusive. Some authors theorize that diabetes alters the arterial remodeling process, which normally involves compensatory enlargement of vessel circumference to maintain intraluminal diameter in the setting of an obstructive atherosclerotic process (Glagov phenomenon). In the diabetic vessel, an altered remodeling process may result in paradoxical shrinkage of the vasculature, with resultant diffusely narrowed distal vessels that lack the capacity for compensatory enlargement (34)

SYMPTOMS

The primary presenting symptom of hemodynamically significant PAD is intermittent claudication, which is defined as lower-extremity pain or discomfort elicited by walking and relieved by rest. Claudication occurs in the setting of mismatched metabolic supply and demand. In the resting state, oxygen delivery and removal of metabolic byproducts, particularly lactic acid, are adequate. However, in the presence of critical stenosis, this process is insufficient, resulting in muscular discomfort. Symptoms of claudication may be described as aching, cramping, tightness, tiredness, or pain that occurs with ambulation. Alterations in symptom perception, particularly in diabetic patients, may occur as a result of coexisting peripheral neuropathy. Therefore, in diabetic patients, absence of typical claudication symptoms does not exclude the diagnosis of significant PAD. Claudication typically occurs in the muscle group located just distal to the affected artery; therefore, the level of symptoms tends to correlate with the anatomic level of occlusion. Bilateral thigh and buttock claudication suggests aortoiliac disease, while unilateral symptoms suggest iliac disease. Similarly, calf claudication is characteristic of femoral or popliteal involvement (35). Characteristically, claudication symptoms occur at fairly predictable walking distances, resolve after several minutes of rest, and recur at the same level of exertion.

As the disease process continues, the distance traveled before claudication onset decreases. In its most severe form, rest pain occurs. The presence of ischemic rest pain implies severe multilevel vascular disease, which is often severely stenotic or totally occlusive in nature (35). Rest pain is caused by peripheral nerve ischemia and is often persistent in character. Rest pain tends to be worse at night due to supine positioning, and it often awakens the patient from sleep. Characteristically, these symptoms are exacerbated by elevation, heat, or exertion and are relieved by placing the afflicted extremity in the dependent position. The presence of rest or nocturnal symptoms often heralds the development of tissue necrosis and gangrene. In the setting of PAD, such symptoms warrant consideration for either surgical or percutaneous revascularization.

Not all patients have classic claudication symptoms. In a report from Hirsch et al. only 11% of patients with PAD had classic symptoms of claudication, highlighting the need for clinical vigilance with respect to diagnosis and management of PAD.

DIFFERENTIAL DIAGNOSES

Vascular claudication must be distinguished from pseudoclaudication caused by lumbar radiculopathy or stenosis of the lumbar canal. Because these two conditions may coexist, it is essential to determine which disease process is causing symptoms. Pseudoclaudication is often characterized as "neuropathic" pain. In contrast to claudication, in which the degree of activity required to bring about symptoms is usually constant and predictable, patients with pseudoclaudication have symptoms with variable degrees of exertion. Symptoms due to pseudoclaudication may occur with standing and are typically relieved with sitting or body positions that alleviate weight bearing of the afflicted extremity.

Symptoms of diabetic peripheral neuropathy may often mimic those of vascular claudication. Furthermore, neuropathic ulcerations, which tend to occur on the metatarsal heads on the plantar surface of the foot, may be confused with ischemic ulcerations (36). Often a detailed vascular examination with noninvasive testing modalities is required to differentiate sensory neuropathy from vascular claudication. Reflex sympathetic dystrophy is usually the result of traumatic injury to the foot. The lower extremity is often painful, discolored, and swollen; however, peripheral pulses are usually intact (36). Other considerations in the differential diagnosis of vascular claudication include arteritis (e.g., thromboangiitis obliterans), atheroembolism, and entrapment or cystic disease of the popliteal artery.

PHYSICAL EXAMINATION

Atherosclerotic vascular disease in the diabetic patient is commonly associated with cutaneous changes. Visual inspection of the lower extremities often reveals atrophy of the skin, alopecia, dystrophy of the nails, and coldness of the toes. Due to abnormalities in ischemia-induced autonomic regulation, the ischemic foot tends to display changes in color with elevation and dependency (35). Hypoxemia resulting from chronically insufficient blood flow induces vasodilatation in the dependent position. Hence, the ischemic foot is often ruborous in the dependent position but blanches rapidly with elevation. A thorough evaluation for traumatic and ischemic ulcerations is warranted.

In the evaluation of diabetic patients with suspected lower-extremity PAD, careful assessment of pulses at the femoral, popliteal, and pedal (dorsalis pedis and posterior tibial) locations is essential. Capillary and venous refill time should be assessed. Arterial bruits tend to occur in areas with at least 50% narrowing, but they may be undetectable with more severe degrees of stenosis (i.e., greater than 90%). Careful auscultation for bruits in the carotid, femoral, and aortoiliac areas should be performed.

NONINVASIVE EVALUATION

Noninvasive vascular evaluation for PAD provides physiologic assessment of the degree of circulatory insufficiency. Arteriography is not necessary for the diagnosis of PAD, but it should be performed if surgical or percutaneous revascularization is planned, to assess the anatomic nature of the disease. Published guidelines regarding the assessment and follow-up of peripheral vascular disease in diabetic patients are given in Table 21-2.

Ankle-brachial Index

The ankle-brachial index (ABI) is a simple and readily applicable test to assess lower-extremity circulation. Using a blood pressure cuff and a Doppler ultrasound probe, the clinician measures systolic pressures in the brachial arteries of both arms and in the posterior tibial and dorsalis pedis arteries of both lower extremities. The ankle pressure is determined by the higher of the two readings between the dorsalis pedis and posterior tibial arteries. The ABI is a ratio calculated by dividing the ankle systolic pressure by the higher of the two brachial artery pressures. The degree of severity of PAD can be estimated from the ABI (Table 21-3).

In some patients, particularly those with isolated iliac stenoses, typical symptoms of claudication are present with normal peripheral pulses and a normal ABI. In such patients, it is useful to measure ABI before and after exercise testing. If exercise does not result in a significant decrease in ABI, causes other than a vascular etiology of the symptoms should be investigated.

TABLE 21-2. *Summary of recommendations for detection, management, and follow-up of lower extremity arterial disease in diabetic patients*

Test	Diabetic patients	Frequency	Action
Claudication	All adults (>18 yr)	Annually	If present, do ABI annually. If ABI <0.90, start risk factor modification. If present and lifestyle-limiting, consider vascular invasive study, CTA, or angiography.
Signs of critical ischemia	All adults (>18 yr)	Annually	If present (i.e., gangrene, ulcer, skin changes, or ischemic rest pain), refer for SVA and start IRFM.
Peripheral pulses/femoral bruits	All adults (>18 yr)	Annually	If abnormal, do ABI annually. If ABI <0.90, start IRFM.
Ankle-brachial index (ABI)	T2DM adults (>35 yr or with >20 yr diabetes duration)	Depends on baseline result	If ABI <0.50, refer for SVA and start IRFM. If ABI 0.50–0.89, repeat within 3 mo. If confirmed to be <0.90, start IRFM and do ABI annually. If confirmed to be >0.90, repeat every 2–3 yr.
	T2DM adults (>40 yr)		If ABI >0.90, repeat every 2–3 yr. If ankle BP ≥75 mm Hg greater than arm BP, repeat within 3 mo. If confirmed, refer for risk factor modification and consider vascularization. If not confirmed, repeat every 2–3 yr. If ankle BP ≥300 mm Hg, refer for SVA and start IRFM.

CTA, computed tomography angiography; IRFM, intensive risk factor modification; SVA, specialist in vascular assessment; T2DM, type 2 diabetes mellitus.

From Orchard TJ, et al. Assessment of peripheral vascular disease in diabetes. *Diabetes Care* 1993;16:1199–1209, with permission of American Diabetes Association.

In the diabetic patient, the arteries are often calcified and noncompressible due to medial calcification of the vasculature (Monckeberg's sclerosis), rendering measurement of ankle pressures unreliable. This phenomenon should be suspected if ankle pressures are significantly higher (more than 200 to 250 mm Hg) than brachial artery pressures, resulting in an ABI of 1.3 or higher. In such situations, arterial duplex ultrasound, pulse volume waveform analysis, or determination of the toe-brachial index is required to accurately assess lower-extremity circulation.

TABLE 21-3. *Severity of peripheral artery disease and ankle-brachial index (ABI)*

ABI	Severity
0.90–1.30	Normal
0.70–0.89	Mild
0.40–0.69	Moderate
≤0.40	Severe

Segmental Pressures

Determination of segmental lower-extremity pressures is performed by measuring blood pressure at the thigh, calf, and ankle. This technique adds additional information to the ABI by allowing determination of the level of occlusive disease. This type of evaluation is often performed in combination with segmental volume plethysmography or analysis of Doppler-derived waveforms.

Several caveats exist in the measurement of segmental pressures in diabetic patients, who often have diffuse, multilevel disease. Physiologically elevated pressures in the thigh may be measured as normal to low in the presence of an occluded proximal superficial femoral artery. Significant pressure gradients between the proximal and distal thigh may be missed in the presence of superficial femoral disease in combination with aortoiliac disease. Obstructive disease in arteries below the knee may go unrecognized unless all three vessels are involved or the degree of obstruction is quite severe (37).

Segmental Volume Plethysmography

In segmental volume plethysmography, a pulse volume recorder is used to perform plethysmographic measurements of blood flow through the peripheral vasculature. Using blood pressure cuffs, the clinician records plethysmographic tracings at predefined positions throughout the periphery. The normal waveform is similar to that of an arterial waveform and consists of a rapid systolic upstroke, a prominent dicrotic notch, and a brisk downslope. With worsening degrees of obstructive disease, the systolic amplitude of the waveform decreases and the downsloping portion widens (38).

Doppler Ultrasound

Because this modality combines the ability to obtain cross-sectional images with color flow and spectral Doppler information, Doppler ultrasound can be used to assess arterial anatomy and hemodynamic physiology. Velocity changes at particular vascular sites can be quantified, so that hemodynamically significant stenoses can be localized. The sensitivity and specificity of duplex ultrasound in detecting stenosis of the peripheral vasculature are 92% and 97%, respectively. Duplex ultrasound is especially accurate at the aortoiliac and femoral-popliteal levels, but more technical skill is required to accurately identify and assess stenoses at the level of the tibial vessels and below (39).

Other useful information can be derived by analyzing the characteristics of the Doppler waveform. Together with segmental blood pressure determinations, Doppler waveform analysis can add incremental information with regard to determining the extent and location of occlusive disease (38). The normal waveform typically has three components, consisting of a rapid systolic component and a prominent biphasic diastolic component. As the degree of obstruction worsens, the diastolic reversal component of the waveform is lost, resulting in a biphasic waveform. With more severe disease, significant attenuation of the waveform amplitude with eventual dampening occurs (Fig. 21-1).

Magnetic Resonance Angiography

Magnetic resonance imaging of the peripheral vasculature is not currently commonly used, but the technique is rapidly evolving. Rather than imaging the vasculature itself, magnetic resonance angiography (MRA) characterizes intraarterial blood flow. Whereas mild to moderate stenoses may appear as narrowed areas, severely stenotic lesions or complete occlusions may be visualized as signal voids (40). One advantage of MRA is that very distal arteries that may not

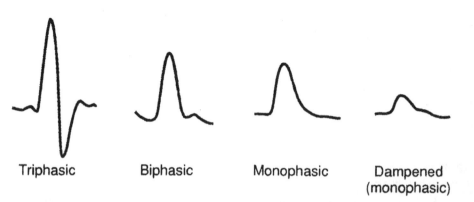

Triphasic   Biphasic   Monophasic   Dampened (monophasic)

FIG. 21-1. Doppler waveforms for normal and diseased arteries. A normal, triphasic arterial waveform is demonstrated on the far left of the figure. There is continued disease progression in the subsequent waveforms. A monophasic, dampened waveform such as that shown on the far right, demonstrates severe arterial disease. (From Crawford MH, Rajagopalan S, Stanley JC, et al. *Cardiology clinics: peripheral vascular disease.* Philadelphia: W.B. Saunders, 2002:493, with permission.)

be demonstrated with other imaging techniques, including contrast angiography, can be well visualized with MRA. MRA has been demonstrated to be very sensitive in identifying distal pedal arteries in diabetic patients with occlusion of the tibial arteries (41,42).

Two types of magnetic resonance imaging techniques are used to visualize the peripheral vasculature: two-dimensional time-of-flight imaging and gadolinium-enhanced MRA. Time-of-flight imaging uses a non-contrast based method to presaturate blood flow directed toward the heart, effectively eliminating venous flow while imaging only arterial flow (40). This method is limited in terms of image processing time and its inaccuracy in imaging complex, multilevel PAD (38). Gadolinium-enhanced MRA (three-dimensional contrast MRA) uses a peripheral venous injection of gadolinium, a nonnephrotoxic contrast agent. This method uses the T1 relaxation properties of gadolinium to provide contrast between blood and the surrounding tissues, rendering this modality less sensitive to motion or blood flow artifacts (38). Several studies have suggested that this method is as accurate as contrast angiography (43). Furthermore, it may be possible to derive hemodynamic data about lesion severity from existing algorithms (38). As this imaging method evolves, MRA may ultimately prove to be the preferred imaging modality for the peripheral vasculature.

Computed Tomographic Angiography

Computed tomographic (CT) angiography is commonly used for vascular imaging, particularly in the pulmonary vasculature and aorta. Advantages of CT angiography in imaging vessels of the periphery include speed of scanning and the ability to generate three-dimensional images from overlapping transaxial images (44). The applicability of three-dimensional imaging techniques has proved to be most useful in imaging the large arteries, such as the thoracic and abdominal aorta, especially in the setting of aneurysmal disease. However, recent advances have greatly facilitated the imaging of lower-extremity arteries. Figure 21-2A depicts a CT angiogram of a person with essentially normal lower-extremity arteries. In contradistinction, Figure 21-2B demonstrates an angiogram of a person with a history of diabetes mellitus and severe below-the-knee disease. There is moderate calcification throughout the lower-extremity arteries and there are severe narrowings in most of the below-the-knee vessels. This technology will probably continue to evolve and may supplant the need for many diagnostic angiography studies.

Limitations of this technique include the need to administer a contrast agent, the inability to image the smaller vessels, particularly infrainguinal vessels (44), and significant imaging artifact from calcification. The latter is especially germane to the diabetic patient, because this population characteristically has diffuse, calcified obstructive lesions, particularly in the smaller vessels.

Contrast Angiography

Contrast angiography is currently considered the gold standard for imaging of the peripheral vasculature. Although this a relatively benign procedure, mortality rates of up to 3% have occurred in elderly patients with severe peripheral vascular disease (45). Complications from this procedure include intraarterial thrombosis (particularly at the access site), pseudoaneurysm formation, arteriovenous fistulae, dissection, contrast-induced nephropathy, and allergic reactions.

The sensitivity of contrast angiography can be significantly enhanced with digital subtraction imaging. However, digital subtraction angiography may fail to visualize the distal peripheral arteries, especially in the setting of severe peripheral vascular disease, a situation that is often present in diabetic patients.

Contrast angiography is most commonly performed via the transfemoral retrograde approach, but alternative access sites include the brachial artery and the radial artery. Once intraarterial access is obtained, the technique of contrast angiography involves intravascular administration of an iodinated radiocontrast medium to opacify the arterial system from the aorta to the ankle. Multiple views, including oblique views, may be obtained to characterize the degree and

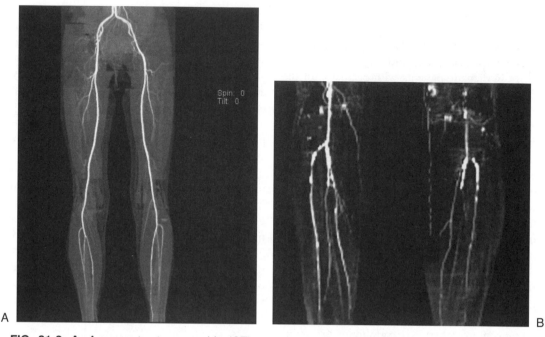

FIG. 21-2. A: A computer tomographic (CT) angiogram of a person with normal lower-extremity arteries. **B:** A CT angiogram of a person with severe diabetic arteriopathy, demonstrating severe disease in below-the-knee arteries. There is a moderate degree of calcification bilaterally. There is also a severe narrowing in the right anterior tibular artery. Similarly, there is severe below-the-knee disease with respect to the left lower extremity.

location of stenoses (40). Due to the association between diabetes and renal insufficiency, the operator should consider the use of low-osmolar contrast agents and must be especially vigilant in limiting the contrast volume.

Metformin and Contrast Angiography

The use of metformin, a commonly used oral hypoglycemic agent, in patients undergoing any procedure involving the use of intravenous contrast material deserves particular attention. Several reports have demonstrated a small but significant incidence of lactic acidosis in patients treated with metformin (46–50). Metformin is renally excreted and is associated with an incidence of lactic acidosis of 0.03 cases per 1,000 patients per year (46). In those patients who do develop lactic acidosis in the setting of metformin use, the mortality rate is 50%. Several reports have highlighted the increased risk of lactic acidosis after contrast administration in patients treated

with metformin (48,50). Current guidelines stipulate that metformin should be discontinued before or at the time of the procedure, withheld for 48 hours after the procedure, and restarted only after renal function is measured and found to be normal (51).

TREATMENT OF PERIPHERAL ARTERY DISEASE IN DIABETIC PATIENTS

The mainstays of conservative therapy for PAD are aggressive risk factor modification, a rigorous walking program, and medical therapy with antiplatelet agents and vasodilators.

Smoking Cessation

Smoking is perhaps the most prevalent risk factor in patients with PAD. In diabetic patients, the presence of smoking confers a marked risk of development of incident PAD (OR = 2.9; 95% confidence interval, 1.46 to 5.73) (4). Furthermore, patients with PAD who stop smoking have a twofold increase in their 5-year survival rate compared with those patients who continue to smoke (52). Therefore, cessation of smoking is of vital importance in the treatment of diabetic patients with PAD and should be of paramount importance in the treatment strategy for PAD.

Glycemic Control

Although tight glycemic control has been shown to reduce microvascular events, the evidence concerning its effect on macrovascular end points is less well established. The Diabetes Control and Complications Trial (DCCT) demonstrated that intensive blood glucose control was associated with a 42% risk reduction in cardiovascular events among patients with insulin-dependent (type 1) diabetes mellitus; however, no reduction in the risk of PAD was observed (53). The United Kingdom Prospective Diabetic Study (UKPDS) demonstrated that intensive glycemic management among patients with non-insulin-dependent (type 2) diabetes mellitus conferred a trend toward reduction of myocardial infarction but had no effect on amputations due to PAD (54). Cautious interpretation of these results has been recommended, because the prevalence of PAD in this population was undefined. The outcome with respect to complications due to PAD might have been different if a predefined population of diabetic patients with documented PAD had been studied (55). Therefore, although the value of intensive glycemic control has been proved in microvascular arteriopathy, the beneficial effects of optimal glycemic control in affecting outcome from macrovascular disease have yet to be demonstrated. Nevertheless, the presence of microvascular disease in patients with PAD imposes a significantly worse prognosis in terms of disease progression, eventual amputation, and, ultimately, mortality (9). Therefore, glycemic control remains an important aspect of the treatment of diabetic patients with PAD.

Dyslipidemia

Diabetes is associated with an atherogenic lipid profile with characteristically low HDL; increased small, dense low-density lipoproteins (LDL); and elevated triglycerides. Dyslipidemia is an important risk factor for the development and progression of atherosclerosis and is commonly found in patients with diabetes and PAD. In the Framingham Study, a total cholesterol concentration greater than 270 mg/dL was associated with twice the risk of developing symptoms of intermittent claudication (56). Similarly, other studies have suggested a link between elevated triglycerides and incidence of PAD (57,58).

Numerous studies have demonstrated that primary and secondary therapy with lipid-lowering agents is beneficial in reducing cardiovascular risk in patients with diabetes and coronary artery disease. However, in diabetic patients with PAD, risk reduction in terms of hard end points such as mortality and cardiovascular events has yet to be definitively demonstrated. In a recent meta-analysis of patients with PAD, lipid-lowering therapy was associated with a nonsignificant mortality reduction and no change in nonfatal cardiovascular events. Despite these findings, lipid-lowering therapy did improve symptoms of claudication (59). Similar findings were found in subgroup analysis of the Scandinavian Simvastatin Survival Study (4S), which demonstrated a 38% risk reduction for the development of new or worsening symptoms of intermittent claudication in patients treated with lipid-lowering therapy (60,61). Given these data, the National Cholesterol Education Program (NCEP) guidelines recommend that patients with PAD should have lifestyle modification and/or pharmacologic therapies aimed at achieving an LDL cholesterol of less than 100 mg/dL (62).

Hypertension

Hypertension is associated with an increased risk of developing atherosclerosis. Several studies have demonstrated the relationship between hypertension and lower-extremity peripheral vascular disease. The presence of hypertension is associated with a twofold to threefold increase in the risk of claudication (63). Although specific data regarding the benefits of treating hypertension in patients with PAD are lacking, consensus statements regarding treatment of hypertension recognize the strong association between PAD and cardiovascular disease (64). Therefore, a target blood pressure of less than 130/85 mm Hg is warranted in these patients.

Current Status of Risk Factor Modification in Patients with Peripheral Artery Disease

The majority of therapies for PAD are directed at reducing the significant attendant cardiovascular risk, the major cause of mortality in patients with PAD. Recent data from Nass et al. (65) underscores the undertreatment of modifiable risk factors in patients undergoing peripheral revascularization procedures. In this study, 58% of patients had a blood pressure greater than 140/90 mm Hg, 23% were active smokers, and, among diabetic patients, 46% had random blood glucose concentrations greater than 140 mg/dL. Of additional concern among these high-risk patients, only 50% were taking aspirin, 35% were taking lipid-lowering medications, and 30% were taking β-blockers. A similar study by Mukherjee et al. (66) found that, 6 months after peripheral vascular intervention, 23% of patients still smoked and only half of the patients had made lifestyle modifications. Medical therapy in this cohort of patients was also clearly suboptimal, with only 77% use of antiplatelet agents, 36% use of angiotensin-converting enzyme inhibitors, 42% use of β-blockers, and 50% use of statins. Importantly, the use of appropriate medical therapy was associated with a significant reduction in the composite end point of death, myocardial infarction, or stroke at 6 months. These sobering data indicate that an enormous opportunity exists to improve the secondary preventive measures in patients with PAD.

EXERCISE THERAPY

In combination with intensive risk factor modification, a supervised walking exercise program is one of the cornerstones of therapy for patients with intermittent claudication. Multiple studies have consistently demonstrated that exercise improves walking ability (67–69), qual-

ity of life (70–72), and functional capacity (73–75) in patients with claudication. A recent metaanalysis by Leng et al. (68) demonstrated that exercise training improved pain free walking time by 180% and maximal walking time by 120% in patients with claudication. Others have suggested that a formal walking program may confer benefits greater than those observed with medications such as pentoxifyline and cilostazol (76).

Guidelines regarding the exercise prescription were outlined by Stewart et al. (76). Exercise should consist of walking on a treadmill or track, because resistance training does not confer the same benefits (77). The patient should be encouraged to initially exercise to a level that elicits claudication within 3 to 5 minutes. Patients should exercise at this level until moderate claudication occurs, rest for a moment until symptoms subside, and then continue in this "exercise-rest-exercise" pattern. Initial duration of exercise should be 35 minutes. With each session, duration should be increased by 5 minutes, until a total of 50 minutes of intermittent walking can be accomplished. The patient should participate in such a program three to five times per week at a level that ensures that claudication symptoms occur during the workout. The importance of a formal exercise regimen has been emphasized in several studies (71,78,79). Data indicate that a supervised, structured exercise program is more beneficial than a less structured, home-based program in relieving symptoms of claudication (78,80). A recent metaanalysis of 21 studies by Gardner and Poehlman (67) determined which components of an exercise rehabilitation program were most effective in improving claudication symptoms in patients with PAD. Characteristics of rehabilitation programs associated with greatest improvement in claudication distances were at least 30 minutes in session duration, exercise at least three times per week, at least 6 months of program duration, walking as the primary mode of exercise, and near-maximal pain during training as the claudication pain end point. Independent predictors for improvement in claudication distances included claudication pain end point, program length, and mode of exercise.

PHARMACOTHERAPY OF PERIPHERAL ARTERY DISEASE

Although aspirin remains the most commonly prescribed medication among patients with PAD, both cilostazol and clopidogrel have emerged as promising new therapies for patients with PAD.

Cilostazol

Cilostazol, a phosphodiesterase III inhibitor, is an arterial vasodilator and inhibitor of platelet aggregation that has demonstrated beneficial effects in the treatment of PAD. Several large, randomized trials have demonstrated that treatment with cilostazol is associated with significant improvements in walking ability, functional status, and quality of life (81–83). Other data have indicated that the beneficial effects of cilostazol are lost after discontinuation of the medication, providing further evidence of significant medication-dependent symptomatic improvement (84). Recent pooled data from eight phase III trials specifically examined the effects of cilostazol in diabetic patients with intermittent claudication. In this analysis, treatment with cilostazol, 100 mg b.i.d., was associated with a significant increase in maximal walking distance, initial claudication distance, and absolute claudication distance, compared with placebo (9).

The beneficial effects of cilostazol may extend beyond its properties as an arterial vasodilator and antiplatelet agent. Cilostazol has been shown to have favorable effects on plasma lipids. In patients with PAD and claudication, therapy with cilostazol has been shown to increase HDL by 10% and to decrease triglyceride levels by 15% (85). Several studies indicated that cilostazol may be beneficial in treatment of diabetic peripheral neuropathy by promoting axonal regeneration (86–88). and increasing small-vessel perfusion, thereby preventing ischemic injury to the nerves of the lower limb (89,90). Another study indicated that cilostazol may have renal protective effects by reducing urinary albumin excretion via reduction in local production of thromboxane A_2 (91). Cilostazol also possesses several potentially advantageous antiinflammatory activities. The compound has been shown to decrease circulating levels of soluble adhesion molecules and platelet-derived microparticles in patients with type 2 diabetes (92). Cilostazol inhibits the cytokine-induced expression of monocyte chemoattractant protein-1 (MCP-1), an important mediator of monocyte recruitment in the atherosclerotic plaque (93,94). Finally, cilostazol possesses several antimitogenic properties that may be beneficial in modulating the propensity for restenosis after intravascular intervention. In addition to inhibiting the aggregation of platelets, cilostazol blocks surface expression of the glycoprotein IIb/IIIa receptor and inhibits α-granule secretion of P-selectin, an important factor in platelet-mediated mitogenesis (93,95). Cilostazol inhibits cyclic adenosine monophosphate (AMP)-dependent vascular smooth muscle proliferation (96). Furthermore, cilostazol inhibits heparin-binding epidermal growth factor-like growth factor (HB-EGF) a potent mitogen for vascular smooth muscle cell proliferation (97). Clinically, cilostazol therapy has been associated with inhibition of neointimal proliferation after percutaneous coronary intervention (98–100).

Pentoxifyline

Pentoxifyline is a methylxanthine derivative that improves red cell deformability, lowers fibrinogen, and inhibits platelet aggregation (101). Although early studies suggested some beneficial effect of pentoxifyline in treating intermittent claudication (102), the treatment effect in other studies was often minimal and nonsignificant (103,104). In a recent randomized, controlled trial (104), cilostazol was found to be more effective than pentoxifyline in improving walking distances. Pentoxifyline had effects similar to placebo. Although it was once the only medication approved by the U. S. Food and Drug Administration (FDA) for the treatment of claudication, its use has been supplanted by more effective therapeutic agents such as cilostazol (104).

Clopidogrel

Clopidogrel, a thienopyridine derivative, is an adenosine diphosphate (ADP)-dependent inhibitor of platelet aggregation. Clopidogrel is indicated for secondary prevention of ischemic events in patients with a known atherosclerotic disease manifested as myocardial infarction, stroke, or symptomatic PAD. In the large, multinational Clopidogrel versus Aspirin in Patients at Risk of Ischaemic Events (CAPRIE) trial, patients with documented atherosclerotic cardiovascular disease who were randomly assigned to clopidogrel had a significant reduction in atherosclerotic events, including vascular death, myocardial infarction, and stroke, compared with those randomly assigned to aspirin (105). In a *post hoc* analysis, patients with documented PAD who received clopidogrel had the greatest percent reduction in events, compared with patients with coronary artery or cerebrovascular disease. Although clopidogrel is not indicated for the treatment of intermittent claudication, its usefulness in the secondary prevention of future events has been proven. Therefore, clopidogrel therapy should be considered in PAD patients who are at high risk for future cardiovascular events.

Novel Pharmacologic Therapies for Peripheral Artery Disease

There are numerous novel pharmacologic therapies being actively investigated in patients with PAD. These include glycoprotein IIb/IIIa receptor antagonists, prostaglandins such as iloprost and beraprost, angiogenic gene therapy, and metabolic agents such as L-propionyl carnitine (106) and L-arginine (107,108).

LOWER-EXTREMITY REVASCULARIZATION

Percutaneous Peripheral Intervention

The technique of percutaneous transluminal angioplasty (percutaneous peripheral intervention, or PPI) for the treatment of iliac and femoral stenoses was first described by Dotter and Judkins in 1964 (109). The first successful PPI procedure was performed by Dotter in 1965 using a Fogarty balloon (110). In 1974, Gruntzig (137) developed an inflatable balloon catheter system, which served as the prototype for today's current angioplasty technology.

There has been a burgeoning of PPI procedures performed (111). As techniques and technology for PPI have evolved, therapeutic strategies are transitioning from a conservative approach to an aggressive revascularization strategy. The most common indications for PPI are symptomatic relief of claudication, limb salvage in the setting of critical limb ischemia, and as adjunctive therapy to improve inflow before surgical bypass of distal vessel of the lower extremity (44). Compared with surgical revascularization, PPI is less invasive; reduces morbidity, mortality, and length of stay; and preserves the saphenous veins for future distal extremity or coronary artery bypass grafting.

The mechanism of angioplasty-induced intraluminal enlargement involves several processes, including plaque fracture and compression, localized dissection, and concomitant stretching of the arterial wall (112). Angioplasty is, in effect, a controlled injury to the vessel wall, which subsequently heals and remodels with a larger luminal diameter (44). This reparative process occurs at the cellular level and involves a complex interplay between neointimal proliferation and remodeling due to macrophage activity at the injury site (40).

In a significant number of patients, particularly diabetic patients, this response to injury is particularly aggressive, leading to luminal renarrowing and failure of PPI. Restenosis is the major limitation of PPI, particularly in diabetic patients. Numerous mechanisms of increased restenosis in diabetic patients may be a direct result of the hyperglycemic state. Chronic hyperglycemia induces vascular endothelial cell damage with resultant vasomotor dysfunction, excessive extracellular matrix formation, and increased cellular proliferation. Furthermore, accumulation of advanced glycation end products (AGEs) in the vessel wall leads to decreased vascular compliance, enhanced smooth muscle proliferation, and augmentation of the inflammatory response after vascular damage from intravascular

TABLE 21-4. *Biologic factors predisposing diabetic patients to increased rates of restenosis*

Endothelial Dysfunction
↓endothelium-derived relaxing factor (nitric oxide)
↓prostacyclin formation
↑endothelin-1 formation
↓vascular endothelial cell proliferation
Enhanced Extracellular Matrix Formation
↑type IV collagen
↑fibronectin
↑laminin
↑growth factor production (platelet-derived growth factor, insulin-like growth factor-1, basic fibroblast growth
  factor, transforming growth factor-β, endothelium-derived relaxing factor, heparin sulfate)
Hemostatic Abnormalities
Platelet abnormalities
  ↑adhesiveness (thromboxane A$_2$, platelet factor-4, β-thromboglobulin)
  ↑larger platelets
  ↑glycoprotein IIb/IIIa receptors
  ↑hypersensitivity to agonists (epi, collagen, thrombin, arachidonic acid)
Enhanced coagulation
  ↑fibrinogen, factor VII, antithrombin III, von Willebrand factor, fibrinopeptide A
Proinflammatory State
↑interleukin-6
↑tumor necrosis factor-α (TNF-α), TNF-α-receptor
↑PAI-1 (mediated by proinflammatory transcription factors NF-κB and Egr-1)

interventions. Other factors that predispose diabetic patients to restenosis include a proinflammatory state, intrinsic coagulation and thrombotic abnormalities, and endothelial dysfunction (Table 21-4).

Aortic Percutaneous Peripheral Intervention

Isolated stenoses in the infrarenal abdominal aorta are rare in diabetic patients, who often have multilevel disease, particularly of the distal vasculature. However, focal stenoses of the abdominal aorta are readily treated with PPI (113), which affords results comparable to those of surgical bypass (114). Lesions of the distal abdominal aorta often involve the bifurcation of the iliac arteries and may be successfully treated with a "kissing balloon technique," which involves simultaneous bilateral balloon inflations and often placement of stents in each iliac artery.

Iliac Percutaneous Peripheral Intervention

Focal stenoses of the common and external iliac arteries are also readily treated with percutaneous modalities with patency rates comparable to those of bypass surgery. Patency rates

between 50% and 90% have been reported, with an average rate of approximately 70% (44,115). Whereas the use of intravascular stents has improved the acute outcome after PPI, the practice of routine (i.e., primary) stenting for iliac disease has not demonstrated long-term clinical superiority, compared with angioplasty alone (116). In a randomized trial, 2-year clinical outcome was similar between patients treated with primary stenting and those treated with selective stenting as an adjunct for suboptimal angioplasty (117). Chiang and Tripp (44) suggested that primary stenting may be considered in total occlusions, in long segment disease, in severely calcified lesions, and in those vessels in which combined angioplasty with distal surgical bypass is contemplated. Although the field continues to evolve, stenting is emerging as a commonplace therapy.

Femoropopliteal Percutaneous Peripheral Intervention

Femoropopliteal PPI may be performed alone as a limb salvage procedure or in combination with percutaneous or surgical procedures to facilitate reperfusion of more distal vasculature.

Femoropopliteal lesions that are well suited for PPI are those that are focal (less than 2 to 3 cm), concentric, and free of significant calcification (44,118). The status of the runoff vessels is an important prognostic factor in determining long-term patency after femoropopliteal PPI. Jeans et al. (119) demonstrated that vessels with at least two patent runoff vessels have at least two times greater patency after PPI than do vessels with one or no patent runoff vessels (119). Femoropopliteal PPI is associated with success rates similar to those of iliac PPI. Clinical patency rates of 60% to 80% at 1 year and 50% to 60% at 5 years are comparable to those achieved with femoropopliteal bypass (118,120). In the setting of critical limb ischemia and unfavorable anatomy for PPI, angioplasty may restore distal perfusion long enough to facilitate healing and the development of a collateral circulation (121). As with iliac PPI, primary stenting is evolving as the reference standard.

Infrapopliteal Percutaneous Peripheral Intervention

With improvements in endovascular technology came the introduction of low-profile catheters and balloons that have made the practice of infrapopliteal PPI technically feasible. Due to the nature of diabetic peripheral arteriopathy, the majority of patients undergoing infrapopliteal PPI are diabetic patients (122). Many diabetic patients have long, complex stenoses or severely compromised runoff, or both, making infrapopliteal PPI technically challenging. In suitable lesions (i.e., those with short, focal stenoses [less than 1 cm] and good distal runoff [44]), angioplasty of the tibial arteries has a technical success rate of greater than 95% with a 2-year limb salvage rate of 75% to 83% (118). The use of infrapopliteal PPI in combination with femoropopliteal PPI has been shown to improve the durability of the latter (120).

Percutaneous Peripheral Intervention in Surgical Bypass Grafts

Percutaneous angioplasty of lesions in saphenous vein or synthetic peripheral bypass grafts are more commonly being performed. Synthetic femoropopliteal grafts, especially polytetrafluoroethylene (PTFE) grafts, have a higher propensity toward thrombosis. Percutaneous treatment of such lesions often requires adjunctive thrombolytic therapy to resolve the occlusive thrombus, followed by angioplasty and/or stenting of residual stenosis.

Novel Approaches to Percutaneous Peripheral Intervention

Earlier interest in mechanical atherectomy and laser-assisted PPI has waned due to trials demonstrating no improvement in long-term patency with these devices (123). Newer therapies aimed at prevention of restenosis are actively being investigated. Gene therapy, intravascular brachytherapy, and drug-eluting stents are emerging new adjunctive therapies that have shown great promise in attenuating the restenotic response after PPI.

SURGICAL TREATMENT OF PERIPHERAL ARTERY DISEASE

Aortoiliac Disease

The incidence of isolated aortoiliac disease in diabetic patients is significantly lower than that in nondiabetic patients, reflecting the propensity of diabetic patients to develop distal peripheral arteriopathy. In a series of approximately 1,800 patients, Hu demonstrated that the occurrence of symptomatic arterial obstruction due to aortoiliac obstruction was markedly higher in nondiabetics than in diabetics (79.4% versus 20.6%) (33). It has been estimated that the incidence of diabetes in patients undergoing aortoiliofemoral surgery is between 11% and 17% (124–126).

Surgical options for the treatment of aortoiliac occlusive disease include endarterectomy, bypass grafting (aortoiliac and aortofemoral), and construction of extra-anatomic conduits (axillofemoral and femorofemoral) (33). Although outcomes after surgical revascularization for aortoiliac disease tend to be similar in terms of graft patency and amputation (127), in the diabetic patient the presence of diabetes markedly increases the long-term mortality rate (73% versus 36%) at 9 years (126).

In the diabetic patient, the more common finding is that of multilevel occlusive disease that involves the aortoiliac (inflow) arteries. In the setting of multilevel disease, treatment of inflow occlusion alone may be sufficient to relieve claudication symptoms; however, in the setting of critical limb ischemia, limb salvage rates of only 70% to 85% are expected with this approach (33). In a series of aortofemoral bypass procedures, Brewster et al. (128) demonstrated that the need for combined inflow and outflow (infrainguinal) bypass is 30% in the setting of critical limb ischemia and 10% in the treatment for claudication. The impact of diabetes on the need for future revascularization after aortoiliac bypass was described by Faries et al. (129). In this study of more than 500 patients undergoing inflow bypass operations for lower-extremity ischemia, diabetic patients were no more likely than nondiabetic patients to require multiple levels of revascularization, leading to the conclusion that the need for simultaneous inflow and outflow procedures was not justified based on diabetic status alone.

Femoropopliteal Disease

The prevalence of diabetes in reports of surgical femoropopliteal revascularization is estimated at between 15% and 40% (33). As in aortoiliac disease, symptomatic arterial obstruction due to femoropopliteal disease is more common in nondiabetic patients than in diabetic patients (33). However, in most cases, infrapopliteal disease coexists with femoropopliteal disease, thus complicating revascularization strategies. The most commonly used surgical procedure for treatment of femoropopliteal stenosis is saphenous vein bypass from the common femoral artery to the popliteal artery. Several studies have documented the superiority of saphenous vein bypasses compared to synthetic conduits such as PTFE and Dacron (130,131).

The influence of diabetes on graft patency has been examined in several studies. Cutler et al. found a 5-year patency rate of 70% in diabetic patients and 75% in nondiabetic patients undergoing femoropopliteal bypass grafting (138). Similar graft patency rates between diabetic and nondiabetic patients also were reported by Szilagyi (132) and Bergan (133) and their colleagues.

Infrapopliteal Disease

The incidence of infrapopliteal disease is significantly higher in diabetics than in nondiabetics, making consideration of the issue of surgical revascularization particularly germane to this subset of patients. Among patients presenting for surgical revascularization for infrapopliteal atherosclerotic obstructive disease, the reported incidence of diabetes is between 47% and 88% (33). The most common method for surgical bypass is *in situ* saphenous vein bypass rather than placement of synthetic conduits. Success rates for infrapopliteal bypass operations are lower than those for suprapopliteal bypass operations. However, infrapopliteal bypass in diabetic patients is as successful or more successful than it is in nondiabetic patients. Rosenblatt et al. (134) demonstrated patency rates at 1 and 4 years of 95% and 89%, respectively, in diabetic patients and 85% and 80%, respectively, in nondiabetic patients. Shah et al. (135) reported no difference in patency rates at 1, 5, and 10 years after *in situ* saphenous vein bypass grafting in diabetic versus nondiabetic patients. In a series of infrainguinal surgical bypass operations, the majority of which (more than 75%) were infrapopliteal, Akbari et al. reported similar rates for 5-year graft patency (76% versus 72%), limb salvage (87% versus 85%), and overall mortality (41.8% versus 42%) in diabetic patients compared with nondiabetic patients (19). These data suggest that aggressive revascularization strategies should not be withheld from diabetic patients with infrapopliteal disease based on diabetic status alone.

CONCLUSION

In diabetic patients, PAD is extremely prevalent and confers enormous physiologic, psychological, and economic burdens on those afflicted with this disease. The presence of PAD is an indicator of systemic atherosclerosis, and for this reason efforts directed at lowering cardiovascular risk (the major cause of mortality in this patient population) are warranted. Intensive risk factor modification, smoking cessation, and exercise therapy form the cornerstones of conservative therapy for PAD. Medications such as cilostazol and clopidogrel hold promise in improving symptoms of claudication in addition to improving cardiovascular prognosis. However, despite numerous therapeutic guidelines, therapy for PAD is clearly suboptimal and requires immediate remediation. Although surgical revascularization has been used successfully in patients with medically refractory claudication and limb-threatening ischemia, improvements in endovascular technology have made percutaneous revascularization a viable alternative in additional appropriate situations. Clearly, aggressive medical, surgical, and/or percutaneous therapies in addition to continued basic and clinical research are indicated for this progressive and debilitating disease.

REFERENCES

1. Weitz JI, Byrne J, Clagett GP, et al. Diagnosis and treatment of chronic arterial insufficiency of the lower extremities: a critical review. *Circulation* 1996;94:3026–3049.
2. Newman AB, Siscovick DS, Manolio TA, et al. Ankle-arm index as a marker of atherosclerosis in the Cardiovascular Health Study. Cardiovascular Heart Study (CHS) Collaborative Research Group. *Circulation* 1993;88:837–845.
3. *National diabetes fact sheet: national estimates and general information on diabetes in the United States.* Atlanta: U.S. Department of Health and Human Services, Centers for Disease Control and Prevention, 1997.
4. Adler AI, Stevens RJ, Neil A, et al. UKPDS 59: hyperglycemia and other potentially modifiable risk factors for peripheral vascular disease in type 2 diabetes. *Diabetes Care* 2002;25:894–899.
5. Katsilambros NL, Tsapogas PC, Arvanitis MP, et al. Risk factors for lower extremity arterial disease in non-insulin-dependent diabetic persons. *Diabetes Med* 1996;13:243–246.
6. Beckman JA, Creager MA, Libby P. Diabetes and atherosclerosis: epidemiology, pathophysiology, and management. *JAMA* 2002;287:2570–2581.
7. Dolan NC, Liu K, Criqui MH, et al. Peripheral artery disease, diabetes, and reduced lower extremity functioning. *Diabetes Care* 2002;25:113–120.
8. Jude EB, Oyibo SO, Chalmers N, et al. Peripheral arterial disease in diabetic and nondiabetic patients: a comparison of severity and outcome. *Diabetes Care* 2001;24:1433–1437.

9. Hittel N, Donnelly R. Treating peripheral arterial disease in patients with diabetes. *Diabetes Obes Metab* 2002;4[Suppl 2]:S26–S31.
10. Palumbo PJ, Melton LJ. Peripheral vascular disease and diabetes. In: Harris MI, Hamman RF, eds. *Diabetes in America.* Washington, DC: Government Printing Office, 1985:1–21.
11. Levin ME, Sicard GA, Rubin BG. Peripheral vascular disease and the diabetic patient. In: Porte D Jr, Sherwin RS, eds. *Ellenberg and Rifken's diabetes mellitus.* Stanford, CT: Appleton & Lange, 1997:1127–1158.
12. Criqui MH. Peripheral arterial disease: epidemiological aspects. *Vasc Med* 2001;6:3–7.
13. Currie CJ, Morgan CL, Peters JR. The epidemiology and cost of inpatient care for peripheral vascular disease, infection, neuropathy, and ulceration in diabetes. *Diabetes Care* 1998;21:42–48.
14. Goldenberg SG, Alex M, Joshi RA, et al. Nonatheromatous peripheral vascular disease of the lower extremity in diabetes mellitus. *Diabetes* 1959;8:261–273.
15. Irwin ST, Gilmore J, McGrann S, et al. Blood flow in diabetic patients with foot lesions due to "small vessel disease." *Br J Surg* 1988;75:1201–1206.
16. Barner HB, Kaiser GC, Willman VL. Blood flow in the diabetic leg. *Circulation* 1971;43:391–394.
17. Wyss CR, Matsen FA 3rd, Simmons CW, et al. Transcutaneous oxygen tension measurements on limbs of diabetic and nondiabetic patients with peripheral vascular disease. *Surgery* 1984;95:339–346.
18. Searles JM Jr, Colen LB. Foot reconstruction in diabetes mellitus and peripheral vascular insufficiency. *Clin Plast Surg* 1991;18:467–483.
19. Akbari CM, LoGerfo FW. Diabetes and peripheral vascular disease. *J Vasc Surg* 1999;30:373–384.
20. Ross R. Atherosclerosis: an inflammatory disease. *N Engl J Med* 1999;340:115–126.
21. Quyyumi AA. Endothelial function in health and disease: new insights into the genesis of cardiovascular disease. *Am J Med* 1998;105:32S–39S.
22. Chen NG, Holmes M, Reaven GM. Relationship between insulin resistance, soluble adhesion molecules, and mononuclear cell binding in healthy volunteers. *J Clin Endocrinol Metab* 1999;84:3485–3489.
23. Steinberg HO, Chaker H, Leaming R, et al. Obesity/insulin resistance is associated with endothelial dysfunction: implications for the syndrome of insulin resistance. *J Clin Invest* 1996;97:2601–2610.
24. Schaper NC, Nabuurs-Franssen MH, Huijberts MS. Peripheral vascular disease and type 2 diabetes mellitus. *Diabetes Metab Res Rev* 2000;16[Suppl 1]:S11–S15.
25. Kern PA, Ranganathan S, Li C, et al. Adipose tissue tumor necrosis factor and interleukin-6 expression in human obesity and insulin resistance. *Am J Physiol Endocrinol Metab* 2001;280:E745–E751.
26. Nilsson J, Jovinge S, Niemann A, et al. Relation between plasma tumor necrosis factor-alpha and insulin sensitivity in elderly men with non-insulin-dependent diabetes mellitus. *Arterioscler Thromb Vasc Biol* 1998;18:1199–1202.
27. Hauner H, Bender M, Haastert B, et al. Plasma concentrations of soluble TNF-alpha receptors in obese subjects. *Int J Obes Relat Metab Disord* 1998;22:1239–1243.

28. Bierhaus A, Hofmann MA, Ziegler R, et al. AGEs and their interaction with AGE-receptors in vascular disease and diabetes mellitus: I. The AGE concept. *Cardiovasc Res* 1998;37:586–600.

29. Schmidt AM, Hori O, Cao R, et al. RAGE: a novel cellular receptor for advanced glycation end products. *Diabetes* 1996;45[Suppl 3]:S77–S80.

30. Schmidt AM, Yan SD, Wautier JL, et al. Activation of receptor for advanced glycation end products: a mechanism for chronic vascular dysfunction in diabetic vasculopathy and atherosclerosis. *Circ Res* 1999;84:489–497.

31. Conrad MC. Large and small artery occlusion in diabetic patients and nondiabetic patients with severe vascular disease. *Circulation* 1967;36:83–91.

32. Strandness DE Jr, Priest RE, Gibbons GE. Combined clinical and pathological study of diabetic and nondiabetic peripheral arterial disease. *Diabetes* 1964;13:366–372.

33. Hu MY, Allen BT. The role of vascular surgery in the diabetic patient. In: Bowker JH, Pfeifer MA, eds. *Levin and O'Neal's the diabetic foot.* St. Louis: Mosby, 2001:374–394.

34. van der Feen C, Neijens FS, Kanters SD, et al. Angiographic distribution of lower extremity atherosclerosis in patients with and without diabetes. *Diabetes Med* 2002;19:366–370.

35. Hurley JJ, Jung M, Woods JJ, et al. Noninvasive vascular testing: basis, application, and role in evaluating diabetic peripheral arterial disease. In: Bowker JH, Pfeifer MA, eds. *Levin and O'Neal's the diabetic foot.* St. Louis: Mosby, 2001:355–373.

36. Hiatt WR, Nehler MR. Peripheral arterial disease. *Adv Intern Med* 2001;47:89–110.

37. Strandness DE Jr, McCutcheon EP, Rushmer RF. Application of a transcutaneous Doppler flowmeter in evaluation of occlusive arterial disease. *Surg Gynecol Obstet* 1966;122:1039–1045.

38. Jaff MR. Lower extremity arterial disease: diagnostic aspects. *Cardiol Clin* 2002;20:491–500.

39. Edwards JM, Coldwell DM, Goldman ML, et al. The role of duplex scanning in the selection of patients for transluminal angioplasty. *J Vasc Surg* 1991;13:69–74.

40. Dyet JF, Nicholson AA, Ettles DF. Vascular imaging and intervention in peripheral arteries in the diabetic patient. *Diabetes Metab Res Rev* 2000;16[Suppl 1]:S16–S22.

41. Carpenter JP, Baum RA, Holland GA, et al. Peripheral vascular surgery with magnetic resonance angiography as the sole preoperative imaging modality. *J Vasc Surg* 1994;20:861–869; discussion, 869–871.

42. Carpenter JP, Golden MA, Barker CF, et al. The fate of bypass grafts to angiographically occult runoff vessels detected by magnetic resonance angiography. *J Vasc Surg* 1996;23:483–489.

43. Koelemay MJ, Lijmer JG, Stoker J, et al. Magnetic resonance angiography for the evaluation of lower extremity arterial disease: a meta-analysis. *JAMA* 2001;285:1338–1345.

44. Chiang KS, Tripp MD. Radiological intervention in diabetic peripheral vascular disease. In: Bowker JH, Pfeifer MA, eds. *Levin and O'Neal's the diabetic foot.* St. Louis: Mosby, 2001:374–394.

45. Rubin GD, Dake MD, Napel S, et al. Spiral CT of renal artery stenosis: comparison of three-dimensional rendering techniques. *Radiology* 1994;190:181–189.

46. Dachman AH. New contraindication to intravascular iodinated contrast material. *Radiology* 1995;197:545.

47. Hornsby VP. Intravascular injection of iodinated contrast media. *Clin Radiol* 1996;51:820.

48. Nugent RA, Flak B. Contrast-enhanced imaging studies contraindicated in patients receiving Glucophage. *Can Assoc Radiol J* 1996;47:225.

49. Pond GD, Smyth SH, Roach DJ, et al. Metformin and contrast media: genuine risk or witch hunt? *Radiology* 1996;201:879–880.

50. Rasuli P, French G, Hammond DI. New contraindication to intravascular contrast material. *Radiology* 1996;201:289–290.

51. American College of Radiology. *Manual on contrast media,* 4th ed. Reston, VA: American College of Radiology 1998;17–18.

52. Faulkner KW, House AK, Castleden WM. The effect of cessation of smoking on the accumulative survival rates of patients with symptomatic peripheral vascular disease. *Med J Aust* 1983;1:217–219.

53. Hiatt WR. Medical treatment of peripheral arterial disease and claudication. *N Engl J Med* 2001;344:1608–1621.

54. United Kingdom Prospective Diabetes Study (UKPDS) Group. Effect of intensive blood-glucose control with metformin on complications in overweight patients with type 2 diabetes (UKPDS 34). *Lancet* 1998;352:854–865.

55. Regensteiner JG, Hiatt WR. Current medical therapies for patients with peripheral arterial disease: a critical review. *Am J Med* 2002;112:49–57.

56. Kannel WB, Skinner JJ Jr, Schwartz MJ, et al. Intermittent claudication: incidence in the Framingham Study. *Circulation* 1970;41:875–883.

57. Beach KW, Bedford GR, Bergelin RO, et al. Progression of lower-extremity arterial occlusive disease in type II diabetes mellitus. *Diabetes Care* 1988;11:464–472.

58. Hughson WG, Mann JI, Garrod A. Intermittent claudication: prevalence and risk factors. *Br Med J* 1978;1:1379–1381.

59. Belch JJ. Metabolic, endocrine and haemodynamic risk factors in the patient with peripheral arterial disease. *Diabetes Obes Metab* 2002;4[Suppl 2]:S7–S13.

60. Heart Protection Study Collaborative Group. MRC/BHF Heart Protection Study of cholesterol lowering with simvastatin in 20,536 high-risk individuals: a randomised placebo-controlled trial. *Lancet* 2002;360:7–22.

61. Aronow WS, Ahn C. Frequency of new coronary events in older persons with peripheral arterial disease and serum low-density lipoprotein cholesterol > or = 125 mg/dl treated with statins versus no lipid-lowering drug. *Am J Cardiol* 2002;90:789–791.

62. Summary of the second report of the National Cholesterol Education Program (NCEP) Expert Panel on Detection, Evaluation, and Treatment of High Blood Cholesterol in Adults (Adult Treatment Panel II). *JAMA* 1993;269:3015–3023.

63. Murabito JM, D'Agostino RB, Silbershatz H, et al. Intermittent claudication: a risk profile from the Framingham Heart Study. *Circulation* 1997;96:44–49.

64. The sixth report of the Joint National Committee

on prevention, detection, evaluation, and treatment of high blood pressure. *Arch Intern Med* 1997;157:2413–2446.

65. Nass CM, Allen JK, Jermyn RM, et al. Secondary prevention of coronary artery disease in patients undergoing elective surgery for peripheral arterial disease. *Vasc Med* 2001;6:35–41.

66. Mukherjee D, Lingam P, Chetcuti S, et al. Missed opportunities to treat atherosclerosis in patients undergoing peripheral vascular interventions: insights from the University of Michigan Peripheral Vascular Disease Quality Improvement Initiative (PVD-QI2). *Circulation* 2002;106:1909–1912.

67. Gardner AW, Poehlman ET. Exercise rehabilitation programs for the treatment of claudication pain: a meta-analysis. *JAMA* 1995;274:975–980.

68. Leng GC, Fowler B, Ernst E. Exercise for intermittent claudication. *Cochrane Database Syst Rev* 2000;(2):CD000990.

69. Regensteiner JG. Exercise in the treatment of claudication: assessment and treatment of functional impairment. *Vasc Med* 1997;2:238–242.

70. Doxandabaratz Ilundain J, Ferro Mugica J, Iriarte Arotzarena I. [Cardiac rehabilitation results at the physical, psychological, sexual and work levels]. *Rev Esp Cardiol* 1995;48:79–84.

71. Patterson RB, Pinto B, Marcus B, et al. Value of a supervised exercise program for the therapy of arterial claudication. *J Vasc Surg* 1997;25:312–318; discussion, 318–319.

72. Gartenmann C, Kirchberger I, Herzig M, et al. Effects of exercise training program on functional capacity and quality of life in patients with peripheral arterial occlusive disease: evaluation of a pilot project. *Vasa* 2002;31:29–34.

73. Regensteiner JG, Steiner JF, Hiatt WR. Exercise training improves functional status in patients with peripheral arterial disease. *J Vasc Surg* 1996;23:104–115.

74. Clifford PC, Davies PW, Hayne JA, et al. Intermittent claudication: is a supervised exercise class worth while? *Br Med J* 1980;280:1503–1505.

75. Gardner AW, Katzel LI, Sorkin JD, et al. Improved functional outcomes following exercise rehabilitation in patients with intermittent claudication. *J Gerontol A Biol Sci Med Sci* 2000;55:M570–M577.

76. Stewart KJ, Hiatt WR, Regensteiner JG, et al. Exercise training for claudication. *N Engl J Med* 2002;347:1941–1951.

77. Hiatt WR, Wolfel EE, Meier RH, et al. Superiority of treadmill walking exercise versus strength training for patients with peripheral arterial disease: implications for the mechanism of the training response. *Circulation* 1994;90:1866–1874.

78. Regensteiner JG, Meyer TJ, Krupski WC, et al. Hospital vs home-based exercise rehabilitation for patients with peripheral arterial occlusive disease. *Angiology* 1997;48:291–300.

79. Nehler MR, Hiatt WR. Exercise therapy for claudication. *Ann Vasc Surg* 1999;13:109–114.

80. Savage P, Ricci MA, Lynn M, et al. Effects of home versus supervised exercise for patients with intermittent claudication. *J Cardiopulm Rehabil* 2001;21:152–157.

81. Mohler ER 3rd, Beebe HG, Salles-Cuhna S, et al. Effects of cilostazol on resting ankle pressures and

exercise-induced ischemia in patients with intermittent claudication. *Vasc Med* 2001;6:151–156.

82. Beebe HG, Dawson DL, Cutler BS, et al. A new pharmacological treatment for intermittent claudication: results of a randomized, multicenter trial. *Arch Intern Med* 1999;159:2041–2050.

83. Regensteiner JG, Ware JE Jr, McCarthy WJ, et al. Effect of cilostazol on treadmill walking, community-based walking ability, and health-related quality of life in patients with intermittent claudication due to peripheral arterial disease: meta-analysis of six randomized controlled trials. *J Am Geriatr Soc* 2002;50:1939–1946.

84. Dawson DL, DeMaioribus CA, Hagino RT, et al. The effect of withdrawal of drugs treating intermittent claudication. *Am J Surg* 1999;178:141–146.

85. Elam MB, Heckman J, Crouse JR, et al. Effect of the novel antiplatelet agent cilostazol on plasma lipoproteins in patients with intermittent claudication. *Arterioscler Thromb Vasc Biol* 1998;18:1942–1947.

86. Yamamoto Y, Yasuda Y, Komiya Y. Cilostazol prevents impairment of slow axonal transport in streptozotocin-diabetic rats. *Eur J Pharmacol* 2000;409:1–7.

87. Yamamoto Y, Yasuda Y, Kimura Y, et al. Effects of cilostazol, an antiplatelet agent, on axonal regeneration following nerve injury in diabetic rats. *Eur J Pharmacol* 1998;352:171–178.

88. Suh KS, Oh SJ, Woo JT, et al. Effect of cilostazol on the neuropathies of streptozotocin-induced diabetic rats. *Korean J Intern Med* 1999;14:34–40.

89. Okuda Y, Mizutani M, Ikegami T, et al. Hemodynamic effects of cilostazol on peripheral artery in patients with diabetic neuropathy. *Arzneimittelforschung* 1992;42:540–542.

90. Uehara K, Sugimoto K, Wada R, et al. Effects of cilostazol on the peripheral nerve function and structure in STZ-induced diabetic rats. *J Diabetes Complications* 1997;11:194–202.

91. Watanabe J, Sako Y, Umeda F, et al. Effects of cilostazol, a phosphodiesterase inhibitor, on urinary excretion of albumin and prostaglandins in non-insulin-dependent diabetic patients. *Diabetes Res Clin Pract* 1993;22:53–59.

92. Nomura S, Shouzu A, Omoto S, et al. Effect of cilostazol on soluble adhesion molecules and platelet-derived microparticles in patients with diabetes. *Thromb Haemost* 1998;80:388–392.

93. Schror K. The pharmacology of cilostazol. *Diabetes Obes Metab* 2002;4[Suppl 2]:S14–S19.

94. Nishio Y, Kashiwagi A, Takahara N, et al. Cilostazol, a cAMP phosphodiesterase inhibitor, attenuates the production of monocyte chemoattractant protein-1 in response to tumor necrosis factor-alpha in vascular endothelial cells. *Horm Metab Res* 1997;29:491–495.

95. Inoue T, Sohma R, Morooka S. Cilostazol inhibits the expression of activation-dependent membrane surface glycoprotein on the surface of platelets stimulated in vitro. *Thromb Res* 1999;93:137–143.

96. Takahashi S, Oida K, Fujiwara R, et al. Effect of cilostazol, a cyclic AMP phosphodiesterase inhibitor, on the proliferation of rat aortic smooth muscle cells in culture. *J Cardiovasc Pharmacol* 1992;20:900–906.

97. Kayanoki Y, Che W, Kawata S, et al. The effect of cilostazol, a cyclic nucleotide phosphodiesterase III inhibitor, on heparin-binding EGF-like growth factor expression in macrophages and vascular smooth muscle cells. *Biochem Biophys Res Commun* 1997;238:478–481.

98. Tsuchikane E, Katoh O, Sumitsuji S, et al. Impact of cilostazol on intimal proliferation after directional coronary atherectomy. *Am Heart J* 1998;135:495–502.

99. Tsuchikane E, Fukuhara A, Kobayashi T, et al. Impact of cilostazol on restenosis after percutaneous coronary balloon angioplasty. *Circulation* 1999;100:21–26.

100. Kubota Y, Kichikawa K, Uchida H, et al. Pharmacologic treatment of intimal hyperplasia after metallic stent placement in the peripheral arteries: an experimental study. *Invest Radiol* 1995;30:532–537.

101. Schainfeld RM. Management of peripheral arterial disease and intermittent claudication. *J Am Board Fam Pract* 2001;14:443–450.

102. Hood SC, Moher D, Barber GG. Management of intermittent claudication with pentoxifylline: meta-analysis of randomized controlled trials. *CMAJ* 1996;155:1053–1059.

103. Porter JM, Cutler BS, Lee BY, et al. Pentoxifylline efficacy in the treatment of intermittent claudication: multicenter controlled double-blind trial with objective assessment of chronic occlusive arterial disease patients. *Am Heart J* 1982;104:66–72.

104. Dawson DL, Cutler BS, Hiatt WR, et al. A comparison of cilostazol and pentoxifylline for treating intermittent claudication. *Am J Med* 2000;109:523–530.

105. A randomized, blinded, trial of clopidogrel versus aspirin in patients at risk of ischaemic events (CAPRIE). CAPRIE Steering Committee. *Lancet* 1996;348:1329–1339.

106. Conti CR. Current status of medical therapy of peripheral arterial disease. *Clin Cardiol* 1999;22:331–332.

107. Eberhardt RT, Coffman JD. Drug treatment of peripheral vascular disease. *Heart Dis* 2000;2:62–74.

108. Boger RH, Bode-Boger SM, Thiele W, et al. Restoring vascular nitric oxide formation by L-arginine improves the symptoms of intermittent claudication in patients with peripheral arterial occlusive disease. *J Am Coll Cardiol* 1998;32:1336–1344.

109. Dotter CT, Judkins MP. Transluminal treatment of atherosclerotic obstruction: description of a new technique and preliminary report of its application. *Circulation* 1964;30:654.

110. Dotter CT. Transluminal angioplasty: a long view. *Radiology* 1980;135:561–564.

111. Pell JP, Whyman MR, Fowkes FG, et al. Trends in vascular surgery since the introduction of percutaneous transluminal angioplasty. *Br J Surg* 1994;81:832–835.

112. Vesely TM. General percutaneous transluminal angioplasty techniques: clinical aspects. In: Darcy MD, LaBerge JM, eds. *Peripheral vascular interventions.* Fairfax, VA: Society of Cardiovascular and Interventional Radiology, 1994.

113. d'Othee BJ, Haulon S, Mounier-Vehier C, et al. Percutaneous endovascular treatment for stenoses and occlusions of infrarenal aorta and aortoiliac bifurcation: midterm results. *Eur J Vasc Endovasc Surg* 2002;24:516–523.

114. Odurny A, Colapinto RF, Sniderman KW, et al. Percutaneous transluminal angioplasty of abdominal aortic stenoses. *Cardiovasc Intervent Radiol* 1989;12:1–6.

115. Becker GJ, Katzen BT, Dake MD. Noncoronary angioplasty. *Radiology* 1989;170:921–940.

116. Hassen-Khodja R, Sala F, Declemy S, et al. Value of stent placement during percutaneous transluminal angioplasty of the iliac arteries. *J Cardiovasc Surg (Torino)* 2001;42:369–374.

117. Tetteroo E, DeGraaf YV, Bosch JL. Randomized comparison of primary stent placement versus angioplasty with selective stent placement in patients with iliac artery obstruction disease. *Radiology* 1997;205[Suppl]:254.

118. Marks MV. Superficial femoral and popliteal angioplasty: techniques and results. In: Darcy MD, LaBerge JM, eds. *Peripheral vascular interventions.* Fairfax, VA: Society of Cardiovascular and Interventional Radiology, 1994.

119. Jeans WD, Armstrong S, Cole SE, et al. Fate of patients undergoing transluminal angioplasty for lower-limb ischemia. *Radiology* 1990;177:559–564.

120. Rajagopalan S, Grossman PM. Management of chronic critical limb ischemia. *Cardiol Clin* 2002;20:535–545.

121. Dyet JF, Duncan FE, Nicholson AA. The role of radiology in the assessment and treatment of the diabetic foot. In: Boulton AJM, Connor H, Cavanaugh PR, eds. *The foot in diabetes.* New York: John Wiley & Sons, 2000:193–213.

122. Bakal CW. Subtrifurcation percutaneous transluminal angioplasty: techniques and results. In: Darcy MD, LaBerge JM, eds. *Peripheral vascular interventions.* Fairfax, VA: Society of Cardiovascular and Interventional Radiology, 1994.

123. Baum S, Pentecost MJ, eds. *Abrams' angiography: interventional radiology,* Vol. III. Boston: Little, Brown, 1997.

124. Crawford ES, Bomberger RA, Glaeser DH, et al. Aortoiliac occlusive disease: factors influencing survival and function following reconstructive operation over a twenty-five-year period. *Surgery* 1981;90:1055–1067.

125. Brewster DC, Darling RC. Optimal methods of aortoiliac reconstruction. *Surgery* 1978;84:739–748.

126. Malone JM, Moore WS, Goldstone J. The natural history of bilateral aortofemoral bypass grafts for ischemia of the lower extremities. *Arch Surg* 1975;110:1300–1306.

127. Bartlett FF, Gibbons GW, Wheelock FC Jr. Aortic reconstruction for occlusive disease: comparable results in diabetic patients. *Arch Surg* 1986;121:1150–1153.

128. Brewster DC, Perler BA, Robison JG, et al. Aortofemoral graft for multilevel occlusive disease: predictors of success and need for distal bypass. *Arch Surg* 1982;117:1593–1600.

129. Faries PL, LoGerfo FW, Hook SC, et al. The impact of diabetes on arterial reconstructions for multilevel arterial occlusive disease. *Am J Surg* 2001;181:251–255.

130. Veith FJ, Gupta SK, Wengerter KR, et al. Changing arteriosclerotic disease patterns and management strategies in lower-limb-threatening ischemia. *Ann Surg* 1990;212:402–412; discussion, 412–414.

131. Whittemore AD, Kent KC, Donaldson MC, et al. What is the proper role of polytetrafluoroethylene grafts in

infrainguinal reconstruction? *J Vasc Surg* 1989;10:299–305.

132. Szilagyi DE, Hageman JH, Smith RF, et al. Autogenous vein grafting in femoropopliteal atherosclerosis: the limits of its effectiveness. *Surgery* 1979;86:836–851.

133. Bergan JJ, Veith FJ, Bernhard VM, et al. Randomization of autogenous vein and polytetrafluorethylene grafts in femoral-distal reconstruction. *Surgery* 1982;92:921–930.

134. Rosenblatt MS, Quist WC, Sidawy AN, et al. Results of vein graft reconstruction of the lower extremity in diabetic and nondiabetic patients. *Surg Gynecol Obstet* 1990;171:331–335.

135. Shah DM, Darling RC 3rd, Chang BB, et al. Long-term results of in situ saphenous vein bypass: analysis of 2058 cases. *Ann Surg* 1995;222:438–446; discussion, 446–448.

136. Hirsch AT, Criqui MH, Treent-Jacobsen D, et al. Peripheral arterial disease, detection, awareness, and treatment in primary care. *JAMA* 2001;286(11):1317–1324.

137. Gruntzig A, Hoff H. Perkutane rekanalisation chronoischer arterieller verschlusse mit einem neven kilatioskatheter: modifikation der dotter-techniq. *Dtsh Med Wochenschr* 1974;99:2502.

138. Cutler BS, Thompson JE, Kleinsasser LJ, et al. Autologous saphenous vein femeropopliteal bypass. Analysis of 298 cases. *Surgery* 1976;79:325–331.

Diabetes and Cardiovascular Disease
edited by Steven P. Marso and David M. Stern
Lippincott Williams & Wilkins, Philadelphia © 2004

Appendix A

Adjunctive Pharmacology of Diabetes: Chain of Evidence

Maureen E. Knell, Jared T. Lurk, and Jennifer M. Roth

Clinical Assistant Professor, Division of Pharmacy Practice, University of Missouri–Kansas City, Clinical Pharmacist, Multi-specialty Clinic, Saint Luke's Hospital; Adjunct Clinical Assistant Professor, Division of Pharmacy Practice, University of Missouri–Kansas City, Pharmacy Practice Resident, Department of Pharmacy, Saint Luke's Hospital; Adjunct Clinical Assistant Professor, Division of Pharmacy Practice, University of Missouri–Kansas City, Pharmacy Practice Resident, Department of Pharmacy, Saint Luke's Hospital; Kansas City, Missouri

This appendix includes reference tables for most of the available diabetes and cardiovascular drugs used in outpatient clinical practice. The information is arranged in four separate tables: Oral Agents for Treatment of Type 2 Diabetes (Table A-1), Insulin Therapy (Table A-2), Oral Agents for Cardiovascular Risk Factor Management (Table A-3), and Common Combination Products for Cardiovascular Risk Factor Management (Table A-4). Within each table, the information is categorized alphabetically by therapeutic class, then alphabetically by generic drug name. Each entry contains, where applicable, the generic and brand name of the drug; initial, usual and maximum doses, if available; mechanism of action; labeled and unlabeled indications; common

and/or serious adverse reactions; approximate cost of 1 month of therapy (based on the Average Wholesale Price); and a comment section including the therapeutic utility, clinical pearls, and dosing/administration recommendations for the therapeutic class or specific agent. The comment section also includes information on drug interactions; however, this information is not intended as a complete resource on drug interactions. It is important to note that many of the medications used for diabetes and cardiovascular indications have significant drug interactions. One should be aware of this potential when prescribing or recommending new medications and should consult a specific drug interaction reference to obtain more complete drug interaction information.

TABLE A-1. *Oral agents for treatment of type 2 diabetes*

Drug	Dose	Mechanism of action	Indication	Adverse reactions	Cost[a] ($) based on usual dose for 1 mo	Comments
α-GLUCOSIDASE INHIBITORS						
General information		Inhibits α-glucosidase found in the small intestines Delays gut carbohydrate absorption, resulting in a smaller rise in plasma glucose after meals		Gastrointestinal (GI): flatulence, abdominal pain, diarrhea Contraindicated: inflammatory bowel disease, partial intestinal obstruction		Therapeutic utility: elevated postprandial glucose Titrate dose slowly (q.d. dosing initially) to reduce GI adverse effects Administer glucose (avoid complex sugars/ carbohydrates) in patients who develop hypoglycemia
Acarbose (Precose)	Initial: 25 mg q.d.–t.i.d. with meals Usual: 50–100 mg t.i.d. with meals Maximum: 150 mg/day if ≤60 kg, 300 mg/ day if >60 kg	See General Information	Labeled: monotherapy or with sulfonylurea, metformin, or insulin Unlabeled: in combination with other antidiabetic agents	See General Information Elevated serum transaminases (asymptomatic and reversible)	60–70	See General Information
Miglitol (Glyset)	Initial: 25 mg q.d. with a meal Usual: 50–100 mg t.i.d. with meals Maximum: 300 mg/day	See General Information	Labeled: monotherapy or with sulfonylurea Unlabeled: in combination with other antidiabetic agents	See General Information	60–70	See General Information

	Dosage	Mechanism of action	Labeled/unlabeled use		Adverse reactions/contraindications	Comments
BIGUANIDES				90–110		
Metformin (Glucophage)	Initial: 500 mg b.i.d. or 850 q.d. with meals Usual: 1,000 mg b.i.d. or 850 mg b.i.d.–t.i.d. with meals Maximum: 2,500–2,550 mg/day (2–3 divided doses with meals)	Decreases hepatic glucose production, improves insulin sensitivity in hepatic and peripheral tissues, decreases intestinal absorption of glucose	Labeled: monotherapy or with sulfonylurea or insulin Unlabeled: in combination with other antidiabetic agents Prevention of diabetes in patients with impaired fasting glucose or impaired glucose tolerance Weight loss		Black box warning: *lactic acidosis* Contraindicated in renal disease or dysfunction (serum creatinine ≥1.5 mg/dL [males], ≥1.4 mg/dL [females] or abnormal creatinine clearance) Decompensated congestive heart failure Acute or chronic metabolic acidosis GI: diarrhea, nausea/vomiting, flatulence, abnormal stools	Therapeutic utility: overweight, insulin resistance, children (approved for patients >10 yr) Clinically significant responses usually seen at 1,500–2,000 mg/day with little benefit beyond this range; lower starting doses with gradual increases (1–2 wk) recommended to minimize GI symptoms May cause lactic acidosis (see Adverse Reactions): hold at least 48 hours in patients receiving iodinated radiocontrast agents and resume only after renal function has been evaluated as normal after procedure May result in ovulation in previously anovulatory premenopausal women; adequate contraception should be recommended Glycemic efficacy and improved lipid profile with the extended-release formulation may not be equivalent to that achieved with the immediate-release product
(Glucophage XR)	Initial: 500 mg q.d. with evening meal Usual: 1,500–2,000 mg q.d. with evening meal Maximum: 2,000 mg/day (1–2 doses with meals)					

continued

425

TABLE A-1. *Continued*

Drug	Dose	Mechanism of action	Indication	Adverse reactions	Cost[a] ($) based on usual dose for 1 mo	Comments
MEGLITINIDES General information		Stimulates pancreatic insulin secretion from pancreatic beta cells, similar to sulfonylureas but with shorter binding time to receptor	Monotherapy or with metformin	Hypoglycemia Weight gain Upper respiratory tract infections		Therapeutic utility: elevated postprandial glucose, recent type 2 diabetes (requires functioning beta cells to produce endogenous insulin), patients at increased risk for hypoglycemia (e.g., elderly, renal dysfunction) No additional benefit when combined with sulfonylureas due to similar mechanism of action; patients whose hyperglycemia is not adequately controlled with sulfonylureas or other insulin secretagogues should not be switched to meglitinides
Nateglinide (Starlix)	Initial and usual: 60–120 mg with meals Maximum: 360 mg/day	See General Information	See General Information	See General Information	90–95	Hepatically metabolized by CYP2C9 and CYP3A4, and a potential inhibitor of CYP2C9, but no clinically significant drug interactions have been reported Omit if meals are skipped Shorter-acting than repaglinide

Drug	Dosage	Mechanism	Uses	Adverse effects		Comments
Repaglinide (Prandin)	Initial: 0.5 mg with meals Usual: 0.5–4 mg with meals Maximum: 16 mg/day	See General Information	See General Information	See General Information	90–170	CYP3A4 hepatic metabolism; concentrations may be increased by CYP3A4 inhibitors such as ketoconazole, miconazole, erythromycin, and simvastatin; concentrations may be decreased by CYP3A4 inducers such as rifampin, barbiturates, and carbamazepine Skip dose if meal is skipped; add dose if meal is added

SULFONYLUREAS—FIRST GENERATION

Drug	Dosage	Mechanism	Uses	Adverse effects		Comments
General information		Stimulates pancreatic insulin secretion from pancreatic beta cells	Labeled: monotherapy Unlabeled: in combination with other antidiabetic agents	Hypoglycemia Weight gain GI: nausea, epigastric fullness, heartburn Photosensitivity		Therapeutic utility: generally not used due to lower potencies, longer half-lives, and higher incidences of adverse effects and drug interactions compared with second-generation sulfonylureas
Acetohexamide (Dymelor)	Initial: 250 mg q.d. Usual: 250–750 mg q.d.–b.i.d. Maximum: 1,500 mg/day	See General Information	See General Information	See General Information	10–40	See General Information

continued

TABLE A-1. *Continued*

Drug	Dose	Mechanism of action	Indication	Adverse reactions	Cost[a] ($) based on usual dose for 1 mo	Comments
Chlorpropamide (Diabinese)	Initial: 100–250 mg q.d. Usual: 100–500 mg q.d. Maximum: 750 mg/day	See General Information	See General Information	See General Information	10–35	See General Information Can cause SIADH and disulfiram-like reaction if taken with alcohol Greatest risk for profound hypoglycemia due to long half-life
Tolazamide (Tolinase)	Initial: 100–250 mg q.d. Usual: 100–1,000 mg q.d. or divided b.i.d. (divide doses >500 mg/day) Maximum: 1,000 mg/day	See General Information	See General Information	See General Information	10–75	See General Information
Tolbutamide (Orinase)	Initial: 1,000–2,000 mg q.d. Usual: 250–2,000 mg q.d. (or b.i.d.–t.i.d.) if GI intolerance Maximum: 3,000 mg/day	See General Information	See General Information	See General Information	5–30	See General Information
SULFONYLUREAS—SECOND GENERATION						
General information		Stimulates pancreatic insulin secretion from pancreatic beta cells	Labeled: monotherapy Unlabeled: in combination with other antidiabetic agents	Hypoglycemia Weight gain GI: nausea, epigastric fullness, heartburn Photosensitivity		Dosage reductions recommended for the elderly and those with renal or hepatic dysfunction
Glimepiride (Amaryl)	Initial: 0.5–2 mg q.d. Usual: 1–4 mg q.d. Maximum: 8 mg/day	See General Information	See General Information	See General Information	10–30	Little benefit to increasing dose >4 mg/day
Glipizide (Glucotrol)	Initial: 2.5–5 mg q.d. Usual: 2.5–20 mg q.d. or b.i.d. (divide doses >15 mg/day) Maximum: 40 mg/day	See General Information	See General Information	See General Information	5–35	Little benefit to increasing dose >20 mg/day

428

Drug	Dose	(mg/day)	Mechanism/General Information	Adverse effects	Comments
(Glucotrol XL)	Initial: 5 mg q.d. Usual: 5–20 mg q.d. Maximum: 20 mg/day	10–50	See General Information		Little benefit to increasing dose >10 mg/day Active metabolites renally eliminated; may accumulate, predisposing patients with renal dysfunction to hypoglycemia
Glyburide (Micronase, DiaBeta)	Initial: 2.5–5 mg q.d. Usual: 1.25–20 mg q.d. or divide b.i.d. (divide dose if >10 mg/day) Maximum: 20 mg/day	10–80	See General Information		See General Information
Micronized (Glynase)	Initial: 0.75–3 mg q.d. Usual: 0.75–12 mg q.d. or divided (divide if >6 mg/day) Maximum: 12 mg/day	10–75			
THIAZOLIDINEDIONES General information			Activates PPARγ receptor to increase insulin sensitivity in muscle and adipose tissue and decrease hepatic glucose production	Use caution in patients with congestive heart failure; may cause fluid retention; see Comments Weight gain Hemodilution, causing decreases in Hgb and Hct Liver dysfunction (rare); see Comments	Weight gain and fluid retention may be increased, particularly when combined with insulin or insulin secretagogues Not recommended for patients with active liver disease or an ALT >2.5 times upper limit of normal; use caution in patients with ALT 1–2.5 times upper limit of normal Monitor LFTs at baseline, then every 2 mo for 1 yr, then periodically May result in ovulation in previously anovulatory premenopausal women; adequate contraception should be recommended (see Comments for pioglitazone)

continued

429

TABLE A-1. *Continued*

Drug	Dose	Mechanism of action	Indication	Adverse reactions	Cost^a ($) based on usual dose for 1 mo	Comments
Pioglitazone (Actos)	Initial: 15–30 mg q.d. Usual: 15–45 mg q.d. Maximum: 45 mg/day or 30 mg/day when combined with other agents	See General Information	Labeled: monotherapy or with sulfonylurea, metformin, or insulin Unlabeled: other combinations with antidiabetic agents	See General Information	100–170	Metabolized by CYP enzymes, primarily 3A4 and 2C8 Due to an interaction with troglitazone (removed from market) decreasing plasma concentrations of oral contraceptives containing ethinyl estradiol and norethindrone, the manufacturer of pioglitazone recommends additional caution regarding contraception in patients receiving oral contraceptives
Rosiglitazone (Avandia)	Initial: 4 mg q.d. or divided b.i.d. Usual: 4–8 mg q.d. or divided b.i.d. Maximum: 8 mg/day or 4 mg when used with sulfonylurea	See General Information	Labeled: monotherapy or with sulfonylurea or metformin Unlabeled: other combinations with antidiabetic agents	See General Information	85–170	Metabolized by CYP enzymes, primarily 2C8 No clinically relevant interaction with oral contraceptives containing ethinyl estradiol and norethindrone

COMBINATION PRODUCTS[b]

Glipizide + metformin (Metaglip)	2.5 mg/250 mg 2.5 mg/500 mg 5 mg/500 mg	1–4 tablets q.d.–b.i.d.	Not available	FDA-approved, fall 2002 See individual components
Glyburide + metformin (Glucovance)	1.25 mg/250 mg 2.5 mg/500 mg 5 mg/500 mg	q.d.–b.i.d.	30–120	See individual components Glyburide is more bioavailable in combination product than as monotherapy
Rosiglitazone + metformin (Avandamet)	1 mg/500 mg 2 mg/500 mg 4 mg/500 mg	q.d.–b.i.d.	Not available	FDA-approved See individual components

[a]Cost based on Average Wholesale Price 2002 range of "usual dose" for a 30-day supply. Generic price provided if available. Price does not include dispensing fees charged by pharmacies. Patients' costs may vary considerably.

[b]Combination drugs are usually reserved for use after titration to similar or identical doses of at least one of the individual agents first, and doses of the combination product should be adjusted accordingly. After titration of individual agents, there may be cases in which the combination product is less costly or improves compliance with the therapeutic regimen.

ALT, alanine aminotransferase; CYP, cytochrome P-450 enzyme; FDA, U. S. Food and Drug Administration; Hct, hematocrit; Hgb, hemoglobin; PPARγ, peroxisome proliferator-activated receptor-γ; SIADH, syndrome of inappropriate secretion of antidiuretic hormone.

TABLE A-2. *Insulin therapy*

Drug	Onset of action	Peak of action	End of action	Appearance	Cost per vial[a] ($)	Comments
General information						Insulin and its analogs lower blood glucose levels by stimulating peripheral glucose uptake, especially by skeletal muscle and fat, and by inhibiting hepatic glucose production; insulin inhibits lipolysis in the adipocyte, inhibits proteolysis, and enhances protein synthesis; insulin secreted by the beta cells of the pancreas is the principal hormone required for proper glucose use in normal metabolic processes When mixing two types of insulin, always draw clear regular insulin into the syringe first The concentration of insulin vials is 100 U/mL, and they are available as 10-mL vials Insulin glargine (Lantus) should not be mixed with other insulins
RAPID-ACTING						
Aspart (NovoLog)	5–10 min	40–50 min	3–5 hr	Clear	55	See General Information
Lispro (Humalog)	5 min	30–90 min	2–4 hr	Clear	45	Generally not given at night; if given at night (h.s.), blood glucose should be checked at midnight and 3 AM.

432

Insulin	Onset	Peak	Duration	Appearance	Cost[a]	Comments
SHORT-ACTING						
Regular (Humulin R, Novolin R)	30 min	2–5 hr	6–8 hr	Clear	30	See General Information. Generally not given at night; if given at night (h.s.), blood sugar should be checked at midnight and 3 AM
INTERMEDIATE-ACTING						
NPH (Humulin N, Novolin N)	2–4 hr	6–10 hr	14–18 hr	Cloudy	30	See General Information
Lente (Humulin L, Novolin L)	3–4 hr	6–12 hr	16–20 hr	Cloudy	30	
LONG-ACTING						
Glargine (Lantus)	1 hr	Peakless	24 hr	Clear	55	See General Information. Glargine (Lantus) cannot be mixed with any other insulins
Ultralente (Humulin U)	6–10 hr	8–20 hr	20–24 hr	Cloudy	30	
MIXTURES						
NPH-70/Regular-30	30 min	Dual	14–18 hr	Cloudy	30	See individual components and General Information
NPH-50/Regular-50	30 min	Dual	14–18 hr	Cloudy	30	
Humalog mix (75-NPH/25-Humalog)	5 min	Dual	14–18 hr	Cloudy	55	

[a]Cost based on Average Wholesale Price 2002 for one vial (10 mL) and rounded to the nearest $5. Price does not include dispensing fees charged by pharmacies if filled by prescription. Patients' costs may vary considerably.

TABLE A-3. *Oral agents for cardiovascular risk factor management*

Drug	Dose	Mechanism of action	Indication	Adverse reactions	Cost[a] ($, based on usual dose for 1 mo)	Comments
ADRENERGIC ANTAGONISTS—PERIPHERAL						
General information		Inhibits vasoconstriction, most likely by initially decreasing the release of norepinephrine from neuronal storage sites and then causing depletion of neuronal norepinephrine		*Contraindications:* Pheochromocytoma Heart failure Patients taking MAOIs Orthostatic hypotension (severe) Edema (see Contraindications) Depression Diarrhea Drowsiness/fatigue Dry mouth Angina Sexual dysfunction		Therapeutic utility: reserved as last-line antihypertensives in most cases Significant sodium and water retention occurs May aggravate asthma Exaggerates response to vasopressors
Guanadrel (Hylorel)	Initial: 5 mg b.i.d. Usual: 20–75 mg divided b.i.d. Maximum: 150 mg/day	See General Information	Labeled: Hypertension (in addition to a thiazide-type diuretic)	See General Information	110	Discontinue 2–3 days before surgery to reduce the possibility of vascular/ cardiovascular collapse during anesthesia
Reserpine (various)	Initial: 0.1–0.5 mg q.d. Usual: reduce to 0.1–0.25 mg q.d. Maximum: (long-term) 0.25 mg/day (see Comments)	Binds to and depletes stores of catecholamines and 5-hydroxytryptamine in central and peripheral adrenergic neurons resulting in decreased sympathetic outflow	Labeled: Hypertension Psychotic states (decreases agitation)	Depression (see Comments) Drowsiness Nasal congestion Weight gain Abdominal cramps Increased gastric acid production Diarrhea Edema Sexual dysfunction	<10	Therapeutic utility: rarely used due to high incidence of side effects Possible circulatory instability during surgery, even with preoperative withdrawal

α-ADRENERGIC AGONSITS—CENTRAL

Drug	Dosing	Mechanism	Indications	Side effects		Comments
General information		Central α_2 stimulation results in decreased sympathetic outflow		Dry mouth Sedation Hypotension Dizziness Bradycardia Constipation Sexual dysfunction Nausea Headache Urinary retention		Therapeutic utility: not considered first-line antihypertensive agents Abrupt withdrawal causes rebound hypertension Rebound hypertension may be more severe with concurrent administration of β-blockers
Clonidine (Catapres)	Initial: 0.1 mg b.i.d. Usual: 0.2–0.8 mg (divided b.i.d.) Maximum: 2.4 mg/day		Labeled: Hypertension Unlabeled: Hypertensive urgency Alcohol and opiate withdrawal Menopausal hot flashes Smoking cessation Tourette's syndrome	See General Information Depression	5–15	See General Information Patches are replaced weekly When initiating patches, full effects are not achieved until 2–3 days after application; if replacing another antihypertensive agent, the prior antihypertensive therapy may need gradual tapering over 2–3 days
Catapres TTS (transdermal patch)	Initial: TTS-1, 0.1-mg/24 hr patch weekly; add another patch or use a larger system in 1–2 wk Maximum: 0.6 mg/day (two TTS-3 patches)			Contact dermatitis/rash with patches	50–200	
Guanfacine (Tenex)	Initial: 1 mg h.s. Usual: 1 mg h.s. Maximum: 3 mg/day	See General Information	Labeled: Hypertension Unlabeled: Opiate withdrawal Migraine headache prophylaxis	See General Information Constipation	<10	See General Information Risk of rebound hypertension usually less severe and delayed 2–4 days due to long half-life
Guanabenz (Wytensin)	Initial: 4 mg b.i.d. Maximum: 32 mg/day	See General Information	Labeled: Hypertension	See General Information	10–45	See General Information

continued

TABLE A-3. *Continued*

Drug	Dose	Mechanism of action	Indication	Adverse reactions	Cost[a] ($, based on usual dose for 1 mo)	Comments
Methyldopa (Aldomet)	Initial: 250 mg b.i.d.–q.i.d. Usual: 500 mg–2 g daily (divided b.i.d.–q.i.d.) Maximum: 3 g/day	See General Information	Labeled: Hypertension	See General Information Positive Coombs test: 10–20% of patients within 6–12 mo Hemolytic anemia (rare) Hepatitis (rare) Lupus-like syndrome Urine discoloration	5–15	See General Information Traditional antihypertensive agent used in pregnancy
α_1-ADRENERGIC ANTAGONISTS—PERIPHERAL						
General information		Peripherally acting α_1 receptor antagonist; selectively blocks postsynaptic receptors, resulting in arteriolar and venous dilation		Orthostatic hypotension (especially with first dose) Dizziness Lightheadedness Drowsiness Headache Dry mouth Fatigue		Therapeutic utility: not recommended as first-line antihypertensive agents, but may be useful as a second-line agent in patients with hypertension and benign prostatic hyperplasia Give first doses and incremental dosing increases at bedtime to limit orthostatic hypotension
Doxazosin (Cardura)	Initial: 1 mg q.d. Usual: 1–4 mg q.d. Maximum: 16 mg/day	See General Information	Labeled: Hypertension Benign prostatic hyperplasia	See General Information	<10	See General Information Doses >4 mg q.d. increase risk of orthostatic hypotension
Prazosin (Minipress)	Initial: 1 mg b.i.d.–t.i.d. Usual: 6–15 mg/day (divided b.i.d.–t.i.d.) Maximum: 20 mg/day	See General Information	Labeled: Hypertension Unlabeled: Benign prostatic hyperplasia Raynaud's syndrome	See General Information	<10	See General Information A few patients may benefit from 40 mg/day
Terazosin (Hytrin)	Initial: 1 mg q.d. Usual: 1–5 mg q.d. Maximum: 20 mg/day	See General Information	Labeled: Hypertension Benign prostatic hyperplasia	See General Information	<10	See General Information

ANGIOTENSIN-CONVERTING ENZYME (ACE) INHIBITORS

	Action	Dosage	Indications	Contraindications/Adverse Effects		Comments
General information	Inhibits conversion of angiotensin I to angiotensin II by blocking ACE, resulting in suppression of the renin-angiotensin-aldosterone system			Contraindications: Pregnancy Bilateral renal artery stenosis or unilateral in patients with one kidney Cough Hyperkalemia Renal function impairment Angioedema Hypotension Dizziness Headache Rash Neutropenia/agranulocytopenia		Therapeutic utility: reduce risk of progression of diabetic nephropathy in hypertensive and normotensive patients; antihypertensive of choice in diabetic patients; first-line therapy for heart failure Beneficial effects in diabetic neuropathy and heart failure are believed to be drug class effects Angioedema occurrence is rare; it usually occurs with the first dose but may develop at any time Hypotensive effects worsened by volume depletion; use smaller initial doses in patients taking diuretics Antacids decrease bioavailability (particularly with captopril); separate administration times by 1–2 hr
Benazepril (Lotensin)	See General Information	Initial: 5–10 mg q.d. Usual: 20–40 mg q.d.–b.i.d. Maximum: 80 mg/day	Labeled: Hypertension Unlabeled: (see General Information)	See General Information	35–70	See General Information May be more effective with b.i.d. dosing to control hypertension Lower doses recommended for renal insufficiency
Captopril (Capoten)	See General Information	Initial: 6.25–25 mg b.i.d.–t.i.d. Usual: 25–100 mg b.i.d.–t.i.d. (see Comments) Maximum: 150–450 mg/day	Labeled: Hypertension Heart failure Asymptomatic dysfunction LV after myocardial infarction Diabetic nephropathy	See General Information Associated with higher rate of rashes than other ACE inhibitors Altered taste	<10	See General Information Target dose for heart failure: 50 mg t.i.d. Administer 1 hr before meals Lower doses recommended for renal insufficiency

continued

TABLE A-3. *Continued*

Drug	Dose	Mechanism of action	Indication	Adverse reactions	Cost[a] ($, based on usual dose for 1 mo)	Comments
Enalapril (Vasotec)	Initial: 2.5 mg q.d.–b.i.d. Usual: 10–40 mg q.d. or divided b.i.d. (see Comments) Maximum: 40 mg/day	See General Information	Labeled: Hypertension Heart failure Asymptomatic LV dysfunction Unlabeled: (see General Information)	See General Information Altered taste	5–20	See General Information Target dose for heart failure: 10 mg b.i.d. May be more effective with b.i.d. dosing to control hypertension Lower doses recommended for renal insufficiency Available in intravenous form
Fosinopril (Monopril)	Initial: 10 mg q.d. Usual: 20–40 mg q.d. (see Comments) Maximum: 80 mg/day	See General Information	Labeled: Hypertension Heart failure Unlabeled: (see General Information)	See General Information	45	See General Information Target dose for heart failure: 40 mg q.d. Dosage adjustment not required in renal insufficiency Consider dosing reduction in hepatic failure
Lisinopril (Prinivil, Zestril)	Initial: 2.5–10 mg q.d. Usual: 20–40 mg q.d. (see Comments) Maximum: 40 mg/day	See General Information	Labeled: Hypertension Heart failure Acute MI Unlabeled: Migraine headache prophylaxis (see General Information)	See General Information	<10	See General Information Target dose for heart failure: 20–40 mg q.d. Lower doses recommended for renal insufficiency
Moexipril (Univasc)	Initial: 3.75–7.5 mg q.d. Usual: 7.5–30 mg q.d. or divided b.i.d. Maximum: 60 mg/day	See General Information	Labeled: Hypertension Unlabeled: (see General Information)	See General Information	30–60	See General Information May be more effective with b.i.d. dosing to control hypertension Administer 1 hr before meals Consider dosing reduction in hepatic failure

438

Drug	Dosage		Indications	Elimination half-life (hr)		Comments
Perindopril (Aceon)	Initial: 2–4 mg q.d. Usual: 4–8 mg/day q.d. or divided b.i.d. Maximum: 16 mg/day (<8 mg/day advised for elderly)	See General Information	Labeled: Hypertension Unlabeled: (see General Information)	See General Information	40–60	See General Information May be more effective with b.i.d. dosing to control hypertension Lower doses recommended for renal insufficiency; safety and efficacy not established for CrCl <30 mL/min
Quinapril (Accupril)	Initial: 5–10 mg q.d. Usual: 20–80 mg q.d. or divided b.i.d. (see Comments) Maximum: 80 mg/day	See General Information	Labeled: Hypertension Heart failure Unlabeled: (see General Information)	See General Information	40–80	See General Information Target dose for heart failure: 20 mg b.i.d. May be more effective with b.i.d. dosing to control hypertension Lower doses recommended for renal insufficiency
Ramipril (Altace)	Initial: 1.25–2.5 mg q.d. Usual: 2.5–20 mg q.d. or divided b.i.d. (see Comments) Maximum: 10 mg/day	See General Information	Labeled: Reduction in risk of MI, stroke, and CV death in patients at high risk for CV disease Hypertension Heart failure after MI Unlabeled: (see General Information)	See General Information	40–100	See General Information Target dose for heart failure: 5 mg b.i.d. May be more effective with b.i.d. dosing to control hypertension Lower doses recommended for renal insufficiency Consider dosing reduction in hepatic failure Can sprinkle capsule contents on 4 oz apple sauce, apple juice, or water
Trandolapril (Mavik)	Initial: 0.5–2 mg q.d. Usual: 2–4 mg q.d. (see Comments) Maximum: 8 mg/day	See General Information	Labeled: Hypertension Heart failure LV dysfunction after MI Unlabeled: (see General Information)	See General Information	30	See General Information Target dose for heart failure: 4 mg q.d. May be more effective with b.i.d. dosing above 4 mg/day to control hypertension Lower doses recommended for renal insufficiency Initial recommended dose for patients with hepatic cirrhosis: 0.5 mg/day

continued

439

TABLE A-3. *Continued*

Drug	Dose	Mechanism of action	Indication	Adverse reactions	Cost[a] ($, based on usual dose for 1 mo)	Comments
ANGIOTENSIN II RECEPTOR BLOCKERS (ARBs)						
General information		Selectively binds to the angiotensin I receptor in the vascular smooth muscle and adrenal cortex, blocking the binding of angiotensin II, thus diminishing its effects		*Contraindications:* Pregnancy (see Comments) Hypotension Dizziness Headache Facial edema		Therapeutic utility: usually considered the second-line option in patients who can not tolerate ACE inhibitors (ACE inhibitors cost less and have better outcomes evidence) Use with caution in patients with prior angioedema caused by ACE inhibitors; use of ARBs in these patients may increase the risk for this recurrent angioedema Use with caution in patients with renal artery stenosis and/or renal dysfunction Use smaller initial doses for patients taking diuretics and/or with volume depletion
Candesartan (Atacand)	Initial: 8–16 mg q.d. Usual: 8–32 mg q.d. or divided b.i.d. Maximum: 32 mg/day	See General Information	Labeled: Hypertension Unlabeled: Microalbuminuria in type 2 diabetes mellitus Heart failure	See General Information	50–150	See General Information Consider dosing reductions in hepatic impairment
Eprosartan (Teveten)	Initial: 400–600 mg q.d. Usual: 400–800 mg q.d. or divided b.i.d. Maximum: 800 mg/day	See General Information	Labeled: Hypertension	See General Information	35–70	See General Information

440

Drug	Dosage		Indications			Comments
Irbesartan (Avapro)	Initial: 150 mg q.d. Usual: 300 mg q.d. Maximum: 300 mg/day	See General Information	Labeled: Hypertension Slow progression of kidney disease in type 2 diabetes mellitus and hypertension Unlabeled: Delay progression of diabetic nephropathy	See General Information	65	See General Information
Losartan (Cozaar)	Initial: 25–50 mg q.d. Usual: 25–100 mg q.d. or divided b.i.d. Maximum: 100 mg/day	See General Information	Labeled: Hypertension Slow progression of kidney disease in type 2 diabetes mellitus and hypertension Unlabeled: Heart failure in patients intolerant to ACE inhibitors or after MI Delay progression of diabetic nephropathy Stroke prevention in patients with hypertension and LV hypertrophy	See General Information Elevations in liver function tests and serum bilirubin have been reported	55–145	See General Information Consider dosing reductions in hepatic impairment
Olmesartan (Benicar)	Initial: 20 mg q.d. Usual: 40 mg q.d. Maximum: 40 mg/day	See General Information	Labeled: Hypertension	See General Information	45	See General Information

continued

TABLE A-3. *Continued*

Drug	Dose	Mechanism of action	Indication	Adverse reactions	Cost[a] ($, based on usual dose for 1 mo)	Comments
Telmisartan (Micardis)	Initial: 40 mg q.d. Usual: 20–80 mg q.d. Maximum: 80 mg/day	See General Information	Labeled: Hypertension Unlabeled: Delay progression of diabetic nephropathy Prevention of CV morbidity and mortality in high-risk patients	See General Information	50	See General Information
Valsartan (Diovan)	Initial: 40–80 mg q.d. Usual: 160–320 mg q.d. Maximum: 320 mg/day	See General Information	Labeled: Hypertension Heart failure in patient intolerant to ACE inhibitors Unlabeled: Delay progression of diabetic nephropathy	See General Information Hepatotoxicity has been reported	75	See General Information Consider dosing reductions in hepatic impairment and renal dysfunction
β-ADRENERGIC ANTAGONISTS General information		Block β receptors in heart (β_1) and/or peripheral vasculature, lung, pancreas, kidney and liver (β_2), resulting in vasodilation and decreased heart rate, force of contraction and output, and renin secretion		*Contraindications:* Bradycardia, >1st degree heart block Cardiogenic shock Acute heart failure Fatigue Dizziness Bradycardia Bronchospasms in predisposed patients Depression Hypotension Sexual dysfunction Dyslipidemia (usually transient) Exacerbation of heart failure		Therapeutic utility: effective antihypertensive agents for diabetic patients, particularly those with angina or after MI; benefits often outweigh the dyslipidemia and/or blunting of hypoglycemic effects associated with this drug class β_1-selective β-blockers lose selectivity with high doses High degree of interpatient variability between dose and effect Abrupt withdrawal may cause rebound hypertension and/or precipitate angina in patients with coronary heart disease

442

Drug	Dosage	Pharmacology	Indications		Comments
				Blunted hypoglycemic reactions	
Acebutolol (Sectral)	Initial: 200 mg q.d.–b.i.d. Usual: 400–800 mg q.d. or divided b.i.d. Maximum: 1,200 mg/day	See General Information β_1 selective with ISA and membrane-stabilizing activity	Labeled: Hypertension Ventricular arrhythmia	See General Information — 10–20	Rebound hypertension with clonidine withdrawal may be made more severe with concurrent administration of β-blockers See General Information Resting heart rate may be increased because of ISA
Atenolol (Tenormin)	Initial: 25 mg q.d. Usual: 50–100 mg q.d. (see Comments) Maximum: 200 mg/day	See General Information β_1 selective	Labeled: Hypertension Angina pectoris Acute MI Unlabeled: Alcohol withdrawal Migraine headache prophylaxis Ventricular arrhythmias	See General Information Low lipid solubility leads to low penetration in CNS and lower incidence of CNS adverse events — <10	See General Information Doses >100 mg q.d. are unlikely to produce additional antihypertensive benefits Lower doses are recommended for renal insufficiency Available in IV form
Betaxolol (Kerlone)	Initial: 10 mg q.d. Usual: 10–20 mg q.d. (see Comments) Maximum: 40 mg/day	See General Information β_1 selective with ISA and membrane-stabilizing activity	Labeled: Hypertension Reduction in ocular hypertension (ophthalmic drops)	See General Information — 40–60	See General Information Therapeutic utility: eye drops for glaucoma Systemic effects may be seen with ophthalmic administration Oral doses >20 mg are unlikely to produce additional antihypertensive benefits
Bisoprolol (Zebeta)	Initial: 2.5–5 mg q.d. Usual: 5–10 mg q.d. (see Comments) Maximum: 20 mg/day	See General Information β_1 selective	Labeled: Hypertension Unlabeled: Mild to moderate (NYHA class II–III) stable heart failure Angina pectoris Supraventricular arrhythmias Ventricular premature complexes	See General Information — 30	See General Information Lower doses recommended for renal and/or hepatic insufficiency

continued

TABLE A-3. *Continued*

Drug	Dose	Mechanism of action	Indication	Adverse reactions	Cost^a ($, based on usual dose for 1 mo)	Comments
Carteolol (Cartrol)	Initial: 2.5 mg q.d. Usual: 2.5–10 mg q.d. (see Comments) Maximum: 10 mg/day	See General Information Nonselective β-blocker with ISA	Labeled: Hypertension Reduction in ocular hypertension (ophthalmic drops) Unlabeled: Angina pectoris	See General Information	50–100	See General Information Lower doses recommended for renal insufficiency
Metoprolol (Lopressor) (Toprol-XL)	Initial: 12.5–50 mg divided b.i.d. Usual: 50–450 mg divided b.i.d. Maximum: 450 mg/day Heart failure: Initial: 12.5–25 mg q.d. Usual: 25–200 mg q.d. Maximum: 200 mg/day (see Comments) Hypertension: Initial: 25–100 mg q.d. Usual: 50–400 mg q.d. Maximum: 400 mg/day	See General Information β_1 selective	Labeled: Hypertension Angina pectoris Mild to moderate (NYHA class II–III), stable heart failure Unlabeled: Ventricular arrhythmias, supraventricular arrhythmias Migraine headache prophylaxis Essential tremor Aggressive behavior Antipsychotic-induced akathisia	See General Information	<10	See General Information Before initiating for heart failure, patients should be stabilized on ACE inhibitors, diuretic, and digoxin (if used) Lower dosing range and slow titration recommended in treatment of heart failure; dose should be titrated no sooner than every 2 wk Available in IV form

Drug	Dose		Indications			Comments
Nadolol (Corgard)	Initial: 40 mg q.d. Usual: 40–80 mg q.d. (see Comments) Maximum: 240–320 mg/day	See General Information Nonselective β-blocker	Labeled: Hypertension Angina pectoris Unlabeled: Ventricular arrhythmias Migraine headache prophylaxis Essential tremor and other tremors Aggressive behavior Antipsychotic induced akathisia Esophageal varices rebleeding Reduce intraocular pressure	See General Information	<10	See General Information Lower doses recommended for renal insufficiency
Penbutolol (Levatol)	Initial: 20 mg q.d. Usual: 20 mg q.d. (see Comments) Maximum: 80 mg/day	See General Information Nonselective β-blocker with ISA	Labeled: Hypertension	See General Information High lipid solubility leads to increased CNS penetration and depression	45	See General Information Doses >20 mg q.d. are unlikely to produce additional antihypertensive benefits Maximal effects may not be seen for several weeks, so titrate dose slowly
Pindolol (Visken)	Initial: 5 mg b.i.d. Usual: 20–60 mg divided b.i.d. (see Comments) Maximum: 60 mg/day	See General Information Nonselective β-blocker with ISA and membrane stabilizing activity	Labeled: Hypertension Unlabeled: Ventricular arrhythmias Anxiety Antipsychotic induced akathisia	See General Information	10–25	See General Information Maximal effects may not be seen for several weeks, so titrate dose slowly Lower doses recommended for severe renal and/or hepatic insufficiency

continued

TABLE A-3. *Continued*

Drug	Dose	Mechanism of action	Indication	Adverse reactions	Cost[a] ($, based on usual dose for 1 mo)	Comments
Propranolol (Inderal) (Inderal LA)	Initial: 10 mg t.i.d.–q.i.d. or 40 mg b.i.d. Usual: 120–240 mg divided b.i.d.–t.i.d. Maximum: 640 mg/day Initial: 80 mg q.d. Usual: 160 mg q.d. Maximum: 640 mg/day	See General Information Nonselective β-blocker with membrane-stabilizing activity	Labeled: Hypertension Angina pectoris Cardiac arrhythmias MI Pheochromocytoma Migraine headache prophylaxis Hypertrophic obstructive cardiomyopathy Essential tremor Unlabeled: Alcohol withdrawal Esophageal varices rebleeding Anxiety Thyrotoxicosis	See General Information High lipid solubility leads to increased CNS penetration and depression	<10	See General Information Therapeutic utility: more often used for noncardiovascular indications Lower doses recommended for hepatic insufficiency and in geriatric patients IV form available Recommended IV doses are much smaller than oral due to high first-pass effect
Timolol (Blocadren)	Initial: 10 mg b.i.d. Usual: 20–40 mg divided b.i.d. (see Comments) Maximum: 60 mg/day	See General Information Nonselective β-blocker	Labeled: Hypertension MI Migraine headache prophylaxis Glaucoma (ophthalmic drops) Unlabeled: Ventricular arrhythmia Essential tremor Anxiety	See General Information	40–85	See General Information Therapeutic utility: eye drops for glaucoma Systemic effects may be seen with ophthalmic administration Maximal systemic effects may not be seen for at least 1 week, so titrate dose slowly

446

β+α ADRENERGIC ANTAGONISTS

Drug	Dosage		Indications			Comments
Carvedilol (Coreg)	Heart failure: Initial: 3.125 mg b.i.d. Usual: 6.25–50 mg b.i.d. Maximum: 100 mg/day (see Comments) Hypertension: Initial: 6.25 mg b.i.d. Usual: 6.25–25 mg b.i.d. Maximum: 50 mg/day	See General Information for β-blocker Nonselective β-blocker and α₁-adrenergic blocker	Labeled: Mild to moderate (NYHA class II–III), stable heart failure Hypertension	See General Information for β-blocker	120–240	See General Information for β-blocker Before initiating for heart failure, patients should be stabilized on ACE inhibitors, diuretic, and digoxin (if used) Lower initial dosing range and slow titration recommended in treatment of heart failure; dose should be titrated no sooner than every 2 wk For patients weighing <85 kg, maximum dose is 25 mg b.i.d.
Labetalol (Normodyne, Trandate)	Initial: 100 mg b.i.d. Usual: 200–400 mg b.i.d. Maximum: 1,200–2,400 mg/day	See General Information for β-blocker Nonselective β-blocker and α₁-adrenergic blocker	Labeled: Hypertension Unlabeled: Hypertensive crisis Pheochromocytoma Acute aortic dissection Clonidine withdrawal	See General Information for β-blocker Nausea, particularly at higher doses	10–20	See General Information for β-blocker Available in IV form Oral labetalol has 3:1 β to α₁ activity; IV labetalol has 7:1 β to α₁ activity

continued

447

TABLE A-3. *Continued*

Drug	Dose	Mechanism of action	Indication	Adverse reactions	Cost[a] ($, based on usual dose for 1 mo)	Comments
CALCIUM CHANNEL BLOCKING AGENTS (CCBs)—DIHYDROPYRIDINES						
General information		Inhibits movement of calcium ions across cell membrane; result is decreased contraction of smooth muscle and depression of impulse formation and conduction velocity Dihydropyridines have greater effects on vascular smooth muscle compared to cardiac smooth muscle than do nondihydropyridines		Peripheral edema Exacerbation of heart failure Palpitations Dizziness Headache Flushing Arrhythmias (rare) Atrioventricular block (rare)		Therapeutic utility: not considered as first-line antihypertensive agents for diabetic patients but may be useful as add-on therapy for patients with comorbid conditions with indications for CCBs Preliminary data from controlled trials shows possible increased risk of MI after treatment of hypertension with CCBs; SR products should be used when possible; only SR doses are included in this table, except where noted Do not stop therapy abruptly Limit caffeine and alcohol intake Unless noted, sustained-release formulations should not be crushed *Warning:* risk of bradycardia is increased when used concurrently with β-blockers or digoxin Unless noted, all agents are CYP3A3/4 substrates with numerous related drug interactions

448

Drug	Dosage		Indications			Comments
Amlodipine (Norvasc)	Initial: 2.5–5 mg q.d. Usual: 5–10 mg q.d. (see Comments) Maximum: 10 mg/day	See General Information	Labeled: Angina pectoris—chronic stable and vasospastic Hypertension	See General Information	50–75	See General Information Titrate over 7–14 days unless more rapid clinical outcome is warranted Lower doses recommended in hepatic dysfunction and in geriatric patients
Felodipine (Plendil)	Initial: 5 mg q.d. Usual: 5–10 mg q.d. (see Comments) Maximum: 10 mg/day	See General Information	Labeled: Hypertension Unlabeled: Heart failure Raynaud's syndrome	See General Information	45–77	See General Information Titrate over 2 wk Grapefruit juice increases bioavailability and should be avoided Lower doses recommended in hepatic dysfunction and in geriatric patients
Isradipine (DynaCirc)	Initial: 2.5 mg b.i.d. Usual: 2.5–10 mg b.i.d. Maximum: 20 mg/day	See General Information	Labeled: Hypertension	See General Information	90–140	See General Information Doses >10 mg/day are unlikely to produce additional antihypertensive benefits Capsule may be opened; do not crush contents
(DynaCirc CR)	Initial: 5 mg q.d. Usual: 5–10 mg q.d. Maximum: 20 mg/day				50–80	
Nicardipine (Cardene)	Initial: 20 mg t.i.d. Usual: 20–40 mg t.i.d. Maximum: 120 mg/day	See General Information	Labeled: Angina pectoris—chronic stable (immediate release only) Hypertension Unlabeled: Heart failure	See General Information	50–100	See General Information Lower initial doses recommended in hepatic dysfunction Take with food Available in IV formulation
(Cardene SR)	Initial: 30 mg b.i.d. Usual: 30–60 mg b.i.d. Maximum: 120 mg/day					

continued

TABLE A-3. *Continued*

Drug	Dose	Mechanism of action	Indication	Adverse reactions	Cost[a] ($, based on usual dose for 1 mo)	Comments
Nifedipine SR (Adalat CC, Procardia XL)	Initial: 30–60 mg q.d. Usual: 30–60 mg q.d. Maximum: 90 mg/day	See General Information	Labeled: Angina pectoris—vasospastic Hypertension Unlabeled: Migraine headache Primary pulmonary hypertension Lower esophageal sphincter spasm	See General Information Dyspnea Muscle cramping Nausea Gingival hyperplasia (rare)	40–80	See General Information Currently no indication for immediate-release nifedipine Negative inotropic effects can worsen congestive heart failure Adalat CC should be taken with food Lower doses recommended in cirrhosis CYP3A3/4 and CYP3A5-7 substrate—cimetidine, quinidine, and grapefruit juice may increase nifedipine concentrations; nifedipine may increase theophylline, vincristine, digoxin, and warfarin concentrations
Nimodipine (Nimotop)	Usual: 60 mg q 4 h for 21 days	See General Information Has greatest effect on cerebral arteries due to high lipophilicity	Labeled: Subarachnoid hemorrhage (SAH) Unlabeled: Migraine headache	See General Information Hypotension	1,000 (21-day supply)	See General Information Begin therapy within 96 hr of SAH and continue for 21 days Reduce dose to 30 mg q 4 h in patients with liver failure If capsule cannot be swallowed, liquid may be removed from capsules with an 18-gauge needle; contents should be drawn into a syringe and given via nasogastric tube Shown to reduce severity of neurologic deficits caused by cerebral vasospasm after SAH

CALCIUM CHANNEL BLOCKING AGENTS—NONDIHYDROPYRIDINES

Drug	Dosage	General Information	Labeled		Comments
Nisoldipine (Sular)	Initial: 20 mg q.d. Usual: 20–40 mg q.d. Maximum: 60 mg/day	See General Information	Labeled: Hypertension	40	See General Information Grapefruit juice and high-fat meals increase bioavailability and should be avoided Lower doses recommended in hepatic dysfunction

General information

Inhibits movement of calcium ions across cell membrane; result is decreased contraction of smooth muscle and depression of impulse formation and conduction velocity

Nondihydropyridines are more selective for cardiac smooth muscle compared with vascular smooth muscle than are dihydropyridines

See General Information

Therapeutic utility: not considered as first-line antihypertensive agents for diabetic patients but may be useful in reducing progression of diabetic nephropathy; patients unable to tolerate ACE inhibitors or ARBs, or as add-on therapy for comorbid conditions with indications for CCBs

Preliminary data from controlled trials shows possible increased risk of MI after treatment of hypertension with CCBs; SR products should be used if possible; only SR doses are included in this table, except where noted

Do not stop therapy abruptly

Limit caffeine and alcohol intake

Unless noted, SR formulations should not be crushed

Warning: risk of bradycardia is increased when used concurrently with β-blockers or digoxin

continued

TABLE A-3. *Continued*

Drug	Mechanism of action	Indication	Adverse reactions	Cost[a] ($, based on usual dose for 1 mo)	Comments
Bepridil (Vascor)	See General Information Also inhibits fast sodium channels (antiarrhythmic effect) Dose Initial: 200 mg q.d. Usual: 300 mg q.d. Maximum: 400 mg/day	Labeled: Angina pectoris—chronic stable	Palpitations Dizziness Nervousness Headache Asthenia Tinnitus Tremor Gastrointestinal: nausea, diarrhea, abdominal pain Dyspnea Anorexia	120	See General Information Therapeutic utility: limited use except for antiarrhythmic properties *Warning:* Bepridil has class I antiarrhythmic properties, can cause prolonged QT interval, and can induce ventricular tachycardia and fibrillation Monitor electrocardiographic changes during therapy Hypokalemia can potentiate arrhythmias CYP3A3/4 substrate—bepridil may increase concentrations of cyclosporine and digoxin
Diltiazem (Cardizem CD, Cartia XT, Dilacor XR, Tiazac)	See General Information Dose Initial: 180–240 q.d. Usual: 240–360 mg q.d. Maximum: Cardizem CD—360 mg/day, Cartia XT—480 mg/day, Dilacor XR or Tiazac—540 mg/day (see Comments)	Labeled: Angina pectoris—chronic stable and vasospastic Hypertension Arrhythmias Unlabeled: Raynaud's syndrome	Atrioventricular block Bradycardia Peripheral edema Exacerbation of heart failure Hypotension Flushing Dizziness Headache	50–120	See General Information Available in IV formulation Various products are not bioequivalent or therapeutically equivalent Lower doses are recommended in hepatic dysfunction CYP3A3/4 substrate: CYP1A2, CYP2D6, and CYP3A3/4 inhibitor—diltiazem may increase the effect of amiodarone, cimetidine, moricizine, cyclosporine, digoxin, theophylline, and carbamazepine

Verapamil (Calan SR, Covera, Isoptin SR, Verelan)	Initial: 120–240 mg q.d. Usual: 240 mg q.d. Maximum: 480 mg	See General Information	Labeled: Angina pectoris— vasospastic, chronic stable, and unstable Hypertension Arrhythmias Unlabeled: Migraine headache Cardiomyopathy	Constipation Atrioventricular block Bradycardia Peripheral edema Exacerbation of heart failure Dizziness Headache	15	See General Information SR capsules should be taken with food Available in IV formulation Lower doses are recommended in hepatic dysfunction CYP1A2 and CYP3A4 substrate; CYP3A3/4 inhibitor—may decrease the effect of phenobarbital, phenytoin, and rifampin; may increase the effect of amiodarone, aspirin, cimetidine, carbamazepine, cyclosporine, lithium, and theophylline
DIURETICS—LOOP General information		Block chloride, sodium, and water reabsorption in the loop of Henle, with possible additional effects on proximal and/or distal tubules		Electrolyte imbalances (↓K, Cl, Mg, Ca, Phos, Na) Dehydration Azotemia Ototoxicity (especially with rapid IV infusion) Tinnitus Hyperuricemia Hyperglycemia Rash, photosensitivity Dyslipidemia Sexual dysfunction		Therapeutic utility: primarily beneficial in treating edema; agents do not have beneficial cardiovascular evidence found with thiazides diuretics Useful in patients with renal insufficiency because not reliant on glomerular filtration

continued

453

TABLE A-3. *Continued*

Drug	Dose	Mechanism of action	Indication	Adverse reactions	Cost[a] ($, based on usual dose for 1 mo)	Comments
Bumetanide (Bumex)	Initial: 0.5 mg q.d.–b.i.d. Usual: 0.5–2 mg q.d.–t.i.d. Maximum: 10 mg/day	See General Information	Labeled: Edema	See General Information	5–15	See General Information Contains sulfhydryl group; cross-reaction in sulfonamide-allergic patients may occur Available in IV form IV/PO conversion 1:1 IV furosemide/IV bumetanide: 40:1
Furosemide (Lasix)	Initial: 20 mg q.d.–t.i.d. Usual: 20–80 mg q.d.–b.i.d. (wide variability) Maximum: 600 mg/day (see Comments)	See General Information	Labeled: Edema Hypertension Unlabeled: Hypercalcemia	See General Information	<10	See General Information Bioavailability may be decreased in patients with heart failure Contains sulfhydryl group; cross-reaction in sulfonamide-allergic patients may occur Available in IV form IV/PO conversion 1:2 IV furosemide/IV bumetanide: 40:1 Oral and IV doses of 2–2.5 gm/day or higher have been well tolerated

DIURETICS—THIAZIDES AND RELATED AGENTS

Drug	Dosage	Mechanism	Indications	Adverse Effects		Comments
Torsemide (Demadex)	Initial: 5 mg q.d. Usual: 10–20 mg q.d. Maximum: 200 mg/day	See General Information	Labeled: Edema Hypertension	See General Information	30–35	See General Information Contains sulfhydryl group; cross-reaction in sulfonamide-allergic patients may occur Available in IV form IV/PO conversion 1:1 ~20 mg IV furosemide ~5–10 mg IV torsemide
General Information		Increase urinary excretion of sodium and chloride by inhibiting sodium ion transport in the distal tubule	Labeled: Edema Hypertension Unlabeled: Diabetes insipidus Prevention of calcium nephrolithiasis associated with hypercalcemia Osteoporosis	Electrolyte imbalances (↓K, Cl, Mg, Na; ↑Ca and uric acid) Dehydration Rash/photosensitivity Nausea Hypersensitivity reactions Dyslipidemia (usually transient) Hyperglycemia Sexual dysfunction Hematologic abnormalities (rare)		Therapeutic utility: recommended as first-line therapy for hypertension or as second agent of choice; minimal effects on lipids and glycemic control at lower dosing ranges Contain sulfhydryl group; cross-reaction in sulfonamide-allergic patients may occur Not effective in patients with CrCl <30 mL/min (except for metolazone)
Chlorothiazide (Diuril)	Initial: 500 mg q.d.–b.i.d. Usual: 500 mg q.d.–b.i.d. Maximum 2,000 mg/day	See General Information	See General Information	See General Information	<10	See General Information Available in IV form

continued

TABLE A-3. *Continued*

Drug	Dose	Mechanism of action	Indication	Adverse reactions	Cost[a] ($, based on usual dose for 1 mo)	Comments
Chlorthalidone (Hydroton)	Initial: 25 mg q.d. Usual: 25 mg q.d. Maximum: 200 mg/day	See General Information	See General Information	See General Information	<10	See General Information Doses >25 mg are associated with continued reductions in potassium, but provide no additional benefit in diuresis or blood pressure reduction
Hydrochloro-thiazide (Hydro-DIURIL)	Initial: 12.5–25 mg q.d. Usual: 12.5–25 mg q.d. Maximum: 50 mg/day	See General Information	See General Information	See General Information	<10	See General Information Doses >50 mg are associated with marked reductions in potassium; doses >25 provide little additional benefit in blood pressure reduction
Indapamide (Lozol)	Initial: 1.25–2.5 mg q.d. Usual: 1.25–2.5 mg q.d. Maximum: 5 mg/day	See General Information	See General Information	See General Information	<10	See General Information Doses >5 mg are associated with continued reductions in potassium but provide no additional benefit in diuresis or blood pressure reduction Not associated with causing dyslipidemia
Metolazone (Zaroxolyn) (Mykrox)	Initial: 2.5–5 mg q.d. Usual: 5–20 mg q.d. Maximum: 20 mg/day Initial: 0.5 mg q.d. Usual: 0.5–1 mg q.d. Maximum: 1 mg/day	See General Information		See General Information	40–100 45–90	See General Information Zaroxolyn and Mylrox are not bioequivalent or therapeutically equivalent May be useful in patients with CrCl <30 mL/min Long half-life may cause prolonged diuresis Hypokalemia is common and may limit duration of therapy

456

DIURETICS—POTASSIUM-SPARING

Drug	Mechanism	Dosage	Indications	Side effects		Comments
Amiloride (Midamor)	Act directly at the distal convoluted tubule and collecting ducts to decrease active transport of sodium and potassium	Initial: 5 mg q.d. Usual: 10 mg q.d. Maximum: 20 mg/day	Labeled: Adjunctive treatment with thiazide or loop diuretics in heart failure and hypertension Unlabeled: Reduction of lithium-induced polyuria without increasing lithium levels as seen with other diuretics Hyperaldosteronism	Headache Gastrointestinal: nausea/vomiting, anorexia, diarrhea Hyperkalemia Dizziness Rash Gynecomastia Sexual dysfunction Hyperchloremic metabolic acidosis Hyponatremia	25	Therapeutic utility: restore or prevent serum potassium in patients who are taking kaliuretic diuretics May cause hyperkalemia in diabetics, even those without evidence of nephropathy; use in diabetic patients is cautioned, and close serum electrolyte and renal function monitoring is recommended, if used Use with caution in patients with renal dysfunction due to potential risk for hyperkalemia
Spironolactone (Aldosterone)	Competitive inhibitor of aldosterone in the distal convoluted tubule	Heart failure: Initial: 12.5–25 mg q.d. Usual: 25 mg q.d. Other indications: Initial: 50 mg q.d.–b.i.d. Usual: 50–200 mg q.d. or divided b.i.d. Maximum: 400 mg/day	Labeled: Primary aldosteronism Edema Hypertension Hypokalemia associated with kaliuretic diuretics Unlabeled: Heart failure (see Comments)	Hyperkalemia Drowsiness Mental confusion Fatigue Headache Gastrointestinal: cramping, diarrhea, nausea/vomiting Rash Menstrual abnormalities Gynecomastia Breast tenderness Sexual dysfunction Hyperchloremic metabolic acidosis Hyponatremia	20–80	Therapeutic utility: edema and ascites due to hepatic impairment and heart failure (NYHA class IV) in patients taking diuretics, ACE inhibitors, β-blockers and digoxin Use with caution in patients with renal dysfunction due to potential risk for hyperkalemia In treatment of heart failure, patients who experience hyperkalemia may be able to continue therapy and reduce serum potassium with dosing reductions to 12.5 mg q.d. or 25 mg q.o.d.

continued

457

TABLE A-3. *Continued*

Drug	Dose	Mechanism of action	Indication	Adverse reactions	Cost[a] ($, based on usual dose for 1 mo)	Comments
Triamterene (Dyrenium)	Initial: 50 mg q.d. Usual: 50–100 mg q.d. Maximum: 300 mg/day	Act directly at the distal convoluted tubule and collecting ducts to decrease active transport of sodium and potassium	Labeled: Edema Hypokalemia associated with kaliuretic diuretics			Therapeutic utility: common agent in combination diuretic products to restore or prevent serum potassium in patients who are taking kaliuretic diuretics
SELECTIVE ALDOSTERONE RECEPTOR BLOCKER						
Eplerenone (Inspra)	Initial: 25–50 mg q.d. Usual: 50 mg q.d.–b.i.d. Maximum: 100 mg/day	Binds to the mineralocorticoid receptor in epithelial tissue (kidney) and nonepithelial tissue (heart, blood vessels and brain) to selectively block the effects of aldosterone	Labeled: Hypertension Unlabeled: Heart failure Delay progression of diabetic proteinuria	Dizziness Hyperkalemia Fatigue Flu-like symptoms Diarrhea Cough Gynecomastia Abnormal vaginal bleeding	Not available	FDA approved, fall 2002 Contraindicated in patients with type 2 diabetes mellitus microalbuminuria Metabolized by CYP3A4 enzyme system Contraindicated with strong CYP3A4 inhibitors (ketoconazole, itraconazole) Use with caution with weak CYP3A4 inhibitors (erythromycin, saquinavir, verapamil and fluconazole); a lower initial dose of 25 mg q.d. is recommended Use with caution with other drugs that cause hyperkalemia including ACE inhibitors, ARBs, potassium supplements, and salt substitutes containing potassium

DYSLIPIDEMIC AGENTS—BILE ACID RESINS

Drug	Dosage	Mechanism	Indications	Cost ($)	Contraindications/Adverse Effects	Comments
Cholestyramine (Questran, Questran Light)	Initial: 4 g q.d.–b.i.d. Usual: 4–8 g q.d.–b.i.d. Maximum: 16–24 g/day	Forms a nonabsorbable complex with bile acids in the intestines; inhibits enterohepatic reuptake of bile salts and thereby increasing fecal loss of bile salt-bound LDL cholesterol	Labeled: Hyperlipidemia	20–55	*Contraindications:* Complete biliary obstruction, Bowel obstruction; Abdominal pain, Bloating, Constipation, Flatulence, Gastrointestinal discomfort, Diarrhea, Hypertriglyceridemia	Therapeutic utility: adverse effects limit use, but may have a role as add-on therapy in patients not achieving goal with monotherapy. Numerous drug interactions due to binding with other medications: digoxin, fat-soluble vitamins, thyroid hormone medications, warfarin, and others. Take other medications 1 hr before or 4–6 hr after cholestyramine. Do not administer the powder in its dry form; mix with fluids. Not systemically absorbed. Cholestyramine may ↑triglyceride levels. See Cholestyramine
Colestipol (Colestid)	Initial: 5 g q.d. Usual: 5–30 g b.i.d.–q.i.d. Maximum: 30 g/day	See Cholestyramine	Labeled: Hyperlipidemia	65–195	See Cholestyramine	
Colesevelam (Welchol)	Usual: 3 tablets b.i.d. with meals or 6 tablets q.d. with a meal Maximum: 7 tabs/day	Colesevelam binds bile acids in the intestines, impeding their reabsorption, thus increasing the fecal loss of bile salt-bound LDL cholesterol	Labeled: Hyperlipidemia	145	*Contraindications:* Bowel obstruction, Constipation, Dyspepsia, Myalgia	When used in combination with the HMG-CoA reductase inhibitors, the maximum recommended dose is 6 tablets/day. Give with meals. Should be used with caution or avoided in patients with elevated triglycerides

continued

TABLE A-3. *Continued*

Drug	Dose	Mechanism of action	Indication	Adverse reactions	Cost[a] ($, based on usual dose for 1 mo)	Comments
DYSLIPIDEMIC AGENTS—CHOLESTEROL ABSORPTION INHIBITORS						
Ezetimibe (Zetia)	Usual: 10 mg q.d.	Reduces cholesterol by inhibiting absorption of cholesterol by the small intestine; this reduces total cholesterol, LDL-cholesterol, and triglycerides and increases HDL-cholesterol in patients with hypercholesterolemia	Labeled: Hypercholesterolemia	*Contraindications:* Combination with an HMG-CoA reductase inhibitor in patients with active liver disease or unexplained persistent elevations in serum transaminases Abdominal pain Diarrhea Musculoskeletal system disorders Arthralgia Back pain	60	Therapeutic utility: newly FDA-approved medication; usefulness and application in clinical practice are yet to be determined The effects of ezetimibe, given either alone or in addition to an HMG-CoA reductase inhibitor, on cardiovascular morbidity and mortality have not been established
DYSLIPIDEMIC AGENTS—FIBRIC ACID DERIVATIVES						
Gemfibrozil (Lopid)	Usual: 600 mg b.i.d., 30 min before morning and evening meal Maximum: 1,200 mg/day	Inhibits peripheral lipolysis and decreases the hepatic extraction of free fatty acids; also, ↓serum triglycerides and VLDL and ↑HDL cholesterol	Labeled: Hypertriglyceridemia types IV and V hyperlipidemia	*Contraindications:* Significant hepatic or renal dysfunction Primary biliary cirrhosis Preexisting gallbladder disease Abdominal/epigastric pain Dyspepsia Diarrhea Rash Hepatotoxicity	15	Increased risk of rhabdomyolysis when given with the HMG-CoA reductase inhibitors Use in combination with statins produces a dose-dependent reduction in LDL-cholesterol

460

			Labeled/Unlabeled	Contraindications		Notes
Fenofibrate (Tricor)	Initial: 54- or 160-mg tab q.d. with meals Usual: 160 mg tab q.d. with meals Maximum: 160 mg/day	↑VLDL catabolism, resulting in ↓VLDL levels and reduction of plasma triglycerides by 30–60% Also see a modest ↑ in HDL	Labeled: Types IV and V Hyperlipidemia	*Contraindications:* Significant hepatic or renal dysfunction Preexisting gallbladder disease Gastrointestinal disturbances -Liver function tests Dyspepsia	30–95	Increased risk of rhabdomyolosis when given with the HMG-CoA reductase inhibitors Contraindicated in patients with severe hepatic or renal impairment or preexisting gallbladder disease

DYSLIPIDEMIC AGENTS—HMG-CoA REDUCTASE INHIBITORS

General information		Inhibits HMG-CoA, the enzyme that catalyzes the rate-limiting step in cholesterol biosynthesis	Labeled: Hypercholesterolemia and mixed lipidemias Unlabeled: Reduce proteinuria in hypertensive patients	*Contraindications:* Active liver disease Unexplained persistent elevations of serum transaminase Pregnancy Heartburn/flatulence Rash/pruritus ↑Creatinine phosphokinase Myalgia Hepatotoxicity	Therapeutic utility: after diet and exercise, the statins are considered first-line therapy to achieve desired LDL reductions Monitor liver function tests at baseline and after 12 wk of therapy, then annually thereafter Statins produce a dose-dependent reduction in LDL-cholesterol and fluvastatin Statins (except pravastatin) are metabolized by the CYP3A4 enzyme system; watch for interactions with other drugs metabolized by this system Rhabdomyolysis is a rare but limiting adverse event associated with this class of medications, and the risk increases when concomitant medications cyclosporine, gemfibrozil, niacin, erythromycin, itraconazole, or ketoconazole are used

continued

461

TABLE A-3. *Continued*

Drug	Dose	Mechanism of action	Indication	Adverse reactions	Cost[a] ($, based on usual dose for 1 mo)	Comments
Atorvastatin (Lipitor)	Initial: 10 mg q.d. Usual: 10–80 mg q.d. Maximum: 80 mg/day	See General Information	See General Information	See General Information	80–130	Greatest dose-dependent reduction of LDL-cholesterol LDL percentage reduction is 38–54%
Fluvastatin (Lescol, Lescol XL)	Initial: 20 mg h.s. Usual: 40–80 mg h.s. Maximum: 80 mg/day		See General Information	See General Information	60–75	Weakest dose dependent reduction in LDL cholesterol LDL percentage reduction is 17–33%; metabolized by CYP2C9 isoenzyme; less likely to be involved in drug interactions
Lovastatin (Mevacor) (Altocor)	Initial: 10–20 mg qPM with meal Usual: 20–80 mg qPM with meal Maximum: 80 mg/day	See General Information	See General Information	See General Information	25–90	LDL percentage reduction is 29–45% Must be taken with evening meal to facilitate absorption Altocor is formulated as extended-release lovastatin
Pravastatin (Pravachol)	Initial: 10–20 h.s. Usual: 10–80 mg h.s. Maximum: 80 mg/day	See General Information	See General Information	See General Information	100–150	LDL percentage reduction is 19–40% Not significantly metabolized by the CYP3A4 enzyme system; less likely to be involved in drug interactions
Simvastatin (Zocor)	Initial: 10 mg h.s. Usual: 10–80 mg h.s. Maximum: 80 mg/day	See General Information	See General Information	See General Information	90–155	LDL percentage reduction is 28–48%

DYSLIPIDEMIC AGENTS—NICOTINIC ACID

Drug	Usual dosage	Mechanism of action		Contraindications/adverse effects	Therapeutic utility
Nicotinic acid (Niacin)	Immediate-release: Initial (start low to minimize adverse effects): 500 mg b.i.d. Usual: 1 g b.i.d.–t.i.d. with meals Maximum: 3–6 g/day	Mechanism of action is not entirely understood; involves partial inhibition of release of free fatty acids from adipose tissue and increased lipoprotein lipase activity, which increases the rate of triglyceride removal from plasma; decreases the rate of hepatic synthesis of VLDL and LDL-cholesterol and does not affect fecal excretion of fats, sterols, or bile acids	Labeled: Hyperlipidemia and mixed lipidemias	10–30	*Contraindications:* Severe liver disease Active peptic ulcer disease Severe hypotension Arterial hemorrhage Facial flushing Hepatic dysfunction Hyperglycemia Hyperuricemia Gastric irritation	Aspirin or NSAID administration 30 min before dose minimizes the risk of flushing
(Niaspan)	Extended-release: Initial: 500 mg h.s. Usual: 1–2 g h.s. Maximum: 2 g/day			40–90		

PLATELET INHIBITORS

Drug	Usual dosage	Mechanism of action		Adverse effects	Therapeutic utility
Aspirin (Ascriptin, Bayer, Ecotrin, St. Joseph)	Usual: 75–325 mg q.d. with food	Acetylates cyclooxygenase, leading to inhibition of prostaglandins and thromboxane A_2, thereby inhibiting vasoconstriction and release and aggregation of platelets	Labeled: Myocardial infarction prophylaxis (300–325 mg q.d.) Transient ischemic attack prophylaxis in males (1,300 mg/day in 2–4 divided doses)	<1 Rash Gastrointestinal bleeding Dyspepsia Tinnitus Prolonged bleeding time	Therapeutic utility: recommended for primary prevention in diabetes mellitus patients >40 yr with one or more other CV risk factors unless contraindicated; consider in diabetes mellitus patients 30–40 yr with one or more other CV risk factors

continued

TABLE A-3. *Continued*

Drug	Dose	Mechanism of action	Indication	Adverse reactions	Cost[a] ($, based on usual dose for 1 mo)	Comments
						Discontinue 7 days before elective surgery Use with caution in asthmatics: hypersensitivity may occur Available in buffered and enteric-coated tablets; however, these do not improve gastrointestinal toxicity; do not crush these formulations Administer with food and a full glass of water
Cilostazol (Pletal)	Usual: 100 mg b.i.d. 1 hr before or 2 hr after a meal	Inhibits cAMP phosphodiesterase III, resulting in vasodilation and inhibition of platelet aggregation	Labeled: Reduction of signs and symptoms of intermittent claudication, indicated by increased walking distance	*Black box warning:* Increased mortality in patients with congestive heart failure Headache Palpitations Diarrhea Peripheral edema Dizziness	100	Concentration of cilostazol increased by strong inhibitors of CYP3A4 (diltiazem, erythromycin, itraconazole, grapefruit juice) and CYP2C19 (omeprazole) Dose should be reduced to 50 mg b.i.d. if used concurrently with strong inhibitors of CYP3A4 and CYP2C19 Contraindicated in patients with congestive heart failure May take up to 12 wk for peak effect
Clopidogrel (Plavix)	Usual: 75 mg q.d.	Inhibits ADP-induced platelet aggregation by directly inhibiting binding of ADP to its receptor; thereby prevents glycoprotein IIb/IIIa complex activation	Labeled: Reduction of thrombotic events secondary to MI, stroke, and peripheral artery disease; ACS (including those managed with PCI or CABG)	Bleeding Neutropenia Agranulocytosis Gastrointestinal abdominal pain, constipation Rash Headache Dizziness	120	In ACS, use concomitantly with aspirin May be administered without regard to meals Discontinue 5 days before elective surgery May be used concomitantly with heparin Use caution when taken concomitantly with NSAIDs or warfarin Load with 300 mg before PCI

464

Drug	Usual dose	Mechanism of action	Labeled indication	Adverse effects	Cost	Comments
Dipyridamole (Persantine)	Usual: 75–100 mg q.i.d. 1 hr before meals	Inhibits platelet adhesion, possibly by inhibition of red blood cell reuptake of adenosine, phosphodiesterase activity, or thromboxane A_2 formation	Labeled: Adjunct to coumarin anticoagulants in prevention of postoperative thromboembolic complications of cardiac valve replacement	Dizziness Abdominal distress Hypotension	75–100	Available in IV formulation Should be taken with water 1 hr before meals
Ticlopidine (Ticlid)	Usual: 250 mg b.i.d. with food	Interferes with platelet membrane function, ADP-induced platelet-fibrinogen binding, and subsequent platelet-platelet interactions	Labeled: Decreases risk of thrombotic stroke	*Black box warning:* Neutropenia Agranulocytosis Thrombotic thrombocytopenic purpura Elevated cholesterol and triglycerides Elevated liver function tests Gastrointestinal diarrhea Rash	150	Therapeutic utility: use limited due to rare but serious adverse events Food increases absorption Discontinue 10–14 days before elective surgery if possible CBC needed every 2 wk for first 3 mo of therapy Discontinue if absolute neutrophil count is <1,200/ mm^3 or platelet count is <80,000/mm^3 CYP2C19 inhibitor-decreases effect of digoxin and cyclosporine; increases effect of cimetidine and theophylline Antacids decrease absorption

[a] Cost based on Average Wholesale Price 2002 of "usual dose" range for a 30-day supply and rounded to the nearest $5. Generic price provided if available. Price does not include dispensing fees charged by pharmacies. Patients' costs may vary considerably.

ACS, acute coronary syndromes; ADP, adenosine diphosphate; cAMP, cyclic adenosine monophosphate; CABG, coronary artery bypass grafting; CBC, complete blood count; CNS, central nervous system; CV, cardiovascular; FDA, U.S. Food and Drug Administration; HDL, high-density lipoprotein; HMG-CoA, 3-hydroxy-3-methylglutaryl coenzyme A; ISA, intrinsic sympathomimetic activity; IV, intravenous; LDL, low-density lipoprotein; LV, left ventricular; MAOIs, monoamine oxidase inhibitors; MI, myocardial infarction; NSAIDs, nonsteroidal antiinflammatory drugs; NYHA, New York Heart Association; PCI, percutaneous coronary intervention; PO, by mouth; VLDL, very-low-density lipoprotein.

TABLE A-4. *Common combination products for cardiovascular risk factor management*

Drug	Strength	Dose[a]	Cost[b] based on usual dose for 1 mo ($)	Comments
ANGIOTENSIN-CONVERTING ENZYME INHIBITOR/CALCIUM CHANNEL BLOCKER				
Benazepril/Amlodipine (Lotrel)	10 mg/2.5 mg 10 mg/5 mg 20 mg/5 mg 20 mg/10 mg	q.d.	70–85	See individual components
Enalapril/Felodipine (Lexxel)	5 mg/2.5 mg 5 mg/5 mg	q.d.	50	See individual components
Trandolapril/Verapamil (Tarka)	1 mg/240 mg 2 mg/180 mg 2 mg/240 mg 4 mg/250 mg	q.d.	65–70	See individual components
ANGIOTENSIN-CONVERTING ENZYME INHIBITOR/DIURETIC				
Enalapril/HCTZ (Vaseretic)	5 mg/12.5 mg 10 mg/25 mg	1–2 tabs q.d.	10–20	See individual components
Fosinopril/HCTZ (Monopril-HCT)	10 mg/12.5 mg 20 mg/12.5 mg	1–2 tabs q.d.	45–90	See individual components
Lisinopril/HCTZ (Prinzide, Zestoretic)	10 mg/12.5 mg 20 mg/12.5 mg 20 mg/25 mg	1–2 tabs q.d.	10–20	See individual components
Moexipril/HCTZ (Uniretic)	7.5 mg/12.5 mg 15 mg/12.5 mg 15 mg/25 mg	1–2 tabs q.d.	35–70	See individual components
Quinapril/HCTZ (Accuretic)	10 mg/12.5 mg 20 mg/12.5 mg 20 mg/25 mg	1–2 tabs q.d.	40–80	See individual components
ANGIOTENSIN II RECEPTOR BLOCKER/DIURETIC				
Candesartan/HCTZ (Atacand HCT)	16 mg/12.5 mg 32 mg/12.5 mg	q.d.	60	See individual components
Eprosartan/HCTZ (Teveten HCT)	600 mg/12.5 mg 600 mg/25 mg	q.d.	35	See individual components FDA approved, fall 2002
Irbesartan/HCTZ (Avalide)	150 mg/12.5 mg 300 mg/12.5 mg	1–2 tabs q.d.	70–130	See individual components
Losartan/HCTZ (Hyzaar)	50 mg/12.5 mg 100 mg/25 mg	1–2 tabs q.d. q.d.	50–150	See individual components

466

Drug (Brand)	Dose	Frequency	Cost[a],[b]	Price
Telmisartan/HCTZ (Micardis HCT)	40 mg/12.5 mg 80 mg/12.5 mg	1–2 tabs q.d.	50–100	See individual components
Valsartan/HCTZ (Diovan HCT)	80 mg/12.5 mg 160 mg/12.5 mg 160 mg/25 mg	q.d.	60–75	See individual components
β-BLOCKER/DIURETIC				
Atenolol/Chlorthalidone (Tenoretic)	Tenoretic 50: 50 mg/25 mg Tenoretic 100: 100 mg/25 mg	q.d.	<10	See individual components
Bisoprolol/HCTZ (Ziac)	2.5 mg/6.25 mg 5 mg/6.25 mg 10 mg/6.25 mg	1–2 tabs q.d.	<10	See individual components
Metoprolol/HCTZ (Lopressor HCT)	50 mg/25 mg 100 mg/25 mg 100 mg/50 mg	q.d.	35–60	See individual components
COMBINATION DIURETICS				
HCTZ/Spironolactone (Aldactazide)	Aldactazide 25: 25 mg/25 mg Aldactazide 50: 50 mg/50 mg	q.d.	10–25	See individual components
HCTZ/Triamterene (Various) (Dyazide [cap]) (Maxzide-25, [cap]) (Maxzide [tab])	50 mg/25 mg cap 25 mg/37.5 mg cap 25 mg/37.5 mg tab 50 mg/75 mg tab	q.d.	<10	See individual components
NICOTINIC ACID/HMG-CoA REDUCTASE INHIBITOR				
Niacin ER/Lovastatin (Advicor)	500 mg/20 mg 750 mg/20 mg 1,000 mg/20 mg	1–2 tabs q.h.s.	40–65	See individual components
PLATELET INHIBITORS				
Dipyridamole/Aspirin (Aggrenox)	200 mg/25 mg	b.i.d.	100	See individual components

FDA, U. S. Food and Drug Administration; HCTZ, hydrochlorothiazide; HMG-CoA, 3-hydroxy-3-methylglutaryl coenzyme A.

[a]Combination drugs are generally reserved for use after titration to similar or identical doses of the individual agents first, and doses of the combination product should be adjusted accordingly. After titration of individual agents, there may be cases in which the combination product is less costly or improves compliance with the therapeutic regimen.

[b]Cost based on Average Wholesale Price 2002 of "usual dose" range for a 30-day supply and rounded to the nearest $5. Generic price provided if available. Price does not include dispensing fees charged by pharmacies. Patients' costs may vary considerably.

Diabetes and Cardiovascular Disease
edited by Steven P. Marso and David M. Stern
Lippincott Williams & Wilkins, Philadelphia © 2004

Appendix B

Synopsis of Major Cardiovascular Trials Involving Diabetic Patients

Avinash Khanna

Mid America Heart Institute, Saint Luke's Hospital, Kansas City, Missouri

The following text highlights selected clinical trials with relevant findings regarding diabetes mellitus and cardiovascular diseases.

I. EPIDEMIOLOGY

Economic Costs of Diabetes in the US in 2002. *Diabetes Care* **2003;26:917–932.**

Clinical Relevance: The prevalence of diabetes continues to grow, as does its impact on the U. S. economy. This study estimated future diabetes prevalence rates, direct medical and indirect productivity-related costs of diabetes, and total and per capita medical expenditures for individuals with and without diabetes.

Findings: According to the results of this study, there were 12.1 million persons with diagnosed diabetes in the United States in 2002. Based on population projections from the U. S. Census Bureau, the number of diagnosed cases of diabetes in the United States will increase to approximately 14 million in 2010 and 17.4 million in 2020. Direct and indirect medical expenditures related to diabetes totaled $132 billion in 2002, translating into a per capita cost of $13,243 for people with diabetes and $2,560 for people without diabetes. However, because prevalence rates were based on self-reported cases of diabetes and did not include increasing rates of obesity and type 2 diabetes in children, the actual prevalence rates and costs are likely to be understated.

Reduction in the Incidence of Type 2 Diabetes with Lifestyle Intervention or Metformin. *N Engl J Med* **2002;346:393–403.**

Clinical Relevance: Persons who are overweight, lead a sedentary lifestyle, and have elevated plasma glucose levels in the fasting state and after a glucose load are at high risk for development of diabetes. This study compared the effects of metformin and intensive lifestyle modification in decreasing the risk of developing diabetes in a cohort of persons at risk for type 2 diabetes mellitus.

Findings: In this study, 3,234 nondiabetic patients with a mean body mass index of more than 24, fasting glucose level of 95 to 125 mg/dL, and a 2-hour plasma glucose concentration of 140 to 199 mg/dL after a 75-mg load of glucose were randomly assigned to one of three interventions: standard lifestyle modification plus metformin at a dose of 850 mg twice daily, standard lifestyle modification plus placebo, or an intensive program of lifestyle modification with goals of at least 7% weight loss and at least 150 minutes of physical activity per week. The mean age of participants was 51 years, and the mean body mass index was 34. After an average follow-up of 2.8 years, intensive lifestyle intervention reduced the incidence of diabetes by 58%, and metformin reduced the incidence by 31%, compared with placebo. The estimated number of persons who would need to be treated for 3 years to prevent one case of diabetes during this period was 6.9 for the intensive lifestyle intervention and 13.9

for metformin. Both strategies are effective at reducing the incidence of type 2 diabetes, but lifestyle intervention is superior.

Prevalence of the Metabolic Syndrome among US Adults: Findings from the Third National Health and Nutrition Examination Survey. *JAMA* **2002;287:356–359.**

Clinical Relevance: Metabolic syndrome is characterized by the presence of three or more of the following abnormalities: waist circumference greater than 102 cm in men or 88 cm in women; serum triglyceride level of at least 150 mg/dL; high-density-lipoprotein (HDL) level of less than 40 mg/dL in men or less than 50 mg/dL in women; blood pressure of at least 130/85 mm Hg; and serum glucose level of at least 110 mg/dL. Patients with metabolic syndrome are at high risk for development of type 2 diabetes. This study was done to estimate the prevalence of metabolic syndrome in the adult U. S. population.

Findings: The unadjusted and age-adjusted prevalence rates of metabolic syndrome were 21.8% and 23.7%, respectively. The prevalence was equal among men and women and was highest in the age group of 60 to 69 years. Mexican-Americans had the highest age-adjusted prevalence of the metabolic syndrome (31.9%). Women had a higher prevalence than men among African-Americans and Mexican-Americans. Application of these data suggests that there are 47 million U. S. residents (almost one fourth of the total population) with the metabolic syndrome.

Prevalence of Impaired Glucose Tolerance among Children and Adolescents with Marked Obesity. *N Engl J Med* **2002;346:802–810.**

Clinical Relevance: The prevalence of obesity is increasing among children and adolescents in the United States at an unprecedented rate. Because obesity is an important risk factor for the development of type 2 diabetes, these investigators sought to determine the prevalence of impaired glucose tolerance in a cohort of obese children and adolescents.

Findings: In the study, 55 children (4 to 10 years of age) and 112 adolescents (11 to 18 years of age) were recruited. All patients were obese, with a body mass index that was greater than the 95th percentile for age and sex. All subjects underwent a 2-hour oral glucose tolerance test. Impaired glucose tolerance, defined as a fasting plasma glucose level lower than 126 mg/dL and a 2-hour plasma glucose level between 140 and 200 mg/dL, was detected in 25% of obese children and 22% of obese adolescents. Fasting proinsulin levels were almost twice as high in patients with impaired glucose tolerance as in those with normal glucose tolerance, and these patients also had a higher incidence of insulin resistance. Impaired glucose tolerance, which is a precursor of type 2 diabetes, is highly prevalent among obese children and adolescents.

Treatment of Cardiac Risk Factors in Diabetic Patients: How Well Do We Follow the Guidelines? *Am Heart J* **2001;142:857–863.**

Clinical Relevance: Patients with type 2 diabetes mellitus have a cluster of cardiovascular risk factors. Because there is also a significant increase in cardiovascular morbidity and mortality with increasing numbers of risk factors, tight control of risk factors is an important goal of therapy. This study sought to assess the degree of control of numerous risk factors in a sample of diabetic patients undergoing elective coronary angiography.

Findings: This was a prospective, observational study of 235 treated diabetic patients undergoing elective cardiac catheterization. Patients were observed for 2 years; 85% had angiographic evidence of coronary artery disease (CAD), and only a minority of patients achieved the targeted goal. Only 21% of patients achieved a hemoglobin A_{1C} level of less than 7%, 52% had a low-density-lipoprotein (LDL) cholesterol concentration lower than 100 mg/dL, 76% had a triglyceride level lower than 200 mg/dL, 18% of the male patients had an HDL cholesterol level greater than 45 mg/dL, and 22% of the female patients had an HDL cholesterol level greater than 55 mg/dL. Only 10% of the patients had appropriate blood pressure control (less than 130/85 mm Hg). Of the 191 patients with documented CAD, only 51% were taking lipid-lowering agents, 39% were taking angiotensin-converting enzyme (ACE) inhibitors, 56% were taking β-blockers, and 82% were taking aspirin.

In this group of diabetic patients undergoing elective cardiac catheterization, risk factors were not adequately treated according to current guidelines.

Variation and Trends in Incidence of Childhood Diabetes in Europe. *Lancet* **2000;355: 873–876.**

Clinical Relevance: The prevalence of type 2 diabetes mellitus appears to be increasing among children. This study examined the trends and variation of incidence of diabetes mellitus in children in Europe.

Findings: This report was based on 16,362 patients registered from 1989 through 1994 by 44 centers across Europe. The annual rate of increase in the incidence of diabetes was 3.4%. The rates of increase were 6.3% for children between the ages of 0 and 4 years, 3.1% for those between 5 and 9 years, and 2.4% for those between 10 and 14 years. There was a wide range of annual incidence rates across Europe, from 3.2 (in Macedonia) per 10,000 per year to 40.2 (in Finland) per 10,000 per year. There was a steady increase in the incidence of diabetes in European children, especially among those younger than 5 years of age. These data support the concept that type 2 diabetes is more prevalent among children than previously observed.

Diabetes Trends in the US: 1990–1998. *Diabetes Care* **2000;23:1278–1283.**

Clinical Relevance: This study estimated the prevalence of diabetes in U. S. adults by means of a standardized telephone survey in states that participated in the Behavioral Risk Factor Surveillance System from 1990 to 1998.

Findings: The study reported that 149,806 individuals completed the telephone survey. They were asked whether they had been diagnosed with diabetes by a physician. Information regarding body mass index was also collected. The prevalence of diabetes increased from 4.9% in 1990 to 6.5% in 1998, a 33% increase. This increase was seen in both sexes and across all age groups, all education levels, all ethnic groups, and almost all states. There was a large variation by state in diabetes prevalence and in percentage increase. In 1998, Oklahoma had the highest prevalence (9.1%), and Arizona had the lowest rate (2.9%). Individuals between the ages of 30

and 39 years and those with higher education had the highest increase in diabetes prevalence. The prevalence of diabetes was highly correlated with the prevalence of obesity.

Nontraditional Risk Factors for Coronary Heart Disease Incidence among Persons with Diabetes: The Atherosclerosis Risk in Communities (ARIC) Study. *Ann Intern Med* **2000;133:81–91.**

Clinical Relevance: This study examined the association of traditional and nontraditional risk factors with CAD in patients with type 2 diabetes.

Findings: Included in the total cohort were 1,676 patients with type 2 diabetes who were between the ages of 45 and 64 years and had no prior history of CAD. Multiple risk factors were recorded at baseline. Follow-up between 1987 and 1995 identified 186 patients who had developed CAD. As expected, the risk of developing CAD was related to traditional risk factors such as increased LDL cholesterol levels, low HDL cholesterol levels, hypertension, and smoking. After adjustment for these traditional factors, the risk of developing CAD was negatively associated with albumin levels and positively associated with levels of fibrinogen, factor VIII, and von Willebrand factor and with the leukocyte count. All of these factors are markers for inflammation, supporting the idea of an inflammatory basis for atherosclerosis.

Glucose Tolerance and Mortality: Comparison of WHO and American Diabetes Association Diagnostic Criteria. The DECODE Study Group. European Diabetes Epidemiology Group. Diabetes Epidemiology: Collaborative Analysis Of Diagnostic Criteria in Europe. *Lancet* **1999;354:617–621.**

Clinical Relevance: The American Diabetes Association (ADA) and World Health Organization (WHO) have different recommendations as to the diagnostic criteria for diabetes and impaired glucose tolerance. The ADA recommends solely the use of fasting plasma glucose levels, and the WHO recommends coupling fasting glucose levels with results of a 2-hour glucose tolerance test in patients with blood sugar concentrations in the uncertain range of 5.5 to 11.1 mmol/L (100 to 205 mg/dL). This study assessed the mortality associated with the ADA fasting glucose criteria compared with the WHO 2-hour post-challenge glucose criteria.

Findings: This metaanalysis examined data for more than 25,000 patients from 13 prospective European studies. Compared with patients who had normal fasting glucose levels (less than 6.1 mmol/L or 110 mg/dL), the hazard ratio (HR) for death was 1.81 for men and 1.79 for women with newly diagnosed diabetes (fasting glucose level greater than 7.0 mmol/L or 126 mg/dL by the ADA criteria). For impaired glucose tolerance (fasting glucose level of 6.1 to 6.9 mmol/L or 111 to 125 mg/dL), the HR was 1.21 for men and 1.08 for women. For the WHO criteria (plasma glucose level greater than 11.1 mmol/L or 205 mg/dL), the HR for death was 2.02 for men and 2.77 for women with newly diagnosed diabetes; and for impaired glucose tolerance (7.8 to 11.1 mmol/L or 140 to 205 mg/dL), it was 1.51 and 1.60 for men and women, respectively. Overall, the fasting glucose level was not independently related to mortality after adjustment for the 2-hour glucose concentration; however, the 2-hour glucose tolerance result was independently related to mortality after adjustment for the fasting glucose concentration. Patients with normal fasting glucose levels and impaired 2-hour glucose tolerance, which included one third of the men and one half of the women with any degree of glucose abnormality, had the highest number of excess deaths. A 2-hour glucose tolerance test provides additional prognostic information and may be a more useful predictor of mortality than a lone fasting glucose level.

Global Burden of Diabetes, 1995–2025: Prevalence, Numerical Estimates, and Projections. *Diabetes Care* **1998;21:1414–1431.**

Clinical Relevance: This study estimated the prevalence of diabetes in all countries of the world in 1995, 2000, and 2025.

Findings: Age-specific diabetes prevalence estimates were applied to the United Nations' population estimates and projections for the number of adults age 20 years or older in all countries of the world. The prevalence of diabetes is expected to increase from 4.0% in 1995 to 5.4% in 2025, a 35% increase. Prevalence is higher in the developed countries and will remain so in 2025; however, the proportional increase will be greater in developing countries. The number of adults with diabetes is expected to increase by 122%, from 135 million in 1995 to 300 million in 2025. There will be a 42% increase, from 51 million to 72 million, in developed countries. In developing countries, there will be a 170% increase, from 84 million to 228 million. The greatest increase will be seen in India (195%, from 19 million to 57 million). By the year 2025, more than 75% of adults with diabetes will live in the developing countries. The first quarter of the 21st century is expected to see an epidemic of diabetes globally, and urgent steps are needed to control and prevent the disease.

Diabetes, Other Risk Factors, and 12-yr Cardiovascular Mortality for Men Screened in the Multiple Risk Factor Intervention Trial. *Diabetes Care* **1993;16:434–444.**

Clinical Relevance: The study compared the risk of cardiovascular disease (CVD) death in men with and without diabetes and assessed predictors of CVD mortality.

Findings: Participants were men age 35 to 57 years. There were 347,978 participants, of whom 5,163 were taking medications for diabetes. After an average follow-up of 12 years, there were 1,092 deaths (160.1 per 10,000 person-years) among men with diabetes and 20,867 deaths (53.2 per 10,000 person-years) among men without diabetes. After adjustment for age, race, systolic blood pressure, serum cholesterol level, and cigarettes smoked per day, the relative risk of CVD mortality was three times higher for diabetic men than for nondiabetic men. At every level of cholesterol, systolic blood pressure, and cigarette use, the rate of CVD death was higher for diabetic men than for nondiabetic men. The steep increase in CVD mortality in the diabetic cohort correlated with increasing numbers of risk factors. The presence of these risk factors, singly or in combination, was associated with a steeper increase in CVD mortality for diabetic men.

II. DIABETES AND LIPID-LOWERING THERAPY

Prevention of Coronary and Stroke Events with Atorvastatin in Hypertensive Patients

Who Have Average or Lower-than-Average Cholesterol Concentrations, in the Anglo-Scandinavian Outcomes Trial—Lipid Lowering Arm (ASCOT-LLA): A Multicentre Randomized Controlled Trial. *Lancet* 2003;361:1149–1158.

Clinical Relevance: This study evaluated the efficacy of lipid lowering using atorvastatin in patients with a history of hypertension and at least three other cardiovascular risk factors.

Findings: This trial involved 19,242 hypertensive patients age 40 to 79 years who were randomly assigned to one of two antihypertensive regimens in the ASCOT trial. There were 10,305 patients with nonfasting total cholesterol concentrations of 6.5 mmol/L (250 mg/dL) or less. The mean follow-up period was 5 years. The primary end point was nonfatal myocardial infarction (MI) or fatal coronary heart disease. For the overall cohort, there was a significant reduction in the primary end point for the atorvastatin-treated patients, 1.9% compared with 3.0% for the placebo-treated cohort (unadjusted hazard ratio [HR] = 0.64; 95% CI, 0.50 to 0.83; p = .0005). This benefit was noted early and persisted through follow up. There were 2,532 patients with a reported history of diabetes in this study. There did not appear to be a similar reduction in end points for patients with a history of diabetes. There was a 3% incidence of the primary end point in the atorvastatin-treated cohort, compared with 3.6% for the placebo-treated cohort (unadjusted HR = 0.84; 95% CI, 0.55 to 1.29; p = .43). Statin therapy has been consistently shown to benefit patients with a reported history of diabetes. However, this study included a significant number of patients with diabetes and did not find a similar risk reduction in diabetic patients treated with atorvastatin compared with placebo, an effect that was seen in the nondiabetic cohort. Results of this subset analysis should be considered in the setting of the overall trial findings and the multitude of other studies that have shown a marked benefit in cardiovascular risk reduction in diabetic patients treated with a 3-hydroxy-3-methylglutaryl coenzyme A (HMG-CoA) reductase inhibitor.

MRC/BHF Heart Protection Study of Cholesterol Lowering with Simvastatin in 20,536 High-Risk Individuals: A Randomised Placebo-Controlled Trial. *Lancet* 2002;360:7–22.

Clinical Relevance: This landmark trial assessed the effects of lowering the cholesterol level on cardiovascular events in high-risk patients irrespective of baseline cholesterol levels.

Findings: The 20,536 patients (age 40 to 80 years) were randomly assigned to receive 40 mg of simvastatin or placebo. Almost 6,000 patients with diabetes were included in this report. Patients were deemed to be at high risk for cardiovascular disease based on the presence of prior CAD, other occlusive arterial disease, or diabetes. The average follow-up period was 5 years. There was a significant reduction of vascular events in persons with diabetes, regardless of whether there was a history of coronary heart disease treated with simvastatin (20.2% versus 25.1%, p < .001).

Effect of Fenofibrate on Progression of Coronary-Artery Disease in Type 2 Diabetes: The Diabetes Atherosclerosis Intervention Study, a Randomised Study. *Lancet* 2001;357:905–910.

Clinical Relevance: This study assessed the effect of fenofibrate on lipoprotein abnormalities and coronary atherosclerosis in persons with type 2 diabetes.

Findings: In this study, 418 patients with type 2 diabetes were randomly assigned to receive fenofibrate or placebo. Baseline angiograms and lipid profiles were obtained for all patients, who were included if they had at least one visible coronary lesion. Lipid entry criteria were as follows: a total cholesterol to HDL cholesterol ratio of 4 or more, plus an LDL cholesterol concentration of 3.5 to 4.5 mmol/L (135 to 174 mg/dL) and a triglyceride concentration of 5.2 mmol/L (200 mg/dL) or less or a triglyceride concentration of 1.7 to 5.2 mmol/L (65 to 200 mg/dL) and an LDL cholesterol level of 4.5 mmol/L (174 mg/dL) or less. After treatment for 36 to 55 months, fenofibrate had predictable effects on the plasma lipids, with moderate but significant decreases in total and LDL cholesterol concentrations, a more substantial and significant decrease in the plasma concentrations of triglycerides, and a significant increase in HDL cholesterol levels. There was no significant change in lipid levels in the placebo group. In terms of the primary end points, fenofibrate resulted in a 40% smaller decrease in minimum lumen diameter and a 42% smaller increase in percentage diameter stenosis than did placebo ($p = .02$).

Reduced Coronary Events in Simvastatin Treated Patients with Coronary Heart Disease and Diabetes or Impaired Fasting Glucose Levels: Subgroup Analysis in the Scandinavian Simvastatin Survival Study. *Arch Intern Med* **1999;159:2661–2667.**

Clinical Relevance: This study sought to determine the effects of simvastatin on coronary events in patients with coronary heart disease and diabetes or impaired fasting glucose levels in patients with a baseline cholesterol level between 213 and 309 mg/dL.

Findings: This was a randomized, double-blind, prospective trial in which patients age 35 to 70 years were randomly assigned to receive 20 to 40 mg of simvastatin or placebo. The study group included 483 patients with diabetes and 678 patients with impaired glucose tolerance. The mean follow-up period was 5.4 years. Diabetic patients treated with simvastatin had a 42% reduction in major coronary events and a 48% reduction in revascularization procedures. There was a nonsignificant decrease in total and coronary mortality rates. For patients with impaired glucose tolerance, there was a significant decrease in major coronary events, coronary deaths, and all-cause mortality rates.

Cardiovascular Events and Their Reduction with Pravastatin in Diabetic and Glucose-Intolerant Myocardial Infarction Survivors with Average Cholesterol Levels: Subgroup Analyses in the Cholesterol and Recurrent Events (CARE) Trial. The CARE Investigators. *Circulation* **1998;98:2513–2519.**

Clinical Relevance: This study sought to assess the effect of lowering cholesterol levels on coronary events in diabetic patients with prior MI.

Findings: This was a substudy of the CARE trial, which included 4,159 patients with a history of MI (occurring 3 to 20 months before randomization), total cholesterol level less than 240 mg/dL, LDL cholesterol level between 115 and 174 mg/dL, and triglyceride level less than 350 mg/dL. The incidence of an adverse cardiovascular event (including coronary heart disease, death, MI, stroke, or revascularization) was 36.8% for the placebo group and 28.7% for the pravastatin group ($p < .05$). Five hundred eighty-six diabetic patients were randomly assigned to pravastatin (40 mg/day) or placebo. The average follow-up period was 5 years. Baseline LDL and total cholesterol levels were 136 mg/dL and 206 mg/dL, respectively.

Prevention of Cardiovascular Events and Death with Pravastatin in Patients with Coronary Artery Heart Disease and a Broad Range of Initial Cholesterol Levels. The Long-Term Intervention with Pravastatin in Ischemic Disease (LIPID) Study Group. *N Engl J Med* **1998;339:1349–1357.**

Clinical Relevance: In patients with CAD and a broad range of cholesterol levels (baseline, 155 to 271 mg/dL), cholesterol-lowering therapy may decrease mortality.

Findings: This randomized, prospective, double-blind trial compared treatment with pravastatin (40 mg/day) and placebo in 9,014 patients. The average follow-up period was 6.1 years. There was a 24% risk reduction in death from coronary heart disease and a 22% risk reduction in overall mortality. In the diabetic subgroup, which included 782 patients, there was a 19% risk reduction in the composite end point of death from coronary heart disease and nonfatal MI. The investigators found a consistent reduction in death from coronary heart disease and in the nonfatal MI rate for patients receiving pravastatin compared with other subgroups in this trial.

III. DIABETES AND ANTIHYPERTENSIVE AGENTS

Major Outcomes in High-Risk Hypertensive Patients Randomized to Angiotensin-Converting Enzyme Inhibitor or Calcium Channel Blocker vs. Diuretic: The Antihypertensive and Lipid-Lowering Treatment to Prevent Heart Attack Trial (ALLHAT). *JAMA* **2002;288:2981–2997.**

Clinical Relevance: This study compared the effects of an ACE inhibitor or calcium channel blocker and a thiazide diuretic on cardiovascular outcomes in high-risk patients.

Findings: There were more than 11,000 type 2 diabetic patients among the 33,357 study participants. Patients were randomly assigned to receive amlodipine, lisinopril, or chlorthalidone. Patients were given other open-label drugs, including atenolol, reserpine, clonidine, or hydralazine, to achieve blood pressure control. The follow-up period was 4 to 8 years. The risks of all-cause death, stroke, nonfatal MI, plus CAD, death, and combined coronary heart disease were similar in the three treatment arms, including the diabetic subgroup. Compared with amlodipine and lisinopril, patients (including those with type 2 diabetes) receiving chlorthalidone had a lower rate of heart failure.

Cardiovascular Mortality and Morbidity in Patients with Diabetes in the Losartan Intervention for Endpoint Reduction in Hypertension Study (LIFE): A Randomized Trial against Atenolol. *Lancet* **2002;359:1004–1010.**

Clinical Relevance: The study assessed whether the angiotensin receptor blocker, losartan, is superior to atenolol in decreasing cardiovascular end points.

Findings: In this trial, 1,195 hypertensive diabetic patients were randomly assigned to receive losartan or atenolol. The patients were monitored for 4 years. The primary end point was a composite of cardiovascular morbidity and mortality (i.e., cardiovascular death, MI, or stroke). The primary end point occurred in 17.6% of patients receiving losartan and 22.8% of those receiving atenolol therapy (RR = 0.76, p = .01). Losartan was associated with a 36.6% lower relative risk for cardiovascular mortality. At the end of the study, the mean blood pressure was equal in both groups; however, patients receiving losartan had a greater decrease in left ventricular hypertrophy by electrocardiographic criteria.

Microalbuminuria Reduction with Valsartan in Patients with Type 2 Diabetes Mellitus: A Blood Pressure-Independent Effect. *Circulation* **2002;106:672–678.**

Clinical Relevance: Microalbuminuria has been associated with adverse cardiovascular outcomes. This study was performed to assess the efficacy of valsartan in decreasing urine albumin excretion rate (UAER) in patients with diabetes, independent of its blood pressure-lowering effect.

Findings: There were 332 patients with type 2 diabetes and microalbuminuria, with or without hypertension, randomly assigned to valsartan (80 mg/day) or amlodipine (5 mg/day) for 24 weeks. At 24 weeks, the UAER was 56% of baseline with valsartan and 92% of baseline with amlodipine. More patients reversed to normoalbuminuria with valsartan (29.9% versus 14.5%, p = .001). Blood pressure reductions were similar in both groups.

Reduced Cardiovascular Mortality and Morbidity in Hypertensive Diabetic Patients on First-Line Therapy with an ACE Inhibitor Compared with a Diuretic/Beta-Blocker-Based Treatment Regimen: A Subanalysis of the Captopril Prevention Project. *Diabetes Care* **2001;24:2091–2096.**

Clinical Relevance: The Captopril Prevention Project (CAPP) trial evaluated the effect of captopril versus conventional therapy with β-blockers and diuretics in hypertensive patients. This substudy assessed the cardiovascular outcomes of diabetic patients in these two groups.

Findings: There were 10,985 hypertensive patients in the CAPP trial, of whom 572 had a diagnosis of diabetes. At baseline, patients (age 25 to 66 years) with a diastolic blood pressure of more than 100 mm Hg were randomly assigned to receive captopril or conventional antihypertensive treatment (i.e., diuretic, β-blocker, or both). Patients were monitored for an average of 6.1 years. The treatment goal was a supine diastolic blood pressure of less than 100 mm Hg. In diabetic patients, the primary end point of fatal and nonfatal MI and stroke, as well as other cardiovascular death, was significantly lower in the captopril group compared with the conventional therapy group (11.3% versus 17.5%, RR = 0.59, p = .018). MI was less frequent in the captopril group than in the conventional therapy group (3.9% versus 10.3%, RR = 0.34, p = .002). Among the nondiabetic population, captopril decreased the incidence of new-onset diabetes by 21%. Captopril was superior to conventional agents (i.e., β-blockers and diuretics) in decreasing cardiovascular end points in diabetic patients.

Effects of Losartan on Renal and Cardiovascular Outcomes in Patients with Type 2 Diabetes and Nephropathy. *N Engl J Med* 2001;345:861–869.

Clinical Relevance: Diabetic nephropathy is the leading cause of end-stage renal disease and is associated with adverse cardiovascular outcomes. This study evaluated the effects of losartan in patients with type 2 diabetes and nephropathy.

Findings: A total of 1,513 patients with type 2 diabetes were randomly assigned to receive either losartan (50 to 100 mg daily) or placebo, coupled with conventional antihypertensive treatment. The primary end point was doubling of the baseline serum creatinine level, development of end-stage renal disease, or death. Secondary end points included a composite of morbidity and mortality from cardiovascular disease. Patients were monitored for a mean of 3.4 years. Losartan decreased the incidence of doubling of the serum creatinine concentration (risk reduction, 25%; $p = .006$) and the incidence of end-stage renal disease (risk reduction, 28%; $p = .002$) but had no effect on the rate of death. The benefit exceeded that attributable to changes in blood pressure. The composite of mortality and morbidity from cardiovascular causes was similar in both groups, although the rate of first hospitalization for heart failure was significantly lower with losartan (risk reduction, 32%; $p = .005$). Losartan conferred significant renal protection in patients with type 2 diabetes. There was no significant reduction in cardiovascular end points except in the incidence of first admissions for heart failure.

Renoprotective Effects of the Angiotensin-Receptor Antagonist Irbesartan in Patients with Nephropathy Due to Type 2 Diabetes. *N Engl J Med* 2001;345:851–860.

Clinical Relevance: The Irbesartan Diabetic Nephropathy Trial (IDNT) compared the effect of irbesartan and amlodipine on progression of nephropathy and cardiovascular outcomes in hypertensive diabetic patients.

Findings: In the IDNT, 1,715 diabetic patients with established nephropathy (serum creatinine concentration between 1.0 and 3.0 mg/dL and urinary protein excretion of at least 900 mg/24 hours) were randomly assigned to treatment with irbesartan, amlodipine, or placebo. The target blood pressure was less than 135/85 mm Hg in all groups. The mean follow-up period was 2.6 years. Treatment with irbesartan was associated with a 33% reduction in risk of doubling of the serum creatinine level compared with the placebo group, and a 37% reduction compared with the amlodipine group. Treatment with irbesartan was associated with a relative risk of end-stage renal disease that was 23% lower than that in other groups. These differences were not explained by blood pressure differences in the groups. There was no difference among treatment groups in terms of cardiovascular end points, although the patients receiving irbesartan had lower rates of hospitalization for congestive heart failure.

The Effect of Irbesartan on the Development of Diabetic Nephropathy in Patients with Type 2 Diabetes. *N Engl J Med* 2001;345:870–878.

Clinical Relevance: Hypertension and microalbuminuria are risk factors for the development of diabetic nephropathy and adverse cardiovascular outcomes. This study evaluated whether the angiotensin receptor blocker irbesartan could decrease the rate of progression of microalbuminuria to overt nephropathy.

Findings: A total of 590 hypertensive patients with diabetes and microalbuminuria, defined as a urinary microalbumin excretion rate of 20 to 200 μg per minute, were randomly assigned to receive placebo, 150 mg of irbesartan, or 300 mg of irbesartan. Patients with serum creatinine concentrations greater than 1.5 mg/dL were excluded. Use of additional antihypertensive agents was allowed in all three groups to achieve blood pressure goals. The primary outcome of overt nephropathy, defined as urinary albumin rate of greater than 200 μg per minute, was reached in 15% of the placebo group, 9.7% of the 150-mg irbesartan group, and 5.2% of the 300-mg irbesartan group. After adjustment for the baseline level of microalbuminuria and blood pressure achieved during the study, the hazard ratio for diabetic nephropathy was 0.56 in the 150-mg group ($p = .05$) and 0.32 in the 300-mg group ($p < .001$). Irbesartan was renoprotective independent of its blood pressure-lowering effect in patients with type 2 diabetes and microalbuminuria. The Irbesartan and Microalbuminuria (IRMA) study and Irbesartan Diabetic Nephropathy Trial (IDNT) demonstrated that irbesartan can delay the development of overt diabetic nephropathy (IRMA) and delay its progression to end-stage renal disease (IDNT).

Effect of Ramipril on Cardiovascular and Microvascular Outcomes in People with Diabetes Mellitus: Results of the HOPE Study and the MICRO-HOPE Study. *Lancet* 2000;355:253–259.

Clinical Relevance: The presence of diabetes increases the risk of developing cardiovascular and renal disease. This substudy of the Heart Outcomes Prevention Evaluation (HOPE) trial investigated the effects of ramipril on the incidence of adverse cardiovascular and renal outcomes.

Findings: The 3,577 patients with diabetes (age 55 years or older) who were not taking ACE inhibitors were randomly assigned to ramipril (10 mg/day) or placebo and monitored for 4.5 years. Patients with heart failure and proteinuria were excluded. Ramipril reduced the combined outcome of MI, stroke, or death by 25%, total mortality by 24%, and overt nephropathy by 24%. This benefit was greater than that attributable to the decrease in blood pressure.

Effects of Calcium-Channel Blockade in Older Patients with Diabetes and Systolic Hypertension. Systolic Hypertension in Europe Trial Investigators. *N Engl J Med* 1999;340: 677–684.

Clinical Relevance: The study ascertained whether nitrendipine-based antihypertensive therapy could decrease cardiovascular outcomes in patients with diabetes and systolic hypertension. Before publication of this study, there was concern regarding the use of long-acting calcium channel blockers in diabetic patients.

Findings: This was a multicenter, randomized, controlled trial in which 4,695 patients older than 60 years of age and with a systolic blood pressure of 160 to 219 mm Hg and a diastolic pressure of less than 95 mm Hg were assigned to receive active treatment or placebo. The treatment arm consisted of nitrendipine with possible addition of or substitution with enalapril or hydrochlorothiazide. Baseline use of antihypertensive drugs was similar in both groups. There were 492 diabetic patients in the study. After a mean follow-up period of 2 years, systolic and diastolic blood pressures differed by 8.6 and 3.9 mm Hg, respectively, in the treatment and placebo group. In the diabetic population, active treatment decreased mortality by 55%, mortality from cardiovascular disease by 76%, and strokes by 73%.

Outcome Results of the Fosinopril versus Amlodipine Cardiovascular Events Randomized Trial (FACET) in Patients with Hypertension and NIDDM. *Diabetes Care* 1998;21:597–603.

Clinical Relevance. The primary aim of this trial was to compare the effects of fosinopril and amlodipine on serum lipids and diabetic control in patients with type 2 diabetes and hypertension. Cardiovascular events were assessed as secondary outcomes.

Findings: In the FACET, 380 hypertensive diabetic patients were assigned to open-label fosinopril (20 mg/day) or amlodipine (10 mg/day) and monitored for up to 3.5 years. Patients with known CAD or stroke were excluded. Both treatments resulted in similar reductions in blood pressure. There were no significant differences in total cholesterol, hemoglobin A_{1C}, or fasting serum glucose levels in the two groups. Patients receiving fosinopril had a significantly lower risk of the combined outcome of acute MI, stroke, or angina requiring hospitalization than did those receiving amlodipine (hazard ratio = 0.49, 95% CI, 0.26 to 0.95).

Tight Blood Pressure Control and the Risk of Macrovascular and Microvascular Complications in Type 2 Diabetes: UKPDS 38. UK Prospective Diabetes Group. *BMJ* 1998;317:703–720.

Clinical Relevance: The study determined the effects of tight blood pressure control to a target of less than 150/85 mm Hg on microvascular and macrovascular complications in patients with type 2 diabetes mellitus and compared the effects of captopril versus atenolol on these outcomes.

Findings: In this randomized, controlled trial, 1,148 patients were randomly assigned to tight blood pressure control (less than 150/85 mm Hg) with captopril (400 patients) or atenolol (358 patients) or to less tight control (less than 180/105 mm Hg). Other antihypertensive agents were used if target blood pressure was not reached. The median follow-up period was 8.4 years. The total mortality rate was 22.4% in the tight control group and 27.2% in the less tight control group (RR = 0.82, p = .17). Tight blood pressure control reduced the risk for stroke (RR = 0.56, p = .013), heart failure (RR = 0.44, p = .0043), and microvascular complications (RR = 0.63, p = .009). However, the investigators found no difference in terms of risk reduction or blood pressure reduction between the captopril and atenolol groups, suggesting that intensive blood pressure control may be more important than the drugs used to achieve it.

Effects of Intensive Blood-Pressure Lowering and Low-Dose Aspirin in Patients with Hypertension: Principal Results of the Hypertension Optimal Treatment (HOT) Randomised Trial. HOT Study Group. *Lancet* **1998;351:1755–1762.**

Clinical Relevance: The HOT study determined the optimal diastolic blood pressure in treated hypertensive patients and assessed the role of low-dose aspirin (75 mg) in the prevention of cardiovascular events.

Findings: Almost 19,000 patients with hypertension and diastolic blood pressure between 100 and 115 mm Hg were randomly assigned to a spectrum of target diastolic blood pressures. There were 1,501 diabetic patients in the HOT study. All patients received felodipine (5 mg/day). Additional therapy in the form of ACE inhibitors, β-blockers, or diuretics or an increase in the dose of felodipine was given to reach target blood pressures. Patients were also randomly assigned to receive either low-dose aspirin or placebo. The average follow-up period was 3.8 years. In the diabetic subgroup, there was a significant decrease in major cardiovascular events in the lower target pressure group. There was a more than 50% reduction in major cardiovascular events in the less than 80 mm Hg group compared with the less than 90 mm Hg group (24.4 events per 1,000 patient-years versus 11.9 events per 1,000 patient-years, p = .005). Im-

portantly, the cardiovascular mortality rate was also significantly reduced, from 11.1 to 3.7 events per 1,000 patient-years for the less than 90 mm Hg and less than 80 mm Hg groups, respectively (p = .02).

Effect of Diuretic-Based Antihypertensive Treatment on Cardiovascular Disease Risk in Older Diabetic Patients with Isolated Systolic Hypertension. Systolic Hypertension in the Elderly Program Cooperative Research Group. *JAMA* **1996;276:1886–1892.**

Clinical Relevance: The Systolic Hypertension in the Elderly Program (SHEP) evaluated the effect of diuretic-based therapy (i.e., chlorthalidone) in older patients with isolated systolic hypertension.

Findings: Patients were randomly assigned to placebo or chlorthalidone. The goal for systolic blood pressure was less than 160 mm Hg. Atenolol was added, if needed, to achieve the target blood pressure. There were 583 patients with type 2 diabetes in the study. The 5-year outcome for all major cardiovascular events was 35% lower in the treatment group. Absolute risk reduction with active therapy compared with placebo was twice as great for diabetic patients as for nondiabetic patients (101 versus 51 per 1,000 randomized participants at the 5-year follow-up). In summary, treating older diabetic patients who have systolic hypertension with diuretic-based therapy is effective in reducing major cardiovascular events.

IV. REVASCULARIZATION IN STABLE CORONARY ARTERY DISEASE

A. Coronary Artery Bypass Graft Surgery Versus Percutaneous Coronary Intervention

Percutaneous Coronary Intervention versus Coronary Artery Bypass Graft Surgery for Diabetic Patients with Unstable Angina and Risk Factors for Adverse Outcomes with Bypass: Outcome of Diabetic Patients in the AWESOME Randomized Trial and Registry. *J Am Coll Cardiol* **2002;40:1555–1566.**

Clinical Relevance: The Angina with Extremely Serious Operative Mortality Evaluation (AWESOME) trial compared the results of coronary artery bypass graft surgery (CABG) and percutaneous coronary intervention (PCI) in a diabetic subgroup. Participants were patients with medically refractory angina and at least one of five high-risk characteristics: prior CABG, MI within 7 days, left ventricular ejection fraction less than 0.35, age older than 70 years, or the use of an intraaortic balloon pump.

Findings: There was a total of 758 patients with type 2 diabetes in the study, and 233 patients were eligible for CABG or PCI, 144 of whom consented to be randomized. The patients who refused to be randomized constituted the patient-choice registry, and the 525 patients who were not acceptable for CABG or PCI constituted the physician-directed registry. The CABG and PCI 36-month survival rates for diabetic patients were 72% and 81% for randomized patients, 85% and 89% for patient-choice registry patients, and 73% and 71% for the physician-directed registry patients, respectively. These differences were not statistically different. Although the study was underpowered, PCI may be a safe alternative to CABG in high-risk patients with medically refractory unstable angina.

Clinical and Economic Impact of Diabetes Mellitus on Percutaneous and Surgical Treatment of Multivessel Coronary Disease Patients: Insights from the Arterial Revascularization Therapy Study (ARTS) Trial. *Circulation* **2001;104:533–538.**

Clinical Relevance: The ARTS trial compared CABG and stenting for the treatment of diabetic patients with multivessel CAD.

Findings: There were 1,205 patients with multivessel CAD (208 with a history of diabetes) randomly assigned to stent implantation or CABG. Patients with left main coronary artery disease or an ejection fraction less than 30% were excluded. In the diabetic population, the 1-year, event-free survival rate for MI, death, cerebrovascular events, or any repeat revascularization was 84.4% for patients undergoing CABG and 63.4% for patients undergoing stent placement. The 1-year mortality rate was more than twofold greater in the stent group than in the CABG group (6.3% versus 3.1%). However, diabetic patients undergoing CABG had a higher risk of cerebrovascular events compared with non-

diabetic patients undergoing CABG (6.3% versus 2.4%). Only 3.5% of the patients undergoing stenting received a glycoprotein IIb/IIIA inhibitor.

Seven-Year Outcome in the Bypass Angioplasty Revascularization Investigation (BARI) by Treatment and Diabetic Status. *J Am Coll Cardiol* **2000;35:1122–1129.**

Clinical Relevance: This substudy of BARI sought to compare long-term outcomes of percutaneous transluminal coronary angioplasty (PTCA) and coronary artery bypass grafting (CABG) in diabetic patients with multivessel disease.

Findings: Patients were included if they had multivessel disease that was amenable to revascularization with the CABG or PTCA strategy. Of the 1,829 patients enrolled, 353 had diabetes. All results were based on the intention-to-treat principle. At 5 years, diabetic patients assigned to CABG had an increased survival rate of 80.6%, compared with 65.5% in the PTCA group (*p* = 0.003). The 7-year follow-up assessment also demonstrated an increased survival rate for CABG over PTCA (76.4% versus 55.7%, respectively). This survival benefit was limited to the diabetic patients who received at least one internal mammary artery graft. Diabetic patients undergoing PTCA also had increased requirements for repeat revascularization compared with diabetic patients undergoing CABG or nondiabetic patients undergoing PTCA.

Eight-Year Mortality in the Emory Angioplasty versus Surgery Trial (EAST). *J Am Coll Cardiol* **2000;35:1116–1121.**

Clinical Relevance: EAST compared the strategy of PTCA with that of CABG in treating patients with multivessel disease. Of the 392 patients enrolled, 59 were diabetic.

Findings: Results of the randomized, controlled trial in which patients were assigned to bypass surgery or coronary angioplasty were initially published after a 3-year follow-up period. Results from an extended follow-up period of 8 years were subsequently published. Patients with left main coronary artery disease and an ejection fraction of less than 25% were excluded. At 3 years' follow-up, the survival rate was essentially the same for diabetic patients treated with surgery or PTCA (90% versus 93.1%). After 5 years, the curves began to diverge, and by 8 years, they favored surgery, although this difference was not statistically significant (surgical survival, 75.5%; angioplasty survival, 60.1%; $p = .23$).

B. Diabetes and Percutaneous Coronary Intervention

Diabetes Mellitus is Associated with a Shift in the Temporal Risk Profile of In-Hospital Death after Percutaneous Coronary Intervention: An Analysis of 25,223 Patients over 20 Years. *Am Heart J* 2003;145:270–277.

Clinical Relevance: Patients with a history of diabetes have a higher event rate after percutaneous coronary revascularization. This cohort of patients is more likely to have restenosis, a higher incidence of late MI, and late mortality after percutaneous coronary revascularization procedures. The risk of in-hospital mortality has previously been undescribed.

Findings: There were 25,223 patients analyzed in this registry between 1980 and 1999. Diabetes was associated with a twofold increased risk of in-hospital mortality in the elective cohort. The in-hospital mortality rates for nondiabetics and diabetics were 0.8% and 1.4%, respectively ($p < .001$). The mortality rate after urgent percutaneous coronary intervention for acute MI was 6.9% for the nondiabetic patients and 12.7% for the diabetic patients ($p < .001$). A time analysis suggested that the in-hospital mortality rate has been decreasing in recent years for the elective PCI cohort among both nondiabetic and diabetic patients; however, there does not appear to be a significant downward trend in the in-hospital mortality rate for diabetic patients presenting with an acute MI.

Effects of Coronary Stenting on Vessel Patency and Long-Term Clinical Outcome after Percutaneous Coronary Revascularization in Diabetic Patients. *J Am Coll Cardiol* 2002;40:410–417.

Clinical Relevance: The study assessed whether coronary stenting improves angiographic and clinical outcomes in diabetic patients.

Findings: This retrospective study matched 157 diabetic patients who had undergone stenting with a similar number of diabetic patients who underwent balloon angioplasty. Patients were matched with respect to gender, antidiabetic regimen, stenosis location, reference diameter, and minimal luminal diameter. At 6-month angiographic follow-up, the rate of restenosis was lower in the stent group than in the balloon angioplasty group (27% versus 62%, $p < .0001$). At 4 years, the combined clinical end point of cardiac death and nonfatal MI was lower in the stent group (14.8% versus 26.0%). The need for target vessel revascularization was also lower in the stent group (35.4% versus 52.1%).

Impact of Different Platelet Glycoprotein IIb/IIIa Receptor Inhibitors among Diabetic Patients Undergoing Percutaneous Coronary Intervention. Do Tirofiban and ReoPro Give Similar Efficacy Outcomes Trial (TARGET): 1-Year Follow-up. *Circulation* 2002;105;2730–2736.

Clinical Relevance: This study compared the efficacy of abciximab with that of tirofiban among patients undergoing percutaneous coronary intervention (PCI) and assessed whether the benefits of glycoprotein IIb/IIIA inhibition were derived from a class effect.

Findings: In this randomized, controlled trial, a total of 1,117 diabetic patients received tirofiban or abciximab at the time of PCI. Patients were monitored for 1 year. Among patients randomly assigned to tirofiban, the incidence of death, MI, or urgent target vessel revascularization was 6.2%, and for those randomly assigned to abciximab, the rate was 5.4% ($p = .54$). The 1-year mortality rate was 2.1% for the tirofiban group and 2.9% for the abciximab group ($p = .436$). Among diabetic patients undergoing PCI, abciximab and tirofiban were associated with similar outcomes over periods of 6 months and 1 year.

Patency of Percutaneous Transluminal Coronary Angioplasty Sites at 6-Month Angiographic Follow-up: A Key Determinant of Survival in Diabetics after Coronary Balloon Angioplasty. *Circulation* 2001;103:1218–1224.

Clinical Relevance: This study analyzed the determinants of long-term mortality in diabetic patients undergoing balloon angioplasty.

Specifically, the effects of restenosis on mortality were studied.

Findings: The 513 diabetic patients who were successfully treated by standard balloon angioplasty underwent repeat angiography at 6 months and long-term clinical follow-up (mean follow-up, 6.5 ± 2.4 years). On the basis of the 6-month angiographic findings, patients were subdivided into three groups: group 1, 162 patients (32%) without restenosis; group 2, 257 patients (50%) with nonocclusive restenosis; and group 3, 94 patients (18%) with coronary occlusion. At the end of the clinical follow-up period, six variables were found to be independently associated with mortality: coronary occlusion at 6 months, age at initial procedure, a lower left ventricular ejection fraction (LVEF) at baseline, end-organ damage, decrease in LVEF at the 6-month angiographic study, and hypertension. The mortality rate for patients with coronary occlusion was 45%, compared with 26% and 17% in patients with nonocclusive restenosis and no restenosis, respectively ($p < .001$).

Abciximab Reduces Mortality in Diabetic Patients Following Percutaneous Coronary Intervention. *J Am Coll Cardiol* **2000;35:922–928.**

Clinical Relevance: The study evaluated the effect of abciximab, a glycoprotein IIb/IIIa inhibitor, at the time of percutaneous intervention on patients with diabetes. This was a subgroup analysis of diabetic patients from the Early Postmenopausal Intervention Cohort (EPIC), Evaluation in PTCA to Improve Long-Term Outcome with Abciximab GP IIb/IIIa Blockade (EPILOG), and Evaluation of Platelet IIb/IIIa Inhibition in Stenting Trial (EPISTENT) trials.

Findings: There were 5,072 nondiabetic and 1,462 diabetic patients enrolled in the study. The overall 1-year mortality rate for diabetic patients was higher than for nondiabetic patients (3.3% versus 2.1%, $p = .012$). For patients with diabetes, abciximab decreased the 1-year mortality rate from 4.5% to 2.5% ($p = .099$). Among patients undergoing multivessel angioplasty, abciximab reduced the mortality rate from 7.7% to 0.9% ($p = 0.018$). Diabetic patients receiving abciximab at the time of intervention had 1-year mortality rates similar to those of nondiabetic patients receiving

placebo. Patients with insulin resistance also derived a 1-year mortality rate reduction with the use of abciximab compared with placebo (5.1% versus 2.3%, $p = .044$).

Optimizing the Percutaneous Interventional Outcomes for Patients with Diabetes Mellitus: Results of the EPISTENT (Evaluation of Platelet IIb/IIIA Inhibition in Stenting Trial) Diabetic Substudy. *Circulation* **1999;100:2477–2484.**

Clinical Relevance: Diabetic patients are known to be at a higher risk after percutaneous intervention. This substudy of EPISTENT determined whether abciximab plus stenting was associated with improved events compared with stenting alone or PTCA plus abciximab in diabetic patients within the EPISTENT trial.

Findings: The 491 diabetic patients were randomly assigned to stent plus placebo, stent plus abciximab, or PTCA plus abciximab. Patients in all three groups received aspirin and heparin. The follow-up period was 6 to 12 months. The composite end point of death, MI, or target vessel revascularization was reached in 25.2% of the stent-placebo group, 23.4% of the balloon-abciximab group, and 13.0% of the stent-abciximab group ($p = 0.05$). The 6-month death or MI rates were 7.8% in the balloon plus abciximab group, 6.2% in the stent plus abciximab group, and 12.7% in the stent plus placebo group. The composite end point of 6-month death, MI, and target vessel revascularization was lowest when abciximab was combined with stenting, compared with placebo plus stenting or PTCA plus abciximab.

Restenosis, Late Vessel Occlusion and Left Ventricular Function Six Months after Balloon Angioplasty in Diabetic Patients. *J Am Coll Cardiol* **1999;34:476–485.**

Clinical Relevance: This study assessed the 6-month angiographic outcomes of diabetic patients treated by balloon angioplasty. The effect of restenosis on left ventricular function was also assessed.

Findings: The 485 diabetic patients who were treated by traditional balloon angioplasty without stent implantation underwent clinical follow-up evaluation at 6 months. The procedure was successful in 455 (94%) of the patients, and angiographic follow-up was available for 377 (84%) of these patients. The presence of restenosis, defined as more than 50% stenosis in the dilated segment at follow-up, was observed in 257 (68%) of the 377 patients. Of these patients, 55 (15%) had at least one dilated lesion occluded at follow-up. By multivariate analysis, five independent predictors of restenosis were identified: the presence of end-organ damage, angioplasty at a saphenous venous graft, a bifurcation lesion, a lesion with a Thrombolysis in Myocardial Infarction (TIMI) grade flow of less than 3 before the procedure, and the degree of residual stenosis after angioplasty ($p < .05$). During follow-up, there was a decrease in the left ventricular ejection fraction (LVEF) in patients with occlusion ($-6.2\% \pm 9.9\%, p = .0001$), whereas no significant change in LVEF was observed in patients without restenosis or in those with nonocclusive restenosis.

V. ISCHEMIC HEART DISEASE

Processes and Outcomes of Care for Diabetic Acute Myocardial Infarction Patients in Ontario: Do Physicians Undertreat? *Diabetes Care* 2003;26:1427–1434.

Clinical Relevance: It is well established that patients with diabetes presenting with acute MI are at increased short-term and long-term risk for major cardiovascular end points.

Findings: This study compared the use of health care services by diabetic and nondiabetic patients with a history of acute MI. A total of 25,697 patients were enrolled in the Ontario area between April 1992 and December 1993, including 6,052 diabetics and 19,645 nondiabetics. Although diabetic patients had a higher cardiovascular event rate in the follow-up period, they were less likely to be seen by a cardiologist within 90 days of follow-up (22.2% versus 25.6%, $p < .001$), less likely to receive aspirin therapy (59.7% versus 63.5%, $p < .001$), and less likely to receive β-blocker therapy (34.2% versus 44.0%, $p < .001$). They were also less likely to be referred for coronary angiography (20.3% versus 24.7%, $p < .001$). In this study, the presence of diabetes was associated with an increase in 5-year morbidity and 5-year mortality rates.

Ventricular Remodeling Does Not Accompany the Development of Heart Failure in Diabetic Patients after Myocardial Infarction. *Circulation* 2002;106:1251–1255.

Clinical Relevance: Diabetic patients are at heightened risk for long-term mortality after acute MI and generally are at increased risk for congestive heart failure.

Findings: In this echocardiographic substudy of the Survival And Ventricular Enlargement (SAVE) trial, 412 nondiabetic and 100 diabetic patients underwent echocardiographic evaluation at baseline, at 3 months, and at 1 and 2 years after MI. As expected, the prevalence of heart failure was substantially higher in the diabetic cohort (30% versus 17%, $p < .001$). Maladaptive ventricular remodeling was associated with heart failure in the nondiabetic cohort. For example, the left ventricular diastolic area was substantially greater in nondiabetic patients who developed heart failure than in nondiabetic patients in whom heart failure did not develop. There was an 11.0 cm^2 increase in diastolic cavity area over 2 years in the nondiabetic patients who developed heart failure, compared with a decrease of 2.9 cm^2 in cavity area in the diabetic patients in whom heart failure developed ($p = .018$). These data suggest that the increased instance of heart failure after MI is not explained by a tendency for left ventricular remodeling in the diabetic cohort.

Amplified Benefit of Clopidogrel versus Aspirin in Patients with Diabetes Mellitus. *Am J Cardiol* 2002;90:625–628.

Clinical Relevance: Diabetic patients with arteriosclerotic disease have higher rates of vascular events than nondiabetic patients. This subanalysis determined whether clopidogrel was more effective than aspirin in preventing these events.

Findings: Of a total of 19,185 patients in the Clopidogrel versus Aspirin in Patients at Risk of Ischemic Events (CAPRIE) study, 3,866 had diabetes. Inclusion criteria were recent ischemic stroke, MI, and symptomatic peripheral artery disease. Patients were randomly assigned to receive either aspirin or clopidogrel. The average follow-up period was 1.9 years. The event rate (i.e., vascular death, MI, stroke, rehospitalization, or bleeding) per year was 15.6% for the diabetic patients receiving clopidogrel and 17.7% for patients receiving aspirin, with a relative risk reduction of 13.1% ($p = .032$). Clopidogrel was more effective than aspirin in preventing vascular events in diabetic patients with known atherosclerotic disease.

Influence of Diabetes Mellitus on Clinical Outcomes across the Spectrum of Acute Coronary Syndromes. Findings from the GUSTO IIb Study. GUSTO IIb Investigators. *Eur Heart J* **2000;21:1750–1758.**

Clinical Relevance: The study assessed the outcomes of the 2,175 diabetic patients in the GUSTO-IIb study, the primary aim of which was to evaluate the efficacy of hirudin versus heparin. The study included patients with unstable angina, non-ST-elevation MI, and ST-elevation MI.

Findings: Patients were monitored for 6 months. Diabetic patients had an overall higher incidence of death or reinfarction at 30 days compared with nondiabetic patients (13.1% versus 8.5%). This rate of death or reinfarction remained higher in the diabetic group (18.8% versus 11.4%) at the end of a 6-month follow-up period. Diabetes was associated with a 1.8-fold increased risk of death or reinfarction. Use of hirudin resulted in a nonsignificant decrease in these end points compared with heparin.

Glycoprotein IIb/IIIa Receptor Blockade Improves Outcomes in Diabetic Patients Presenting with Unstable Angina/Non-ST-Elevation Myocardial Infarction: Results from the Platelet Receptor Inhibition in Ischemic Syndrome Management in Patients Limited by Unstable Signs and Symptoms (PRISM-PLUS) Study. *Circulation* **2000;102:2466–2472.**

Clinical Relevance: This study assessed whether the diabetic subset from the PRISM-PLUS study benefited from treatment with the glycoprotein IIb/IIIa inhibitor tirofiban in the setting of acute coronary syndrome.

Findings: Patients with unstable angina or non-ST-elevation MI were randomly assigned to receive heparin or heparin plus tirofiban. Of the total 1,915 patients, 23% had a history of diabetes. The primary end point of death, new MI, or refractory ischemia within 7 days of randomization was not significantly lower (14.8% versus 21.8%) in patients receiving tirofiban. The risk of death or MI was significantly lower at 7, 30, and 180 days for patients receiving tirofiban plus heparin compared with those receiving heparin alone (1.2% versus 9.3% at 7 days, $p = .005$; 4.7% versus 15.5% at 30 days, $p = .02$; 11.2% versus 19.2% at 180 days, $p = .03$). This effect of tirofiban in reducing death or MI was more pronounced in diabetic patients than in nondiabetic patients. Patients in the tirofiban arm had a slight but not statistically significant increase in bleeding.

Effect of the Angiotensin-Converting Enzyme Inhibitor Trandolapril on Mortality and Morbidity on Diabetic Patients with Left Ventricular Dysfunction after Acute Myocardial Infarction. TRACE Study Group. *J Am Coll Cardiol* **1999;34:83–89.**

Clinical Relevance: Clinical trials have shown a reduction in cardiovascular events with the use of ACE inhibitors in patients with postinfarction heart failure. This substudy assessed the effect of the ACE inhibitor trandolapril on diabetic patients with left ventricular dysfunction after acute MI.

Findings: The Trandolapril Cardiac Evaluation (TRACE) study was a randomized, placebo-controlled trial. There were 237 diabetic patients among the 1,749 trial participants. The left ventricular ejection fraction was less than 35%, and the average follow-up period was 26 months. Fifty-one (45%) of the diabetic patients randomly assigned to trandolapril died, compared with 75 (61%) of those assigned to placebo (RR = 0.64; 95% CI, 0.45 to 0.91). Treatment with trandolapril significantly decreased the incidence of the end points of sudden death, cardiovascular death, and reinfarction.

Effects of the ACE Inhibitor Lisinopril on Mortality in Diabetic Patients with Acute Myocardial Infarction: Data from the GISSI-3 Study. *Circulation* **1997;96:4239–4245.**

Clinical Relevance: Diabetic patients have a high mortality rate after acute MI. This *post hoc* analysis assessed the benefits of the ACE inhibitor lisinopril on mortality and morbidity in diabetic patients with acute MI.

Findings: Patients were randomly assigned to receive lisinopril with or without nitroglycerin, in an open-label, 2×2 fashion, within 24 hours after being diagnosed with acute MI. There were 2,790 diabetic patients among the 18,895 patients enrolled in the study. Treatment with lisinopril decreased the 6-week mortality rate (8.7% versus 12.4%), and the survival benefit was maintained at 6 months (12.9% versus 16.1%). Nitroglycerin had no effect on mortality. The treatment effect of lisinopril was significantly higher in diabetic patients than nondiabetic patients.

Effect of Beta-Blockade on Mortality among High-Risk and Low-Risk Patients after Myocardial Infarction. *N Engl J Med* 1998;339:489–497.

Clinical Relevance: This study assessed the incidence and benefits of β-blocker administration to patients after MI.

Findings: The study was organized by the Cooperative Cardiovascular Project and funded by the Health Care Finance Administrator. The medical records of 201,752 patients were abstracted, identifying 59,445 patients with a diagnosis of diabetes. Mortality among patients treated with β-blockers was compared over a 2-year period with mortality among untreated patients. The study evaluated the efficacy of β-blocker therapy across numerous subgroups of patient cohorts with acute MI. Thirty percent of diabetic patients received β-blockers, compared with 35% of nondiabetic patients. Among diabetic patients, the 2-year mortality rate was 17% for those receiving treatment with β-blockers and 26.6% for those not receiving them (RR = 0.64, 95% CI, 0.60 to 0.68). β-Blockers, which appear to be underused, are effective in decreasing mortality after acute MI in patients with diabetes.

Prospective Randomised Study of Intensive Insulin Treatment on Long Term Survival after Acute Myocardial Infarction in Patients with Diabetes Mellitus. DIGAMI (Diabetes Mellitus, Insulin Glucose Infusion in Acute Myocardial Infarction) Study Group. *BMJ* 1997;314:1512–1515.

Clinical Relevance: The DIGAMI study group assessed whether insulin glucose infusion followed by multidose insulin therapy would decrease mortality among patients with acute MI.

Findings: The study enrolled 620 patients with diabetes (blood glucose level greater than 11 mmol/L or 200 mg/dL) and acute MI. They were randomly assigned to receive either insulin glucose infusion or placebo infusion for at least 24 hours. Patients in the insulin infusion group then received subcutaneous insulin four times each day for at least 3 months. Thrombolytic therapy and β-blockers were given unless contraindicated. At 1 year, the insulin infusion group had a mortality rate of 19%, compared with 26% for the control group. At 3 years, this difference in mortality persisted (33% versus 44%, respectively).

VI. DIABETIC CONTROL AND CARDIOVASCULAR EVENTS

Intensive Blood Glucose Control with Sulfonylureas or Insulin Compared with Conventional Treatment and Risk of Complications in Patients with Type 2 Diabetes (UKPDS 33). UK Prospective Diabetes Study (UKPDS) Group. *Lancet* 1998;352:837–853.

Clinical Relevance: This randomized, controlled trial compared the effects of blood glucose control with the intensive use of sulfonylurea agents or insulin versus conventional therapy on microvascular and macrovascular events in patients with type 2 diabetes.

Findings: The 3,867 newly diagnosed patients with type 2 diabetes (age 25 to 65 years) were randomly assigned to intensive treatment with a sulfonylurea (i.e., chlorpropamide, glibenclamide, or glipizide) or with insulin or to conventional treatment with diet. The aim of treatment in the intensive group was a fasting plasma glucose concentration of less than 6 mmol/L (110 mg/dL). In the conventional group, drugs were added only if the fasting plasma glucose level was greater than 15 mmol/L (270 mg/dL). The median follow-up period was 10 years. There was a 25% reduction in microvascular end points in the intensive treatment group, including the need for retinal photocoagulation; however, the incidence of macrovascular complications was similar in the conventional and intensive groups. There was no difference for any end point in the sulfonylurea and insulin groups. None of the drugs had adverse effects on cardiovascular outcomes. Hypoglycemia was more common in the intensive treatment group.

Effect of Intensive Blood-Glucose Control with Metformin on Complications in Overweight Patients with Type 2 Diabetes (UKPDS 34). UK Prospective Diabetes Study (UKPDS) Group. *Lancet* 1998;352:854–865.

Clinical Relevance: In patients with type 2 diabetes, intensive glucose control with sulfonylurea or insulin decreases microvascular events. This study assessed whether intensive glucose control with metformin has any additional benefits.

Findings: In this trial, 753 overweight patients (i.e., more than 120% of ideal body weight) newly diagnosed with type 2 diabetes were randomly assigned to receive either conventional treatment with diet ($n = 411$) or intensive treatment with metformin ($n = 342$). The patients allocated to metformin were also compared with 951 overweight patients who received intensive glucose control with sulfonylureas or insulin. The patients in the metformin group had a risk reduction of 42% ($p = .017$) for diabetes-related death and 36% ($p = .011$) for all-cause mortality, compared with patients in the conventional treatment group. Compared with patients in the sulfonylurea or insulin intensive treatment arm, patients in the metformin group had significantly lower incidence of any diabetes-related end point (i.e., diabetes-related death, all-cause mortality, MI, stroke, peripheral vascular disease, and microvascular events), all-cause mortality, and stroke. Metformin was also associated with a lower incidence of hypoglycemia compared with insulin or sulfonylurea agents. Metformin should be the initial treatment of choice for overweight patients with type 2 diabetes provided there are no contradictions to its use.

Effect of Intensive Diabetes Management on Macrovascular Events and Risk Factors in the Diabetes Control and Complications Trial. *Am J Cardiol* 1995:894–903.

Clinical Relevance: This study evaluated the efficacy of intensive insulin treatment versus conservative treatment in patients with insulin-dependent (type 1) diabetes.

Findings: The 1,441 patients (age 13 to 39 years) were randomly assigned to one of the two treatment groups. Patients with cardiovascular disease, hypertension, hypercholesterolemia, or obesity were excluded. The average follow-up period was 6.5 years. Major macrovascular events occurred two times more frequently in the conventional group than in the intensive treatment group (40 versus 23 events), although this difference did not reach statistical significance ($p = .08$). Intensive treatment also resulted in lower levels of total cholesterol, LDL cholesterol, and triglycerides, which are known risk factors for atherosclerosis ($p < .01$). This study suggests that intensive treatment of type 1 diabetic patients can decrease the incidence of macrovascular complications and the development of certain cardiovascular risk factors.

Potent Inhibitory Effect of Troglitazone on Carotid Arterial Wall Thickness in Type 2 Diabetes. *J Clin Endocrinol Metab* 1998;83:1818–1820.

Clinical Relevance: Insulin resistance may be related to atherosclerosis, which can be assessed noninvasively by measuring carotid artery intimal-medial thickness with B-mode ultrasound. This study assessed the effect of troglitazone, an insulin sensitizer, on carotid arterial intimal and medial complex thickness (IMT).

Findings: A total of 135 type 2 diabetic patients were randomly assigned to receive either troglitazone (400 mg daily) or placebo. After 3 months, the troglitazone group showed a significant decrease in IMT (−0.080 mm) compared with the placebo group (+0.027 mm). This study suggests that troglitazone (no longer available in the United States because of adverse hepatic effects) may cause regression of atherosclerosis.

Subject Index

Note: Page numbers followed by f indicate figures; those followed by t indicate tables.